NURSE'S
5-MINUTE
CLINICAL
CONSULT

Multisystem
Disorders

 Wolters Kluwer | Lippincott Williams & Wilkins
Health

Philadelphia · Baltimore · New York · London
Buenos Aires · Hong Kong · Sydney · Tokyo

STAFF

Executive Publisher
Judith A. Schilling McCann, RN, MSN

Editorial Director
H. Nancy Holmes

Clinical Director
Joan M. Robinson, RN, MSN

Art Director
Elaine Kasmer

Clinical Project Manager
Kate Stout, RN, MSN, CCRN

Editors
Christiane L. Brownell, ELS, Jennifer Kowalak

Copy Editors
Leslie Dworkin, Linda Hager, Janet P. Carroll

Designers
Linda Jovinelly Franklin

Digital Composition Services
Diane Paluba (manager), Joyce Rossi Biletz,
Donna S. Morris

Associate Manufacturing Manager
Beth J. Welsh

Editorial Assistants
Karen Kirk, Jeri O'Shea, Linda Ruhf

Indexer
Barbara E. Hodgson

RNEGC010707

Library of Congress

Nurse's 5-minute clinical consult. Multisystem disorders.
  p. ; cm.
  Includes bibliographical references and index.
  1. Catastrophic illness—Nursing—Handbooks, manuals, etc. I. Title: Nurse's five-minute clinical consult. Multisystem disorders. II. Title: Multisystem disorders.
  [DNLM: 1. Nursing Assessment—methods—Handbooks. 2. Acute Disease—nursing—Handbooks. 3. Wounds and Injuries—nursing—Handbooks. WY 49 N974277 2008]
  RT42.N826 2008
  610.73—dc22
ISBN-13: 978-1-58255-698-7 (alk. paper)
ISBN-10: 1-58255-698-9 (alk. paper)   2007027837

Contents

Contributors and consultants

Timothy L. Hudson, RN, CCRN, MS, MEd, FACHE
Performance Improvement Coordinator
Womack Army Medical Center
Ft. Bragg, N.C.

Todd Isbell, RN, CCRN-CSC, BSN
Director, Critical Care
MountainView Hospital
Las Vegas

Fiona K. S. Johnson, RN, CCRN, MSN
Clinical Education Specialist
Memorial Health University Medical
Center
Savannah, Ga.

Jill Johnson, RN, FNP, CCRN, CEN, CFRN, MSN
BSN Nursing Faculty
Midway (Ky.) College

Barbara Selvek, RN, CCRN, MS
Assistant Professor
Finger Lakes Community College
Canandaigua, N.Y.

Jennifer Sofie, RN, APRN, MSN
Adjunct Assistant Professor
College of Nursing
Montana State University
Bozeman

Belinda L. Spencer, RN, CCRN, ACNP-BC, MSN
Chief Inspections, Medical Command
MEDCOM
Fort Sam Houston, Tex.

Kathy L. Stallcup, RN, BSN, CCRN
Clinical Consultant
Integris Southwest Medical Center
Oklahoma City

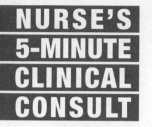

Multisystem Disorders

Abdominal trauma LIFE-THREATENING DISORDER

OVERVIEW

- May occur as a singular injury or as a part of combined multisystem and multiorgan trauma
- Morbidity and mortality of patients with abdominal trauma directly affected by early diagnosis and prompt treatment
- No outward signs of trauma in one-third of patients with abdominal trauma
- In some patients, delayed organ rupture or hemorrhage hours or days after the initial traumatic event
- Classified as blunt or penetrating
- Blunt abdominal trauma: Carries a higher mortality risk than penetrating trauma because of possible severe internal damage with little external evidence of injury, resulting in delayed diagnosis and treatment
- Penetrating trauma: Appearance of entrance and exit wounds doesn't determine extent of internal injury
- Motor vehicle accidents leading cause of blunt abdominal trauma
- Usually occurs in patients younger than age 50; half are involved in motor vehicle accidents

CAUSES

- Motor vehicle accident
- Sports
- Fall
- Physical altercation
- Gunshot or stab wounds
- Impalement by various objects
- May be associated with spinal, thoracic, or pelvic injuries, such as acceleration-deceleration injuries and seat belt injuries

PATHOPHYSIOLOGY

- Abdominal trauma may cause extensive damage to the abdominal organs, possibly resulting in massive blood loss.
- Generally, blunt trauma causes greater injury to solid organs (lungs, liver, spleen, pancreas, and kidneys), whereas penetrating trauma causes greater injury to hollow organs (stomach, small intestine, large intestine, and urinary bladder).
- When a blunt object strikes a person's abdomen, it raises intra-abdominal pressure. Depending on the force of the blow, the trauma can lacerate the liver and spleen, rupture the stomach, bruise the duodenum, and even damage the kidneys.
- Trauma to solid organs typically results in bleeding from lacerations or fractures; trauma to hollow organs results in rupture and release of organ contents into the abdominal cavity, which causes inflammation and infection.
- The greater the speed or force behind the injury, the greater the degree of trauma sustained and the greater the risk of complications. (See *Disorders affecting management of abdominal trauma*, pages 6 and 7.)

RESPIRATORY SYSTEM

- The intrathoracic abdomen is the upper part of the abdomen that lies beneath the rib cage. Trauma to this area of the abdomen may cause injury to the diaphragm, causing respiratory difficulty and compromised gas exchange.
- Blood and fluid may accumulate, causing a hemothorax.
- Accumulation of air or gas between the parietal and visceral pleurae may cause a tension pneumothorax, which may be life-threatening.

CARDIOVASCULAR SYSTEM

- After abdominal trauma, massive fluid shifts can occur (for example, fluid shifts to the bowel wall or irritated peritoneum), resulting in decreased vascular volume.
- Blood and fluid may be lost from an open penetrating abdominal wound, further decreasing vascular volume and increasing fluid loss.
- Injury to the spleen or the abdominal aorta or inferior vena cava can lead to massive hemorrhage and fluid loss. If left untreated, hypovolemic shock can occur. If prolonged, hypovolemia can lead to organ ischemia and failure.

GASTROINTESTINAL SYSTEM

- Rupture of the stomach, bowel, or liver can lead to spillage or leakage of organ contents and secretions into the normally sterile peritoneal cavity, which initiates an inflammatory response.
- The release of bacteria and intestinal contents into the peritoneum leads to peritonitis. If peritonitis progresses, sepsis may occur.
- Electrolyte imbalances occur because of the disruption in the GI tract's integrity.

RENAL SYSTEM

- Blunt or penetrating abdominal trauma may injure the kidneys or ureters or bladder, causing a hematoma and potential renal dysfunction, based on the precise area and extent of injury.
- Renal function may also be compromised if abdominal trauma results in massive blood loss, causing decreased renal perfusion.

HEMATOLOGIC SYSTEM

- Major abdominal trauma can result in the loss of massive amounts of blood and body fluid.
- The body experiences systemic inflammation and metabolic changes secondary to the stress and the release of catecholamines that ultimately affect the vasculature.
- Coagulation factors are mobilized in response to blood loss and become depleted, upsetting the delicate balance among the components needed for hemostasis.

- If massive blood transfusions are necessary, hemostasis may be further disrupted. Subsequently, disseminated intravascular coagulation can occur.

ASSESSMENT

HISTORY
- Trauma
- Determination of mechanism of injury (if possible) including:
- if a fall, the height and point of impact
- if a motor vehicle accident, the patient's placement in the car, use of a seat belt, speed and type of impact, and internal damage to the vehicle
- if a gunshot wound, the caliber of gun and range of fire (as reported by the authorities)
- if a stab wound, the length and type of object and the sex of the attacker (males more likely to stab upward, whereas females tending to stab downward)
- Location and quality of pain, any history of abdominal surgeries, and presence of nausea and vomiting

PHYSICAL FINDINGS
- Clinical manifestations of abdominal trauma dependent on specific organs injured (see *Assessing for abdominal organ injuries*)
- Obvious signs of trauma, such as stab, puncture, or gunshot wounds; bruising; or lacerations
- Masses
- Pulsations
- Asymmetry
- Discoloration
- Abdominal distention
- Decreased or absent bowel sounds (possibly caused by an irritant, such as blood or intestinal contents outside the bowel)
- Hyperactive bowel sounds (possibly the result of irritants inside the bowel)
- Bruits over the abdominal aorta, renal arteries, and femoral arteries

Assessing for abdominal organ injuries

Specific organ injuries associated with abdominal trauma and their assessment findings are outlined below.

ORGAN	ASSESSMENT FINDINGS
Colon	- Possible rectal bleeding - Peritoneal irritation due to perforation - Signs of obstruction
Diaphragm	- Bowel sounds in chest - Decreased breath sounds - Chest pain
Duodenum	- Fever - Jaundice - Vomiting - Pain - Peritoneal signs
Esophagus	- Pain that radiates to the neck, chest, or shoulders - Possible diffuse abdominal pain - Dysphagia
Liver	- Tenderness of right upper quadrant with guarding - Peritoneal irritation - Right shoulder pain when lying flat or in Trendelenburg's position - Positive Kehr's sign - Positive Ballance's sign
Pancreas	- Positive Grey Turner's sign (ecchymosis in the flank area, suggesting retroperitoneal bleeding) - Ileus - Epigastric pain radiating to the back, or pain in the left upper quadrant - Nausea and vomiting - Positive Kehr's sign (pain in the left shoulder secondary to diaphragmatic irritation by blood)
Small intestine	- Ileus - Peritoneal irritation - Abdominal pain and tenderness - Guarding - Decreased or absent bowel sounds
Spleen	- Left-upper-quadrant pain radiating to the left shoulder - Shock - Positive Kehr's sign - Positive Ballance's sign - Peritoneal irritation - Rigidity
Stomach	- Blood in nasogastric aspirate or hematemesis - Epigastric pain and tenderness - Signs of peritonitis due to release of acidic gastric contents - Guarding - Decreased or absent bowel sounds - Shock

(continued)

WARNING *If bruits are auscultated, don't perform percussion or palpation because there's a risk of rupturing the aorta.*

◆ Dullness on percussion, suggesting fluid
◆ Tympany, indicating air
◆ Rebound tenderness and guarding, indicating inflammation of the peritoneum
◆ Blood and possible anterior tenderness with peritoneal irritation on rectal palpation
◆ Possible coexisting injuries, such as head, thoracic, or orthopedic injuries, and their associated signs and symptoms

DIAGNOSTIC TEST RESULTS

◆ Complete blood count reveals an increase in the white blood cell (WBC) count. Early, mild elevation in WBC count results from the neuroendocrine stress response; extreme elevation later on may indicate peritoneal inflammation. Hemoglobin and hematocrit levels are reduced with hemorrhage.
◆ Serum amylase level may be elevated with injuries to the duodenum or pancreas.
◆ Serum bilirubin level may be increased with duodenal or liver injuries.
◆ Serum lipase level may be increased with pancreatic injury.
◆ Chest X-ray may reveal lower rib fractures, raising the risk of injury to the liver or spleen. Abdominal contents in the chest cavity indicate a diaphragmatic tear. Right diaphragm elevation may be seen in injury to the liver.
◆ Abdominal X-ray may reveal foreign bodies or free air in the abdomen, which indicates perforation of abdominal organs.

◆ Abdominal ultrasound may detect free intraperitoneal fluid and evaluates the heart, liver, spleen, and pelvis to detect bleeding. (See *The FAST exam.*)
◆ Diagnostic peritoneal lavage may be positive for blood, bile, or bacteria; WBC count is greater than 500/µl; red blood cell count is greater than 100,000/µl; and amylase is greater than 175 units/dl.
◆ Computed tomography detects bleeding, organ contusion, laceration, or rupture.

The FAST exam

The Focused Assessment with Sonography for Trauma (FAST) exam is part of the secondary survey of the Advanced Trauma Life Support protocol for patients with significant abdominal injuries. This ultrasound examines four major areas: pericardiac, perihepatic, perisplenic, and pelvic.

The pericardiac view examines the four chambers of the heart to detect a hemopericardium. The perihepatic view examines portions of the liver, diaphragm, and right kidney to detect fluid. The perisplenic view examines the spleen and left kidney for fluid in the splenorenal recess, left pleural space, and the subphrenic space. The pelvic view examines the bladder. Positive FAST findings may require a follow-up computed tomography scan for more specific identification of injuries.

The advantage of using the FAST exam over a diagnostic peritoneal lavage is that it's quick, noninvasive, portable, and accurate. It's also the test of choice in evaluating clinically unstable patients with possible abdominal injury.

TREATMENT

GENERAL
◆ The primary goals of treatment for the patient with abdominal trauma are to maintain hemodynamic stability, maintain organ function, and prevent major complications.

WARNING *Perform emergency interventions, including maintaining airway, breathing, and circulation and a patent airway.*

WARNING *Never remove an object that has penetrated the abdomen. The object may provide a tamponade effect to the surrounding tissues or organ; its removal could result in massive hemorrhage.*

WARNING *If dressings become saturated or require changing more than twice in 24 hours, or if drainage appears bright red, report these findings immediately.*

DIET
◆ Nothing by mouth until assessment rules out surgery
◆ After surgery, clear liquids initially; then solid food as tolerated, once bowel sounds have returned and per surgeon's order
◆ If intestinal damage occurs, possible total parenteral nutrition

ACTIVITY
◆ As tolerated

MEDICATIONS
◆ Analgesics
◆ Antibiotics

SURGERY
◆ Laparoscopy for diagnostic purposes (possible)
◆ Thoracotomy (used for extreme injury)
◆ Laparotomy

NURSING DIAGNOSES

◆ Acute pain
◆ Anxiety
◆ Risk for activity intolerance
◆ Risk for decreased cardiac output
◆ Risk for deficient fluid volume
◆ Risk for infection
◆ Risk for injury

EXPECTED OUTCOMES

The patient will:
◆ express feelings of increased comfort and decreased pain
◆ demonstrate adequate coping behavior and report less anxiety
◆ maintain mobility and tolerate activity within confines of injury
◆ maintain adequate cardiac perfusion and be hemodynamically stable
◆ achieve a balanced fluid level
◆ remain free from signs and symptoms of infection
◆ remain free from injury.

NURSING INTERVENTIONS

◆ Administer I.V. fluid replacement therapy and blood components.
◆ Monitor intake and output; report if urine output is less than 30 ml/hour.
◆ Monitor heart rate and rhythm, heart sounds, and blood pressure every hour for changes; use continuous cardiac monitoring to detect possible arrhythmias.
◆ Perform hemodynamic monitoring, including central venous pressure, pulmonary capillary wedge pressure, and cardiac output.
◆ Auscultate breath sounds at least every 2 hours, reporting a decrease in or absence of breath sounds or signs of congestion or fluid accumulation.
◆ Monitor oxygen saturation levels; administer supplemental oxygen.
◆ Assist with endotracheal intubation and mechanical ventilation, if indicated.
◆ Assess pain level and administer analgesics, as ordered.
◆ Assess dressings over penetrating trauma sites; provide appropriate wound care.
◆ Monitor and maintain a nasogastric tube.
◆ Monitor hemoglobin level and hematocrit.
◆ Perform pulmonary hygiene measures, including coughing and deep breathing and splinting the abdomen.
◆ Provide emotional support.

Be sure to cover:
◆ disorder, diagnostic testing, and treatment
◆ preoperative and postoperative teaching, as indicated
◆ medication administration, dosage, and possible adverse effects
◆ deep-breathing and coughing exercises and use of incentive spirometry
◆ wound care and signs and symptoms of infection
◆ importance of follow-up care.

RESOURCES

Organizations

National Center for Injury Prevention and Control (NCICP): *www.cdc.gov/ncipchm.htm*

Selected references

Franklin, G., and Casos, S. "Current Advances in the Surgical Approach to Abdominal Trauma," *Injury* 37(12):1143-156, December 2006.

Radwan, M., and Abu-Zidan, F. "Focused Assessment Sonograph Trauma (FAST) and CT scan in Blunt Abdominal Trauma; Surgeon's Perspective," *African Health Sciences* 6(3):187-90, September 2006.

Yegiyants, S., et al. "The Management of Blunt Abdominal Trauma Patients with Computed Tomography Scan Findings of Free Peritoneal Fluid and No Evidence of Solid Organ Injury," *The American Surgeon* 72(10):943-46, October 2006.

(continued)

Disorders affecting management of abdominal trauma

This chart highlights disorders that affect the management of abdominal trauma.

DISORDER	SIGNS AND SYMPTOMS	DIAGNOSTIC TEST RESULTS	TREATMENT AND CARE
Disseminated intravascular coagulation (complication)	◆ Abnormal bleeding without a history of a hemorrhagic disorder ◆ Bleeding into the skin, such as cutaneous oozing, petechiae, ecchymoses, and hematomas ◆ Bleeding from surgical or invasive procedure sites, such as incisions or venipuncture sites ◆ Nausea and vomiting ◆ Severe muscle, back, and abdominal or chest pain ◆ Hemoptysis and epistaxis ◆ Seizures ◆ Oliguria ◆ Diminished peripheral pulses ◆ Hypotension ◆ Mental status changes, including confusion	◆ Platelet count is decreased. ◆ Fibrinogen level is less than 150 mg/dl. ◆ Prothrombin time is greater than 15 seconds. ◆ Partial thromboplastin time is greater than 60 seconds. ◆ Fibrin degradation products are increased, often greater than 45 mcg/ml. ◆ D-dimer test is positive at less than 1:8 dilution. ◆ Fibrin monomers are positive; levels of factors V and VIII are diminished with fragmentation of red blood cells (RBCs). ◆ Hemoglobin is less than 10 g/dl. ◆ Urine studies reveal blood urea nitrogen (BUN) greater than 25 mg/dl. ◆ Serum creatinine level is greater than 1.3 mg/dl.	◆ Ensure a patent airway, and assess breathing and circulation. Monitor vital signs and cardiac and respiratory status closely, at least every 30 minutes, or more frequently, depending on the patient's condition. ◆ Observe skin color and check peripheral circulation, including color, temperature, and capillary refill. ◆ Administer supplemental oxygen, and monitor oxygen saturation with continuous pulse oximetry and serial ABG analysis; anticipate the need for endotracheal intubation and mechanical ventilation should the patient's respiratory status deteriorate. ◆ Assess neurologic status frequently—at least every hour, or more often, as indicated—for changes. ◆ Assess the extent of blood loss, and begin fluid replacement. Obtain a blood type, and crossmatch for blood component therapy. ◆ If hypotension occurs, administer vasoactive drugs, such as amrinone (Inocor), dobutamine (Dobutrex), dopamine (Intropin), epinephrine, and nitroprusside (Nitropress). ◆ Assess hemodynamic parameters. ◆ Institute continuous cardiac monitoring to evaluate for possible arrhythmias, myocardial ischemia, or adverse effects of treatment. ◆ Administer heparin I.V. in low doses, antifibrinolytic agents cautiously, and vitamin K and folate (to correct deficiencies). ◆ Assess urine output hourly; check all stools and drainage for occult blood. ◆ Inspect skin and mucous membranes for signs of bleeding; assess all invasive insertion sites and dressings for evidence of frank bleeding or oozing. Weigh the dressings that are wet or saturated to determine the extent of blood loss. Watch for bleeding from the GI and genitourinary tracts. ◆ Institute bleeding precautions. Limit all invasive procedures, such as venipunctures and I.M. injections, as much as possible. Apply pressure for 3 to 5 minutes over venous insertion sites and for 10 to 15 minutes over arterial sites. ◆ Institute safety precautions to minimize the risk of injury.
Hypovolemic shock (complication)	*Minimal volume loss (10% to 15%)* ◆ Slight tachycardia ◆ Normal supine blood pressure ◆ Positive postural vital signs, including a decrease in systolic blood pressure that's greater than 10 mm Hg or an increase in pulse rate that's greater than 20 beats/minute ◆ Increased capillary refill time (longer than 3 seconds) ◆ Urine output more than 30 ml/hour ◆ Cool, pale skin on arms and legs ◆ Anxiety	◆ Complete blood count reveals low hematocrit and decreased hemoglobin level, RBC count, and platelet counts. ◆ Metabolic studies reveal elevated serum potassium, sodium, lactate dehydrogenase, creatinine, and BUN levels. ◆ Urine studies reveal increased urine specific gravity (greater than 1.020) and urine osmolality and urine sodium levels less than 50 mEq/L. ◆ Urine creatinine levels may be decreased.	◆ Assess the extent of blood loss, and begin fluid replacement. ◆ Obtain a blood type, and crossmatch for blood component therapy. ◆ Assess airway, breathing, and circulation, and institute emergency resuscitative measures. ◆ Administer supplemental oxygen, and monitor oxygen saturation. ◆ Monitor vital signs and hemodynamic status continuously for changes. Observe skin color and check capillary refill. ◆ Institute continuous cardiac monitoring to evaluate for possible arrhythmias, myocardial ischemia, or adverse effects of treatment. ◆ Assess neurologic status frequently—about every 30 minutes until the patient stabilizes, and then every 2 to 4 hours. ◆ Monitor urine output at least hourly.

DISORDER	SIGNS AND SYMPTOMS	DIAGNOSTIC TEST RESULTS	TREATMENT AND CARE
Hypovolemic shock (complication) *(continued)*	*Moderate volume loss (about 25%)* ◆ Rapid, thready pulse ◆ Supine hypotension ◆ Cool truncal skin ◆ Urine output of 10 to 30 ml/hour ◆ Severe thirst ◆ Restlessness, confusion, or irritability *Severe volume loss (40% or more)* ◆ Marked tachycardia ◆ Marked hypotension ◆ Weak or absent peripheral pulses ◆ Cold, mottled, or cyanotic skin ◆ Urine output less than 10 ml/hour ◆ Unconsciousness	◆ Arterial blood gas (ABG) analysis may reveal decreased pH and partial pressure of arterial oxygen and increased partial pressure of arterial carbon dioxide. ◆ Gastroscopy, X-rays, and aspiration of gastric contents through a nasogastric tube may reveal evidence of frank or occult bleeding. ◆ Coagulation studies may show evidence of coagulopathy.	◆ Administer dopamine or norepinephrine (Levophed) I.V. to increase cardiac contractility and renal perfusion. ◆ During therapy, assess skin color and temperature, and note changes. ◆ Watch for signs of impending coagulopathy, such as petechiae, bruising, and bleeding or oozing from gums or venipuncture sites. ◆ Prepare the patient for surgery, as appropriate.
Peritonitis (complication)	◆ Vague or localized abdominal pain or diffuse pain over abdomen that becomes increasingly severe and unremitting; increases with movement and respirations; may be referred to the shoulder or the thoracic area ◆ Abdominal distention ◆ Anorexia, nausea, and vomiting ◆ Inability to pass feces and flatus ◆ Fever, tachycardia, and hypotension ◆ Lying still in bed with knees flexed to try to alleviate abdominal pain ◆ Shallow breathing ◆ Excessive sweating ◆ Cool, clammy skin ◆ Pallor ◆ Signs of dehydration ◆ Diminished to absent bowel sounds ◆ Abdominal rigidity and rebound tenderness	◆ White blood cell count shows leukocytosis (commonly more than 20,000/mm^3). ◆ Serum electrolyte levels may be abnormal; albumin levels may be decreased, suggesting bacterial peritonitis. ◆ Abdominal X-rays show edematous and gaseous distention of the small and large bowel. With perforation of a visceral organ, the X-ray shows air in the abdominal cavity. ◆ Chest X-ray may reveal elevation of the diaphragm. ◆ Abdominal ultrasound may reveal fluid collections. ◆ Paracentesis discloses the nature of the exudate and permits bacterial culture so appropriate antibiotic therapy can be started.	◆ Ensure a patent airway, and assess the patient's respiratory status at least every hour, or more frequently, as indicated; auscultate lungs bilaterally for adventitious or diminished breath sounds. ◆ Assess oxygen saturation continuously with pulse oximetry or mixed venous oxygen saturation through a pulmonary artery catheter (if in place). ◆ Monitor serial ABG levels. ◆ If the patient's respiratory status deteriorates, assist with endotracheal intubation and mechanical ventilation. ◆ Place the patient in a comfortable position that maximizes air exchange. ◆ Closely monitor the patient's heart rate and blood pressure at least every hour, or more frequently, as indicated; institute continuous cardiac monitoring, observe for arrhythmias, and prepare to treat. ◆ Monitor the patient's temperature every 1 to 2 hours; administer antipyretics, and use measures to reduce the patient's temperature, such as a hypothermia blanket and tepid sponge baths. ◆ Assess hemodynamic status closely—at least every hour, or more frequently, as indicated. ◆ Insert or assist with intubation with a nasogastric or nasoenteric tube, if not already in place. Monitor tube drainage every 1 to 2 hours for color, amount, and characteristics. ◆ Assess the abdomen for evidence of bowel sounds and distention. Maintain nothing-by-mouth status until bowel function returns. Expect to administer histamine-2 receptor antagonists to reduce the risk of gastric ulcer formation. ◆ Administer I.V. fluid and electrolyte replacement; prepare to administer blood component therapy if hemorrhage occurs. ◆ Administer I.V. antimicrobial agents. ◆ Monitor intake and output closely; assess urine output hourly. ◆ Assess neurologic status for changes. ◆ Assess patient's complaints of pain, and administer analgesics based on patient's degree of pain. ◆ Prepare the patient for surgery, as appropriate.

AIDS and HIV

OVERVIEW

- Human immunodeficiency virus (HIV) type I: retrovirus that causes acquired immunodeficiency syndrome (AIDS)
- Renders patients susceptible to opportunistic infections, unusual cancers, and other abnormalities
- Marked by progressive failure of the immune system
- Transmitted by contact with infected blood or body fluids and associated with identified high-risk behaviors
- Average time between exposure to virus and diagnosis of AIDS usually 8 to 10 years, but shorter and longer incubation times recorded

CAUSES

- Infection with HIV

RISK FACTORS

- Sharing of I.V. drug needles or syringes
- Unprotected sexual intercourse
- Placental transmission
- History of sexually transmitted disease
- Contact with infected blood
- Blood transfusion from infected donor

PATHOPHYSIOLOGY

- HIV strikes helper T cells bearing the CD4+ antigen. Normally a receptor for major histocompatibility complex molecules, the antigen now serves as a receptor for the retrovirus and allows it to enter the cell.
- Viral binding also requires the presence of a coreceptor (believed to be the chemokine receptor CCR5) on the cell surface.
- Through the action of reverse transcriptase, HIV produces deoxyribonucleic acid (DNA) from its viral ribonucleic acid (RNA). Transcription is usually poor, leading to mutations, some of which make HIV resistant to antiviral drugs.
- The viral DNA enters the nucleus of the cell and is incorporated into the host cell's DNA, where it's transcribed into more viral RNA. If the host cell reproduces, it duplicates the HIV DNA along with its own and passes it on to the daughter cells.
- If activated, the host cell carries this information and replicates the virus. Viral enzymes—proteases—arrange the structural components and RNA into viral particles that move to the periphery of the host cell, where the virus buds and emerges. The virus is now free to travel and infect other cells. (See *How HIV replicates*.)
- HIV replication may lead to cell death or may become latent.
- HIV infection leads to profound changes, either directly through destruction of CD4+ cells or other immune cells and neuroglial cells, or directly through the secondary effects of CD4+ T-cell destruction and resulting immunosuppression. (See *Disorders affecting management of AIDS,* pages 11 to 13.)
- The HIV infectious process takes three forms:
- immunodeficiency: causing opportunistic infections and unusual cancers
- autoimmunity: causing lymphoid interstitial pneumonitis, arthritis, hypergammaglobulinemia, and the production of autoimmune antibodies
- neurologic dysfunction: causing AIDS dementia complex, HIV encephalopathy, and peripheral neuropathies.

IMMUNE SYSTEM

- As the immune system begins to compromise, opportunistic infections may develop.
- The risk of cancer increases, most likely because HIV stimulates existing cancer cells or because the immune deficiency allows cancer-causing substances, such as viruses, to transform susceptible cells into cancer cells.

GASTROINTESTINAL SYSTEM

- GI signs and symptoms may be related to the effect of HIV on the cells lining the intestine.
- Oral candidiasis—a fungal infection—is a common manifestation in patients with AIDS.
- Dehydration, altered skin integrity, and poor nutrition can also contribute to the development of candidiasis, which, in some patients, may spread to other body systems.
- Involuntary weight loss, chronic diarrhea, and chronic fatigue may lead to a hypermetabolic state, in which calories are burned at an excessively high rate and lean body mass is lost, possibly leading to organ failure.

INTEGUMENTARY SYSTEM

- The overall effects of HIV infection, including weight loss, altered nutrition, weakness, and decreased mobility, predispose the patient to skin breakdown, which, along with the patient's immunodeficiency, increases the risk of infection.

NEUROLOGIC SYSTEM

- Neurologic system dysfunction is directly related to the effect of HIV on nervous system tissue, opportunistic infections, primary or metastatic neoplasms, cerebrovascular changes, metabolic encephalopathy, or complications secondary to therapy.
- Central nervous system responses to HIV infection include atrophy, demyelination, inflammation, degeneration, and necrosis.

RESPIRATORY SYSTEM

- Advanced and persistent immunosuppression allows opportunistic respiratory infections, such as *Pneumocystis carinii (jiroveci)* pneumonia, to develop.
- Tuberculosis may also be a presenting illness in patients infected with HIV.

How HIV replicates

This flowchart shows the steps in human immunodeficiency virus (HIV) cell replication.

HIV enters the bloodstream.

↓

HIV attaches to the surface of the CD4+ T lymphocyte.

↓

Proteins on the HIV cell surface bind to the protein receptors on the host cell's surface.

↓

HIV penetrates the host cell membrane and injects its protein coat into the host cell's cytoplasm.

↓

HIV's genetic information, ribonucleic acid (RNA), is released into the cell after its protective coat is partially dissolved.

↓

The single-stranded viral RNA, via the action of reverse transcriptase, is converted (transcribed) into double-stranded deoxyribonucleic acid (DNA).

↓

Viral DNA integrates itself into the host cell's nucleus.

↓

Integrase, an enzyme, inserts HIV's double-stranded DNA into the host cell's DNA.

↓

When the host cell is activated, the viral DNA takes over, telling the host cell to produce RNA (now viral RNA).

↓

Two strands of RNA are produced and transported out of the nucleus.

↓

One strand becomes the subunit of the HIV (that is, enzymes and structural proteins); the other becomes the genetic material for new viruses.

↓

Cleavage occurs (viral subunits are separated) through the action of protease, a viral enzyme.

↓

HIV subunits combine to make up new viral particles and begin to break down the host cell membrane.

↓

The genetic material in the new viral particles merges with the cell membrane that has been changed, forming a new viral envelope (outer covering).

↓

Viral budding occurs, in which the new HIV is released to enter the circulation.

ASSESSMENT

HISTORY
◆ Mononucleosis-like syndrome after a high-risk exposure and inoculation; possibly remaining asymptomatic for years
◆ In latent stage, laboratory evidence of seroconversion only sign of HIV infection

PHYSICAL FINDINGS
◆ Persistent generalized adenopathy
◆ Nonspecific symptoms (weight loss, fatigue, night sweats, fevers)
◆ Neurologic symptoms, resulting from HIV encephalopathy
◆ Opportunistic infection or cancer (Kaposi's sarcoma)

DIAGNOSTIC TEST RESULTS
◆ CD4+ T-cell count of 200 cells/μl or more confirms HIV infection.
◆ Screening test (enzyme-linked immunosorbent assay) and confirmatory test (Western blot) detect the presence of HIV antibodies, which indicate HIV infection.

TREATMENT

GENERAL
◆ Variety of therapeutic options for opportunistic infections (leading cause of morbidity and mortality in patients infected with HIV)
◆ Disease-specific therapy for a variety of neoplastic and premalignant diseases and organ-specific syndromes
◆ Symptom management (fatigue and anemia)

DIET
◆ Well-balanced

ACTIVITY
◆ Regular exercise, as tolerated, with adequate rest periods

(continued)

MEDICATIONS
- Immunomodulatory agents
- Anti-infectives
- Antidiarrheals
- Antineoplastics
- Highly active antiretroviral therapy

Primary therapy
- Protease inhibitors
- Nucleoside reverse transcriptase inhibitors
- Nonnucleoside reverse transcriptase inhibitors

NURSING CONSIDERATIONS

NURSING DIAGNOSES
- Activity intolerance
- Anxiety
- Compromised family coping
- Disturbed body image
- Fatigue
- Fear
- Hopelessness
- Imbalanced nutrition: Less than body requirements
- Impaired skin integrity
- Ineffective coping
- Ineffective sexuality patterns
- Powerlessness
- Risk for deficient fluid volume
- Risk for infection
- Social isolation

EXPECTED OUTCOMES
The patient will:
- perform activities of daily living without fatigue
- report feelings of decreased anxiety
- seek support systems and exhibit adequate coping behaviors
- verbalize feelings about changed body image
- express feelings of energy and decreased fatigue
- express feelings and concerns
- seek out available support systems
- consume required caloric intake
- exhibit improved or healed wounds or lesions
- demonstrate effective coping skills
- voice feelings about disease implications and social response to disease, and follow safer sex practices

Adverse effects of commonly used HIV medications

This chart shows some of the adverse effects of commonly used human immunodeficiency virus (HIV) medications. These adverse effects may be confused with signs and symptoms of disease process complications or opportunistic infections.

MEDICATION	ASSESSMENT FINDINGS
Delavirdine (Rescriptor)	Rash, headache, fatigue, increased liver enzymes
Didanosine (ddl, Videx)	Upper abdominal pain, diarrhea, persistent nausea and vomiting, pain, tingling or numbness, difficulty breathing, mental confusion
Indinavir (Crixivan)	Nephrolithiasis, asymptomatic hyperbilirubinemia, hyperglycemia, anemia, elevated cholesterol and triglycerides
Lamivudine (3TC, Epivir)	Headache, fever, rash, severe abdominal pain, shortness of breath, fatigue, muscle pain, mania, psychosis, confusion, lactic acidosis, pancreatitis
Nevirapine (Viramune)	Thrombocytopenia, rash, fever, anemia, stomatitis
Ritonavir (Norvir)	Diarrhea, nausea, vomiting, anorexia, abdominal pain, body fat redistribution, hyperglycemia, hyperlipidemia
Saquinavir (Fortovase)	Diarrhea (if formulated with lactose), body fat redistribution, hyperglycemia
Stavudine (Zerit)	Numbness, pain or tingling of the extremities, neutropenia, thrombocytopenia
Zalcitabine (dideoxycytidine, ddC, Hivid)	Rashes, mouth sores, upper abdominal pain, itching, numbness or tingling, mental confusion, seizures, fever, hyperbilirubinemia
Zidovudine (AZT, Retrovir)	Headache, fever, rash, severe abdominal pain, shortness of breath, fatigue, muscle pain, anemia, leukopenia, cardiomyopathy, cholestatic jaundice

Preventing HIV transmission

- Use precautions in all situations that risk exposure to blood, body fluids, and secretions. Diligently practicing standard precautions can prevent the inadvertent transmission of human immunodeficiency virus (HIV), hepatitis B, and other infectious diseases that are transmitted by similar routes.
- Teach the patient and his family, sexual partners, and friends about the prevention of disease transmission to others.
- Tell the patient not to donate blood, blood products, organs, tissue, or sperm.
- If the patient uses I.V. drugs, caution him not to share needles.
- Inform the patient that unprotected sex that involves exchange of body fluids, such as vaginal or anal intercourse without a condom, increases risk.
- Discuss safer sex practices, such as hugging, petting, mutual masturbation, and protected sexual intercourse. Emphasize that abstinence is the most effective way to prevent transmission.
- Advise women of childbearing age to avoid pregnancy. Explain that an infant may become infected before birth, during delivery, or during breast-feeding.

- express feelings of having greater control over the current situation
- maintain balanced intake and output
- remain free from signs and symptoms of infection
- maintain social interaction.

NURSING INTERVENTIONS
- Monitor vital signs, pulse oximetry, and laboratory values.
- Monitor for adverse effects of medications. (See *Adverse effects of commonly used HIV medications.*)
- Observe caloric intake, offering frequent small meals.
- Avoid using glycerin swabs for mucous membranes; rather, use normal saline or bicarbonate mouthwash for daily oral rinsing.
- Ensure adequate fluid intake during episodes of diarrhea, and provide antidiarrheals, as ordered.
- Monitor skin integrity and provide meticulous skin care, especially in the debilitated patient.
- Encourage the patient to maintain as much physical activity as he can tolerate. However, make sure his schedule includes time for rest periods.
- Monitor for signs of complications.
- Help the patient to cope with an altered body image, the emotional burden of a serious illness, and the threat of death.

PATIENT TEACHING

Be sure to cover:
- disorder, diagnostic testing, and treatment
- medication administration, dosage, and possible adverse effects
- importance of informing potential sexual partners, caregivers, and health care workers of HIV infection (see *Preventing HIV transmission*)
- signs of impending infection and the importance of seeking immediate medical attention
- symptoms of AIDS dementia and its stages and progression
- use of social services to set up home care, as appropriate
- use of local support group or hospice care, as indicated.

RESOURCES
Organizations
Center for AIDS Prevention Studies: *www.caps.ucsf.edu*
Centers for Disease Control and Prevention: *www.cdc.gov*
National AIDS Treatment Advocacy Project: *www.natap.org*

Selected references
Jones, S.G. "A Step-by-Step Approach to HIV/AIDS," *The Nurse Practitioner* 31(6):26-39, June 2006.
Kasper, D.L., et al., eds. *Harrison's Principles of Internal Medicine,* 16th ed. New York: McGraw-Hill Book Co., 2005
Kourtis, A.P., et al. "Mother-to-Child Transmission of HIV-1: Timing and Implications for Prevention," *The Lancet Infectious Diseases* 6(11):726-32, November 2006.
Mahat, G., et al. "Preparing Peer Educators for Teen HIV/AIDS Prevention," *Journal of Pediatric Nursing* 21(5):378-84, October 2006.

Disorders affecting management of AIDS

This chart highlights disorders that affect the management of acquired immunodeficiency syndrome (AIDS).

DISORDER	SIGNS AND SYMPTOMS	DIAGNOSTIC TEST RESULTS	TREATMENT AND CARE
Cryptosporidiosis (complication)	◆ Frequent stools (6 to 26 per day) ◆ Fever ◆ Watery diarrhea ◆ Right-upper-quadrant pain and cramping ◆ Flatulence ◆ Nausea and vomiting ◆ Weight loss ◆ Malaise	◆ Stool testing is positive for ova and parasites.	◆ Closely monitor the patient's fluid and electrolyte balance. ◆ Encourage an adequate intake of fluids, especially those rich in electrolytes. ◆ Monitor the patient's intake and output, and weigh him daily to evaluate the need for fluid replacement. Watch him closely for signs of dehydration, and provide fluid replacement. ◆ Administer analgesics, antidiarrheal and antiperistaltic agents, and antibiotics. Observe the patient for signs of adverse reactions as well as therapeutic effects. ◆ Apply perirectal protective cream to prevent excoriation and skin breakdown. ◆ Encourage small, frequent meals to help prevent nausea. ◆ Administer amphotericin B with or without flucytosine (Ancobon), fluconazole (Diflucan), or itraconazole (Sporonox).
Cytomegalovirus (CMV) (complication)	◆ Blind or dark spots in visual field (scotomas) ◆ Loss of peripheral vision ◆ Visual floaters	◆ Complement fixation studies and hemagglutination inhibition antibody tests isolate the virus.	◆ Institute standard precautions before coming into contact with the patient's blood or other body fluids. Secretion precautions are especially important for infants. ◆ Administer medications to treat symptoms. ◆ Monitor intake and output. Offer nutritionally adequate meals. If the patient has diarrhea, replace fluids.

(continued)

DISORDER	SIGNS AND SYMPTOMS	DIAGNOSTIC TEST RESULTS	TREATMENT AND CARE
Cytomegalo–virus (CMV) (complication) *(continued)*	◆ Chorioretinitis ◆ Difficulty concentrating ◆ Sleepiness ◆ Mouth ulcerations ◆ Dysphagia ◆ Abdominal pain ◆ Bloody diarrhea ◆ Weight loss ◆ Rectal ulcers ◆ Persistent fever ◆ Fatigue ◆ Urine retention ◆ Incontinence	◆ Chest X-ray reveals bilateral, diffuse, white infiltrates.	◆ Provide emotional support and counseling to the parents of a child with severe CMV infection. Help them find support systems, and coordinate referrals to other health care professionals. ◆ Monitor the patient with splenomegaly for signs of rupture, and protect him from excess activity and injury. ◆ For the patient with impaired vision, provide a safe environment and encourage independence. Make referrals to community resources. ◆ For the patient with respiratory involvement, frequently assess ventilation status and administer oxygen, as needed. Position the patient in semi-Fowler's or a sitting position to facilitate ventilation. ◆ Administer ganciclovir (Cytovene), foscarnet (Foscavir), or cidofovir (Vestide).
Kaposi's sarcoma (complication)	◆ Multicentric skin lesions that vary from brown to red to purple ◆ Swelling and pain in the lower extremities, penis, scrotum, or face	◆ With central nervous system involvement, lumbar puncture indicates increased pressure; cerebrospinal fluid analysis demonstrates increased protein levels and, possibly, pleocytosis. ◆ Tissue biopsy determines the lesion's type and stage. ◆ Computed tomography scan may show areas of metastasis.	◆ Inspect the patient's skin every shift, looking for new lesions and skin breakdown. ◆ Administer pain medications. ◆ To help the patient adjust to changes in his appearance, urge him to share his feelings, and give him encouragement. ◆ Plan meals around the patient's treatment. Supply the patient with high-calorie, high-protein meals. If he can't tolerate regular meals, provide frequent, smaller portions. ◆ If the patient can't take food by mouth, administer I.V. fluids. ◆ Give antiemetics and sedatives. ◆ Provide rest periods if the patient tires easily. ◆ Be alert for adverse effects of radiation therapy or chemotherapy—such as anorexia, nausea, vomiting, and diarrhea—and take steps to prevent or alleviate them. ◆ Systemic therapy may include vincristine (Oncovin), vinblastine (Velban), etoposide (VePesid), doxorubicin (Doxil), daunorubicin (Cerubidine), bleomycin (Blenoxane), and interferon alfa (Roferon-A) with or without an HIV-specific antiretroviral agent.
*Mycobacterium avium–*intracellular complex infection (complication)	◆ Weight loss ◆ Night sweats ◆ Persistent fever ◆ Weakness ◆ Diarrhea ◆ Anemia ◆ Fatigue ◆ Abdominal discomfort	◆ Sputum culture, bronchial wash, stool culture, acid-fast bacillus (AFB) blood culture, bone marrow aspiration, and tissue biopsy test positive for the bacteria.	◆ Monitor white blood cell count and differential. ◆ Instruct the patient in how to prevent infection. ◆ Teach the patient and his caregiver about the need to report possible infection. ◆ Monitor the patient for infection; fever, chills, and diaphoresis; cough; shortness of breath; oral pain or painful swallowing; creamy-white patches in the oral cavity; urinary frequency, urgency, or dysuria; redness, swelling, or drainage from wounds; and vesicular lesions on the face, lips, or perianal area. ◆ Administer combination therapy with two to five agents (clarithromycin [Biaxin], azithromycin [Zithromax], rifampin [Rifadin], rifabutin [Mycobutin], clofazimine [Lamprene], ethambutol [Myambutol], ciprofloxacin [Cipro], and amikacin [Amikin]).
Pneumocystis carinii (jiroveci) pneumonia (complication)	◆ Low-grade, intermittent fever ◆ Increasing shortness of breath ◆ Nonproductive cough ◆ Tachypnea ◆ Dyspnea	◆ Gallium scan reveals increased uptake over the lungs. ◆ Bronchoscopy and pleural washing show *P. carinii.* ◆ CD4+ T-cell count is less than 200 cells/µl.	◆ Use standard precautions. ◆ Give prescribed oral or I.V. TMP-SMZ (Bactrim, Septra) and oxygen. ◆ Encourage ambulation and use of incentive spirometry. ◆ Provide adequate rest periods. ◆ Encourage the patient to express his fears, feelings, or concerns. ◆ Provide emotional support. ◆ Assess for altered respiratory status, tachypnea, use of accessory muscles to breathe, cough, sputum color changes, abnormal breath sounds, dusky or cyanotic skin color, restlessness, confusion, or somnolence. Report abnormal findings.

DISORDER	SIGNS AND SYMPTOMS	DIAGNOSTIC TEST RESULTS	TREATMENT AND CARE
Pneumocystis carinii (jiroveci) pneumonia (complication) *(continued)*	◆ Accessory muscle use for breathing ◆ Cyanosis ◆ Dullness on percussion ◆ Crackles ◆ Decreased breath sounds	◆ Sputum specimen is positive for *P. carinii.* ◆ Chest X-ray reveals slowly progressing, fluffy infiltrates; occasional nodular lesions; or spontaneous pneumothorax.	◆ Monitor arterial blood gas values. ◆ Monitor fluid and electrolyte status. ◆ Provide pulmonary care (cough, deep breathing, postural drainage and percussion, and vibration) every 2 hours.
Toxoplasmosis (complication)	◆ Visual changes ◆ Constant dull headache ◆ Disorientation ◆ Seizures ◆ Aphasia ◆ Altered mental status ◆ Cranial nerve palsies ◆ Hemiparesis	◆ *Toxoplasma gondii* antibodies are detected in body fluid, blood, or tissue specimens.	◆ Make sure the patient with fever, vomiting, and sore throat receives sufficient fluid intake. ◆ Provide nutritionally adequate foods and small, frequent feedings. ◆ Promote bed rest during the acute stage. Later, help the patient gradually increase his level of activity. ◆ Frequently assess respiratory status. Provide chest physiotherapy, administer oxygen, and assist with ventilation. ◆ Assess the patient for signs of neurologic involvement and increased intracranial pressure. ◆ Don't palpate the patient's abdomen vigorously; this could cause a ruptured spleen. ◆ Modify the environment to protect a patient with neurologic manifestations or chorioretinitis. ◆ Administer pyrimethamine with sulfadiazine (Fansidar). ◆ Carefully monitor the patient's drug therapy. ◆ Because sulfonamides cause blood dyscrasias and pyrimethamine depresses bone marrow, closely monitor the patient's hematologic values.
Tuberculosis (complication)	◆ Night sweats ◆ Hemoptysis ◆ Fever ◆ Cough ◆ Shortness of breath ◆ Fatigue ◆ Headache ◆ Chills ◆ Nausea and vomiting ◆ Weight loss	◆ Purified protein derivative is positive. ◆ Chest X-ray reveals the penetrating lung parenchyma. ◆ Sputum smear and culture test positive for AFB.	◆ Initiate AFB isolation precautions immediately. ◆ Teach the infectious patient to cough and sneeze into tissues and to dispose of all secretions properly. ◆ Instruct the patient to wear a mask when outside of his room. ◆ Visitors and staff members should wear particulate respirators. ◆ Administer isoniazid (Nydrazid), rifampin, and (either) ethambutol or streptomycin. ◆ Remind the patient to get plenty of rest. Stress the importance of eating balanced meals. Record the patient's weight weekly. ◆ Be alert for adverse effects of medications. Because isoniazid sometimes leads to hepatitis or peripheral neuritis, monitor aspartate aminotransferase and alanine aminotransferase levels. ◆ To prevent or treat peripheral neuritis, give pyridoxine (vitamin B_6). If the patient receives ethambutol, watch for optic neuritis; if it develops, discontinue the drug. If he receives rifampin, watch for hepatitis and purpura. Observe the patient for other complications such as hemoptysis.
Wasting syndrome (complication)	◆ Fever ◆ Nausea and vomiting ◆ Fatigue ◆ Abdominal pain ◆ Pain or discomfort while eating ◆ Diarrhea	◆ No specific diagnostic tests are used; diagnosis is based on evidence of underlying human immunodeficiency virus infection and assessment findings.	◆ Monitor weight; intake and output; and hematocrit, hemoglobin, and ferritin levels to evaluate nutritional status and fluid and electrolyte balance. ◆ Monitor for and report signs and symptoms of dehydration, such as extreme thirst and reduced skin turgor.

Acute coronary syndrome LIFE-THREATENING DISORDER

OVERVIEW

- All-inclusive term that describes the potential for three conditions: unstable angina, non-ST-segment elevation myocardial infarction (NSTEMI), and ST-segment elevation myocardial infarction (STEMI)
- Definition of condition dependent on degree of occlusion
- Involves the rupture or erosion of plaque that results in platelet adhesions, fibrin clot formation, and activation of thrombin
- Symptoms caused by myocardial ischemia, resulting from an imbalance between supply and demand for myocardial oxygen
- Affects approximately one million people in the United States annually
- Higher incidence in males younger than age 70; females having protective effects of estrogen
- Almost one-half of sudden deaths caused by myocardial infarction (MI) occurring before hospitalization or within 1 hour of the onset of symptoms (See "Myocardial Infarction," pages 326 to 335)

CAUSES

- Atherosclerotic plaque disease
- Coronary artery vasospasm
- Ventricular hypertrophy resulting from hypertension, valvular disease, or cardiomyopathy
- Embolic occlusion of the coronary arteries
- Hypoxia from carbon monoxide poisoning or acute pulmonary disorders
- Inflammation of epicardial arteries

RISK FACTORS

- Increased age (40 to 70)
- Diabetes mellitus
- Elevated serum triglyceride and serum low-density lipoprotein levels and decreased serum high-density lipoprotein levels
- Excessive intake of saturated fats, carbohydrates, or salt
- Hypertension
- Obesity
- Family history of coronary artery disease (CAD)

UP CLOSE

Understanding CAD

Coronary artery disease (CAD) results as atherosclerotic plaque fills the lumens of the coronary arteries and obstructs blood flow. The primary effect of CAD is a diminished supply of oxygen and nutrients to myocardial tissue.

PROGRESSION OF CAD IN ATHEROSCLEROSIS

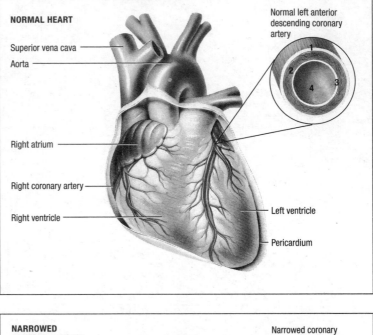

NORMAL HEART

- Superior vena cava
- Aorta
- Right atrium
- Right coronary artery
- Right ventricle
- Left ventricle
- Pericardium

Normal left anterior descending coronary artery

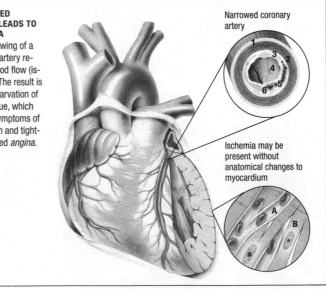

NARROWED ARTERY LEADS TO ISCHEMIA

The narrowing of a coronary artery reduces blood flow (ischemia). The result is oxygen starvation of heart tissue, which causes symptoms of chest pain and tightness, called *angina*.

Narrowed coronary artery

Ischemia may be present without anatomical changes to myocardium

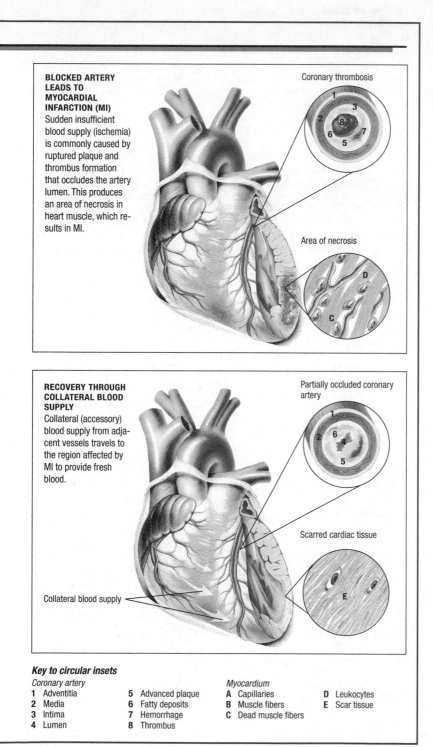

BLOCKED ARTERY LEADS TO MYOCARDIAL INFARCTION (MI)

Sudden insufficient blood supply (ischemia) is commonly caused by ruptured plaque and thrombus formation that occludes the artery lumen. This produces an area of necrosis in heart muscle, which results in MI.

Coronary thrombosis

Area of necrosis

RECOVERY THROUGH COLLATERAL BLOOD SUPPLY

Collateral (accessory) blood supply from adjacent vessels travels to the region affected by MI to provide fresh blood.

Partially occluded coronary artery

Scarred cardiac tissue

Collateral blood supply

Key to circular insets

Coronary artery
1 Adventitia
2 Media
3 Intima
4 Lumen
5 Advanced plaque
6 Fatty deposits
7 Hemorrhage
8 Thrombus

Myocardium
A Capillaries
B Muscle fibers
C Dead muscle fibers
D Leukocytes
E Scar tissue

◆ Sedentary lifestyle
◆ Smoking
◆ Stress or a type A personality
◆ Use of drugs, such as amphetamines or cocaine

PATHOPHYSIOLOGY

◆ For patients with unstable angina, a thrombus full of platelets partially occludes a coronary vessel. The partially occluded vessel may have distal microthrombi that cause necrosis in some myocytes.
◆ The smaller vessels infarct, thus placing the patient at higher risk for a NSTEMI.
◆ If a thrombus fully occludes the vessel for a prolonged time, it's classified as a STEMI. This type of MI involves a greater concentration of thrombin and fibrin.
◆ Occlusion of a vessel progresses through three stages:
– Ischemia occurs first, indicating that blood flow and oxygen demand are imbalanced.
– Injury occurs when the ischemia is prolonged enough to damage the heart area.
– Infarct occurs when myocardial cells die. (See *Disorders affecting management of ACS*, pages 18 and 19.)

CARDIOVASCULAR SYSTEM
◆ An area of viable ischemic tissue surrounds the zone of injury.
◆ With heart muscle damage, integrity of the cell membrane is impaired, and intracellular contents are released. (See *Understanding CAD*.)
◆ The infarcted area becomes edematous and cyanotic and leukocytes infiltrate the necrotic area and begin to remove necrotic cells, thus thinning the ventricular wall.
◆ The scar tissue that forms on the necrotic area inhibits contractility, activating compensatory mechanisms to maintain cardiac output.
◆ Ventricular dilation may also occur in a process called *remodeling*.
◆ Functionally, MI may cause reduced contractility with abnormal wall mo-

(continued)

tion, altered left ventricular compliance, reduced stroke volume, reduced ejection fraction, and elevated left ventricular end-diastolic pressure.

◆ Cardiogenic shock is caused by failure of the heart to perform as an effective pump and can result in low cardiac output, diminished peripheral perfusion, pulmonary congestion, elevated systemic vascular resistance and pulmonary vascular pressures, and renal failure.

◆ Ineffective contractility of the heart leads to accumulation of blood in the venous circulation upstream to the failing ventricle.

◆ Arrhythmias can occur as a result of autonomic nervous system imbalance, electrolyte disturbances, ischemia, and slowed conduction in zones of ischemic myocardium.

NEUROLOGIC SYSTEM

◆ Hypoperfusion of the brain results in altered mental status.

◆ If the decrease in cerebral perfusion continues, stupor or coma may result.

RENAL SYSTEM

◆ Shock and hypoperfusion cause the kidney to conserve salt and water.

◆ Poor perfusion results in diminished renal blood flow; increased afferent arteriolar resistance also occurs, causing a decreased glomerular filtration rate.

◆ Increased amounts of antidiuretic hormone and aldosterone are released to help maintain perfusion; however, urine formation is reduced.

◆ Depletion of renal adenosine triphosphate stores results from prolonged renal hypoperfusion, causing impaired renal function.

RESPIRATORY SYSTEM

◆ Cardiogenic shock with left-sided heart failure results in increased fluid in the lungs. This process can overwhelm the capacity of the pulmonary lymphatics, resulting in interstitial and alveolar edema.

◆ Lung edema occurs when pulmonary capillary pressure exceeds 18 mm Hg.

◆ Pulmonary alveolar edema develops when pressures exceed 24 mm Hg, impairing oxygen diffusion.

◆ Increased interstitial and intra-alveolar fluid causes progressive reduction in lung compliance, increasing the work of ventilation and increasing perfusion of poorly ventilated alveoli.

ASSESSMENT

HISTORY

◆ Possible CAD with increasing anginal frequency, severity, or duration

◆ Persistent, crushing substernal pain or pressure, possibly radiating to the left arm, jaw, neck, and shoulder blades, and possibly persisting for 12 or more hours (cardinal symptom of MI)

◆ Pain possibly absent in elderly patients or those with diabetes; pain possibly mild and presenting as indigestion in others

◆ Feeling of impending doom, fatigue, nausea, vomiting, and shortness of breath

◆ Sudden death (may be the first and only indication of MI)

PHYSICAL FINDINGS

◆ Extreme anxiety and restlessness

◆ Dyspnea

◆ Diaphoresis

◆ Tachycardia

◆ Hypotension or hypertension

◆ Bradycardia and hypotension, in inferior MI

◆ S_4, S_3, and paradoxical splitting of S_2, in ventricular dysfunction

◆ Systolic murmur of mitral insufficiency

◆ Pericardial friction rub, in transmural MI or pericarditis

◆ Low-grade fever

◆ Jugular vein distention

◆ Reduced urine output (secondary to reduced renal perfusion and increased aldosterone and antidiuretic hormone)

◆ Pulmonary congestion, such as crackles and a productive cough

DIAGNOSTIC TEST RESULTS

◆ 12-lead electrocardiogram (ECG) may reveal characteristic changes, such as serial ST-segment depression in non–Q-wave MI and ST-segment elevation in Q-wave MI. The Q waves are considered abnormal when they appear greater than or equal to 0.4 second wide and their height is greater than 25% of the R-wave height in that lead. An ECG can also identify the location of MI, arrhythmias, hypertrophy, and pericarditis. The more combinations of leads affected with ECG changes, the more myocardial damage and the worse the prognosis.

◆ Serial cardiac enzymes and proteins may show a characteristic rise and fall of cardiac enzymes, specifically CK-MB; the proteins troponin, T and I; and myoglobin.

◆ Laboratory testing may reveal elevated white blood cell count and erythrocyte sedimentation rate and changes in electrolytes.

◆ Echocardiography may show ventricular wall motion abnormalities and may detect septal or papillary muscle rupture or identify pericardial effusions.

◆ Chest X-rays may show left-sided heart failure, cardiomegaly, or other noncardiac causes of dyspnea or chest pain.

◆ Nuclear imaging scanning, using thallium 201 and technetium 99m, can be used to identify areas of infarction and areas of viable muscle cells.

◆ Multiple-gated acquisition scanning is used to determine left ventricular function and identify aneurysms, problems with wall motion, and intracardiac shunting.

◆ Cardiac catheterization may identify the involved coronary artery as well as to provide information on ventricular function and pressures and volumes within the heart.

TREATMENT

GENERAL
- Cardiac catheterization, coronary stent placement, balloon angioplasty
- Pacemaker implantation or electrical cardioversion for arrhythmias
- Intra-aortic balloon pump for cardiogenic shock
- Left ventricular assist device

DIET
- Low-fat, low-cholesterol
- Calorie restriction, if indicated

ACTIVITY
- Bed rest with bedside commode
- Gradual increase in activity, as tolerated

MEDICATIONS
- Oxygen
- Aspirin
- Nitrates
- I.V. morphine
- I.V. thrombolytic therapy
- Antiarrhythmics
- Calcium channel blockers
- I.V. heparin
- Inotropic agents
- Beta-adrenergic blockers
- Angiotensin-converting enzyme (ACE) inhibitors
- Glycoprotein IIb/IIIa inhibitors
- Stool softeners

SURGERY
- Surgical revascularization (coronary artery bypass graft)

NURSING CONSIDERATIONS

NURSING DIAGNOSES
- Activity intolerance
- Acute pain
- Anxiety
- Decreased cardiac output
- Excess fluid volume
- Fatigue
- Fear
- Imbalanced nutrition: Less than body requirements
- Ineffective coping
- Ineffective denial
- Ineffective sexuality patterns
- Ineffective tissue perfusion: Cardiopulmonary

EXPECTED OUTCOMES
The patient will:
- perform activities of daily living without excessive fatigue or exhaustion
- express feelings of increased comfort and decreased pain
- verbalize strategies to reduce anxiety and stress
- maintain adequate cardiac output
- develop no complications of fluid volume excess
- verbalize the importance of balancing activity, as tolerated, with rest
- express decreased feelings of fear
- achieve ideal weight
- exhibit adequate coping skills
- recognize his acute condition and accept the lifestyle changes he needs to make
- voice feelings about changes in sexual patterns
- maintain hemodynamic stability and develop no arrhythmias.

NURSING INTERVENTIONS
- Assess pain level and give prescribed analgesics. Record the severity, location, type, and duration of pain. Avoid I.M. injections.
- Check the patient's blood pressure before and after giving nitroglycerin, ACE inhibitors, and beta-adrenergic blockers.
- Obtain ECG during episodes of chest pain.
- Organize patient care and activities to provide uninterrupted rest.
- Provide a low-cholesterol, low-sodium diet with caffeine-free beverages.
- Allow the patient to use a commode.
- Help with range-of-motion exercises.
- Provide emotional support, and help to reduce stress and anxiety.
- If the patient has undergone percutaneous transluminal coronary angioplasty or cardiac catheterization, sheath care is necessary. Watch for bleeding. Keep the leg with the sheath insertion site immobile, and maintain strict bed rest. Check peripheral pulses in affected leg according to facility protocol.
- Monitor serial ECGs, cardiac rhythm, vital signs, heart and breath sounds, daily weight, and laboratory values.

> ⚡ **WARNING** *Watch for crackles, cough, tachypnea, and edema, which may indicate impending left-sided heart failure.*

PATIENT TEACHING

Be sure to cover:
- disorder, diagnostic testing, and treatment
- medication administration, dosage, and possible adverse effects
- dietary restrictions
- information on smoking cessation
- progressive resumption of sexual activity
- appropriate response to symptoms
- types of chest pain to report
- information on a cardiac rehabilitation program
- available weight-reduction programs, if needed.

RESOURCES
Organizations
American Heart Association: *www.americanheart.org*
National Heart, Lung and Blood Institute: *www.nhlbi.nih.gov*

Selected references
Amin, A. "Improving the Management of Patients after Myocardial Infarction, from Admission to Discharge," *Clinical Therapeutics* 28(10):1509-539, October 2006.
Cannon, C. "Evolving Management of ST-Segment Elevation Myocardial Infarction: Update on Recent Data," *American Journal of Cardiology* 98(12S1):S10-S21, December 2006.
Gorjup, V., et al. "Acute ST-Elevation Myocardial Infarction after Successful Cardiopulmonary Resuscitation," *Resuscitation* 72(3):379-85, March 2007.
Yang, E., et al. "Modern Management of Acute Myocardial Infarction," *Current Problems in Cardiology* 31(12):769-817, December 2006.

(continued)

Disorders affecting management of ACS

This chart highlights disorders that affect the management of acute coronary syndrome (ACS).

DISORDER	SIGNS AND SYMPTOMS	DIAGNOSTIC TEST RESULTS	TREATMENT AND CARE
Cardiogenic shock (complication)	*Compensatory stage* ◆ Tachycardia and bounding pulse caused by sympathetic stimulation ◆ Restlessness and irritability related to cerebral hypoxia ◆ Tachypnea to compensate for hypoxia ◆ Reduced urinary output secondary to vasoconstriction ◆ Cool, pale skin associated with vasoconstriction; warm, dry skin in septic shock resulting from vasodilation *Progressive stage* ◆ Hypotension as compensatory mechanisms begin to fail ◆ Narrowed pulse pressure associated with reduced stroke volume ◆ Weak, rapid, thready pulse caused by decreased cardiac output ◆ Shallow respirations as the patient weakens ◆ Reduced urinary output as poor renal perfusion continues ◆ Cold, clammy skin caused by vasoconstriction ◆ Cyanosis related to hypoxia *Irreversible (refractory) stage* ◆ Unconsciousness and absent reflexes caused by reduced cerebral perfusion, acid-base imbalance, or electrolyte abnormalities ◆ Rapidly falling blood pressure as decompensation occurs ◆ Weak pulse caused by reduced cardiac output ◆ Slow, shallow, or Cheyne-Stokes respirations secondary to respiratory center depression ◆ Anuria related to renal failure	◆ Arterial blood gas (ABG) analysis may show metabolic acidosis, respiratory acidosis, and hypoxia. ◆ Electrocardiography (ECG) shows possible evidence of acute myocardial infarction (MI), ischemia, or ventricular aneurysm. ◆ Thermodilution catheterization reveals a reduced cardiac index. ◆ Serum enzyme measurements display elevated levels of creatine kinase (CK), lactate dehydrogenase (LD), aspartate aminotransferase, and alanine aminotransferase, which indicate MI or ischemia and suggest heart failure or shock. ◆ CK-MB and LD isoenzyme levels may be elevated, confirming acute MI.	◆ Administer oxygen by face mask or artificial airway to ensure adequate oxygenation of tissues. ◆ Monitor and record blood pressure, pulse, respiratory rate, and peripheral pulses every 1 to 5 minutes until the patient stabilizes. ◆ Monitor cardiac rhythm continuously. ◆ Closely monitor PAP, PAWP, and, if equipment is available, cardiac output. ◆ Record hemodynamic pressure readings every 15 minutes. ◆ Insert an indwelling urinary catheter, if needed, to measure hourly urine output. ◆ Administer dopamine (Intropin), amiodarone (Cordarone), dobutamine (Dobutrex), norepinephrine (Levophed), nitroglycerin (Tridil), and nitroprusside (Nitropress) as well as a vasopressor. ◆ Monitor ABG values, complete blood count, and electrolyte levels. Expect to administer sodium bicarbonate by I.V. push if the patient is acidotic. Administer electrolyte replacement therapy, as indicated by laboratory results. ◆ During therapy, assess skin color and temperature, and note changes. Cold, clammy skin may be a sign of continuing peripheral vascular constriction, indicating progressive shock. ◆ Move the patient with an intra-aortic balloon pump (IABP) as little as possible. Never flex the patient's ballooned leg at the hip because this may displace or fracture the catheter. ◆ Never place the patient on IABP in a sitting position while the balloon is inflated; the balloon will tear through the aorta and result in immediate death. ◆ During IABP use, assess pedal pulses and skin temperature and color to ensure adequate peripheral circulation. ◆ Check the dressing over the insertion site frequently for bleeding. Also check the site for hematoma or signs of infection; culture any drainage.

DISORDER	SIGNS AND SYMPTOMS	DIAGNOSTIC TEST RESULTS	TREATMENT AND CARE
Heart failure (complication)	◆ Cough that produces pink, frothy sputum ◆ Cyanosis of the lips and nail beds ◆ Pale, cool, clammy skin ◆ Diaphoresis ◆ Jugular vein distention ◆ Ascites ◆ Pulsus alternans ◆ Tachycardia ◆ Hepatomegaly ◆ Decreased pulse pressure ◆ Third and fourth heart sounds ◆ Moist, basilar crackles and rhonchi ◆ Expiratory wheezing ◆ Decreased pulse oximetry ◆ Peripheral edema ◆ Decreased urinary output	◆ B-type natriuretic peptide immunoassay may be elevated. ◆ Chest X-ray shows increased pulmonary vascular markings, interstitial edema, or pleural effusions and cardiomegaly. ◆ ECG reveals heart enlargement or ischemia, tachycardia, extrasystole, or atrial fibrillation. ◆ Pulmonary artery pressure (PAP), pulmonary artery wedge pressure (PAWP), and left ventricular end-diastolic pressure are elevated in the presence of left-sided heart failure; right atrial or central venous pressure is elevated in right-sided heart failure.	◆ Administer supplemental oxygen and mechanical ventilation if needed. ◆ Place the patient in Fowler's position. ◆ Administer diuretics, inotropic drugs, vasodilators, angiotensin-converting enzyme inhibitors, angiotensin receptor blockers, cardiac glycosides, beta-adrenergic blockers, or electrolyte supplements. ◆ Initiate cardiac monitoring. ◆ Maintain adequate cardiac output, and monitor hemodynamic stability. ◆ Assess for deep vein thrombosis, and apply antiembolism stockings.

Acute GI bleeding

OVERVIEW

- Bleeding that can occur anywhere in the GI tract and is classified as upper or lower
- Upper GI bleeding above the ligament of Treitz (where the duodenum meets the jejunum); esophagus, stomach, and duodenum common sites
- Lower GI bleeding below the Treitz ligament; colon most common site
- Usually stops spontaneously in most patients; however, acute GI bleeding accounting for significant morbidity and mortality
- Incidence of upper GI bleeding greater (100 patients per 100,000 adults) than that of lower GI bleeding (20 patients per 100,000 adults)
- On average, about 25% of patients who develop upper GI bleeding already hospitalized with another condition, whereas only 5% of these patients affected by lower GI bleeding

CAUSES

Common causes of *upper GI bleeding* include the following:
- Peptic ulcer disease (most common)
- Rupture of esophageal varices
- Esophagitis and esophageal ulcers
- Mallory-Weiss syndrome
- Reflux or infectious esophagitis
- Neoplasms
- Erosive gastritis
- Angiodysplasias
- Arteriovenous malformations

Common causes of *lower GI bleeding* include the following:
- Diverticulitis
- Inflammatory bowel disease
- Polyps
- Neoplasms
- Arteriovenous malformation
- Internal hemorrhoids
- Fissure

PATHOPHYSIOLOGY

- The extensive arterial blood supply near the stomach and esophagus can lead to a rapid loss of large amounts of blood, which may result in hypovolemia and shock. (See *Disorders affecting management of acute GI bleeding,* pages 22 and 23.)

CARDIOVASCULAR SYSTEM

- Loss of circulating blood volume leads to a decrease in venous return.
- Cardiac output and blood pressure decrease, resulting in inadequate tissue perfusion.
- Interstitial fluids shift to the intravascular space as a result of the body's attempt to compensate.
- The sympathetic nervous system is stimulated, resulting in vasoconstriction and an increase in heart rate.

RENAL SYSTEM

- The renin-angiotensin-aldosterone system is activated, causing increased secretion of antidiuretic hormone, thereby leading to fluid retention. These compensatory mechanisms lead to an increase in blood pressure.
- If blood loss continues, the compensatory mechanisms ultimately fail; cardiac output continues to decrease, which leads to cellular hypoxia and a shift from aerobic to anaerobic metabolism (with the subsequent buildup of lactic acid), resulting in metabolic acidosis.
- Eventually, all organs experience hypoperfusion, and fail.

ASSESSMENT

HISTORY

- Alcohol use
- Use of NSAIDs or anticoagulants
- History of hematochezia (bright red blood from the rectum) or melena (black, tarry, sticky stools)
- History of bloody or coffee ground vomitus
- History of weight loss or gain

PHYSICAL FINDINGS

- Asymptomatic, if total blood volume lost is 10% to 15% (500 to 750 ml)
- Anxiety, agitation, confusion
- Tachycardia
- Hypotension
- Oliguria
- Diaphoresis, pallor, and cool, clammy skin, if total blood volume lost is 35% to 50% (1,500 to 2,000 ml)
- Bright red bloody or coffee ground nasogastric (NG) tube drainage or vomitus (hematemesis)
- Crampy lower abdominal pain

DIAGNOSTIC TEST RESULTS

- Stool specimen positive for occult blood.
- Upper GI endoscopy reveals the source of bleeding, such as an ulcer, esophageal varices, or Mallory-Weiss tear.
- Colonoscopy reveals the source of lower GI bleeding, such as polyps.
- Complete blood count shows decreased hemoglobin level and hematocrit (usually 6 to 8 hours after the initial symptoms; hematocrit may be normal initially but can drop dramatically); increased reticulocyte and platelet levels; and a decrease in red blood cells.
- Blood urea nitrogen:creatinine ratio is greater than 30.
- Coagulation studies may be elevated.
- Arterial blood gas analysis reveals low pH and bicarbonate levels, indicating lactic acidosis.
- 12-lead electrocardiogram may reveal evidence of cardiac ischemia secondary to hypoperfusion.
- Abdominal X-ray may indicate air under the diaphragm, suggesting ulcer perforation.
- Angiography may help visualize the site of bleeding if the bleeding is from an artery or large vein.
- Small-bowel follow-through or a wireless capsule endoscope may help diagnose bleeding in the small bowel.

TREATMENT

GENERAL
- Fluid volume replacement with crystalloid solutions, initially, followed by colloids and blood component therapy
- Respiratory support, including supplemental oxygen and, possibly, mechanical ventilation for the patient who experiences respiratory failure
- Gastric intubation with gastric lavage (unless the patient has esophageal varices) and gastric pH monitoring
- Endoscopic therapy; sclerotherapy or cauterization

DIET
- Nothing by mouth during acute bleeding episode

ACTIVITY
- Bed rest during acute bleeding episodes

MEDICATIONS
- Oxygen
- Vasoconstrictors
- Histamine-2 receptor antagonists
- Proton pump inhibitor
- Calcium supplements
- Vitamin K (if International Normalized Ratio is elevated)

SURGERY
- Based on affected area and cause of bleeding

NURSING CONSIDERATIONS

NURSING DIAGNOSES
- Acute pain
- Anxiety
- Decreased cardiac output
- Deficient fluid volume
- Disturbed sleep pattern
- Imbalanced nutrition: Less than body requirements
- Risk for injury

EXPECTED OUTCOMES
The patient will:
- express feelings of increased comfort and decreased pain
- identify strategies to reduce anxiety
- remain hemodynamically stable
- maintain adequate fluid volume
- resume regular sleep patterns
- achieve adequate caloric and nutritional intake
- remain free from injury.

NURSING INTERVENTIONS
- Monitor vital signs, pulse oximetry, intake and output, and laboratory values.
- Give prescribed drugs.
- Maintain nothing-by-mouth status until acute bleeding resolves.
- Administer blood products, as ordered.
- Assess NG drainage for blood or coffee ground fluid.
- Note character and amount of stools.
- Offer emotional support.

PATIENT TEACHING

Be sure to cover:
- disorder, diagnostic testing, and treatment
- medication administration, dosage, and possible adverse effects
- warnings against over-the-counter medications, especially aspirin, aspirin-containing products, and NSAIDs, unless approved by the practitioner
- warnings against caffeine and alcohol intake during exacerbations
- appropriate lifestyle changes
- dietary modifications
- information on smoking cessation, if indicated.

RESOURCES
Organizations
Digestive Disease National Coalition: *www.ddnc.org*
National Digestive Diseases Information Clearinghouse: *www.niddk.nih.gov/health/digest/nddic.htm*

Selected references
Gisbert, J.P., et al. "Risk Assessment and Outpatient Management in Bleeding Peptic Ulcer," *Journal of Clinical Gastroenterology* 40(2):129-34, February 2006.

McGee, M., et al. "Management of Acute Gastrointestinal Hemorrhage," *Advances in Surgery* 40:119-58, 2006.

Tierney, L., et al. *Current Medical Diagnosis & Treatment 2006.* New York: McGraw-Hill Book Co., 2006.

Wong, T. "The Management of Upper Gastrointestinal Haemorrhage," *Clinical Medicine* 6(5): 460-64, September-October 2006.

(continued)

Disorders affecting management of acute GI bleeding

This chart highlights disorders that affect the management of acute GI bleeding.

DISORDER	SIGNS AND SYMPTOMS	DIAGNOSTIC TEST RESULTS	TREATMENT AND CARE
Aspiration pneumonia (complication)	◆ Fever ◆ Crackles ◆ Dyspnea ◆ Tachycardia ◆ Cough with blood-tinged sputum ◆ Cyanosis ◆ Decreased pulse oximetry	◆ Chest X-ray reveals infiltrates. ◆ Sputum for Gram stain and culture and sensitivity may reveal inflammatory cells and possible secondary bacterial infection. ◆ Bronchoscopy or transtracheal aspiration reveals possible secondary bacterial infection.	◆ Maintain a patent airway and adequate oxygenation. Place the patient in Fowler's position to maximize chest expansion, and give supplemental oxygen, as ordered. ◆ Assess respiratory status at least every 2 hours. Auscultate the lungs for abnormal breath sounds. If respiratory status deteriorates, anticipate the need for endotracheal intubation and mechanical ventilation. ◆ Encourage coughing and deep breathing. ◆ Monitor cardiac rhythm to detect arrhythmias secondary to hypoxemia. ◆ Monitor pulse oximetry and arterial blood gas (ABG) results to detect deteriorating oxygenation. ◆ Administer respiratory treatments and assess response to treatment. ◆ Reposition the patient every 2 hours. Maintain upright position (if possible) if patient has frequent vomiting episodes.
Hypovolemic shock (complication)	◆ Pale skin ◆ Decreased level of consciousness (LOC) ◆ Hypotension ◆ Tachycardia ◆ Urine output less than 25 ml/hour ◆ Cold, clammy skin	◆ Central venous pressure, right atrial pressure, pulmonary artery wedge pressure, and cardiac output are decreased. ◆ Hematocrit, hemoglobin, red blood cell count, and platelet count are decreased. ◆ Serum potassium, sodium, lactate dehydrogenase, blood urea nitrogen, and creatinine levels are elevated. ◆ Urine specific gravity is increased. ◆ ABG analysis reveals respiratory acidosis.	◆ Assess extent of fluid loss. ◆ Immediately administer fluid and blood replacement. ◆ Administer supplemental oxygen. ◆ Monitor respiratory status and pulse oximetry. ◆ Monitor vital signs continuously for changes. ◆ Anticipate the need for intubation and mechanical ventilation ◆ Prepare the patient for surgery to control bleeding, if indicated.
Myocardial infarction (complication)	◆ Pressure, squeezing, pain, or fullness in the center of the chest lasting several minutes ◆ Pain radiating to the shoulders, neck, arms, or jaw ◆ Pain in the back between the shoulder blades ◆ Light-headedness ◆ Fainting ◆ Sweating ◆ Nausea ◆ Shortness of breath ◆ Palpitations ◆ Feeling of impending doom	◆ Serial electrocardiogram may reveal ST-segment depression or ST-segment elevation. ◆ Serial cardiac enzymes (CK-MB) and proteins (troponin T and I) and myoglobin show a characteristic rise and fall. ◆ Nuclear imaging scanning may identify areas of infarction. ◆ Cardiac catheterization may show involved coronary and ventricular function. ◆ Chest X-rays may show left-sided heart failure or cardiomegaly. ◆ White blood cell count may be elevated. ◆ Echocardiography may show ventricular wall abnormalities.	◆ Percutaneous coronary intervention may be used; however, the patient with GI bleeding shouldn't receive heparin after the procedure. ◆ Administer morphine, as prescribed, to relieve chest pain. ◆ Administer oxygen, as needed. ◆ Administer nitroglycerin cautiously to relieve chest pain and reduce blood pressure. ◆ Administer beta-adrenergic blockers to decrease the heart's workload. ◆ Fibrinolytics, anticoagulants, and antiplatelet drugs, such as aspirin, are contraindicated in patients with GI bleeding.

Disorders affecting management of acute GI bleeding *(continued)*

DISORDER	SIGNS AND SYMPTOMS	DIAGNOSTIC TEST RESULTS	TREATMENT AND CARE
Stroke (complication)	◆ Sudden onset of hemiparesis or hemiplegia ◆ Dizziness ◆ Seizures ◆ Aphasia ◆ Dysphagia ◆ Decreased LOC ◆ Hypertension	◆ Cardiac catheterization may identify the involved coronary artery. ◆ Computed tomography identifies ischemic stroke within 72 hours and hemorrhagic stroke immediately. ◆ Magnetic resonance imaging identifies the area of ischemia, infarction, or edema. ◆ Angiography reveals disruption of cerebral circulation.	◆ Fibrinolytics, anticoagulants, and antiplatelet drugs, such as aspirin, are contraindicated in patients with GI bleeding. ◆ Percutaneous transluminal angioplasty or stent insertion may be used to open occluded vessels. ◆ Manage intracranial pressure with osmotic diuretics and corticosteroids. ◆ Administer anticonvulsants to treat or prevent seizures. ◆ Carotid endarterectomy may be indicated to open partially occluded carotid arteries.

Acute pancreatitis

- Inflammation of the pancreas
- Occurs in acute and chronic forms
- Acute form in 2 out of every 10,000 people, with 10% mortality rate
- Chronic form in 2 out of every 25,000 people, with irreversible tissue damage, which tends to progress to significant pancreatic function loss
- May be idiopathic but is sometimes associated with biliary tract disease, alcoholism, trauma, and certain drugs
- Affects more men than women
- Four times more common in Blacks than in Whites

CAUSES

- Abnormal organ structure
- Alcoholism
- Biliary tract disease
- Metabolic or endocrine disorders
- Pancreatic cysts or tumors
- Penetrating peptic ulcers
- Penetrating trauma
- Viral or bacterial infection

RISK FACTORS

- Use of glucocorticoids, sulfonamides, thiazides, and hormonal contraceptives
- Renal failure and kidney transplantation
- Endoscopic retrograde cholangiopancreatography (ERCP)
- Heredity
- Emotional or neurogenic factors

Acute pancreatitis occurs in two forms:
- Edematous (interstitial), which causes fluid accumulation and swelling
- Necrotizing (hemorrhagic), which causes cell death and tissue damage.

GASTROINTESTINAL SYSTEM

- Inflammation is caused by premature activation of enzymes (elastase and phospholipase A), which causes tissue damage. (See *Why enzymes activate prematurely.*) Enzymes back up and spill out into the pancreatic tissue, resulting in autodigestion of the pancreas.
- Elastase, which is activated by trypsin, digests the elastic tissue of the blood vessel walls, causing hemorrhage.
- Phospholipase A, which may be activated by trypsin or bile acids, digests the phospholipids contained in the cell membranes.
- Large amounts of fluid shift from the intravascular space to the peritoneal and interstitial spaces.

Why enzymes activate prematurely

Normally, the acini in the pancreas secrete enzymes in an inactive form. Sometimes, however, the enzymes are activated prematurely. Two theories attempt to explain why this occurs.

One theory suggests that a toxic agent, such as alcohol, alters the way the pancreas secretes enzymes. Increased pancreatic secretion then alters the metabolism of the acinar cells and encourages duct obstruction by causing pancreatic secretory proteins to precipitate.

Another theory suggests that reflux of duodenal contents containing activated enzymes enters the pancreatic duct, activating other enzymes and setting up a cycle for more pancreatic damage. This reflux may occur if atony and edema of the sphincter of Oddi occur, or if pancreatic duct obstruction or pancreatic ischemia is present.

- Additional fluid loss may occur because of vomiting, diarrhea, hemorrhage, and nasogastric suction.
- Third-space fluid shifting may occur because of hypoalbuminemia.
- Fluid losses eventually lead to hypovolemic shock.

CARDIOVASCULAR SYSTEM

- Trypsin activates kallikrein, which is thought to cause local damage and systemic hypotension. In turn, kallikrein causes vasodilation and increased vascular permeability, invasion of white blood cells, and pain.
- Tachycardia occurs as a result of hypotension, pain, and fever.

HEMATOLOGIC SYSTEM

- Pancreatic inflammation interferes with the absorption of vitamin K, resulting in vitamin K deficiency.
- Vitamin K deficiency, in turn, impairs clotting mechanisms, causing disseminated intravascular coagulation. (See *Disorders affecting management of acute pancreatitis,* page 27.)

IMMUNE SYSTEM

- The necrosed pancreatic tissue or tissue surrounding the pancreas may become infected/inflamed, resulting in leukocytosis and fever.
- Secondary infections occur as microorganisms, typically from other body areas such as the colon, move to the necrosed pancreas.
- As pancreatic enzymes cause further tissue necrosis, purulent drainage collects within the pancreas, which may erode through the retroperitoneum into the bowel, pleural space, mediastinum, or pelvis, subsequently leading to sepsis.

RESPIRATORY SYSTEM

◆ Severe pain interferes with the patient's ability to breathe deeply and expand his lungs adequately, commonly resulting in pneumonia.
◆ Pancreatic enzymes released into the circulation damage the pulmonary vessels, stimulate inflammation, and cause alveolocapillary leakage, resulting in intrapulmonary shunting, hypoxemia and, possibly, pleural effusion.

ASSESSMENT

HISTORY

◆ Severity of pancreatitis predicted using Ranson's criteria: if patient meets fewer than three of the criteria, mortality rate less than 1%; if patient meets three or four of the criteria, mortality rate increasing to 15% to 20%; if patient meets five or six criteria, mortality rate increasing to 40% (see *Ranson's criteria*)
◆ History of alcohol abuse, new or recent dietary changes, medications that are known to affect the pancreas, or cholelithiasis
◆ Intense epigastric pain centered close to the umbilicus and radiating to the back, between the 10th thoracic and 6th lumbar vertebrae
◆ Pain aggravated by fatty foods, alcohol consumption, or recumbent position
◆ Weight loss with nausea and vomiting

PHYSICAL FINDINGS

◆ Hypotension
◆ Tachycardia
◆ Fever
◆ Dyspnea, orthopnea
◆ Generalized jaundice
◆ Cullen's sign (bluish periumbilical discoloration)
◆ Turner's sign (bluish flank discoloration)
◆ Steatorrhea (with chronic pancreatitis)
◆ Abdominal tenderness, rigidity, and guarding

DIAGNOSTIC TEST RESULTS

◆ Abdominal and chest X-rays differentiate pancreatitis from other diseases that cause similar symptoms; they also detect pleural effusions.
◆ Computed tomography scans and ultrasonography show increased pancreatic diameter, pancreatic cysts, and pseudocysts.
◆ ERCP shows pancreatic anatomy, identifies ductal system abnormalities, and differentiates pancreatitis from other disorders.
◆ Serum amylase and lipase levels are elevated.
◆ White blood cell count is elevated.
◆ Serum bilirubin level is elevated.
◆ Transient hyperglycemia and glycosuria are present.
◆ Urine amylase level is increased.

Ranson's criteria

Use Ranson's criteria—a set of 11 signs, 5 of which are measured on admission to the health care facility, and 6 in the first 48 hours after admission—to assess the severity of acute pancreatitis. The more criteria met by the patient, the more severe the episode of pancreatitis and, therefore, the greater the risk of mortality.

ON ADMISSION

◆ Age older than 55
◆ White blood cell count greater than 16,000/mm^3
◆ Serum glucose greater than 200 mg/dl
◆ Lactate dehydrogenase greater than 350 IU/L
◆ Aspartate aminotransferase greater than 250 U/L

AFTER ADMISSION

◆ A 10% decrease in hematocrit
◆ Blood urea nitrogen increase greater than 5 mg/dl
◆ Serum calcium less than 8 mg/dl
◆ Base deficit greater than 4 mEq/L
◆ Partial pressure of arterial oxygen less than 60 mm Hg
◆ Estimated fluid sequestration greater than 6L

(continued)

TREATMENT

GENERAL
- Emergency treatment of shock, as needed; vigorous I.V. replacement of fluid, electrolytes, and proteins
- Respiratory support with supplemental oxygen and endotracheal intubation and mechanical ventilation, if necessary
- Blood transfusions (for hemorrhage)
- Nasogastric suctioning

DIET
- Nothing by mouth initially
- Once crisis starts to resolve, oral low-fat, low-protein feedings implemented gradually
- Alcohol and caffeine abstention

ACTIVITY
- As tolerated

MEDICATIONS
- Oxygen
- Analgesics
- Antacids
- Histamine antagonists
- Antibiotics
- Anticholinergics
- Total parenteral nutrition (TPN)
- Pancreatic enzymes
- Insulin
- Albumin

SURGERY
- Not indicated for acute pancreatitis, unless complications occur
- Sphincterotomy for chronic pancreatitis
- Pancreaticojejunostomy

NURSING CONSIDERATIONS

NURSING DIAGNOSES
- Acute pain
- Deficient fluid volume
- Disturbed body image
- Hopelessness
- Imbalanced nutrition: Less than body requirements
- Ineffective breathing pattern
- Risk for impaired skin integrity
- Risk for injury

EXPECTED OUTCOMES
The patient will:
- verbalize feelings of increased comfort and decreased pain
- maintain normal fluid volume
- express positive feelings about self
- participate in decisions about care
- achieve adequate caloric and nutritional intake
- maintain an effective breathing pattern
- maintain skin integrity
- remain free from injury.

NURSING INTERVENTIONS
- Give prescribed drugs and I.V. therapy.
- Encourage the patient to express his feelings.
- Provide emotional support.
- Monitor vital signs, intake and output, and nasogastric tube function and drainage.
- Assess respiratory status, acid-base balance, and oxygenation.
- Monitor capillary glucose levels, and provide appropriate insulin therapy.
- Weigh the patient daily.
- Assess pain level and provide analgesia, as ordered.
- Administer TPN, as ordered.

PATIENT TEACHING

Be sure to cover:
- disorder, diagnostic testing, and treatment
- medication administration, dosage, and possible adverse effects
- identification and avoidance of acute pancreatitis triggers
- dietary needs
- alcohol cessation, if appropriate
- available community resource and support services, as needed.

RESOURCES
Organizations
Alcoholics Anonymous: *www.aa.org*
Digestive Disease National Coalition: *www.ddnc.org*
National Digestive Diseases Information Clearinghouse: *www.niddk.nih.gov/health/digest/nddic.htm*

Selected references
Chowdhury, P., and Gupta, P. "Pathophysiology of Alcoholic Pancreatitis: An Overview," *World Journal of Gastroenterology* 12(46):7421-427, December 2006.

Phillips, R. "Acute Pancreatitis: Inflammation Gone Wild," *Nursing Made Incredibly Easy* 4(5):18-28, September-October 2006.

Shrikhande, S.V., et al. "Management of Pain in Small Duct Chronic Pancreatitis," *Journal of Gastrointestinal Surgery* 10(2):227-33, February 2006.

Tierney, L., et al. *Current Medical Diagnosis & Treatment 2006.* New York: McGraw-Hill Book Co., 2006.

Disorders affecting management of acute pancreatitis

This chart highlights disorders that affect the management of acute pancreatitis.

DISORDER	SIGNS AND SYMPTOMS	DIAGNOSTIC TEST RESULTS	TREATMENT AND CARE
Acute respiratory distress syndrome (ARDS) (complication)	◆ Rapid, shallow breathing ◆ Tachycardia ◆ Cool, clammy skin ◆ Dyspnea ◆ Restlessness ◆ Agitation	◆ Initially, arterial blood gas (ABG) analysis shows respiratory alkalosis; as ARDS worsens, respiratory acidosis. ◆ Pulmonary artery wedge pressure (PAWP) is 12 mm Hg or less. ◆ Chest X-ray shows ground-glass appearance and, eventually, "white-outs" of both lung fields.	◆ Assess respiratory status at least every 2 hours. ◆ Monitor pulse oximetry and ABG results. ◆ Monitor ventilator settings frequently. ◆ Suction only when necessary to maintain positive end-expiratory pressure. ◆ Administer neuromuscular blocking agents and sedation at regular intervals for maximum effect. ◆ Monitor heart rate and blood pressure hourly, or more frequently as indicated. ◆ Administer high-dose corticosteroids early in disease process. ◆ Administer diuretics to reduce interstitial and pulmonary edema.
Disseminated intravascular coagulation (complication)	◆ Bleeding from puncture sites ◆ Petechiae ◆ Ecchymoses ◆ Hematoma ◆ Nausea ◆ Vomiting ◆ Severe muscle, back, and abdominal pain ◆ Chest pain ◆ Hemoptysis	◆ Platelet count is decreased (less than 100,000/mm³). ◆ Fibrinogen is less than 150 mg/dl. ◆ Prothrombin time (PT) is greater than 15 seconds. ◆ Fibrin degradation product level is greater than 45 mcg/ml. ◆ D-dimer is elevated. ◆ Blood urea nitrogen (BUN) and creatinine levels are elevated.	◆ Treat underlying cause. ◆ Administer fresh frozen plasma, platelets, cryoprecipitate, and packed RBCs. ◆ Monitor vital signs at least every 30 minutes. ◆ Administer supplemental oxygen, as indicated. ◆ Assess level of consciousness (LOC) hourly and when the patient's condition changes. ◆ Monitor serial hemoglobin and hematocrit, partial thromboplastin time, PT, fibrinogen levels, fibrinogen degradation products, and platelet counts. ◆ Administer low-dose heparin infusion.
Hypovolemic shock (complication)	◆ Pale skin ◆ Decreased LOC ◆ Hypotension ◆ Tachycardia ◆ Urine output less than 25 ml/hour ◆ Cold, clammy skin	◆ Central venous pressure, right atrial pressure, PAWP, and cardiac output are decreased. ◆ Hematocrit, hemoglobin level, red blood cell (RBC) count, and platelet counts are low. ◆ Serum potassium, sodium, lactate dehydrogenase, BUN, and creatinine levels are elevated. ◆ Urine specific gravity is increased. ◆ ABG analysis reveals respiratory acidosis.	◆ Administer vitamin K and folate. ◆ Institute safety precautions to minimize bleeding. ◆ Assess extent of fluid loss. ◆ Administer fluid and blood replacement immediately. ◆ Administer supplemental oxygen. ◆ Monitor respiratory status and pulse oximetry. ◆ Monitor vital signs continuously for changes. ◆ Anticipate the need for intubation and mechanical ventilation. ◆ Prepare the patient for surgery, if indicated, to control bleeding.
Sepsis (complication)	◆ Agitation ◆ Anxiety ◆ Altered LOC ◆ Tachycardia ◆ Hypotension ◆ Rapid, shallow respirations ◆ Fever ◆ Urine output less than 25 ml/hour	◆ Blood cultures are positive for the infecting organism. ◆ Complete blood count reveals whether anemia, neutropenia, and thrombocytopenia are present. ◆ ABG studies show metabolic acidosis. ◆ BUN and creatinine levels are increased. ◆ Electrocardiogram shows ST-segment depression, inverted T waves, and arrhythmias.	◆ Locate and treat the underlying cause of sepsis. ◆ Monitor vital signs frequently. ◆ Administer antibiotics. ◆ Administer I.V. fluids to replace intravascular volume. ◆ Administer vasopressors if fluid resuscitation doesn't maintain blood pressure. ◆ Assess respiratory status. ◆ Prepare for intubation and mechanical ventilation, if needed. ◆ Monitor lactate levels.

Acute renal failure

OVERVIEW

- Sudden interruption of renal function resulting from obstruction, reduced circulation, or renal parenchymal disease
- Normally occurs in three distinct phases: oliguric, diuretic, and recovery (see *Phases of acute renal failure*)
- Classified as prerenal, intrarenal (also called *intrinsic* or *parenchymal failure*), or postrenal
- Occurs in 5% of hospitalized patients
- Usually reversible with medical treatment
- If not treated, may progress to end-stage renal disease, uremia, and death

CAUSES

Prerenal failure
- Hemorrhagic blood loss
- Hypotension or hypoperfusion
- Hypovolemia
- Loss of plasma volume
- Water and electrolyte losses

Intrarenal failure
- Acute tubular necrosis (ATN)
- Coagulation defects
- Glomerulopathies
- Malignant hypertension

Postrenal failure
- Bladder neck obstruction
- Obstructive uropathies, usually bilateral
- Ureteral destruction

PATHOPHYSIOLOGY

- Oliguria occurs as a result of decreased glomerular filtration rate (GFR).
- Hyperkalemia occurs as a result of decreased GFR and metabolic acidosis.
- Hyperphosphatemia and hypocalcemia occur because the kidney can't excrete phosphorus.

RENAL SYSTEM
Prerenal failure
- Prerenal failure is caused by impaired blood flow.
- The decrease in filtration pressure causes the GFR to decline.
- Failure to restore blood volume or blood pressure may cause ATN or acute cortical necrosis.

Intrarenal failure
- A severe episode of hypotension, commonly associated with hypovolemia, is often a significant contributing event.
- Cell swelling, injury, and necrosis—a form of reperfusion injury that may also be caused by nephrotoxins—results from ischemia-generated, toxic, oxygen-free radicals and anti-inflammatory mediators.

Postrenal failure
- Postrenal failure usually occurs with urinary tract obstruction that affects the kidneys bilaterally such as prostatic hyperplasia. (See *Disorders affecting management of acute renal failure*, page 31.)

CARDIOVASCULAR SYSTEM
- Hypertension and edema occur with fluid accumulation and hypervolemia.
- Fluid overload may cause pulmonary and peripheral edema, possibly leading to heart failure because of how these conditions increase the heart's workload.

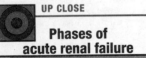

UP CLOSE

Phases of acute renal failure

When acute renal failure occurs, the renal system goes through 3 phases:

OLIGURIC PHASE
- May last a few days or several weeks
- Urine output less than 400 ml/day
- Fluid volume excess, azotemia, and electrolyte imbalance
- Local mediators released, causing intrarenal vasoconstriction
- Medullary hypoxia causing cellular swelling and adherence of neutrophils to capillaries and venules
- Hypoperfusion
- Cellular injury and necrosis
- Reperfusion causing reactive oxygen species to form, leading to further cellular injury

DIURETIC PHASE
- Renal function recovering
- Urine output gradually increasing
- Glomerular filtration rate improving, although tubular transport systems remain abnormal

RECOVERY PHASE
- May last 3 to 12 months, or longer
- Gradual return to normal or near normal renal function

- Acute pulmonary edema and hypertensive crisis may result from nephron dysfunction, causing decreased blood flow to the kidneys.
- Arrhythmias and cardiac arrest may result from hyperkalemia.

ENDOCRINE AND METABOLIC SYSTEMS
- Metabolic acidosis occurs because the kidney can't excrete hydrogen ions and reabsorb sodium and bicarbonate.

GASTROINTESTINAL SYSTEM
- Nausea, vomiting, and anorexia occur with uremia.
- GI bleeding may occur with coagulation abnormalities and uremic gastric irritation.

IMMUNE AND HEMATOLOGIC SYSTEMS
- Infection and sepsis may occur because of decreased white blood cell–mediated immunity.
- A hypercoagulable state results from anticoagulant abnormalities, which leads to bleeding and clotting difficulties.

NEUROLOGIC SYSTEM
- Altered mental status and peripheral neuropathies are related to the effects of uremic toxins on the highly sensitive nerve cells.
- Headache, drowsiness, irritability, and seizures result from central nervous system involvement and, without treatment, may progress to coma.

RESPIRATORY SYSTEM
- Tachypnea and labored breathing result from anemia, causing tissue hypoxia. Respiratory rate and effort also increase to compensate for metabolic acidosis.
- Fluid overload may lead to pulmonary congestion, impaired gas exchange, and ineffective breathing.

ASSESSMENT

HISTORY
- Predisposing disorder
- Recent fever, chills, or central nervous system problem
- Recent GI problems

PHYSICAL FINDINGS
- Oliguria or anuria
- Tachycardia
- Bibasilar crackles
- Irritability, drowsiness, or confusion
- Altered level of consciousness
- Bleeding abnormalities
- Dry, pruritic skin
- Dry mucous membranes
- Uremic breath odor

DIAGNOSTIC TEST RESULTS
- Blood urea nitrogen, serum creatinine, and potassium levels are elevated.
- Hematocrit, blood pH, bicarbonate, and hemoglobin levels are decreased.
- Urine casts and cellular debris are present, and specific gravity is decreased.
- In glomerular disease, proteinuria and urine osmolality are close to serum osmolality level.
- Urine sodium level is less than 20 mEq/L, caused by decreased perfusion in oliguria.
- Urine sodium level is greater than 40 mEq/L, caused by intrarenal problem in oliguria.
- Urine creatinine clearance measures GFR and estimates the number of remaining functioning nephrons.
- Kidney ultrasonography, kidney-ureter-bladder radiography, excretory urography renal scan, retrograde pyelography, computed tomography scan, nephrotomography may show structural cause of renal malfunction.
- Electrocardiography shows tall, peaked T waves; a widening QRS complex; and disappearing P waves, if hyperkalemia is present.

TREATMENT

GENERAL
- Hemodialysis or continuous renal replacement therapy

DIET
- High-calorie, low-protein, low-sodium, and low-potassium
- Fluid restriction

ACTIVITY
- Rest periods when fatigued

MEDICATIONS
- Diuretics
- For hyperkalemia, hypertonic glucose-and-insulin infusions, sodium bicarbonate, and sodium polystyrene sulfonate
- Antiarrhythmics

SURGERY
- Insertion of vascular access for hemodialysis

(continued)

NURSING DIAGNOSES

- Activity intolerance
- Decreased cardiac output
- Fatigue
- Fear
- Imbalanced nutrition: Less than body requirements
- Impaired gas exchange
- Impaired urinary elimination
- Ineffective tissue perfusion: Renal
- Interrupted family processes
- Risk for imbalanced fluid volume
- Risk for infection
- Risk for injury

EXPECTED OUTCOMES

The patient (or family) will:

- perform activities of daily living without excessive fatigue or exhaustion
- maintain hemodynamic stability
- remain free from signs and symptoms of circulatory overload
- express the importance of balancing activities with adequate rest periods
- discuss fears or concerns
- verbalize appropriate food choices
- maintain adequate ventilation and oxygenation
- demonstrate the ability to manage urinary elimination problems
- maintain adequate urine output
- verbalize the effect the patient's condition has on the family unit
- maintain fluid balance
- remain free from signs or symptoms of infection
- remain free from injury.

NURSING INTERVENTIONS

- Give prescribed drugs.
- Encourage the patient to express his feelings.
- Provide emotional support.
- Identify patients at risk for and take steps to prevent ATN. (See *Preventing acute tubular necrosis.*)
- Monitor intake and output, daily weight, renal function studies, and vital signs.
- Observe for effects of excess fluid volume.
- Assess dialysis access site every shift.

Be sure to cover:

- disorder, diagnostic testing, and treatment
- medication administration, dosage, and possible adverse effects
- recommended fluid allowance
- compliance with diet and drug regimen
- importance of immediately reporting weight changes of 3 lb or more
- signs and symptoms of edema and importance of reporting them
- need for follow-up care with nephrologist.

RESOURCES
Organizations

American Association of Kidney Patients: *www.aakp.org*
National Institute of Diabetes & Digestive & Kidney Diseases: *www.niddk.nih.gov*
National Kidney Foundation: *www.kidney.org*

Selected references

Chan, V., et al. "Valve Replacement Surgery Complicated by Acute Renal Failure—Predictors of Early Mortality," *Journal of Cardiac Surgery* 21(2):139-43, March-April 2006.

Diseases, 4th ed. Philadelphia: Lippincott Williams & Wilkins, 2006.

Francisco, A.L., and Pinera, C. "Challenges and Future of Renal Replacement Therapy," *Hemodialysis International* 10(Suppl 1):S19-23, January 2006.

Perkins, C., and Kisel, M. "Utilizing Physiological Knowledge to Care for Acute Renal Failure," *British Journal of Nursing* 14(14):768-73, July-August 2005.

Uchino, S., et al. "Acute Renal Failure in Critically Ill Patients: A Multinational, Multicenter Study," *JAMA* 294(7):813-18, August 2005.

Preventing acute tubular necrosis

Acute tubular necrosis (ATN) occurs mainly in elderly hospitalized patients. Contributing causes include aminoglycoside therapy and exposure to industrial chemicals, heavy metals, and contrast media. Patients who have been exposed must receive adequate hydration; monitor their urinary output closely.

To prevent ATN, make sure every patient is well hydrated before surgery or after X-rays that use a contrast medium. Administer mannitol, as ordered, to a high-risk patient before and during these procedures. Carefully monitor a patient receiving a blood transfusion, and stop the transfusion immediately if signs of transfusion reaction (fever, rash, and chills) occur.

Disorders affecting management of acute renal failure

This chart highlights disorders that affect the management of acute renal failure.

DISORDER	SIGNS AND SYMPTOMS	DIAGNOSTIC TEST RESULTS	TREATMENT AND CARE
Hyperkalemia (complication)	◆ Skeletal muscle weakness ◆ Flaccid paralysis ◆ Decreased heart rate ◆ Irregular pulse ◆ Decreased cardiac output ◆ Hypotension ◆ Cardiac arrest	◆ Electrocardiography (ECG) shows tall, tented T waves (characteristic); flattened P wave; and prolonged PR interval. ◆ Serum potassium levels are greater than 5 mEq/L; however, with severe hyperkalemia, levels are greater than 7 mEq/L.	◆ Administer loop diuretics. ◆ Discontinue medications known to increase potassium, including antibiotics, angiotensin-converting enzyme inhibitors, beta-adrenergic blockers, digoxin, heparin, nonsteroidal anti-inflammatory drugs, and potassium-sparing diuretics. ◆ Administer sodium polystyrene sulfonate (Kayexalate) (for mild hyperkalemia) or sorbitol. Watch for signs of heart failure when administering Kayexalate. Administer I.V. hypertonic glucose, insulin, and sodium bicarbonate (for severe hyperkalemia). ◆ Monitor serum potassium and other electrolytes frequently. ◆ Assess vital signs. ◆ Institute and maintain cardiac monitoring. ◆ Monitor intake and output, reporting an output of less than 30 ml/hour. ◆ Watch for signs of hypokalemia. ◆ Prepare the patient for dialysis if other treatments fail.
Hypertension (complication)	◆ Bounding pulse ◆ Fourth heart sound (S₄) ◆ Dizziness ◆ Fatigue ◆ Palpitations ◆ Chest pain ◆ Dyspnea ◆ Elevated blood pressure on at least two consecutive readings after initial screening	◆ Blood pressure is elevated (intermittent or sustained). ◆ Urinalysis may show protein, red blood cells, white blood cells, or glucose. ◆ Serum potassium levels are less than 3.5 mEq/L, possibly indicating adrenal dysfunction. ◆ Blood urea nitrogen (BUN) and creatinine levels are normal or elevated. ◆ ECG may reveal left ventricular hypertrophy. ◆ Arterial blood gas (ABG) analysis shows hypoxemia, hypercapnia, or acidosis. ◆ Chest X-ray shows diffuse haziness of the lung fields, cardiomegaly, and pleural effusion.	◆ Administer antihypertensives; adjust dosage to manage blood pressure. ◆ Monitor blood pressure. ◆ Monitor BUN and creatinine levels. ◆ Institute a sodium-restricted, low-fat diet. ◆ Encourage stress reduction, an exercise program, and behavior modification related to alcohol or tobacco use. ◆ Assess for bruits over the abdominal aorta and femoral arteries or the carotids. ◆ Assess for peripheral edema, bounding pulse, and respiratory distress related to hypervolemia. ◆ Assess for S₄.
Pulmonary edema (complication)	◆ Restlessness and anxiety ◆ Rapid, labored breathing ◆ Intense, productive cough ◆ Frothy, bloody sputum ◆ Mental status changes ◆ Jugular vein distention ◆ Wheezing ◆ Crackles ◆ Third heart sound (S₃) ◆ Tachycardia ◆ Hypotension ◆ Thready pulse ◆ Peripheral edema ◆ Hepatomegaly	◆ Pulse oximetry may reveal decreased oxygenation of the blood. ◆ Pulmonary artery catheterization may reveal increased pulmonary artery wedge pressures. ◆ ECG may show valvular disease and left ventricular hypokinesis or akinesis.	◆ Identify and attempt to correct or manage the underlying disease. ◆ Closely monitor pulse oximetry and ABG results and hemodynamic values. ◆ Institute energy conservation strategies and space activities, as dictated by respiratory ability. ◆ Provide supplemental oxygen and mechanical ventilation if needed. ◆ Restrict fluids and sodium. ◆ Closely monitor intake and output. ◆ Implement cardiac monitoring. ◆ Administer antiarrhythmics, diuretics, preload and afterload reducing agents, bronchodilators, or vasopressors. ◆ Maintain adequate cardiac output. ◆ Assess weight daily.

Acute respiratory distress syndrome LIFE-THREATENING DISORDER

OVERVIEW

- Severe form of alveolar injury or acute lung injury
- Form of noncardiogenic pulmonary edema; may be difficult to recognize
- Hypoxemia despite increased supplemental oxygen (hallmark sign)
- Four-stage syndrome; may rapidly progress to intractable and fatal hypoxemia
- Little or no permanent lung damage occurring in patients who recover
- May coexist with disseminated intravascular coagulation (DIC) and sepsis
- 85% probability of developing acute respiratory distress syndrome (ARDS) in patients with three concurrent causes
- Also known as *adult respiratory distress syndrome* and *shock lung, stiff lung, white lung, wet lung,* or *Da Nang lung*

CAUSES

- Acute miliary tuberculosis
- Anaphylaxis
- Aspiration of gastric contents
- Diffuse pneumonia (especially viral)
- Drug overdose
- Gestational hypertension
- Hemodialysis
- Idiosyncratic drug reaction
- Indirect or direct lung trauma (most common)
- Inhalation of noxious gases
- Leukemia
- Massive blood transfusion
- Near drowning
- Oxygen toxicity
- Pancreatitis
- Prolonged coronary artery bypass grafting
- Sepsis
- Thrombotic thrombocytopenic purpura
- Uremia
- Venous air embolism

PATHOPHYSIOLOGY

- The alveolar epithelium and the pulmonary capillary epithelium are injured by a specific agent or event, triggering a series of cellular and biochemical changes. (See *How ARDS develops.*)

RESPIRATORY SYSTEM

- Damage to alveolar and pulmonary capillary epithelium triggers neutrophils, macrophages, monocytes, and lymphocytes to produce various cytokines that promote cellular activation, chemotaxis, and adhesion.
- Damage can occur directly (by aspiration of gastric contents and inhalation of noxious gases) or indirectly (from chemical mediators released in response to systemic disease).
- The activated cells produce inflammatory mediators, including oxidants, proteases, kinins, growth factors, and neuropeptides, which initiate the complement cascade, intravascular coagulation, and fibrinolysis.
- Vascular permeability to proteins increases, ultimately affecting the hydrostatic pressure gradient of the capillary. Plasma and blood leak into the alveoli and interstitial space.
- Fluid accumulates in the lung interstitium, the alveolar spaces, and the small airways, causing the lungs to stiffen and thus impairing ventilation and reducing oxygenation of the pulmonary capillary blood.
- Pressure changes and decreased surfactant result in alveolar collapse and atelectasis.
- Interstitial inflammation develops, and epithelial cells proliferate.
- Fluid in the alveoli and alveolar cell damage reduce surfactant production, which increases surface tension in the alveoli.
- Lung surface area is decreased as the lungs become less compliant and the alveoli collapse. (See *Disorders affecting management of ARDS,* pages 36 and 37.)

- Gas exchange is impaired, and respirations increase to address hypoxia.
- Initially, oxygenation is affected and carbon dioxide (CO_2) levels decrease because CO_2 is more easily diffused across the impaired alveolar-capillary membrane. As gas exchange worsens, hypercapnia develops.
- Hyaline membranes form because of the lack of surfactant and the collection of tissue debris and white blood cells in the airway.
- Inflammation leads to fibrosis, further impeding gas exchange, which progressively obliterates alveoli, respiratory bronchioles, and the interstitium. Functional residual capacity decreases, and shunting becomes more serious.
- Increasing partial pressure of arterial carbon dioxide ($Paco_2$) leads to respiratory acidosis.
- Hypoxia further increases acidosis; pH decreases.
- Hypoxia and acidosis result in mental changes.

IMMUNE SYSTEM

- The lung injury causes an inflammatory response, which continues as ARDS progresses.
- Platelets aggregate at the lung injury site and release substances—such as serotonin, bradykinin, and histamine—that attract and activate neutrophils. These substances inflame and damage the alveolar membrane and increase capillary permeability.
- Additional chemotactic factors are released, including endotoxins (such as those present in septic states), tumor necrosis factor, and interleukin-1 (IL-1). The activated neutrophils also release several inflammatory mediators and platelet aggravating factors that damage the alveolar capillary membrane and increase capillary permeability.

How ARDS develops

These diagrams show the process and progress of acute respiratory distress syndrome (ARDS).

Phase 1. Injury reduces normal blood flow to the lungs. Platelets aggregate and release histamine (H), serotonin (S), and bradykinin (B).

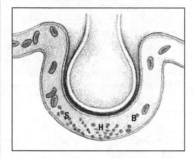

Phase 2. The released substances inflame and damage the alveolar capillary membrane, increasing capillary permeability. Fluids then shift into the interstitial space.

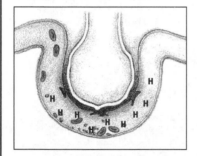

Phase 3. Capillary permeability increases and proteins and fluids leak out, increasing interstitial osmotic pressure and causing pulmonary edema.

Phase 4. Decreased blood flow and fluids in the alveoli damage surfactant and impair the cell's ability to produce more. The alveoli then collapse, thus impairing gas exchange.

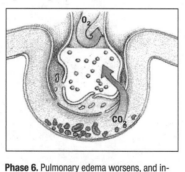

Phase 5. Oxygenation is impaired, but carbon dioxide (CO_2) easily crosses the alveolar capillary membrane and is expired. Blood oxygen (O_2) and CO_2 levels are low.

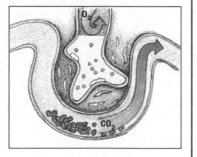

Phase 6. Pulmonary edema worsens, and inflammation leads to fibrosis. Gas exchange is further impeded.

- Histamines and other inflammatory substances also increase capillary permeability, allowing fluids to move into the interstitial space. As capillary permeability increases, proteins, blood cells, and more fluid leak out, increasing interstitial osmotic pressure and causing pulmonary edema.
- Mediators released by neutrophils and macrophages cause varying degrees of pulmonary vasoconstriction, resulting in pulmonary hypertension and causing a ventilation-perfusion mismatch.
- Systemically, neutrophils and inflammatory mediators cause generalized endothelial damage and increased capillary permeability throughout the body.
- Multiple organ dysfunction syndrome (MODS) occurs as the cascade of mediators affects each body system.
- Death may occur from the combined influence of ARDS and MODS.

(continued)

HISTORY
- Causative factor (one or more)
- Dyspnea, especially on exertion

PHYSICAL FINDINGS
Stage I
- Shortness of breath, especially on exertion
- Normal to increased respiratory and pulse rates
- Diminished breath sounds

Stage II
- Respiratory distress
- Use of accessory muscles for respiration
- Pallor, anxiety, and restlessness
- Dry cough with thick, frothy sputum
- Bloody, sticky secretions
- Cool, clammy skin
- Tachycardia and tachypnea
- Elevated blood pressure
- Basilar crackles

Stage III
- Respiratory rate more than 30 breaths/minute
- Tachycardia with arrhythmias
- Labile blood pressure
- Productive cough
- Pale, cyanotic skin
- Crackles and rhonchi (possibly)

Stage IV
- Acute respiratory failure with severe hypoxia
- Deteriorating mental status (may become comatose)
- Pale, cyanotic skin
- Lack of spontaneous respirations
- Bradycardia with arrhythmias
- Hypotension
- Metabolic and respiratory acidosis

DIAGNOSTIC TEST RESULTS
- Arterial blood gas (ABG) analysis initially shows a partial pressure of arterial oxygen (Pao_2) of less than 60 mm Hg and a $Paco_2$ of less than 35 mm Hg.
- ABG analysis later shows increased $Paco_2$ (more than 45 mm Hg), decreased bicarbonate levels (less than 22 mEq/L), and decreased Pao_2 despite oxygen therapy.
- Gram stain and sputum culture and sensitivity show infectious organisms.
- Blood cultures reveal infectious organisms.
- Toxicology tests show drug ingestion (in overdose).
- Serum amylase level is increased (in pancreatitis).
- Chest X-rays show early bilateral infiltrates; in later stages, chest X-rays show a ground-glass appearance and, eventually, "whiteouts" of both lung fields.
- Pulmonary artery catheterization shows a pulmonary artery wedge pressure between 12 and 18 mm Hg.

GENERAL
- Treatment of the underlying cause
- Correction of electrolyte and acid-base imbalances
- Deep vein thrombosis prophylaxis

For mechanical ventilation
- Target low tidal volumes; use of increased respiratory rates
- Target plateau pressures less than or equal to 40 cm H_2O
- Positive end-expiratory pressure (PEEP), as necessary

DIET
- Fluid restriction
- Tube feedings or parenteral nutrition while intubated

ACTIVITY
- Bed rest
- Prone positioning to help with perfusion to the lungs
- Head of bed at 30 degrees, if tolerated

MEDICATIONS
- Humidified oxygen
- Bronchodilators
- Diuretics

With mechanical ventilation
- Sedatives
- Opioids
- Neuromuscular agents
- Short course of high-dose corticosteroids, if fatty emboli or chemical injury is present
- Sodium bicarbonate, if severe metabolic acidosis is identified
- Fluids and vasopressors, if hypotensive
- Antimicrobials, if nonviral infection is identified

SURGERY
- Possible tracheostomy

NURSING DIAGNOSES
◆ Anxiety
◆ Decreased cardiac output
◆ Fatigue
◆ Fear
◆ Imbalanced nutrition: Less than body requirements
◆ Impaired gas exchange
◆ Impaired physical mobility
◆ Ineffective tissue perfusion: Cardiopulmonary
◆ Risk for impaired skin integrity
◆ Risk for infection

EXPECTED OUTCOMES
The patient will:
◆ express feelings of comfort and decreased anxiety
◆ maintain adequate cardiac output
◆ express feelings of energy and decreased fatigue
◆ verbalize feelings of fear
◆ consume required caloric intake
◆ maintain a patent airway
◆ maintain joint mobility and range of motion (ROM)
◆ maintain hemodynamic stability
◆ maintain skin integrity
◆ remain free from signs or symptoms of infection.

NURSING INTERVENTIONS
◆ Give prescribed drugs.
◆ Maintain a patent airway.
◆ Perform tracheal suctioning, only when necessary.
◆ Ensure adequate oxygen humidification.
◆ Reposition the patient every 2 hours.
◆ Apply sequential compression stockings.
◆ Consider prone positioning for alveolar recruitment.
◆ Administer tube feedings or parenteral nutrition, as ordered.
◆ Allow periods of uninterrupted sleep.
◆ Perform passive ROM exercises.
◆ Provide meticulous skin and mouth care.
◆ Reposition the endotracheal tube according to facility policy.
◆ Provide emotional support.

◆ Provide alternative communication means.
◆ Monitor vital signs, pulse oximetry, hemodynamics, and intake and output.

WARNING *Because PEEP may lower cardiac output, check for hypotension, tachycardia, and decreased urine output. To maintain PEEP, suction only as needed.*
◆ Assess respiratory status (breath sounds, ABG results) every 2 to 4 hours, and as needed.
◆ Check mechanical ventilator settings and alarms every shift.
◆ Monitor sputum characteristics, level of consciousness, daily weight, and laboratory studies.
◆ Observe response to treatment.
◆ Watch for complications, such as cardiac arrhythmias, DIC, GI bleeding, infection, malnutrition, and pneumothorax.
◆ Assess nutritional status.

Be sure to cover:
◆ disorder, diagnostic testing, and treatment
◆ medication administration, dosage, and possible adverse effects
◆ when to notify the practitioner
◆ complications, such as GI bleeding, infection, and malnutrition
◆ expected recovery time
◆ available pulmonary rehabilitation program, if indicated.

RESOURCES
Organizations
ARDS Clinical Network: *www.ardsnet.org*
National Heart, Lung, and Blood Institute: *www.nhlbi.nih.gov*

Selected references
Cameron, J.I., et al. "Well-Being in Informal Caregivers of Survivors of Acute Respiratory Distress Syndrome," *Critical Care Medicine* 34(1):81-86, January 2006.
Delong, P., et al. "Mechanical Ventilation in the Management of Acute Respiratory Distress Syndrome," *Seminars in Dialysis* 19(6):517-24, November-December 2006.
Downar, J., and Mehta, S. "Bench to Bedside Review: High Frequency Oscillatory Ventilation in Adults with Acute Respiratory Distress Syndome," *Critical Care* 10(6): 240, December 2006.
Taylor, M. "ARDS Diagnosis and Management; Implications for the Critical Care Nurse," *Dimensions of Critical Care* 24(5):197-207, September-October 2005.

(continued)

Disorders affecting management of ARDS

This chart highlights disorders that affect the management of acute respiratory distress syndrome (ARDS).

DISORDER	SIGNS AND SYMPTOMS	DIAGNOSTIC TEST RESULTS	TREATMENT AND CARE
Metabolic acidosis (complication)	◆ Headache, lethargy progressing to drowsiness, central nervous system depression, Kussmaul's respirations, hypotension, stupor, and coma ◆ Anorexia, nausea, vomiting, diarrhea, and possibly dehydration ◆ Warm, flushed skin ◆ Fruity breath odor	◆ Arterial pH is below 7.35. ◆ Partial pressure of arterial carbon dioxide ($Paco_2$) may be normal or less than 34 mm Hg; bicarbonate level may be less than 22 mEq/L. ◆ Serum potassium level is greater than 5.5 mEq/L. ◆ Anion gap is greater than 14 mEq/L.	◆ Correct the underlying cause. ◆ For severe cases, administer sodium bicarbonate I.V. ◆ Frequently monitor vital signs, laboratory results, and level of consciousness (LOC) because changes can occur rapidly. ◆ Evaluate and correct electrolyte imbalances. ◆ Because metabolic acidosis commonly causes vomiting, position the patient to prevent aspiration. ◆ Record intake and output carefully to monitor renal function.
Multiple organ dysfunction syndrome (complication)	◆ Hypotension ◆ Tachycardia ◆ Weak, thready peripheral pulses ◆ Decreased urine output ◆ Respiratory distress (tachypnea, accessory muscle use) ◆ Lung crackles on auscultation ◆ Peripheral edema ◆ Decreased LOC	◆ Complete blood count may reveal increased white blood cells and decreased hemoglobin. ◆ Serum studies show hyperglycemia in early stages, increased lactate levels, and electrolyte and enzyme abnormalities. ◆ Arterial blood gas (ABG) analysis shows metabolic acidosis with a pH less than 7.35 and a $Paco_2$ less than 32 mm Hg. ◆ Chest X-ray may show pulmonary edema.	◆ Administer oxygen therapy, as needed, to increase oxygen available to tissues. ◆ Monitor blood pressure, heart rate, and peripheral pulses continuously or every hour. ◆ Administer I.V. fluids, inotropic drugs, and vasodilators or vasopressors to maximize cardiac function. ◆ Watch the patient closely for signs of decreased cerebral perfusion (decreased LOC, restlessness) and decreased renal perfusion (urine output less than 0.5 ml/kg/hour, elevated serum blood urea nitrogen, creatinine, and potassium levels). ◆ Administer antibiotic therapy to treat underlying infection. ◆ Assess for interstitial edema, indicated by pretibial, sacral, ankle, and hand edema and lung crackles. ◆ Prepare for endotracheal intubation and mechanical ventilation if the patient exhibits impaired gas exchange. ◆ Maintain a patent airway by assisting with coughing or suctioning, as needed.
Pneumonia (coexisting)	◆ Elevated temperature ◆ Cough with purulent, yellow, or bloody sputum ◆ Dyspnea ◆ Crackles ◆ Decreased breath sounds ◆ Pleuritic pain ◆ Chills ◆ Malaise	◆ Chest X-ray shows infiltrates. ◆ Sputum smear reveals acute inflammatory cells.	◆ Provide humidified oxygen therapy for hypoxia and mechanical ventilation for respiratory failure. ◆ Administer antimicrobial therapy according to the causative organism. ◆ Administer an analgesic to relieve pleuritic chest pain. ◆ Provide a high-calorie diet, adequate fluid intake, and bed rest, as needed.

DISORDER	SIGNS AND SYMPTOMS	DIAGNOSTIC TEST RESULTS	TREATMENT AND CARE
Pneumothorax (coexisting)	◆ Tachypnea ◆ Sudden, sharp pleuritic pain exacerbated by chest movement, breathing, and coughing ◆ Asymmetrical chest wall movement ◆ Shortness of breath ◆ Cyanosis and respiratory distress ◆ Absent breath sounds on the affected side ◆ Chest rigidity ◆ Tachycardia and hypotension ◆ Mediastinal shift and tracheal deviation	◆ Chest X-ray shows air in the pleural space and, possibly, mediastinal shift. ◆ ABG analysis may show hypoxemia, possibly with respiratory acidosis and hypercapnia.	◆ If the lung collapse is less than 30% and the patient shows no signs of dyspnea or other compromise, treatment includes bed rest, blood pressure monitoring, oxygen administration and, possibly, needle aspiration of the chest to remove air. ◆ If more than 30% of the lung is collapsed, treatment to reexpand the lung includes placing a thoracostomy tube and connecting it to an underwater seal or low-pressure suction. ◆ Watch for pallor, gasping respirations, and sudden chest pain. ◆ Carefully monitor vital signs at least every hour for indications of shock, increasing respiratory distress, or mediastinal shift. ◆ Ascultate for breath sounds over both lungs. ◆ Encourage the patient to cough and deep breathe at least once per hour to facilitate lung expansion after the chest tube is in place. ◆ Observe the chest tube site for leakage; change dressings around the chest tube insertion site, as needed. ◆ Prevent potential barotraumas and pneumothorax by using the lowest pressures needed to reduce hypoxemia, or by ventilating with smaller volumes and permitting hypercapnia.

■ Acute respiratory failure LIFE-THREATENING DISORDER

OVERVIEW

- Inadequate ventilation resulting from the inability of the lungs to adequately maintain arterial oxygenation or eliminate carbon dioxide
- Occurs in patients with hypercapnia or hypoxemia and in patients who have an acute deterioration in arterial blood gas (ABG) values

CAUSES

- Accumulated secretions secondary to cough suppression
- Airway irritants
- Any condition that increases the work of breathing and decreases the respiratory drive of patients with chronic obstructive pulmonary disease (COPD)
- Bronchospasm
- Central nervous system depression
- Endocrine or metabolic disorders
- Gas exchange failure
- Heart failure
- Myocardial infarction (MI)
- Pulmonary emboli
- Respiratory tract infection
- Thoracic abnormalities
- Ventilatory failure

PATHOPHYSIOLOGY

- Respiratory failure results from impaired gas exchange. Any condition associated with alveolar hypoventilation, ventilation-perfusion ($\dot{V}/\dot{Q}$) mismatch, and intrapulmonary shunting can cause acute respiratory failure, if left untreated.

RESPIRATORY SYSTEM

- Hypoxemia and hypercapnia stimulate strong compensatory responses by all of the body systems.
- Decreased oxygen saturation may result from alveolar hypoventilation, in which chronic airway obstruction reduces alveolar minute ventilation. Partial pressure of arterial oxygen (Pao_2) levels fall and partial pressure of arterial carbon dioxide ($Paco_2$) levels rise, resulting in hypoxemia. The most common cause of alveolar hypoventilation is airway obstruction, commonly seen with COPD (emphysema or bronchitis).
- Most commonly, hypoxemia—V imbalance—occurs when such conditions as pulmonary embolism or ARDS interrupt normal gas exchange in a specific lung region. Too little ventilation with normal blood flow or too little blood flow with normal ventilation may cause the imbalance, resulting in decreased Pao_2 levels and, thus, hypoxemia.
- Although uncommon, a decreased fraction of inspired oxygen may lead to respiratory failure. Inspired air doesn't contain adequate oxygen to establish an adequate gradient for diffusion into the blood—for example, at high altitudes or in confined, enclosed spaces. As a result, hypoxemia occurs.
- Tissue hypoxemia results in anaerobic metabolism and lactic acidosis. Respiratory acidosis occurs from hypercapnia. (See *Disorders affecting management of acute respiratory failure*, page 41.)
- Cyanosis occurs because of increased amounts of unoxygenated blood. As respiratory failure worsens, intercostal, supraclavicular, and suprasternal retractions may also occur.

CARDIOVASCULAR SYSTEM

- Untreated $\dot{V}/\dot{Q}$ imbalances can lead to right-to-left shunting, in which blood passes from the heart's right side to its left without being oxygenated. This results in unoxygenated blood reaching the arterial system to be distributed to the rest of the body.
- Heart rate and stroke volume increases; heart failure may occur.
- Hypoxemia deprives the myocardial tissue of oxygen and nutrients, possibly resulting in ischemia or MI.

NEUROLOGIC SYSTEM

- In response to hypoxemia, the sympathetic nervous system triggers vasoconstriction, increases peripheral resistance, and increases the heart rate.
- Hypoxemia or hypercapnia (or both) cause the brain's respiratory control center to increase respiratory depth (tidal volume) and then to increase the respiratory rate.

HEMATOLOGIC SYSTEM

- Hypoxia of the kidneys results in release of erythropoietin from renal cells, causing the bone marrow to increase production of red blood cells—an attempt by the body to increase the blood's oxygen-carrying capacity.

HISTORY

Precipitating events

- Infection
- Accumulated pulmonary secretions secondary to cough suppression
- Trauma
- MI
- Heart failure
- Pulmonary emboli
- Exposure to irritants (smoke or fumes)
- Myxedema
- Metabolic acidosis

PHYSICAL FINDINGS

- Cyanosis of the oral mucosa, lips, and nail beds
- Yawning and use of accessory muscles
- Pursed-lip breathing
- Nasal flaring
- Ashen skin
- Rapid breathing
- Cold, clammy skin
- Asymmetrical chest movement
- Decreased tactile fremitus over obstructed bronchi or a pleural effusion
- Increased tactile fremitus over consolidated lung tissue
- Hyperresonance
- Diminished or absent breath sounds
- Wheezes (in asthma)
- Rhonchi (in bronchitis)
- Crackles (in pulmonary edema)

DIAGNOSTIC TEST RESULTS

- ABG analysis reveals hypercapnia and hypoxemia.
- Serum white blood cell count is increased in bacterial infections.
- Serum hemoglobin and hematocrit show decreased oxygen-carrying capacity.
- Serum electrolyte results reveal hypokalemia and hypochloremia.
- Blood cultures, Gram stain, and sputum cultures show the pathogen. (See *Identifying respiratory failure.*)
- Chest X-rays may show underlying pulmonary diseases or conditions, such as emphysema, atelectasis, lesions, pneumothorax, infiltrates, and effusions.
- Electrocardiography may show arrhythmias, cor pulmonale, or myocardial ischemia.
- Pulse oximetry may show decreased arterial oxygen saturation.
- Pulmonary artery catheterization may show pulmonary or cardiovascular causes of acute respiratory failure.

TREATMENT

GENERAL

- Mechanical ventilation with an endotracheal or a tracheostomy tube
- High-frequency ventilation, if the patient doesn't respond to conventional mechanical ventilation
- Deep vein thrombosis prophylaxis

DIET

- Fluid restriction (heart failure)

ACTIVITY

- As tolerated
- Head of bed at 30 degrees, if tolerated

MEDICATIONS

- Cautious oxygen therapy to increase Pao_2
- Antacids
- Histamine-receptor antagonists, as ordered
- Antibiotics
- Bronchodilators
- Corticosteroids
- Positive inotropic agents
- Vasopressors
- Diuretics

SURGERY

- Possible tracheostomy

Identifying respiratory failure

Use these measurements to identify respiratory failure:
- vital capacity less than 15 cc/kg
- tidal volume less than 3 cc/kg
- negative inspiratory force less than -25 cm H_2O
- respiratory rate more than twice the normal rate
- diminished partial pressure of arterial oxygen despite increased fraction of inspired oxygen
- elevated partial pressure of arterial carbon dioxide, with pH lower than 7.25.

(continued)

NURSING CONSIDERATIONS

NURSING DIAGNOSES

- Anxiety
- Fatigue
- Fear
- Imbalanced nutrition: Less than body requirements
- Impaired gas exchange
- Impaired skin integrity
- Impaired verbal communication
- Ineffective breathing pattern
- Ineffective coping
- Ineffective tissue perfusion: Cardiopulmonary

EXPECTED OUTCOMES

The patient will:

- express feelings of increased comfort and decreased anxiety
- express feelings of increased energy and decreased fatigue
- verbalize feelings of fear
- consume required caloric intake
- maintain adequate ventilation and oxygenation
- maintain skin integrity
- develop alternate means of communication to express self
- maintain a patent airway
- identify effective coping strategies
- maintain hemodynamic stability.

NURSING INTERVENTIONS

- Administer oxygen, as ordered.
- Maintain a patent airway.
- Monitor vital signs, pulse oximetry, intake and output, laboratory studies, daily weight, and cardiac rate and rhythm.
- Give prescribed drugs.
- Orient the patient frequently.
- Encourage pursed-lip breathing.
- Encourage the use of an incentive spirometer.
- Reposition the patient every 1 to 2 hours; keep head of bed at 30 degrees, if tolerated.
- Help clear the patient's secretions with postural drainage and chest physiotherapy.
- Assist with or perform oral hygiene.
- Maintain normothermia.
- Schedule care to provide frequent rest periods.

- Assess respiratory status (breath sounds and ABG results) according to facility policy.
- Note chest X-ray results.
- Maintain skin integrity, and provide skin care.
- Observe for complications and sputum quality, consistency, and color.

With mechanical ventilation

- Obtain blood samples for ABG analysis, as ordered.
- Suction the trachea after hyperoxygenation, as indicated.
- Provide humidification.
- Secure the endotracheal (ET) tube according to facility policy.
- Prevent tracheal erosion.
- Provide alternative communication means.
- Provide sedation, as necessary.
- Monitor ventilator settings, cuff pressures, and ET tube position and patency.
- Observe for complications of mechanical ventilation.

PATIENT TEACHING

Be sure to cover:

- disorder, diagnostic testing, and treatment
- medication administration, dosage, and possible adverse effects
- when to notify the practitioner
- smoking cessation, if appropriate
- communication techniques, if intubated
- signs and symptoms of respiratory infection
- available support services.

RESOURCES

Organization

National Lung Health Education Program: *www.nlhep.org*

Selected references

Lippincott Manual of Nursing Practice Pocket Guide: Critical Care Nursing. Philadelphia: Lippincott Williams & Wilkins, 2006.

Rose, L. "Advanced Modes of Mechanical Ventilation: Implications for Practice," *AACN Advanced Critical Care* 17(2): 145-58, April-June 2006.

Swigris, J., and Brown, K. "Acute Interstitial Pneumonia and Acute Exacerbation of Idiopathic Pulmonary Fibrosis," *Seminars in Respiratory and Critical Care Medicine* 27(6):659-76, December 2006.

Disorders affecting management of acute respiratory failure

This chart highlights disorders that affect the management of acute respiratory failure.

DISORDER	SIGNS AND SYMPTOMS	DIAGNOSTIC TEST RESULTS	TREATMENT AND CARE
Myocardial infarction (MI) (complication)	◆ Persistent, crushing substernal chest pain that may radiate to the left arm, jaw, neck, or shoulder blades ◆ Cool extremities, perspiration, anxiety, and restlessness ◆ Blood pressure and pulse initially elevated ◆ Hypotension (if cardiac output is reduced) ◆ Bradycardia (associated with conduction disturbances) ◆ Fatigue and weakness ◆ Nausea and vomiting ◆ Shortness of breath ◆ Lung crackles on auscultation ◆ Jugular vein distension ◆ Reduced urine output	◆ Electrocardiography (ECG) shows ST-segment changes. ◆ Total creatine kinase (CK) and CK-MB isoenzyme levels are elevated over a 72-hour period. ◆ Myoglobin is elevated within 3 to 6 hours. ◆ Echocardiography shows ventricular-wall motion abnormalities. ◆ Multiple-gated acquisition scan or radionuclide ventriculography identifies acutely damaged muscle. ◆ Homocysteine and C-reactive protein levels are elevated.	◆ Be prepared to administer an antiarrhythmic to possibly assist with pacemaker insertion and, rarely, to assist with cardioversion to treat cardiac arrhythmias. ◆ Be prepared to administer thrombolytic therapy (streptokinase or recombinant tissue plasminogen) to preserve myocardial tissue. ◆ Percutaneous transluminal coronary angioplasty may be done to restore blood flow to the heart muscle. ◆ Be prepared to administer other drugs, as needed, including antiplatelet drugs (aspirin) to inhibit platelet aggregation; sublingual or I.V. nitrates (nitroglycerin) to relieve pain, increase cardiac output, and reduce myocardial workload; morphine for pain and sedation; and angiotensin-converting enzyme inhibitors to improve survival rate in large anterior-wall MI. ◆ Administer oxygen at a modest flow rate for 3 to 6 hours. ◆ Assist with pulmonary artery catheterization, which is used to detect left- or right-sided heart failure and to monitor the patient's response to treatment. ◆ Assess and record the severity of chest pain. ◆ During episodes of chest pain, obtain ECG, blood pressure, and pulmonary artery catheter measurements for changes. ◆ Monitor vital signs frequently. ◆ Watch for signs and symptoms of fluid retention (crackles, cough, tachypnea, and edema). ◆ Carefully monitor daily weight, intake and output, and serum enzyme levels.
Pneumonia (complication)	◆ Elevated temperature ◆ Cough with purulent, yellow, or bloody sputum ◆ Dyspnea ◆ Crackles ◆ Decreased breath sounds ◆ Pleuritic pain ◆ Chills ◆ Malaise ◆ Tachypnea	◆ Chest X-ray shows infiltrates. ◆ Sputum specimen reveals acute inflammatory cells.	◆ Provide humidified oxygen therapy for hypoxia and mechanical ventilation for respiratory failure. ◆ Administer antimicrobial therapy according to the causative agent. ◆ Administer an analgesic for pleuritic pain and an antipyretic for increased temperature. ◆ Provide a high-calorie diet, adequate fluid intake, and bed rest, as needed.
Respiratory acidosis (complication)	◆ Restlessness ◆ Confusion ◆ Apprehension ◆ Somnolence ◆ Fine or flapping tremor (asterixis) ◆ Coma ◆ Headaches ◆ Dyspnea and tachypnea ◆ Papilledema ◆ Depressed reflexes ◆ Hypoxemia (unless the patient is receiving oxygen) ◆ Tachycardia ◆ Hypertension ◆ Atrial and ventricular arrhythmias ◆ Hypotension with vasodilation ◆ Bounding pulses and warm periphery (in severe acidosis)	◆ Arterial blood gas (ABG) analysis shows partial pressure of carbon dioxide greater than 45 mm Hg, pH less than 7.35, normal HCO_3^- (bicarbonate) in the acute stage, and elevated HCO_3^- in the chronic stage. ◆ Chest X-ray commonly shows such causes as heart failure, pneumonia, chronic obstructive pulmonary disease (COPD), and pneumothorax. ◆ Serum potassium level is greater than 5 mEq/L, and serum chloride is low. ◆ Urine pH is acidic.	◆ The goal of treatment is to correct the underlying source of alveolar hypoventilation. ◆ Mechanical ventilation may be needed until the underlying condition can be treated. If so, maintain a patent airway and provide adequate humidification, perform tracheal suctioning regularly, and continuously monitor ventilator settings and respiratory status. ◆ Treatment for patients with COPD may include a bronchodilator, oxygen, a corticosteroid and, commonly, an antibiotic. ◆ Closely monitor the patient's ABG values. ◆ Watch for critical changes in the patient's respiratory, central nervous system, and cardiovascular functions. ◆ Maintain adequate hydration.

Acute tubular necrosis

- Injury to the nephron's tubular segment, resulting from ischemic or nephrotoxic injury and causing renal failure and uremic syndrome
- Accounts for about 75% of acute renal failure cases
- Most common cause of acute renal failure in critically ill patients
- Also known as *intrinsic renal azotemia*

CAUSES

- Diseased tubular epithelium
- Ischemic or toxic injury to glomerular epithelial cells or vascular endothelium
- Obstructed urine flow

PATHOPHYSIOLOGY

- Acute tubular necrosis (ATN) is characterized by sloughing of renal tubule epithelial cells and decreased glomerular filtration and waste clearance.
- One theory suggests that the resultant tubule obstruction leads to ischemia, damage to the basement membrane, tubule death, and renal failure.
- Ischemic injury disrupts blood flow to the kidneys. Ischemic ATN can damage the epithelial and basement membranes and cause lesions in the renal interstitium.

RENAL SYSTEM

- Oliguria occurs as a result of decreased glomerular filtration rate (GFR).
- Hyperkalemia occurs as a result of decreased GFR and metabolic acidosis.
- Hyperphosphatemia and hypocalcemia occur because the kidney can't excrete phosphorus.
- Hypotension and dehydration may occur (during the diuretic phase), leading to further kidney ischemia.

CARDIOVASCULAR SYSTEM

- Hypotension may occur early, followed by hypervolemia as the disease progresses.
- Hypertension and peripheral edema occur with hypervolemia.
- Heart failure develops as hypervolemia and anemia increase the heart's workload, resulting in pulmonary edema (complication of heart failure).
- Cardiac arrest and arrhythmias may result from hyperkalemia.

ENDOCRINE AND METABOLIC SYSTEMS

- A hypermetabolic state caused by the energy demands promotes tissue catabolism and altered glucose levels.
- Metabolic acidosis occurs because the kidney can't excrete hydrogen ions and reabsorb sodium and bicarbonate.

GASTROINTESTINAL SYSTEM

- Nausea, vomiting, and anorexia occur with uremia.
- GI bleeding may occur in patients with coagulation abnormalities or uremic gastric irritation.

IMMUNE AND HEMATOLOGIC SYSTEMS

- Anemia may occur related to decreased renal production of erythropoietin, glomerular filtration of erythrocytes, or bleeding associated with platelet dysfunction.
- Platelet dysfunction is related to uremia.
- Infection and sepsis commonly occur because of decreased white blood cell–mediated immunity. (See *Disorders affecting management of ATN*, pages 44 and 45.)
- A hypercoagulable state results from anticoagulant abnormalities, resulting in bleeding and clotting difficulties.

INTEGUMENTARY SYSTEM

◆ Dryness, pruritus, pallor, purpura, and uremic frost may occur because of the accumulation of uremic toxins.

MUSCULOSKELETAL SYSTEM

◆ Muscle weakness is related to hyperkalemia.
◆ Osteoporosis and pathological bone fractures may occur related to hyperphosphatemia and resultant hypocalcemia.

NEUROLOGIC SYSTEM

◆ Altered mental status and peripheral neuropathies are related to the effects of uremic toxins on the highly sensitive nerve cells.
◆ Headache, drowsiness, irritability, and seizures result from central nervous system involvement and may progress to coma without treatment.

RESPIRATORY SYSTEM

◆ Anemia causes tissue hypoxia, which stimulates increased ventilation and work of breathing.
◆ Increased respiratory effort and rate compensate for metabolic acidosis.

◆ Condition typically advanced at time of diagnosis

HISTORY

◆ Ischemic or nephrotoxic injury
◆ Urine output less than 400 ml/24 hours
◆ Fever and chills

WARNING *Fever and chills may signal the onset of an infection, which is the leading cause of death in ATN.*

PHYSICAL FINDINGS

◆ Evidence of bleeding abnormalities, such as petechiae and ecchymosis
◆ Dry, pruritic skin
◆ Dry mucous membranes
◆ Uremic breath
◆ Cardiac arrhythmia (if hyperkalemic)
◆ Muscle weakness

DIAGNOSTIC TEST RESULTS

◆ Urinary sediment contains red blood cells (RBCs) and casts.
◆ Urine specific gravity is 1.010.
◆ Urine osmolality is less than 400 mOsm/kg.
◆ Urine sodium level is 40 to 60 mEq/L.
◆ Blood urea nitrogen and serum creatinine levels are elevated.
◆ Anemia is present.
◆ Platelet adherence is defective.
◆ Metabolic acidosis is present.
◆ Hyperkalemia is present.
◆ Electrocardiography may show arrhythmias and, with hyperkalemia, a widening QRS complex, disappearing P waves, and tall, peaked T waves.
◆ Renal ultrasound, computed tomography scanning, or magnetic resonance imaging measures kidney size and excludes obstruction.

GENERAL
Acute phase

◆ Vigorous supportive measures until normal kidney function resumes
◆ Continuous renal replacement therapy or hemodialysis

Long-term management

◆ Daily replacement of projected and calculated fluid loss (including insensible loss)
◆ Peritoneal dialysis or hemodialysis, if the patient is catabolic or if hyperkalemia and fluid volume overload aren't controlled by other measures
◆ Transfusion of packed RBCs

DIET

◆ Fluid restriction
◆ Low-sodium, low-potassium

ACTIVITY

◆ Bed rest during acute phase
◆ Rest periods when fatigued

MEDICATIONS

◆ Diuretics
◆ Epoetin alfa
◆ Antibiotics
◆ Emergency I.V. administration of 50% glucose, regular insulin, and sodium bicarbonate (for hyperkalemia)
◆ Sodium polystyrene sulfonate with sorbitol by mouth or by enema (for hyperkalemia)

(continued)

NURSING CONSIDERATIONS

NURSING DIAGNOSES
◆ Acute pain
◆ Decreased cardiac output
◆ Excess fluid volume
◆ Fatigue
◆ Imbalanced nutrition: Less than body requirements
◆ Ineffective tissue perfusion: Renal
◆ Risk for infection
◆ Risk for injury

EXPECTED OUTCOMES
The patient will:
◆ express feelings of increased comfort and decreased pain
◆ maintain hemodynamic stability
◆ maintain fluid balance
◆ demonstrate energy conservation skills
◆ consume required caloric intake
◆ maintain urine specific gravity within the designated limits and have improved kidney function
◆ remain free from signs and symptoms of infection
◆ remain free from injury.

NURSING INTERVENTIONS
◆ Monitor intake and output, vital signs, and laboratory studies.
◆ Give prescribed drugs and blood products.
◆ Restrict foods containing high sodium and potassium levels.
◆ Use aseptic technique, particularly when handling catheters.
◆ Perform passive range-of-motion exercises.
◆ Provide meticulous skin care.
◆ Observe for signs and symptoms of complications.

PATIENT TEACHING

Be sure to cover:
◆ disorder, diagnostic testing, and treatment
◆ medication administration, dosage, and possible adverse effects
◆ signs of infection and when to report them to the practitioner
◆ dietary restrictions
◆ how to set goals that are realistic for the patient's prognosis
◆ follow-up care
◆ available supportive resources or social services.

RESOURCES
Organizations
American Association of Kidney Patients: *www.aakp.org*
National Institute of Diabetes & Digestive & Kidney Diseases: *www.niddk.nih.gov*

Selected references
Rennke, H., and Denker, B. *Renal Pathophysiology.* Philadelphia: Lippincott Williams & Wilkins, 2006.
Small, K., and McMullen, M. "Critical Care Extra: When Clear Becomes Cloudy: A Review of Acute Tubular Necrosis, a Form of Renal Failure," *AJN* 105(1):72AA-72GG, January 2005.
Wicklow, B., et al. "Biopsy-Proven Acute Tubular Necrosis in a Child Attributed to Vancomycin Intoxication," *Pediatric Nephrology* 21(8):1194-196, August 2006.

Disorders affecting management of ATN

This chart highlights disorders that affect the management of acute tubular necrosis (ATN).

DISORDER	SIGNS AND SYMPTOMS	DIAGNOSTIC TEST RESULTS	TREATMENT AND CARE
GI hemorrhage (complication)	◆ Anxiety ◆ Agitation ◆ Confusion ◆ Tachycardia ◆ Hypotension ◆ Oliguria ◆ Diaphoresis ◆ Pallor ◆ Cool, clammy skin ◆ Bright red blood in nasogastric tube drainage or vomitus (hematemesis) ◆ Coffee-ground drainage or vomitus ◆ Hematochezia (bright red blood from the rectum) ◆ Melena (black, tarry, sticky stools)	◆ Complete blood count shows decreased hemoglobin level and hematocrit (usually 6 to 8 hours after the initial symptoms); increased reticulocyte and platelet levels; and a decrease in red blood cells. ◆ Arterial blood gas (ABG) analysis reveals low pH and bicarbonate levels. ◆ 12-lead electrocardiogram (ECG) may reveal evidence of cardiac ischemia secondary to hypoperfusion. ◆ Abdominal X-ray may indicate air under the diaphragm, suggesting ulcer perforation. ◆ Angiography may help visualize the site of bleeding if the bleeding is from an artery or large vein.	◆ Begin fluid resuscitation. ◆ Ensure a patent airway, and assess breathing and circulation. ◆ Monitor cardiac and respiratory status closely—at least every 15 minutes or more, depending on the patient's condition. ◆ Administer supplemental oxygen. Monitor oxygen saturation levels (via continuous pulse oximetry) or serial ABG levels for evidence of hypoxemia. ◆ Assist with insertion of a central venous or pulmonary artery catheter to evaluate hemodynamic status. ◆ Assess level of consciousness (LOC) frequently—approximately every 30 minutes until the patient stabilizes, and then every 2 to 4 hours as indicated by the patient's status. ◆ Monitor intake and output closely. ◆ Assist with or insert a nasogastric tube, and perform lavage using room temperature saline to clear blood and clots from the stomach. Assess gastric pH every 2 to 4 hours or continuously, if indicated; maintain gastric pH between 4.0 and 5.0. Administer pharmacologic agents to maintain pH.

DISORDER	SIGNS AND SYMPTOMS	DIAGNOSTIC TEST RESULTS	TREATMENT AND CARE
Hyperkalemia (complication)	◆ Nausea ◆ Muscle weakness ◆ Paresthesia ◆ Diarrhea ◆ Abdominal cramps ◆ Irritability ◆ Hypotension ◆ Irregular heart rate ◆ Possible cardiac arrhythmias	◆ Serum potassium level is greater than 5 mEq/L. ◆ Arterial pH is decreased. ◆ ECG shows tall, peaked T waves, possibly flattened P waves, prolonged PR intervals, widened QRS complexes, and depressed ST segments.	◆ Treat the underlying cause. ◆ Administer a rapid infusion of 100% calcium gluconate to decrease myocardial irritability. ◆ Administer insulin and 10% to 50% glucose I.V. for severe hyperkalemia. ◆ Administer sodium polystyrene sulfate orally or rectally using an enema for mild hyperkalemia. ◆ Initiate dialysis as a final treatment option. ◆ Discontinue medications or I.V. fluids that may contribute to hyperkalemia. ◆ Monitor cardiac rhythm and potassium levels for response to treatment. ◆ Implement a potassium-restricted diet.
Pulmonary edema (complication)	◆ Restlessness and anxiety ◆ Rapid, labored breathing ◆ Intense, productive cough ◆ Frothy, blood-tinged sputum ◆ Mental status changes ◆ Jugular vein distention ◆ Wheezing ◆ Crackles ◆ Third heart sound ◆ Tachycardia ◆ Hypotension ◆ Thready pulse ◆ Peripheral edema	◆ Chest X-ray shows diffuse haziness of the lung fields, cardiomegaly, and pleural effusion. ◆ ABG analysis shows hypoxemia, hypercapnia, or acidosis. ◆ Pulse oximetry may indicate decreased oxygenation of the blood. ◆ Hemodynamic readings may reveal increased pulmonary artery wedge pressures. ◆ ECG may show valvular disease and left ventricular hypokinesis or akinesis.	◆ Treat the underlying cause. ◆ Administer oxygen therapy and be prepared to assist with endotracheal intubation and mechanical ventilation, if necessary. ◆ Closely monitor for changes in the patient's respiratory status. ◆ Institute energy conserving strategies. ◆ Implement fluid and sodium restriction. ◆ Administer diuretics, antiarrhythmics, preload and afterload reducing agents, bronchodilators, and vasopressors. ◆ Measure cardiac output, pulmonary artery pressure, and central venous pressure. ◆ Obtain daily weight. ◆ Monitor vital signs, pulse oximetry, and ABG levels.
Sepsis (complication)	◆ Agitation ◆ Anxiety ◆ Altered LOC ◆ Tachycardia ◆ Hypotension ◆ Rapid, shallow respirations ◆ Fever ◆ Urine output less than 25 ml/hour	◆ Blood cultures are positive for the infecting organism. ◆ Complete blood count reveals whether anemia, neutropenia, and thrombocytopenia are present. ◆ ABG studies show metabolic acidosis. ◆ Blood urea nitrogen and creatinine are increased. ◆ ECG shows ST-segment depression, inverted T waves, and arrhythmias.	◆ Locate and treat the underlying cause of sepsis. ◆ Monitor vital signs frequently. ◆ Administer antibiotics. ◆ Administer I.V. fluids to replace intravascular volume. ◆ Administer vasopressors if fluid resuscitation doesn't maintain blood pressure. ◆ Assess respiratory status. ◆ Prepare the patient for intubation and mechanical ventilation. ◆ Administer recombinant human activated protein (Xigris) and follow protocol for laboratory testing.

Adrenal hypofunction

- Primary adrenal hypofunction or insufficiency (Addison's disease): originates within the adrenal gland and is characterized by decreased secretion of mineralocorticoids, glucocorticoids, and androgens
- Relatively uncommon and can occur in both sexes and at any age, although most people diagnosed between ages 20 and 40
- Secondary adrenal hypofunction caused by a disorder outside the gland, such as impaired pituitary secretion of corticotropin, and characterized by decreased glucocorticoid secretion
- Adrenal crisis (addisonian crisis): critical deficiency of mineralocorticoids and glucocorticoids that generally follows acute stress, sepsis, trauma, surgery, or the omission of steroid therapy in patients who have chronic adrenal insufficiency; a medical emergency that needs immediate, vigorous treatment (see *How acute adrenal crisis develops*)
- Autoimmune Addison's disease: most common in white females (genetic predisposition is likely) and more common in patients with a familial predisposition to autoimmune endocrine diseases

CAUSES
Primary hypofunction
- Autoimmune process, in which circulating antibodies react specifically against the adrenal tissue
- Bilateral adrenalectomy
- Family history of autoimmune disease (may predispose the patient to Addison's disease and other endocrinopathies)
- Hemorrhage into the adrenal gland
- Infection (histoplasmosis, cytomegalovirus)
- Neoplasm
- Tuberculosis (once the chief cause, now responsible for less than 20% of adult cases)

Secondary hypofunction
- Abrupt withdrawal of long-term corticosteroid therapy
- Hypopituitarism
- Removal of a corticotropin-secreting tumor

Adrenal crisis
- Trauma, surgery, or other physiologic stress that exhausts body stores of glucocorticoids in a patient with adrenal hypofunction

- Adrenal hypofunction results from the partial or complete destruction of the adrenal cortex.
- The disorder manifests as a clinical syndrome in which the symptoms are associated with deficient production of the adrenocortical hormones, cortisol, aldosterone, and androgen, which results in high levels of corticotropin and corticotropin-releasing hormone.

UP CLOSE

How acute adrenal crisis develops

Acute adrenal crisis, the most serious complication of Addison's disease, involves a critical deficiency of glucocorticoids and mineralocorticoids. This life-threatening event requires prompt assessment and immediate treatment. The flowchart below highlights the underlying mechanisms responsible for the complication.

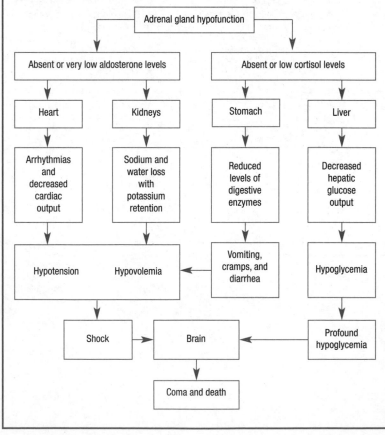

- Secondary adrenal hypofunction involves all zones of the cortex, causing deficiencies of the adrenocortical hormones, glucocorticoids, androgens, and mineralocorticoids.

RENAL SYSTEM
- Aldosterone deficiency causes increased renal sodium loss and enhances potassium reabsorption.
- Sodium excretion causes a reduction in water volume that leads to hypotension.
- Low plasma volume and arteriolar pressure stimulate renin release and a resulting increased production of angiotensin II. (See *Disorders affecting management of adrenal hypofunction,* page 49.)

INTEGUMENTARY SYSTEM
- Androgen deficiency may decrease hair growth in axillary and pubic areas as well as on the extremities of women.
- Abnormal bronze skin coloration results from decreased secretion of cortisol, which causes the pituitary gland to simultaneously secrete excessive amounts of melanocyte-stimulating hormone and corticotropin.

ASSESSMENT

HISTORY
- Synthetic steroid use, adrenal surgery, or recent infection
- Muscle weakness
- Fatigue
- Weight loss
- Craving for salty food
- Decreased tolerance for stress
- GI disturbances
- Dehydration
- Amenorrhea (in women)
- Impotence (in men)

PHYSICAL FINDINGS
- Poor coordination
- Decreased axillary and pubic hair (in women)
- Bronze coloration of the skin and darkening of scars
- Areas of vitiligo
- Increased pigmentation of mucous membranes
- Weak, irregular pulse
- Hypotension

DIAGNOSTIC TEST RESULTS
- Rapid corticotropin stimulation test measures corticotropin levels; low levels indicate a secondary disorder; elevated levels indicate a primary disorder.
- Plasma cortisol level is less than 10 mcg/dl in the morning and even lower in the evening.
- Serum sodium and fasting blood glucose levels are decreased.
- Serum potassium, calcium, and blood urea nitrogen levels are increased.
- Hematocrit is elevated; lymphocyte and eosinophil counts are increased.
- Computed tomography scan of the abdomen shows adrenal calcification (if the cause is infectious).

TREATMENT

GENERAL
- I.V. fluids

DIET
- Small, frequent, high-protein meals

ACTIVITY
- Periods of rest

MEDICATIONS
- Lifelong corticosteroid replacement, usually with cortisone or hydrocortisone
- Oral fludrocortisone
- Hydrocortisone
- I.V. saline and glucose solutions (for adrenal crisis)
- I.V. hydrocortisone replacement (for adrenal crisis)

(continued)

NURSING DIAGNOSES
- Activity intolerance
- Deficient fluid volume
- Disturbed body image
- Imbalanced nutrition: Less than body requirements
- Ineffective coping
- Risk for imbalanced body temperature
- Risk for impaired skin integrity
- Risk for infection

EXPECTED OUTCOMES
The patient will:
- maintain joint mobility and range of motion
- maintain an adequate fluid balance
- verbalize feelings about changed body image
- consume required caloric intake
- develop effective coping skills
- remain normothermic
- maintain skin integrity
- remain free from signs and symptoms of infection.

NURSING INTERVENTIONS
- Monitor vital signs, cardiac rhythm, blood glucose levels, daily weight, and intake and output.
- Until onset of mineralocorticoid effect, encourage fluids to replace excessive fluid loss.
- Arrange for a diet that maintains sodium and potassium balances; if the patient is anorexic, suggest six small meals per day to increase caloric intake.
- Observe for cushingoid signs such as fluid retention around the eyes and face.
- Check for petechiae.
- If the patient receives glucocorticoids alone, observe for orthostatic hypotension or electrolyte abnormalities.
- Observe for signs of shock (decreased level of consciousness and urine output).
- Note potassium levels before and after treatment.

Be sure to cover:
- disorder, diagnostic testing, and treatment
- medication administration, dosage, and possible adverse effects
- symptoms of steroid overdose (swelling, weight gain) and steroid underdose (lethargy, weakness)
- possible need for dosage to be increased during times of stress or illness (when the patient has a cold, for example)
- possibility of adrenal crisis being precipitated by infection, injury, or profuse sweating in hot weather
- importance of carrying a medical identification card that states the patient is on steroid therapy (drug name and dosage should be included on the card)
- how to give a hydrocortisone injection and to keep an emergency kit containing hydrocortisone in a prepared syringe available for use in times of stress
- stress management techniques
- available support services.

RESOURCES
Organization
National Adrenal Diseases Foundation: *www.medhelp.org/nadf*

Selected references
Anglin, R., et al. "The Neuropsychiatric Profile of Addison's Disease: Revisiting a Forgotten Phenomenon," *Journal of Neuropsychiatry* 18(4):450-59, Fall 2006.

Maddox, T., and Parker, D. "Deciphering Diagnostics: Going Up? Rapid ACTH Screening," *Nursing Made Incredibly Easy* 4(3):62-63, May-June 2006.

Richey, T. "A Deceptive Presentation: Addison's Disease," *Advanced Nursing Practice* 14(9):57-58, September 2006.

Disorders affecting management of adrenal hypofunction

This chart highlights disorders that affect the management of adrenal hypofunction.

DISORDER	SIGNS AND SYMPTOMS	DIAGNOSTIC TEST RESULTS	TREATMENT AND CARE
Acute adrenal crisis (complication)	◆ Profound weakness ◆ Fatigue ◆ Nausea, vomiting, cramps, and diarrhea ◆ Hypotension ◆ Dehydration ◆ High fever followed by hypothermia (occasionally) ◆ Hypovolemia ◆ Shock ◆ Coma	◆ Plasma cortisol is less than 10 mcg/dl in the morning; less in the evening. ◆ Serum sodium and glucose levels are decreased. ◆ Serum potassium, blood urea nitrogen, and lymphocyte count are increased. ◆ Hematocrit is decreased. ◆ Eosinophil count is decreased. ◆ X-ray shows adrenal calcification if the cause is infection.	◆ Monitor vital signs closely. ◆ Watch for hypotension, volume depletion, decreased level of consciousness, reduced urine output, and other signs of shock. ◆ Monitor for hyperkalemia before treatment and for hypokalemia (from excessive mineralocorticoid effect) after treatment. ◆ Check for cardiac arrhythmias. ◆ Monitor blood pressure. ◆ Monitor sodium levels. ◆ Prepare prompt I.V. bolus administration of hydrocortisone. Doses are given I.M. or are diluted with dextrose in saline solution and given I.V. until the patient's condition stabilizes. ◆ Know that up to 300 mg/day of hydrocortisone and 3 to 5 L of I.V. saline solution may be required during the acute phase.
Diabetes mellitus (coexisting)	◆ Weight loss despite voracious hunger ◆ Weakness ◆ Vision changes ◆ Frequent skin and urinary tract infections ◆ Dry, itchy skin ◆ Poor skin turgor ◆ Dry mucous membranes ◆ Dehydration ◆ Decreased peripheral pulses ◆ Cool skin temperature ◆ Decreased reflexes ◆ Orthostatic hypotension ◆ Muscle wasting ◆ Loss of subcutaneous fat ◆ Fruity breath odor because of ketoacidosis	◆ At least two occasions of fasting plasma glucose level are ≥ 126 mg/dl, or a random blood glucose level is ≥ 200 mg/dl. ◆ Blood glucose level is ≥ 200 mg/dl 2 hours after ingestion of 75 grams oral dextrose. ◆ An ophthalmologic examination may show diabetic retinopathy.	◆ Keep a snack available in case the patient becomes hypoglycemic. ◆ Keep accurate records of vital signs, weight, fluid intake, urine output, and calorie intake. ◆ Monitor serum glucose and urine acetone levels. ◆ Monitor for acute complications of diabetic therapy, especially hypoglycemia (vagueness, slow cerebration, dizziness, weakness, pallor, tachycardia, diaphoresis, seizures, and coma); immediately give carbohydrates in the form of fruit juice, hard candy, honey or, if the patient is unconscious, glucagon or I.V. dextrose. ◆ Be alert for signs of hyperosmolar coma (polyuria, thirst, neurologic abnormalities, and stupor). This hyperglycemic crisis requires I.V. fluids and insulin replacement. ◆ Monitor the patient for effects on the cardiovascular system, such as cerebrovascular, coronary artery, and peripheral vascular impairment. ◆ Monitor for effects on the peripheral and autonomic nervous systems. ◆ Provide meticulous skin care, especially to the feet and legs. Treat all injuries, cuts, and blisters. ◆ Observe for signs of urinary tract and vaginal infections. ◆ Encourage adequate fluid intake.

Alcoholism

OVERVIEW

- Chronic disorder of uncontrolled intake of alcoholic beverages
- Interferes with physical and mental health, social and familial relationships, and occupational responsibilities
- Affects all social and economic groups
- 50% of all alcohol consumed by 10% of population
- Evidence of alcohol abuse or dependence in about 13% of all adults older than age 18
- Men two to five times more likely to abuse alcohol than women
- Occurs at all stages of the life cycle, beginning as early as elementary school age
- Occurs in 20% of adult hospital inpatients

CAUSES

- Biological factors
- Psychological factors
- Sociocultural factors

RISK FACTORS

- Male gender
- Low socioeconomic status
- Family history
- Depression
- Anxiety
- History of other substance abuse disorders

PATHOPHYSIOLOGY

- Alcohol is soluble in water and lipids and permeates all body tissues.
- The liver, which metabolizes 90% of alcohol absorbed, is the most severely affected organ; hepatic steatosis, followed by hepatic fibrosis, is evident days after heavy drinking.
- Alcoholism causes Laënnec's cirrhosis after inflammatory response (alcoholic hepatitis) or, in the absence of inflammation, from direct activation of lipocytes (Ito cells).
- The condition promotes lactic acidosis and excess uric acid; opposes gluconeogenesis, beta-oxidation of fatty acids, and the Krebs cycle; and results in hypoglycemia and hyperlipidemia.
- Alcoholism results in cell toxicity through reduction of mitochondrial oxygenation, depletion of deoxyribonucleic acid, and other actions. (See *Disorders affecting management of alcoholism*, pages 52 and 53.)

ASSESSMENT

HISTORY

- Need for daily or episodic alcohol use for adequate function
- Inability to discontinue or reduce alcohol intake
- Episodes of anesthesia or amnesia during intoxication
- Episodes of violence during intoxication
- Interference with social and familial relationships and occupational responsibilities
- Malaise, dyspepsia, mood swings or depression, and an increased incidence of infection
- Secretive behavior

PHYSICAL FINDINGS

- Poor personal hygiene
- Unusually high tolerance for sedatives and opioids
- Signs of nutritional deficiency
- Signs of injury
- Withdrawal signs and symptoms
- Major motor seizures

DSM-IV-TR *criteria*

A diagnosis is confirmed when the patient exhibits at least three of these signs and symptoms:

- more alcohol ingested than intended
- persistent desire or efforts to diminish alcohol use
- excessive time spent obtaining alcohol
- frequent intoxication or withdrawal symptoms
- impairment of social, occupational, or recreational activities
- continued alcohol consumption despite knowledge of a social, psychological, or physical problem that's caused or exacerbated by alcohol use
- marked tolerance
- characteristic withdrawal symptoms
- use of alcohol to relieve or avoid withdrawal symptoms
- persistent symptoms for at least 1 month or recurrence over a longer time.

DIAGNOSTIC TEST RESULTS

◆ Blood alcohol tests show levels of 0.10% weight/volume (200 mg/dl) or higher.
◆ Serum electrolyte levels are abnormal.
◆ Serum ammonia levels are increased.
◆ Serum amylase levels are increased.
◆ Urine toxicology may show abuse of other drugs.
◆ Liver function study results are abnormal.
◆ CAGE screening test: Two affirmative responses make patient seven times more likely to be alcohol dependent.
◆ Alcohol Use Disorders Identification Test: Score greater than eight indicates alcohol dependency.
◆ Michigan Alcohol Screening Test: Score greater than five indicates alcohol dependency.

GENERAL
Immediate
◆ Respiratory support
◆ Prevention of aspiration of vomitus
◆ Replacement of fluids
◆ I.V. glucose administration
◆ Correction of hypothermia or acidosis
◆ Treatment of trauma, infection, or GI bleeding

Long-term
◆ Total abstinence
◆ Detoxification, rehabilitation, and aftercare program
◆ Supportive counseling
◆ Individual, group, or family psychotherapy
◆ Ongoing support group participation
◆ Safety precautions, including preventing aspiration of vomitus
◆ Seizure precautions

DIET
◆ Well-balanced

MEDICATIONS
◆ Anticonvulsants
◆ Antiemetics
◆ Antidiarrheals
◆ Tranquilizers, particularly benzodiazepines
◆ Naltrexone
◆ Antipsychotics
◆ Daily oral disulfiram
◆ Vitamin supplements

NURSING DIAGNOSES
◆ Anxiety
◆ Bathing or hygiene self-care deficit
◆ Compromised family coping
◆ Dressing or grooming self-care deficit
◆ Dysfunctional family processes: Alcoholism
◆ Imbalanced nutrition: Less than body requirements
◆ Impaired social interaction
◆ Risk for injury
◆ Risk for other-directed violence

EXPECTED OUTCOMES
The patient (or his family) will:
◆ verbalize feelings of anxiety and fear
◆ demonstrate improved hygiene and other self-care measures
◆ seek counseling and support for family issues
◆ demonstrate improved grooming and other self-care measures
◆ express understanding of the disorder and treatment modality, as will his family
◆ consume required caloric intake
◆ engage in appropriate social interaction with others
◆ remain free from injury
◆ inflict no harm upon others.

NURSING INTERVENTIONS
◆ Monitor vital signs, nutritional and hydration status, and intake and output.
◆ Institute safety measures.
◆ Institute seizure precautions.
◆ Give prescribed drugs.
◆ Orient the patient to reality.
◆ Maintain a calm environment, minimizing noise and shadows.
◆ Avoid restraints, unless necessary for protection.
◆ Use a nonthreatening approach.
◆ Assess mental status.

(continued)

Be sure to cover:

♦ disorder, diagnostic testing, and treatment
♦ medication administration, dosage, and possible adverse effects
♦ alcohol abstinence
♦ plan for relapse prevention
♦ effects of disorder on significant others
♦ available rehabilitation programs
♦ available support services.

RESOURCES
Organizations

Al-Anon: *www.al-anon.alateen.org*
Alateen: *www.al-anon.alateen.org/ alateen.html*
Alcoholics Anonymous: *www.alcoholics-anonymous.org*
National Association for Children of Alcoholics: *www.nacoa.net*

Selected references

Blondell, R.D. "Ambulatory Detoxification of Patients with Alcohol Dependence," *American Family Physician* 71(3):495-502, February 2005.

Fitzpatrick, J. "Alcohol Awareness," *Archives of Psychiatric Nursing* 20(5):203-205, October 2006.

Gerevich, J., and Bacskai, E. "Intimate Partner Violence, Suicidal Intent, and Alcoholism," *Journal of Clinical Psychiatry* 67(12):2033-2034, December 2006.

O'Dowd, A. "Drink Problem," *Nursing Times* 102(34):18-19, August 2006.

Disorders affecting management of alcoholism

This chart highlights disorders that affect the management of alcoholism.

DISORDER	SIGNS AND SYMPTOMS	DIAGNOSTIC TEST RESULTS	TREATMENT AND CARE
Aspiration pneumonia (complication)	♦ Fever ♦ Crackles ♦ Dyspnea ♦ Tachycardia ♦ Cough with blood-tinged sputum ♦ Cyanosis ♦ Decreased pulse oximetry	♦ Chest X-ray reveals infiltrates. ♦ Sputum for Gram stain and culture and sensitivity may reveal inflammatory cells and possible secondary bacterial infection. ♦ Bronchoscopy or transtracheal aspiration reveals possible secondary bacterial infection.	♦ Maintain a patent airway and oxygenation. Place the patient in Fowler's position to maximize chest expansion, and give supplemental oxygen, as ordered. ♦ Assess respiratory status at least every 2 hours. Auscultate the lungs for abnormal breath sounds. If respiratory status deteriorates, anticipate the need for endotracheal intubation and mechanical ventilation. ♦ Encourage coughing and deep breathing. ♦ Monitor cardiac rhythm to detect arrhythmias secondary to hypoxemia. ♦ Monitor pulse oximetry and arterial blood gas (ABG) results to detect deteriorating oxygenation. ♦ Administer respiratory treatments and assess response to treatment. ♦ Reposition the patient every 2 hours. Maintain upright position (if possible) if patient has frequent vomiting episodes.

DISORDER	SIGNS AND SYMPTOMS	DIAGNOSTIC TEST RESULTS	TREATMENT AND CARE
GI hemorrhage (complication)	◆ Anxiety ◆ Agitation ◆ Confusion ◆ Tachycardia ◆ Hypotension ◆ Oliguria ◆ Diaphoresis ◆ Pallor, cool, clammy skin ◆ Hematochezia ◆ Hematemesis ◆ Melena	◆ Upper GI endoscopy reveals the source of bleeding, such as an ulcer, esophageal varices, or Mallory-Weiss tear. ◆ Colonoscopy reveals the source of bleeding, such as polyps. ◆ Complete blood count reveals decrease in hemoglobin level and hematocrit, increase in reticulocyte and platelet levels, and decrease in red blood cell count. ◆ ABG studies reveal low pH and bicarbonate levels, indicating lactic acidosis from massive hemorrhage and possible hypoxemia. ◆ Electrocardiography may reveal cardiac ischemia secondary to hypoperfusion. ◆ Angiography may aid in visualizing the site of bleeding.	◆ Assess the patient for the amount of blood loss; begin fluid resuscitation with crystalloids and blood products. ◆ Ensure a patent airway and assess breathing and circulation. Monitor cardiac and respiratory status. ◆ Administer supplemental oxygen. Monitor oxygen saturation and ABG values for evidence of hypoxemia. ◆ Monitor vital signs for changes indicating hypovolemic shock. ◆ Monitor hemoglobin and hematocrit levels. ◆ Monitor intake and output, including GI losses. Check stool for occult blood. ◆ Administer histamine-2 receptor agonists or other agents, such as sucralfate, misoprostol, and omeprazole. ◆ Prepare the patient for endoscopic or surgical repair of bleeding sites.
Malnutrition (coexisting and complication)	◆ Diarrhea ◆ Steatorrhea ◆ Flatulence and abdominal discomfort ◆ Nocturia ◆ Weakness and fatigue ◆ Edema ◆ Amenorrhea ◆ Glossitis ◆ Peripheral neuropathy ◆ Bruising ◆ Bone pain ◆ Skeletal deformities	◆ Stool specimen for fat reveals excretion of greater than 6 g of fat/day. ◆ D-xylose absorption test shows less than 20% of 25 g of D-xylose in the urine after 5 hours. ◆ Schilling test reveals deficiency of vitamin B_{12} absorption. ◆ Culture of duodenal and jejunal contents confirms bacterial overgrowth. ◆ GI barium studies show characteristic features of the small intestine. ◆ Small intestine biopsy reveals atrophy of the mucosal villi.	◆ Assess nutritional status; monitor daily calorie count and obtain daily weight. ◆ Evaluate the patient's tolerance to foods. ◆ Assess fluid status, and administer fluid replacement, as needed. ◆ Administer dietary supplements and vitamins. ◆ Monitor laboratory values, especially electrolytes and coagulation studies. ◆ Assist with nutritional therapy, such as peripheral parenteral nutrition or total parenteral nutrition.

Amyotrophic lateral sclerosis LIFE-THREATENING DISORDER

OVERVIEW

- Chronic, rapidly progressive, and debilitating neurologic disease that's incurable and invariably fatal
- Attacks neurons responsible for controlling involuntary movements
- Characterized by weakness that begins in upper extremities and progressively involves neck and throat, eventually leading to disability, respiratory failure, and death
- Three times more common in men than in women
- Affects people ages 40 to 70
- Also known as *ALS* or *Lou Gehrig disease*

CAUSES

- Exact cause unknown
- Immune complexes such as those formed in autoimmune disorders
- Inherited as an autosomal dominant trait by 10% of patients
- Virus that creates metabolic disturbances in motor neurons

PRECIPITATING FACTORS THAT CAUSE ACUTE DETERIORATION

- Severe stress such as from myocardial infarction
- Traumatic injury
- Viral infections
- Physical exhaustion

PATHOPHYSIOLOGY

- An excitatory neurotransmitter accumulates to toxic levels, resulting in motor units that no longer innervate.
- Progressive degeneration of axons causes loss of myelin.
- Progressive degeneration of upper and lower motor neurons occurs.
- Progressive degeneration of motor nuclei in the cerebral cortex and corticospinal tracts results. (See *Disorders affecting management of ALS*, page 57.)

ASSESSMENT

HISTORY

- Mental function intact
- Family history of ALS
- Asymmetrical weakness first noticed in one limb
- Easy fatigue and easy cramping in the affected muscles

PHYSICAL FINDINGS

- Location of the affected motor neurons
- Severity of the disease
- Fasciculations in the affected muscles
- Progressive weakness in muscles of the arms, legs, and trunk
- Brisk and overactive stretch reflexes
- Difficulty talking, chewing, swallowing, and breathing
- Shortness of breath and occasional drooling

DIAGNOSTIC TEST RESULTS

- Protein in cerebrospinal fluid (CSF) is increased.
- Computed tomography scan rules out other disorders.
- Muscle biopsy discloses atrophic fibers.
- EEG rules out other disorders.
- Electromyography shows the electrical abnormalities of involved muscles.
- Nerve conduction study results usually appear normal.
- Lumbar puncture may be performed to analyze CSF.

TREATMENT

GENERAL
◆ Oxygen support
◆ Rehabilitative measures
◆ Occupational and physical therapy

DIET
◆ As tolerated; possible tube feedings

ACTIVITY
◆ As tolerated

MEDICATIONS
◆ Muscle relaxants
◆ Antidepressants
◆ Benadryl (for excessive salivation)
◆ Dantrolene
◆ Baclofen
◆ I.V. or intrathecal administration of thyrotropin-releasing hormone
◆ Riluzole (Rilutek) (slows progression)

NURSING CONSIDERATIONS

NURSING DIAGNOSES
◆ Anticipatory grieving
◆ Anxiety
◆ Bathing or hygiene self-care deficit
◆ Compromised family coping
◆ Dressing or grooming self-care deficit
◆ Feeding self-care deficit
◆ Imbalanced nutrition: Less than body requirements
◆ Impaired physical mobility
◆ Impaired verbal communication
◆ Ineffective airway clearance
◆ Ineffective breathing pattern
◆ Ineffective coping
◆ Risk for impaired skin integrity
◆ Risk for infection

EXPECTED OUTCOMES
The patient will:
◆ seek support systems to discuss fear of dying
◆ verbalize feelings of anxiety and fear
◆ perform self-care activities related to bathing and hygiene
◆ develop adequate coping mechanisms and support systems
◆ perform self-care activities related to dressing and grooming
◆ perform self-care activities related to feeding
◆ consume required caloric intake
◆ maintain joint mobility and range of motion (ROM)
◆ develop alternate means of communication to express self
◆ maintain a patent airway and adequate ventilation
◆ maintain effective breathing pattern
◆ exhibit adequate coping behaviors
◆ maintain skin integrity
◆ remain free from signs and symptoms of infection.

NURSING INTERVENTIONS
◆ Provide airway and respiratory management.
◆ Assess muscle weakness, respiratory status, speech, and swallowing ability.
◆ Provide emotional and psychological support.
◆ Promote independence.
◆ Turn and reposition the patient every 2 hours.
◆ Give prescribed drugs.
◆ Promote nutrition.
◆ Maintain aspiration precautions.
◆ Provide skin care and assess skin integrity.
◆ Note nutritional status.
◆ Monitor environment (for safety purposes).
◆ Observe response to treatment.
◆ Watch for signs and symptoms of complications.

(continued)

Be sure to cover:
◆ disorder, diagnostic testing, and treatment
◆ medication administration, dosage, and possible adverse effects
◆ swallowing therapy regimen
◆ skin care
◆ ROM exercises
◆ deep-breathing and coughing exercises
◆ safety in the home (see *Modifying the home for a patient with ALS*)
◆ available support services.

RESOURCES

Organizations

ALS Association: *www.alsa.org*
National Institutes of Health: *www.nih.gov*

Selected references

Choi, A., et al. "Caregiver Time Use in ALS," *Neurology* 67(5):902-904, September 2006.
Handbook of Pathophysiology, 2nd ed. Philadelphia: Lippincott Williams & Wilkins, 2005.
Trueman, C. "ALS and MS Patients: The Role of Long-Term Home Care," *Caring* 25(5):50, May 2006.
Van den Berg, J., et al. "Multidisciplinary ALS Care Improves Quality of Life in Patients with ALS," *Neurology* 65(8):1264-1267, October 2005.

Modifying the home for a patient with ALS

To help the patient with amyotrophic lateral sclerosis (ALS) live safely at home, follow these guidelines:
◆ Explain basic safety precautions, such as keeping stairs and pathways free from clutter; using nonskid mats in the bathroom and in place of loose throw rugs; keeping stairs well lit; installing handrails in stairwells and in the shower, tub, and toilet areas; and removing electrical and telephone cords from traffic areas.
◆ Discuss the need for rearranging the furniture, moving items in or out of the patient's care area, and obtaining a hospital bed, a commode, or oxygen equipment.
◆ Recommend devices to ease the patient's and caregiver's work, such as extra pillows or a wedge pillow to help the patient sit up, a draw sheet to help him move up in bed, a lap tray for eating, and a bell for calling the caregiver.
◆ Help the patient adjust to changes in the environment. Encourage independence.
◆ Advise the patient to keep a suction machine handy to reduce the fear of choking due to secretion accumulation and dysphagia. Teach him how to suction himself when necessary.

Disorders affecting management of ALS

This chart highlights disorders that affect the management of amyotrophic lateral sclerosis (ALS).

DISORDER	SIGNS AND SYMPTOMS	DIAGNOSTIC TEST RESULTS	TREATMENT AND CARE
Aspiration pneumonia (complication)	◆ Fever ◆ Crackles ◆ Dyspnea ◆ Tachycardia ◆ Cough with blood-tinged sputum ◆ Cyanosis ◆ Decreased pulse oximetry	◆ Chest X-ray reveals infiltrates. ◆ Sputum for Gram stain and culture and sensitivity may reveal inflammatory cells and possible secondary bacterial infection. ◆ Bronchoscopy or transtracheal aspiration reveals possible secondary bacterial infection.	◆ Maintain a patent airway and oxygenation. Place the patient in Fowler's position to maximize chest expansion and give supplemental oxygen, as ordered. ◆ Assess respiratory status at least every 2 hours. Auscultate the lungs for abnormal breath sounds. If respiratory status deteriorates, anticipate the need for endotracheal intubation and mechanical ventilation. ◆ Encourage coughing and deep breathing. ◆ Monitor cardiac rhythm to detect arrhythmias secondary to hypoxemia. ◆ Monitor pulse oximetry and arterial blood gas (ABG) results to detect deteriorating oxygenation. ◆ Administer respiratory treatments and assess response to treatment. ◆ Reposition the patient every 2 hours. Maintain upright position (if possible) if patient has frequent vomiting episodes.
Deep vein thrombophlebitis (complication)	◆ Homans' sign elicited ◆ Severe pain in affected extremity ◆ Fever, chills ◆ Malaise ◆ Swelling and cyanosis of the affected extremity ◆ Affected area possibly warm to touch	◆ Doppler ultrasonography identifies reduced blood flow to the area of the thrombus and any obstruction to venous blood flow. ◆ Plethysmography shows decreased circulation distal to the affected area. ◆ Plebography (also called venography) shows filling defects and diverted blood flow.	◆ Administer anticoagulants and monitor for adverse effects, such as bleeding, dark tarry stools, and coffee ground vomitus. ◆ Assess pulses, skin color, and temperature of the affected extremity. ◆ Measure and record the circumference of the affected extremity. ◆ Perform range-of-motion exercises with the unaffected extremities, and turn the patient every 2 hours. ◆ Apply warm soaks to improve circulation and relieve pain and inflammation. ◆ Assess for signs of pulmonary emboli.
Respiratory failure (complication)	◆ Tachypnea ◆ Cyanosis ◆ Crackles, rhonchi, wheezing ◆ Diminished breath sounds ◆ Restlessness ◆ Altered mental status ◆ Tachycardia ◆ Increased cardiac output ◆ Increased blood pressure ◆ Cardiac arrhythmias	◆ ABG values show deteriorating values and a pH below 7.35. ◆ Chest X-ray shows pulmonary disease or condition. ◆ Electrocardiogram may show cardiac arrhythmia or right ventricular hypertrophy. ◆ Pulse oximetry shows decreasing arterial oxygen saturation.	◆ Administer oxygen therapy and monitor respiratory status; assist with endotracheal intubation and mechanical ventilation, if necessary. ◆ Assess breath sounds and note changes. ◆ Monitor ABG values and pulse oximetry. ◆ Monitor vital signs and intake and output. ◆ Monitor cardiac rhythm for arrhythmias. ◆ Administer antibiotics, bronchodilators, corticosteroids, positive inotropic agents, diuretics, vasopressors, or antiarrhythmics.

Aneurysm, abdominal aortic

- Abnormal dilation in the arterial wall of the aorta, commonly between the renal arteries and iliac branches
- Can be fusiform (spindle-shaped), saccular (pouchlike), or dissecting
- Seven times more common in hypertensive men than in hypertensive women
- Most common in whites ages 50 to 80

CAUSES

- Arteriosclerosis or atherosclerosis (95%)
- Syphilis or other infections
- Trauma

PATHOPHYSIOLOGY

- Focal weakness in the tunica media layer of the aorta due to degenerative changes allows the tunica intima and tunica adventitia layers to stretch outward.
- Increasing blood pressure within the aorta progressively weakens vessel walls and enlarges the aneurysm. (See *Disorders affecting management of abdominal aortic aneurysm*, pages 60 and 61.)

CARDIOVASCULAR SYSTEM

- A focal weakness in the muscular layer of the aorta (tunica media) allows the inner layer (tunica intima) and outer layer (tunica adventitia) to stretch outward as a result of pressure in the blood vessel.
- The pressure of a large aneurysm causes damage to adjacent organs.
- If dissection occurs, blood leaks into the space in between the vessel layers. The vessels branching off the aorta become obstructed, causing decreased blood flow and tissue death.
- Nearly all abdominal aortic aneurysms (AAAs) are fusiform, which causes the arterial walls to balloon on all sides. The resulting sac fills with necrotic debris and thrombi. Complications of this type of aneurysm include rupture, obstruction of blood flow to other organs, and embolization to a peripheral artery.
- In the event of rupture, blood supply to vital organs is diminished, and organ failure ensues.
- Free intraperitoneal rupture leads to cardiovascular collapse.

GASTROINTESTINAL SYSTEM

- If AAA ruptures into the duodenum, upper GI bleeding and hemorrhage occur.
- Sigmoid colon ischemia may occur with loss of blood from the hypogastric artery during surgical repair of AAA.

NEUROLOGIC SYSTEM

- AAA rupture causes decreased blood flow to the brain, which alters mental status.

RENAL SYSTEM

- Diminished perfusion of the kidneys may result from obstruction of the renal arteries, rupture of the aneurysm, or surgical repair. Ureteral stents may be placed during surgery as a precaution, causing decreased renal function.
- Retroperitoneal rupture causes a self-limiting hemorrhage to the retroperitoneal space, resulting in pain, hypotension, and flank ecchymosis.

RESPIRATORY SYSTEM

- Rupture of an AAA leads to impaired gas exchange, resulting in diminished perfusion of organs.

HISTORY

- Asymptomatic until aneurysm enlarges and compresses surrounding tissue, or if rupture occurs
- Syncope when aneurysm ruptures
- If clot forms and bleeding stops, patient possibly asymptomatic (again) or may report abdominal pain because of bleeding into the peritoneum

PHYSICAL FINDINGS
Intact aneurysm

- Gnawing, generalized, steady abdominal pain
- Lower back pain unaffected by movement
- Gastric or abdominal fullness
- Sudden onset of severe abdominal or lumbar pain, with radiation to flank and groin
- May note a pulsating mass in the periumbilical area

Ruptured aneurysm

- Severe, persistent abdominal and back pain for rupture into the peritoneal cavity
- GI bleeding with massive hematemesis and melena for rupture into the duodenum
- Mottled skin; poor distal perfusion
- Absent peripheral pulses distally
- Decreased level of consciousness
- Diaphoresis
- Hypotension
- Tachycardia
- Oliguria
- Distended abdomen
- Ecchymosis or hematoma in the abdominal, flank, or groin area
- Paraplegia if aneurysm rupture reduces blood flow to the spine
- Systolic bruit over the aorta
- Tenderness over affected area

DIAGNOSTIC TEST RESULTS

- Abdominal ultrasonography or echocardiography determines the size, shape, and location of the aneurysm.
- Anteroposterior and lateral abdominal X-rays detect aortic calcification,

which outlines the mass, at least 75% of the time.

- Computed tomography scan visualizes an aneurysm's effect on nearby organs.
- Aortography shows condition of vessels proximal and distal to the aneurysm and extent of aneurysm; aneurysm diameter may be underestimated because only the flow channel, and not the surrounding clot, is shown.

TREATMENT

GENERAL
- If the aneurysm is small and asymptomatic, monitoring of condition
- Careful control of hypertension
- Fluid and blood replacement, if rupture occurs
- Deep vein thrombosis prophylaxis

DIET
- Weight reduction, if appropriate
- Low-fat diet

ACTIVITY
- As tolerated

MEDICATIONS
- Beta-adrenergic blockers
- Antihypertensives
- Analgesics
- Antibiotics

SURGERY
- Endovascular grafting or resection of large aneurysms or those that produce symptoms (see *Endovascular grafting for repair of AAA*)
- Bypass procedures for poor perfusion distal to aneurysm
- Repair of ruptured aneurysm with a graft replacement

NURSING CONSIDERATIONS

NURSING DIAGNOSES
- Acute pain
- Anxiety
- Decreased cardiac output
- Deficient fluid volume
- Impaired gas exchange
- Impaired physical mobility
- Impaired skin integrity
- Ineffective tissue perfusion: Cardiopulmonary, renal

EXPECTED OUTCOMES
The patient will:
- express feelings of increased comfort and decreased pain
- express feelings of decreased anxiety
- maintain adequate cardiac output
- maintain adequate urine output (output equivalent to intake)
- maintain adequate ventilation and oxygenation
- maintain optimal mobility within the confines of the disorder
- maintain skin integrity

- maintain palpable pulses distal to the aneurysm site and hemodynamic stability.

NURSING INTERVENTIONS
For an intact aneurysm
- Allow the patient to express his fears and concerns and identify effective coping strategies.
- Offer the patient and his family psychological support.
- Before elective surgery, weigh the patient, insert an indwelling urinary catheter and an I.V. line, and assist with insertion of the arterial line and pulmonary artery catheter to monitor hemodynamic balance.
- Give prescribed prophylactic antibiotics.
- Apply sequential compression stockings.

WARNING *Be alert for signs of rupture, which may quickly progress to death. If rupture does occur, surgery needs to be immediate. Medical antishock trousers may be used while transporting the patient to surgery.*

For a ruptured aneurysm
- Administer fluid and blood products, as ordered.
- Monitor vital signs, pulse oximetry, intake and output, and laboratory values.
- Give prescribed drugs.

After surgery
- Assess peripheral pulses for graft failure or occlusion.
- Watch for signs of bleeding retroperitoneally from the graft site.
- Maintain blood pressure in prescribed range with fluids and medications.

WARNING *Assess the patient for severe back pain, which can indicate that the graft is tearing.*
- Have the patient cough, or suction the endotracheal tube, as needed.
- Provide frequent turning, and assist with ambulation as soon as the patient is able.

Endovascular grafting for repair of AAA

Endovascular grafting is a minimally invasive procedure for the patient who requires repair of an abdominal aortic aneurysm (AAA). Endovascular grafting reinforces the walls of the aorta to prevent rupture and prevents expansion of the size of the aneurysm.

The procedure is performed with fluoroscopic guidance, whereby a delivery catheter with an attached compressed graft is inserted through a small incision into the femoral or iliac artery over a guide wire. The delivery catheter is advanced into the aorta, where it's positioned across the aneurysm. A balloon on the catheter expands the graft and affixes it to the vessel wall. The procedure usually takes 2 to 3 hours to perform. Patients are instructed to walk the first day after surgery and are discharged from the hospital in 1 to 3 days.

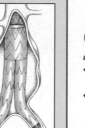
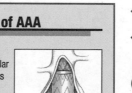

(continued)

- Monitor cardiac rhythm, hemodynamics, vital signs, intake and output hourly, neurologic status, and pulse oximetry.
- Assess respirations and breath sounds at least every hour.
- Obtain arterial blood gases, as ordered.
- Monitor daily weight and laboratory studies.
- Check nasogastric intubation for patency, amount, and type of drainage.
- Perform wound care and assess wound condition and drainage.
- Observe for signs and symptoms of complications.

PATIENT TEACHING

Be sure to cover:
- disorder, diagnostic testing, and treatment
- medication administration, dosage, and possible adverse effects
- surgical procedure and the expected postoperative care
- wound care
- signs and symptoms of complications

- physical activity restrictions until medically cleared by the practitioner
- need for regular examination and ultrasound checks to monitor progression of the aneurysm, if surgery wasn't performed.

RESOURCES
Organizations
American Heart Association: *www.americanheart.org*
National Heart, Lung, and Blood Institute: *www.nhlbi.nih.gov*

Selected references
Alspach, J., ed. *AACN Core Curriculum for Critical Care Nursing,* 6th ed. Philadelphia: W.B. Saunders Co., 2006.
Cole, E., et al. "Assessment of the Patient with Acute Abdominal Pain," *Nursing Standard* 20(38):56-61, May 2006.
Dambro, M.R. *Griffith's Five-Minute Clinical Consult 2006.* Philadelphia: Lippincott Williams & Wilkins, 2006.
Moore, J., et al. "Topics in Progressive Care: Endovascular Aneurysm Repair Targets Silent Killer," *Nursing 2006 Critical Care* 1(6): 13-19, November 2006.

Disorders affecting management of abdominal aortic aneurysm

This chart highlights disorders that affect the management of abdominal aortic aneurysm.

DISORDER	SIGNS AND SYMPTOMS	DIAGNOSTIC TEST RESULTS	TREATMENT AND CARE
Acute renal failure (complication)	◆ Urine output less than 400 ml/day followed by diuresis of up to 5 L/day ◆ Lethargy ◆ Altered mental status ◆ Headache ◆ Costovertebral pain ◆ Numbness around the mouth ◆ Tingling in the extremities ◆ Anorexia ◆ Restlessness ◆ Weight gain ◆ Nausea and vomiting ◆ Pallor ◆ Diarrhea	◆ Blood urea nitrogen (BUN) and serum creatinine are increased. ◆ Potassium levels are increased. ◆ Hematocrit, blood pH, bicarbonate, and hemoglobin levels are decreased. ◆ Urine casts and cellular debris are present; specific gravity is decreased.	◆ Treat the underlying cause. ◆ Monitor fluid balance status, including skin turgor, peripheral edema, and intake and output. Monitor urine output hourly, and assess daily weight. ◆ Monitor central venous and pulmonary artery pressures. ◆ Anticipate the need for insertion of a temporary dialysis catheter for hemodialysis or continuous renal replacement therapy. ◆ Monitor vital signs and laboratory values, especially BUN, creatinine, and electrolytes.

DISORDER	SIGNS AND SYMPTOMS	DIAGNOSTIC TEST RESULTS	TREATMENT AND CARE
Chronic obstructive pulmonary disease (coexisting)	◆ Dyspnea ◆ Abdominal discomfort ◆ Cyanosis	◆ Pulmonary function tests show increased residual volume, total lung capacity, and compliance. ◆ Chest X-ray shows hyperinflation. ◆ Arterial blood gas analysis shows decreased partial pressure of arterial oxygen and normal or increased partial pressure of arterial carbon dioxide (emphysema). ◆ Electrocardiogram (ECG) may show atrial arrhythmias and peaked P waves in leads II, III, and aV_F (chronic bronchitis); tall, symmetrical P waves in leads II, III, and aV_F; and vertical QRS axis (emphysema).	◆ Help the patient adjust to lifestyle changes needed to decrease oxygen demands. ◆ Perform chest physiotherapy to maintain clear airways. ◆ Administer bronchodilators. ◆ Encourage daily activity to maximize lung capacity and promote psychological well-being. ◆ Provide frequent rest periods to minimize oxygen demands. ◆ Provide a high-calorie, protein-rich diet.
Coronary artery disease (coexisting)	◆ Elevated blood pressure ◆ Chest pain that radiates to the left arm, neck, jaw, or shoulder ◆ Nausea and vomiting ◆ Fainting ◆ Cool extremities ◆ Decreased or absent peripheral pulses	◆ Stress echocardiography may show abnormal wall movement. ◆ Coronary angiography reveals the location and degree of coronary artery stenosis or obstruction. ◆ Exercise testing may detect ST-segment changes during exercise. ◆ ECG may show ischemic changes during exercise.	◆ Monitor the patient for chest pain; have the patient grade the severity of his pain on a scale of 1 to 10. ◆ Observe for signs and symptoms that may signify worsening of condition or pain. ◆ Administer calcium channel blockers, beta-adrenergic blockers, or antilipemics. ◆ Advise the patient to follow the prescribed medication regimen to reduce the risk of cardiac disease. ◆ Help the patient identify risk factors and modify his lifestyle, as appropriate.
Hypertension (coexisting)	◆ Headache ◆ Dizziness ◆ Fatigue ◆ Bounding pulse ◆ Pulsating abdominal mass ◆ Elevated blood pressure ◆ Bruits over the abdominal aorta	◆ Urinalysis may show proteinuria, red blood cells, white blood cells, or glucose. ◆ Serum potassium levels are less than 3.5 mEq/L. ◆ BUN is normal or elevated to more than 20 mg/dl. ◆ Serum creatinine levels are normal or elevated to more than 1.5 mg/dl.	◆ Monitor blood pressure for stability. ◆ Help the patient identify risk factors and modify his diet and lifestyle, as appropriate. ◆ Administer thiazide-type diuretics, angiotensin-converting enzyme inhibitors, angiotensin receptor blockers, beta-adrenergic blockers, or calcium channel blockers. ◆ Help the patient identify stress factors and establish effective coping mechanisms.

Anorexia nervosa

OVERVIEW

- Psychological disorder of self-imposed starvation, resulting from a distorted body image and an intense and irrational fear of gaining weight
- Actual loss of appetite (rare)
- May occur simultaneously with bulimia nervosa
- Affects 5% to 10% of the general population; more than 90% of those affected are females
- Occurs primarily in adolescents and young adults, but may also affect older women and, occasionally, males
- Starvation or suicide resulting in a 6% to 20% mortality rate

CAUSES

- Exact cause unknown
- Pressure to achieve
- Dependence and independence issues
- History of sexual abuse
- Social attitudes that equate slimness with beauty
- Stress caused by multiple responsibilities
- Subconscious effort to exert personal control over life or to protect oneself from dealing with issues surrounding sexuality

RISK FACTORS

- Low self-esteem
- Compulsive personality
- High achievement goals

PATHOPHYSIOLOGY

- Decreased caloric intake depletes body fat and protein stores.
- In women, estrogen deficiency occurs due to lack of lipid substrate for synthesis, causing amenorrhea.
- In men, testosterone levels fluctuate, resulting in decreased erectile function and sperm count.
- Ketoacidosis occurs from increased use of fat as fuel for energy. (See *Disorders affecting management of anorexia nervosa,* page 65.)

ASSESSMENT

HISTORY

- 15% or greater weight loss for no organic reason
- Morbid fear of being fat
- Compulsion to be thin
- Angry disposition
- Tendency to minimize weight loss
- Ritualistic behaviors
- Excessive exercise
- Amenorrhea
- Infertility
- Loss of libido
- Fatigue
- Sleep alterations
- Intolerance to cold
- Laxative or diuretic abuse
- Constipation or diarrhea

PHYSICAL FINDINGS

- Hypotension
- Bradycardia
- Emaciated appearance
- Skeletal muscle atrophy
- Loss of fatty tissue
- Atrophy of breast tissue
- Blotchy or sallow skin
- Lanugo on the face and body
- Dryness or loss of scalp hair
- Calluses on the knuckles
- Abrasions and scars on the dorsum of the hand
- Dental caries
- Oral or pharyngeal abrasions
- Painless salivary gland enlargement
- Bowel distention
- Slowed reflexes

DSM-IV-TR *criteria*

These criteria must be documented:
- Refusal to maintain or achieve normal weight for age and height
- Intense fear of gaining weight or becoming fat, even though underweight
- Disturbance in perception of body weight, size, or shape
- Absence of at least three consecutive menstrual cycles when otherwise expected to occur (in females)

DIAGNOSTIC TEST RESULTS

◆ Hemoglobin level, platelet count, and white blood cell count are decreased.
◆ Bleeding time is prolonged.
◆ Erythrocyte sedimentation rate is decreased.
◆ Levels of serum creatinine, blood urea nitrogen, uric acid, cholesterol, total protein, albumin, sodium, potassium, chloride, calcium, and fasting blood glucose are decreased.
◆ Levels of serum alanine aminotransferase and aspartate aminotransferase are elevated in severe starvation.
◆ Serum amylase levels are elevated.
◆ In women, levels of serum luteinizing hormone and follicle-stimulating hormone are decreased.
◆ Triiodothyronine levels are decreased.
◆ Urinalysis shows dilute urine.
◆ Electrocardiogram may show nonspecific ST segment, T-wave changes, and prolonged PR interval; ventricular arrhythmias may also be present.

TREATMENT

GENERAL
◆ Behavior modification
◆ Group, family, or individual psychotherapy (see *Criteria for hospitalizing a patient with anorexia nervosa*)

DIET
◆ Balanced, with a normal eating pattern
◆ Parenteral nutrition, if necessary

ACTIVITY
◆ Gradual increase in physical activity when weight gain and stabilization occur
◆ Curtailed activity for cardiac arrhythmias

MEDICATIONS
◆ Vitamin and mineral supplements
◆ Electrolyte replacement

Criteria for hospitalizing a patient with anorexia nervosa

A patient with anorexia nervosa can be successfully treated on an outpatient basis. However, if the patient displays any of the signs listed here, hospitalization is mandatory:
◆ rapid weight loss equal to 15% or more of normal body mass
◆ persistent bradycardia (50 beats/minute or less)
◆ hypotension with a systolic reading of less than or equal to 90 mm Hg
◆ hypothermia (core body temperature of less than or equal to 97° F (36.5° C)
◆ presence of medical complications; suicidal ideation
◆ persistent sabotage or disruption of outpatient treatment—resolute denial of condition and the need for treatment.

NURSING CONSIDERATIONS

NURSING DIAGNOSES
◆ Chronic low self-esteem
◆ Constipation
◆ Delayed growth and development
◆ Disturbed body image
◆ Imbalanced nutrition: Less than body requirements

EXPECTED OUTCOMES
The patient will:
◆ express positive feelings about self
◆ regain normal bowel function
◆ express understanding of norms for growth and development
◆ acknowledge change in body image
◆ achieve and maintain expected body weight.

NURSING INTERVENTIONS
◆ Support the patient's efforts to achieve target weight.
◆ Negotiate an adequate food intake with the patient.
◆ Supervise the patient one-on-one during meals.

WARNING *Monitor the patient for 1 hour after meals to ensure no self-induced vomiting.*

◆ Monitor vital signs, intake and output, and electrolyte and complete blood count levels.
◆ Measure weight on a regular schedule.
◆ Supervise activity.

(continued)

Be sure to cover:
♦ disorder, diagnostic testing, and treatment
♦ medication administration, dosage, and possible adverse effects
♦ nutritional needs
♦ importance of keeping a food journal
♦ counseling schedule
♦ avoidance of discussions about food between the patient and her family
♦ follow-up care
♦ available support services.

RESOURCES
Organizations
American Anorexia Bulimia Association: *www.nationaleatingdisorders.org*
National Association of Anorexia Nervosa and Associated Disorders: *www.anad.org*

Selected references
Diseases, 4th ed. Philadelphia: Lippincott Williams & Wilkins, 2006.
Nettina, S.M. *Lippincott Manual of Nursing Practice,* 8th ed. Philadelphia: Lippincott Williams & Wilkins, 2006.
Nix, S. *Williams' Basic Nutrition and Diet Therapy,* 12th ed. St. Louis: Mosby–Year Book, Inc., 2005.
Olson, A. "Outpatient Management of Electrolyte Imbalances Associated with Anorexia Nervosa and Bulimia Nervosa," *Journal of Infusion Nursing* 28(2):118-22, March-April 2005.

Disorders affecting management of anorexia nervosa

This chart highlights disorders that affect the management of anorexia nervosa.

DISORDER	SIGNS AND SYMPTOMS	DIAGNOSTIC TEST RESULTS	TREATMENT AND CARE
Cardiac arrhythmia (complication)	◆ Palpitations ◆ Chest pain ◆ Dizziness ◆ Weakness, fatigue ◆ Irregular heart rhythm ◆ Hypotension ◆ Syncope ◆ Altered level of consciousness ◆ Diaphoresis, pallor, cold, clammy skin	◆ Electrocardiogram (ECG) identifies specific waveform changes associated with the arrhythmia. ◆ Laboratory testing reveals electrolyte abnormalities, hypoxemia, or acid-base abnormalities. ◆ Electrophysiologic testing identifies the mechanism of an arrhythmia and the location of accessory pathways.	◆ Assess airway, breathing, and circulation if life-threatening arrhythmia develops; follow advanced cardiac life support protocols for treatment. ◆ Monitor cardiac rhythm continuously, and obtain serial ECGs to evaluate changes and effects of treatment. ◆ Administer antiarrhythmics and monitor for adverse effects. ◆ Assess cardiovascular system for signs of hypoperfusion; monitor vital signs. ◆ Assist with insertion of temporary pacemaker, or apply transcutaneous pacemaker, if appropriate.
Malnutrition (complication)	◆ Diarrhea ◆ Steatorrhea ◆ Flatulence and abdominal discomfort ◆ Nocturia ◆ Weakness and fatigue ◆ Edema ◆ Amenorrhea ◆ Glossitis ◆ Peripheral neuropathy ◆ Bruising ◆ Bone pain ◆ Skeletal deformities	◆ Stool specimen for fat reveals excretion of > 6 g of fat/day. ◆ D-xylose absorption test shows less than 20% of 25 g of D-xylose in the urine after 5 hours. ◆ Schilling test reveals deficiency of vitamin B_{12} absorption. ◆ Culture of duodenal and jejunal contents confirms bacterial overgrowth. ◆ GI barium studies show characteristic features of the small intestine. ◆ Small intestine biopsy reveals atrophy of the mucosal villi.	◆ Assess nutritional status; monitor daily calorie count and obtain daily weight. ◆ Evaluate the patient's tolerance to foods. ◆ Assess fluid status, and administer fluid replacement, as needed. ◆ Administer dietary supplements and vitamins. ◆ Monitor laboratory values, especially electrolytes and coagulation studies. ◆ Assist with nutritional therapy, such as peripheral parenteral nutrition or total parenteral nutrition.
Osteoporosis (complication)	◆ Dowager's hump ◆ Back pain (thoracic and lumbar) ◆ Loss of height ◆ Unsteady gait ◆ Joint pain ◆ Weakness	◆ Dual photon or dual energy X-ray absorptiometry can detect bone loss. ◆ X-rays reveal characteristic degeneration in the lower vertebrae. ◆ Parathyroid levels may be elevated. ◆ Bone biopsy allows direct examination of changes in bone cells and the rate of bone turnover.	◆ Provide supportive devices such as a back brace. ◆ Encourage lifestyle modifications, such as a moderate exercise program and dietary modifications. ◆ Offer analgesics and heat for pain relief. ◆ Administer calcium and vitamin D supplements to stimulate bone formation. ◆ Give sodium fluoride to stimulate bone formation; give calcitonin to reduce bone resorption and slow the decline in bone mass.

Asthma LIFE-THREATENING DISORDER

OVERVIEW

- Chronic reactive airway disorder involving episodic, reversible airway obstruction, resulting from bronchospasms, increased mucus secretions, and mucosal edema
- Signs and symptoms ranging from mild wheezing and dyspnea to life-threatening respiratory failure (see *Determining the severity of asthma*)
- Signs and symptoms of bronchial airway obstruction possibly persisting between acute episodes
- May occur at any age, but about 50% of all patients with asthma under age 10; affects twice as many boys as girls
- Onset between ages 10 and 30 in about one-third of patients; at least one immediate family member with disease
- Extrinsic and intrinsic asthma possibly coexisting in many patients

CAUSES

- Sensitivity to specific external allergens (extrinsic) or related to internal, nonallergenic factors (intrinsic)

Extrinsic asthma (atopic asthma)

- Animal dander
- Food additives containing sulfites and any other sensitizing substances
- House dust or mold
- Kapok or feather pillows
- Pollen

Intrinsic asthma (nonatopic asthma)

- Emotional stress
- Genetic factors

Bronchoconstriction

- Cold air
- Drugs, such as aspirin, beta-adrenergic blockers, and nonsteroidal anti-inflammatory drugs
- Exercise
- Hereditary predisposition
- Psychological stress
- Sensitivity to allergens or irritants such as pollutants
- Tartrazine
- Viral infections

Determining the severity of asthma

Asthma is classified by severity using these features:
- frequency, severity, and duration of symptoms
- degree of airflow obstruction (spirometry measure) or peak expiratory flow (PEF)
- frequency of nighttime symptoms and the degree that the asthma interferes with daily activities.

Severity can change over time, and even milder cases can become severe in an uncontrolled attack. Long-term therapy depends on whether the patient's asthma is classified as mild intermittent, mild persistent, moderate persistent, or severe persistent. For all patients, quick relief can be obtained by using a short-acting bronchodilator (two to four puffs of a short-acting, inhaled beta$_2$-adrenergic agonist, as needed for symptoms). However, the use of a short-acting bronchodilator more than twice a week in patients with intermittent asthma or daily or increasing use in patients with persistent asthma may indicate the need to initiate or increase long-term control therapy.

MILD INTERMITTENT ASTHMA

The signs and symptoms of mild intermittent asthma include:
- daytime symptoms no more than twice a week
- nighttime symptoms no more than twice a month

- lung function testing (either PEF or forced expiratory volume in 1 second) that's 80% of predicted value or higher
- PEF that varies no more than 20%.

Severe exacerbations, separated by long, symptom-free periods of normal lung function, indicate mild intermittent asthma. A course of systemic corticosteroids is recommended for these exacerbations; otherwise, daily medication isn't required.

MILD PERSISTENT ASTHMA

The signs and symptoms of mild persistent asthma include:
- daytime symptoms more than twice a week but less than once a day
- nighttime symptoms more than 2 times per month
- lung function testing that's 80% of predicted value or higher
- PEF that varies between 20% and 30%.

The preferred treatment for mild, persistent asthma is a low-dose, inhaled corticosteroid, with alternative treatments including a cromolyn, leukotriene modifier, nedocromil, or sustained-release theophylline.

MODERATE PERSISTENT ASTHMA

The signs and symptoms of moderate persistent asthma include:
- daily daytime symptoms
- at least weekly nighttime symptoms

- lung function testing that's 60% to 80% of predicted value
- PEF that varies more than 30%.

The preferred treatment for moderate persistent asthma is a low- or medium-dose, inhaled corticosteroid combined with a long-acting, inhaled beta$_2$-adrenergic agonist. Alternative treatments include increasing the dosage on the inhaled corticosteroid so that it's within the medium-dose range or replacing the low- or medium-dose inhaled corticosteroid with either a leukotriene modifier or theophylline.

For recurring exacerbations, the dosage on the inhaled corticosteroid is increased so that it's within the medium-dose range.

SEVERE PERSISTENT ASTHMA

The signs and symptoms of severe persistent asthma include:
- continual daytime symptoms
- frequent nighttime symptoms
- lung function testing that's 60% of predicted value or lower
- PEF that varies more than 30%.

The preferred treatment for severe, persistent asthma includes a high-dose, inhaled corticosteroid combined with a long-acting, inhaled beta$_2$-adrenergic agonist. Long-term administration of corticosteroid tablets or syrup (2 mg/kg/day, not to exceed 60 mg/day) may be used to reduce the need for systemic corticosteroid therapy.

PATHOPHYSIOLOGY

◆ Tracheal and bronchial linings overreact to various stimuli, causing episodic smooth-muscle spasms that severely constrict the airways.
◆ Mucosal edema and thickened secretions further block the airways.

RESPIRATORY SYSTEM

◆ Bronchial linings overreact to various stimuli, causing episodic smooth-muscle spasms that severely constrict the airways. (See *How asthma progresses,* page 68.)
◆ Immunoglobulin (Ig) E antibodies, attached to histamine-containing mast cells and receptors on cell membranes, initiate intrinsic asthma attacks. When exposed to an antigen, such as pollen, the IgE antibody combines with the antigen.
◆ During an attack, the narrowed bronchial lumen can still expand slightly on inhalation, allowing air to reach the alveoli. On exhalation, increased intrathoracic pressure closes the bronchial lumen completely. Air enters but can't escape. The patient develops a barrel chest and hyperresonance to percussion. (See *Disorders affecting management of asthma,* pages 70 and 71.)
◆ Mucus fills the lung bases, inhibiting alveolar ventilation. Blood is shunted to alveoli in other lung parts, but still can't compensate for diminished ventilation.
◆ Hyperventilation is triggered by lung receptors to increase lung volume because of trapped air and obstructions.
◆ Intrapleural and alveolar gas pressures rise, causing decreased perfusion of alveoli.
◆ Increased alveolar gas pressure, decreased ventilation, and decreased perfusion result in uneven ventilation-perfusion ratios and mismatching within different lung segments.
◆ As the airway obstruction increases in severity, more alveoli are affected. Ventilation and perfusion remain inadequate, and carbon dioxide retention develops, resulting in respiratory acidosis.
◆ If status asthmaticus occurs (if the attack continues):
– hypoxemia worsens and expiratory flows and volumes continue to decrease
– obstructed airways impede gas exchange and increase airway resistance
– breathing becomes increasingly labored
– respiratory rate drops to normal (as the patient tires), partial pressure of carbon dioxide ($Paco_2$) levels rise, and the patient hypoventilates from exhaustion (as breathing and hypoxemia tire the patient)
– respiratory acidosis continues as partial pressure of arterial oxygen levels drop and $Paco_2$ levels continue to rise
– situation becomes life-threatening as no air becomes audible upon auscultation (a silent chest) and $Paco_2$ rises to over 70 mm Hg
– patient experiences acute respiratory failure (without treatment).

NEUROLOGIC SYSTEM

◆ Hypoxia that occurs during an asthma attack triggers hyperventilation by respiratory center stimulation, which, in turn, decreases $Paco_2$ and increases pH, resulting in respiratory alkalosis.

ASSESSMENT

HISTORY

◆ Intrinsic asthma often preceded by severe respiratory tract infections, especially in adults
◆ Intrinsic asthma attacks possibly aggravated by irritants, emotional stress, fatigue, endocrine changes, temperature and humidity variations, and exposure to noxious fumes
◆ Attack may begin dramatically, with simultaneous onset of severe, multiple symptoms; or insidiously, with gradually increasing respiratory distress
◆ Exposure to a particular allergen followed by a sudden onset of dyspnea and wheezing and by tightness in the chest, accompanied by a cough that produces thick, clear, or yellow sputum

PHYSICAL FINDINGS

◆ Visible dyspnea
◆ Ability to speak only a few words before pausing for breath
◆ Use of accessory respiratory muscles
◆ Diaphoresis
◆ Increased anteroposterior thoracic diameter
◆ Hyperresonance
◆ Tachycardia; tachypnea; mild systolic hypertension
◆ Inspiratory and expiratory wheezes
◆ Prolonged expiratory phase of respiration
◆ Diminished breath sounds
◆ Cyanosis, confusion, and lethargy that indicate onset of life-threatening status asthmaticus and respiratory failure

DIAGNOSTIC TEST RESULTS

◆ Arterial blood gas (ABG) analysis reveals hypoxemia.
◆ Increased serum IgE levels result from an allergic reaction.
◆ Complete blood count with differential shows increased eosinophil count.
◆ Chest X-rays may show hyperinflation with areas of focal atelectasis.

(continued)

How asthma progresses

In asthma, hyperresponsiveness of the airways and bronchospasms occur. These illustrations show the progression of an asthma attack.

Histamine (H) attaches to receptor sites in larger bronchi, causing swelling of the smooth muscles.

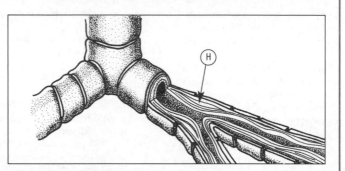

Leukotrienes (L) attach to receptor sites in the smaller bronchi and cause swelling of smooth muscle there. Leukotrienes also cause prostaglandins to travel through the bloodstream to the lungs, where they enhance the histamine's effects.

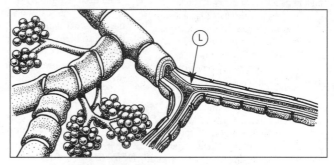

Histamine stimulates the mucous membranes to secrete excessive mucus, further narrowing the bronchial lumen. On inhalation, the narrowed bronchial lumen can still expand slightly; however, on exhalation, the increased intrathoracic pressure closes the bronchial lumen completely.

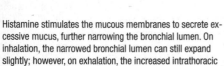

Bronchial lumen on inhalation

Bronchial lumen on exhalation

Mucus fills lung bases, inhibiting alveolar ventilation. Blood is shunted to alveoli in other parts of the lungs, but it still can't compensate for diminished ventilation.

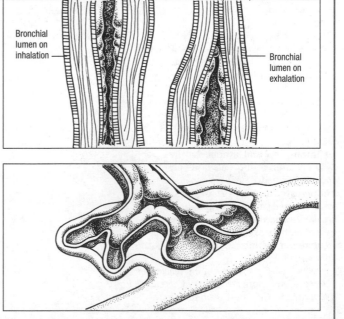

- Pulmonary function studies may show decreased peak flows and forced expiratory volume in 1 second, low-normal or decreased vital capacity, and increased total lung and residual capacities.
- Skin testing may identify specific allergens.
- Bronchial challenge testing shows the clinical significance of allergens identified by skin testing.
- Pulse oximetry measurements may show decreased oxygen saturation.

TREATMENT

GENERAL
- Identification and avoidance of precipitating factors
- Desensitization to specific antigens
- Establishment and maintenance of patent airway

DIET
- Fluid replacement
- Well balanced

ACTIVITY
- As tolerated

MEDICATIONS
- Low-flow oxygen
- Bronchodilators
- Corticosteroids
- Histamine antagonists
- Leukotriene antagonists
- Anticholinergic bronchodilators
- Antibiotics
- Heliox trial (before intubation)
- I.V. magnesium sulfate (controversial)

WARNING *The patient with increasingly severe asthma that doesn't respond to drug therapy is usually admitted for treatment with corticosteroids, epinephrine (Adrenalin), and sympathomimetic aerosol sprays. He may require endotracheal intubation and mechanical ventilation.*

NURSING CONSIDERATIONS

NURSING DIAGNOSES
- Anxiety
- Fear
- Impaired gas exchange
- Ineffective airway clearance
- Ineffective breathing pattern

EXPECTED OUTCOMES
The patient will:
- report feelings of comfort and decreased anxiety
- verbalize feelings of fear
- maintain adequate ventilation
- maintain a patent airway
- maintain an effective breathing pattern.

NURSING INTERVENTIONS
- Administer prescribed humidified oxygen.
- Place the patient in high Fowler's position.
- Encourage pursed-lip and diaphragmatic breathing.
- Adjust oxygen according to the patient's vital signs and ABG values.
- Assist with intubation and mechanical ventilation, if appropriate.
- Monitor ABG results, pulmonary function test results, and pulse oximetry.
- Monitor vital signs and intake and output.
- Give prescribed drugs.
- Perform postural drainage and chest percussion, if tolerated.
- Suction an intubated patient, as needed.
- Administer I.V. fluids, as ordered.
- Anticipate bronchoscopy or bronchial lavage.
- Keep the room temperature comfortable.
- Use an air conditioner or a fan in hot, humid weather.
- Assess response to treatment.
- Note signs and symptoms of theophylline toxicity.
- Assess respiratory status according to facility policy.
- Observe for complications of corticosteroid treatment.
- Provide emotional support.

PATIENT TEACHING

Be sure to cover:
- disorder, diagnostic testing, and treatment
- medication administration, dosage, and possible adverse effects
- when to notify the practitioner
- avoidance of known allergens and irritants
- metered-dose inhaler or dry powder inhaler use
- pursed-lip and diaphragmatic breathing
- use of peak flow meter
- effective coughing techniques
- maintaining adequate hydration
- follow-up care
- available support services.

RESOURCES
Organizations
American Academy of Allergy, Asthma, and Immunology: *www.aaaai.org*
Asthma and Allergy Foundation of America: *www.aafa.org*
National Asthma Education and Prevention Program: *www.nhlbi.nih.gov/about/naepp*

Selected references
Cormier, D., et al. "A Pilot Study of Childhood Health Behaviors and Asthma Using the Health Belief Model," *Journal of Cardiopulmonary Rehabilitation* 26(4):250, July-August, 2006.
MacMullen, N. et al. "Adverse Maternal Outcomes in Women with Asthma: Differences by Race." *MCN,* 31(4):263-68, July/August 2006.
Newell, K., and Hume, S. "Choosing the Right Inhaler for Patients with Asthma," *Nursing Standards,* 21(5):46-8, October 2006.

(continued)

Disorders affecting management of asthma

This chart highlights disorders that affect the management of asthma.

DISORDER	SIGNS AND SYMPTOMS	DIAGNOSTIC TEST RESULTS	TREATMENT AND CARE
Gastroesophageal reflux disease (complication)	◆ Regurgitation without associated nausea or belching ◆ Feeling of fluid accumulation in the throat without a sour or bitter taste ◆ Chronic pain radiating to neck, jaws, and arms	◆ Barium swallow shows evidence of recurrent reflux. ◆ Esophageal acidity test reveals degree of esophageal reflux. ◆ Gastroesophageal scintillation testing shows reflux. ◆ Acid perfusion (Bernstein) test confirms esophagitis. ◆ Esophagoscopy and biopsy confirm pathologic changes in the mucosa.	◆ Assist with diet modifications to decrease reflux activity. ◆ Perform chest physiotherapy to maintain clear airways. ◆ Assist in identifying situations or activities that increase intra-abdominal pressure (such as tight clothing or certain exercises) in order to avoid reflux. ◆ Warn the patient to refrain from using substances that reduce sphincter control (such as alcohol). ◆ Advise the patient to remain in an upright position for at least 2 hours after eating.
Infection (coexisting)	◆ Tachycardia ◆ Fever ◆ Crackles or rhonchi ◆ Rapid, shallow respirations ◆ Malaise	◆ Eosinophil count is increased. ◆ White blood cell (WBC) count and granulocyte count are increased.	◆ Monitor the patient's temperature, and treat elevations. ◆ Encourage increased fluid intake to avoid dehydration from increased metabolism and fever. ◆ Provide frequent rest periods to minimize oxygen demands. ◆ Monitor for complications such as worsening infection. ◆ Monitor WBC count and differential. ◆ Instruct the patient in ways to prevent infection. ◆ Teach the patient and his caregiver about the need to report possible infection.
Pregnancy (coexisting)	◆ Fatigue ◆ Tachypnea ◆ Bronchial wheezing ◆ Use of accessory muscles for breathing	◆ Pulmonary function tests reveal decreased vital capacity and increased total lung and residual capacities. ◆ Peak and expiratory flow rate measurements are less than 60% of baseline. ◆ Pulse oximetry shows arterial oxygen saturation (Sao_2) less than 90%. ◆ Chest X-ray reveals hyperinflation with areas of atelectasis. ◆ Electrocardiogram (ECG) may reveal sinus tachycardia during an attack. ◆ Sputum analysis may indicate increased mucus viscosity and the presence of mucus plugs. ◆ Eosinophil count is increased. ◆ WBC count and granulocyte count are increased (if infection is present).	◆ Advise the patient to follow her prepregnancy asthma therapy and to follow up with her obstetrician or nurse-midwife. ◆ Encourage frequent rest periods. Pregnancy increases oxygen demands and metabolism. ◆ Assist with dietary planning to monitor weight gain of pregnancy. Excess weight gain may increase diaphragmatic elevation and decrease functional residual capacity. ◆ Encourage prompt treatment of asthma attacks to decrease effects of hypoxic damage to the fetus. ◆ If the patient is taking beta-adrenergics to control her asthma, the dose will be tapered close to labor because these drugs have the potential to reduce labor contractions. ◆ Women who have been taking a corticosteroid during pregnancy may need parenteral administration of hydrocortisone during labor because of the added stress during this time. ◆ Advise the patient that corticosteroids should never be abruptly discontinued.

DISORDER	SIGNS AND SYMPTOMS	DIAGNOSTIC TEST RESULTS	TREATMENT AND CARE
Respiratory failure (complication)	◆ Nasal flaring ◆ Restlessness, anxiety, depression, lethargy, agitation, or confusion ◆ Cold, clammy skin ◆ Tachypnea ◆ Tactile fremitus ◆ Diminished breath sounds ◆ Crackles	◆ Chest X-ray shows atelectasis, infiltrates, and effusions. ◆ Arterial blood gas analysis shows decreased partial pressure of arterial oxygen and normal or increased partial pressure of arterial carbon dioxide. ◆ ECG may show arrhythmias. ◆ Pulse oximetry reveals a decreasing Sao_2 and a mixed venous oxygen saturation level of less than 50%. ◆ Electrolyte levels may reflect imbalances from hyperventilation, acidosis, or hypoxia.	◆ Administer antibiotics (if infection is present). ◆ Help the patient adjust to lifestyle changes needed to decrease oxygen demands. ◆ Perform chest physiotherapy to maintain clear airways. ◆ Provide frequent rest periods to minimize oxygen demands. ◆ Provide a high-calorie, protein-rich diet. ◆ Administer diuretics, bronchodilators, vasopressors, positive inotropic agents, or corticosteroids. ◆ Perform incentive spirometry to increase lung volume. ◆ Administer oxygen therapy. ◆ Assist with endotracheal intubation and mechanical ventilation, if needed.

Bronchiectasis

OVERVIEW

- Lung disease that's characterized by abnormal dilation of the bronchi and destruction of the bronchial walls
- Results from chronic inflammatory changes associated with repeated damage to bronchial walls and with abnormal mucociliary clearance, causing a breakdown of supporting tissue adjacent to the airways
- Can occur throughout the tracheobronchial tree, or may be confined to one segment or lobe
- Usually bilateral and involves the basilar segments of the lower lobes
- Three forms: cylindrical (fusiform), varicose, and saccular (cystic) (see *Forms of bronchiectasis*)
- Affects people of both sexes and of all ages
- Incidence dramatically decreased over the past 20 years because of availability of antibiotics to treat acute respiratory infections

CAUSES

- Complications of measles, pneumonia, pertussis, or influenza
- Congenital anomalies (rare) such as bronchomalacia
- Immune disorders
- Inhalation of corrosive gas
- Mucoviscidosis
- Obstruction with recurrent infection
- Recurrent bacterial respiratory tract infections
- Repeated aspiration of gastric juices
- Tuberculosis
- Various rare disorders such as immotile cilia syndrome

PATHOPHYSIOLOGY

- Repeated damage to the bronchial walls and abnormal mucociliary clearance leads to a breakdown in the supporting tissue adjacent to the airways.

RESPIRATORY SYSTEM

- Hyperplastic squamous epithelium that's removed of its cilia replaces ulcerated columnar epithelia, which results in bronchial dilation and inflammatory changes in the walls of the airways.
- Cartilage, muscle, and elastic tissue are gradually destroyed and may be replaced by fibrous tissue.
- Abscess formation involving all layers of the bronchial walls occurs, which produces inflammatory cells and fibrous tissues, resulting in further dilation and narrowing of the airways.
- Sputum stagnates in the dilated bronchi and leads to secondary infection, characterized by inflammation and leukocytic accumulations. Additional debris collects in the bronchi and occludes them.
- Pressure from the retained secretions induces further mucosal injury.
- Inflammatory processes increase the vascularity of the bronchial wall. As vascularity increases, bronchial arteries enlarge and anastomoses form between the bronchial and pulmonary arterial circulations.
- Extensive vascular proliferation of bronchial circulation occurs, producing copious, foul-smelling secretions, commonly occurring with hemoptysis.
- As damage occurs to the bronchial and pulmonary beds, oxygenation is compromised and hypoxia results.
- Airway obstruction can occur from bronchostenosis, impacted retained secretions, or compression by enlarged lymph nodes.

Forms of bronchiectasis

The three types of bronchiectasis are cylindrical, varicose, and saccular. In cylindrical bronchiectasis, bronchioles are usually symmetrically dilated, whereas in varicose bronchiectasis, bronchioles are deformed. In saccular bronchiectasis, large bronchi become enlarged and balloonlike.

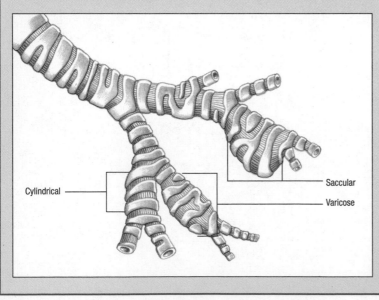

Cylindrical

Saccular

Varicose

CARDIOVASCULAR SYSTEM

◆ Structural changes in the lungs can lead to increased pressure in the pulmonary arteries. This condition (called *pulmonary hypertension*) results in increased workload for the right ventricle, possibly leading to cor pulmonale and heart failure. (See *Disorders affecting management of bronchiectasis*, page 75.)

◆ Because the right side of the heart pumps blood through the lungs under much lower pressure, any condition that leads to prolonged pulmonary hypertension is poorly tolerated by the right ventricle.

IMMUNE SYSTEM

◆ The host inflammatory response includes epithelial injury as a result of mediators released from neutrophils; thus protection against infection is compromised.

◆ Dilated airways and retained secretions are more susceptible to colonization and growth of bacteria. This bacterial growth causes inflammation that produces airway damage, impairs clearance of secretions that harbor the microorganisms, and causes more infection, which then triggers more inflammation.

ASSESSMENT

HISTORY

◆ Frequent bouts of pneumonia
◆ Coughing up of blood or blood-tinged sputum
◆ Chronic cough that produces copious, foul-smelling, mucopurulent secretions
◆ Dyspnea
◆ Weight loss
◆ Malaise

PHYSICAL FINDINGS

◆ Sputum that may show a cloudy top layer, a central layer of clear saliva, and a heavy, thick, purulent bottom layer
◆ Clubbed fingers and toes
◆ Cyanotic nail beds
◆ Dullness over affected lung fields, if pneumonia or atelectasis present
◆ Diminished breath sounds
◆ Inspiratory crackles during inspiration over affected area
◆ Occasional wheezes
◆ Fever

DIAGNOSTIC TEST RESULTS

◆ Computed tomography scan shows bronchiectasis.
◆ Sputum culture and Gram stain may show predominant pathogens.
◆ Complete blood count may reveal anemia and leukocytosis.
◆ Bronchography shows location and extent of disease.
◆ Chest X-rays show peribronchial thickening, atelectatic areas, and scattered cystic changes.
◆ Bronchoscopy may show the source of secretions or the bleeding site in hemoptysis.
◆ Pulmonary function studies show decreased vital capacity, expiratory flow, and hypoxemia.
◆ A sweat electrolyte test may show cystic fibrosis as the underlying cause.

TREATMENT

GENERAL

◆ Postural drainage and chest percussion
◆ Bronchoscopy to remove secretions

DIET

◆ Well-balanced, high-calorie
◆ Adequate hydration

ACTIVITY

◆ As tolerated

MEDICATIONS

◆ Antibiotics
◆ Bronchodilators
◆ Oxygen

SURGERY

◆ Segmental resection
◆ Bronchial artery embolization
◆ Lobectomy
◆ Surgical removal of the affected lung portion

(continued)

NURSING CONSIDERATIONS

NURSING DIAGNOSES
- Anxiety
- Fatigue
- Imbalanced nutrition: Less than body requirements
- Impaired gas exchange
- Ineffective airway clearance
- Ineffective breathing pattern
- Ineffective coping
- Risk for infection

EXPECTED OUTCOMES
The patient will:
- identify strategies to reduce anxiety
- utilize energy conservation techniques
- maintain adequate nutrition and hydration
- maintain adequate ventilation and oxygenation
- maintain a patent airway
- maintain effective breathing pattern
- demonstrate effective coping mechanisms
- remain free from signs and symptoms of infection.

NURSING INTERVENTIONS
- Administer oxygen, as needed.
- Monitor vital signs, intake and output, pulse oximetry, and arterial blood gas results.
- Assess respiratory status, breath sounds, and sputum production.
- Give prescribed drugs.
- Provide supportive care.
- Perform chest physiotherapy.
- Provide a warm, quiet, comfortable environment.
- Alternate rest and activity periods.
- Provide well-balanced, high-calorie meals.
- Offer small, frequent meals.
- Provide adequate hydration.
- Provide frequent mouth care.
- Observe for complications.
- Monitor chest tube drainage after surgery.

PATIENT TEACHING

Be sure to cover:
- disorder, diagnostic testing, and treatment
- medication administration, dosage, and possible adverse effects
- when to notify the physician
- proper disposal of secretions
- infection control techniques
- importance of frequent rest periods
- preoperative and postoperative instructions, if surgery is required
- postural drainage and percussion
- coughing and deep-breathing techniques
- avoidance of air pollutants and people with known upper respiratory tract infections
- immunizations
- balanced, high-protein diet
- avoidance of milk products
- adequate hydration
- available smoking-cessation programs, if indicated.

RESOURCES
Organizations
American Association for Respiratory Care: *www.aarc.org*
American Lung Association: *www.lungusa.org*
National Heart, Lung, and Blood Institute: *www.nhlbi.nih.gov*

Selected references
Kasper, D.L., et al., eds. *Harrison's Principles of Internal Medicine,* 16th ed. New York: McGraw-Hill Book Co., 2005.
King, P.T., et al. "Outcome in Adult Bronchiectasis," *COPD* 2(1):27-34, March 2005.
Sirmali, M., et al. "Surgical Management of Bronchiectasis in Childhood," *European Journal of Cardiothoracic Surgery* 31(1):120-23, January 2007.
Weycker, D., et al. "Prevalence and Economic Burden of Bronchiectasis," *Clinical Pulmonary Medicine* 12(4):205-209, July 2005.

Disorders affecting management of bronchiectasis

This chart highlights disorders that affect the management of bronchiectasis.

DISORDER	SIGNS AND SYMPTOMS	DIAGNOSTIC TEST RESULTS	TREATMENT AND CARE
Acute respiratory failure (complication)	◆ Tachypnea ◆ Cyanosis ◆ Crackles, rhonchi, wheezing ◆ Diminished breath sounds ◆ Restlessness ◆ Altered mental status ◆ Tachycardia ◆ Increased cardiac output ◆ Increased blood pressure ◆ Cardiac arrhythmias	◆ Arterial blood gas (ABG) values show deteriorating values and a pH below 7.35. ◆ Chest X-ray shows pulmonary disease or condition. ◆ Electrocardiogram (ECG) may show cardiac arrhythmia or right ventricular hypertrophy. ◆ Pulse oximetry shows decreasing arterial oxygen saturation.	◆ Administer oxygen therapy and monitor respiratory status; assist with endotracheal intubation and mechanical ventilation, if necessary. ◆ Assess breath sounds and note changes. ◆ Monitor ABG values and pulse oximetry. ◆ Monitor vital signs and intake and output. ◆ Monitor cardiac rhythm for arrhythmias. ◆ Administer antibiotics, bronchodilators, corticosteroids, positive inotropic agents, diuretics, vasopressors, or antiarrhythmics.
Cor pulmonale (complication)	◆ Progressive dyspnea worsening on exertion ◆ Tachypnea and bounding pulse ◆ Orthopnea ◆ Dependent edema ◆ Weakness ◆ Distended neck veins ◆ Enlarged, tender liver ◆ Tachycardia ◆ Enlarged spleen	◆ Pulmonary artery pressure (PAP) shows increased right ventricular pressure. ◆ Echocardiography or angiography indicates right ventricular enlargement. ◆ Chest X-ray suggests right ventricular enlargement. ◆ ABG analysis shows decreased partial pressure of arterial oxygen (less than 70 mm Hg). ◆ ECG may show various arrhythmias.	◆ Encourage bed rest to reduce myocardial oxygen demands. ◆ Administer digoxin, antibiotics, or pulmonary artery vasodilators, such as diazoxide, nitroprusside, hydralazine, angiotensin-converting enzyme inhibitors, calcium channel blockers, or prostaglandins, to reduce pulmonary hypertension. ◆ Provide meticulous respiratory care, including low-dose oxygen therapy, suctioning, and deep-breathing and coughing exercises. ◆ Monitor ABG values, and look for signs of respiratory failure (change in pulse rate, deep labored respirations, and increased fatigue on exertion). ◆ Monitor fluid status carefully; limit fluid intake to 1,000 to 2,000 ml/day, and provide a low sodium diet. ◆ Monitor serum potassium levels if the patient is receiving diuretics; low serum potassium levels can potentiate arrhythmias.
Heart failure (complication)	*Left-sided heart failure* ◆ Dyspnea ◆ Orthopnea ◆ Paroxysmal nocturnal dyspnea ◆ Fatigue ◆ Nonproductive cough ◆ Crackles ◆ Hemoptysis ◆ Tachycardia ◆ Third (S_3) and fourth (S_4) heart sounds ◆ Cool, pale skin ◆ Restlessness and confusion *Right-sided heart failure* ◆ Jugular vein distention ◆ Positive hepatojugular reflex ◆ Right-upper-quadrant pain ◆ Anorexia ◆ Nausea ◆ Nocturia ◆ Weight gain ◆ Edema ◆ Ascites or anasarca	◆ Chest X-rays may show pulmonary vascular markings, interstitial edema, or pleural effusion and cardiomegaly. ◆ ECG may indicate hypertrophy, ischemic changes, infarction, tachycardia, and extrasystoles. ◆ Liver function tests may be abnormal. ◆ Blood urea nitrogen (BUN) and creatinine levels may be elevated. ◆ Prothrombin time may be prolonged. ◆ Brain natriuretic peptide assay may be elevated. ◆ Echocardiography may reveal left ventricular hypertrophy, dilation, and abnormal contractility. ◆ PAP, pulmonary artery wedge pressure, and left ventricular end-diastolic pressure are elevated in the presence of left-sided heart failure; right atrial or central venous pressure is elevated in right-sided heart failure. ◆ Radionuclide ventriculography may reveal ejection fraction less than 40% in diastolic dysfunction.	◆ Place the patient in Fowler's position, and give supplemental oxygen. ◆ Weigh the patient daily, and check for peripheral edema. Monitor intake and output, vital signs, and mental status. ◆ Auscultate for S_3 and S_4 heart sounds and adventitious lung sounds, such as crackles or rhonchi. ◆ Monitor BUN, creatinine, and serum potassium, sodium, chloride, and magnesium levels. ◆ Institute continuous cardiac monitoring to promptly identify and treat arrhythmias. ◆ Administer diuretics, digoxin, beta-adrenergic blockers, inotropics, nesiritide, nitrates, or morphine. ◆ Encourage lifestyle modifications, such as weight loss, limited intake of sodium, smoking cessation, reduced alcohol consumption, and reduced intake of fat. ◆ Prepare the patient for coronary artery bypass grafting or heart transplantation, as appropriate.

Burns

OVERVIEW

- Heat, chemical, or electrical injury to tissue
- May be permanently disfiguring and incapacitating
- May be partial or full thickness
- Classified as first, second, third, or fourth degree (see *Classification of burns*)
- Affect more than 2 million people annually in the United States.
- Cause 70,000 hospitalizations and 20,000 specialized burn unit admissions annually

CAUSES

- Child or elder abuse
- Contact with electrical wiring
- Contact with high-voltage power lines
- Contact, ingestion, inhalation, or injection of acids, alkali, or vesicants
- Friction or abrasion
- Improper handling of firecrackers
- Improper use or handling of matches
- Improperly stored gasoline
- Motor vehicle accidents
- Residential fires
- Scalding accidents
- Space heater or electrical malfunction
- Sun exposure

PATHOPHYSIOLOGY

- The injuring agent denatures cellular proteins. Some cells die because of traumatic or ischemic necrosis.
- Loss of collagen cross-linking also occurs with denaturation, creating abnormal osmotic and hydrostatic pressure gradients, which cause the movement of intravascular fluid into interstitial spaces.
- Cellular injury triggers the release of mediators of inflammation, contributing to local and, in the case of major burns, systemic increases in capillary permeability.
- Specific pathophysiologic events depend upon the severity of the burn. (See *Disorders affecting management of burns,* page 79.)

CARDIOVASCULAR SYSTEM

- Burns may cause fluid shifts or directly injure the heart and blood vessels, leading to impaired circulation.
- The inflammatory response increases capillary permeability. As a result, intravascular fluid shifts to the interstitial spaces, leading to edema, decreased circulating fluid volume, and increased blood viscosity. This hemoconcentration places the patient at risk for thrombus formation.

GASTROINTESTINAL SYSTEM

- As blood is shunted away from the abdominal area and GI tract, peristalsis is slowed or absent altogether.
- Gastric dilation and vomiting may occur, possibly increasing the risk of aspiration.
- Curling's ulcers may result (stomach and intestinal ulcerations and hemorrhage).

INTEGUMENTARY SYSTEM

- Impaired skin integrity increases the risk of infection and causes hypothermia and rapid fluid losses.

Classification of burns

The depth of skin and tissue damage determines burn classification. This illustration shows the four degrees of burn classifications.

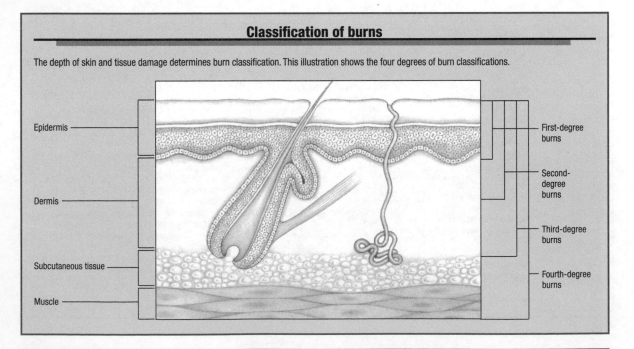

Epidermis

Dermis

Subcutaneous tissue

Muscle

First-degree burns

Second-degree burns

Third-degree burns

Fourth-degree burns

- Contractures and impaired range of motion in extremities may result from hypertrophic scar formation.
- Edema associated with circumferential burns constricts underlying blood vessels, tissue, and muscle, impairing circulation to the affected area or extremity.

IMMUNE AND HEMATOLOGIC SYSTEMS
- One theory suggests burn cells release a toxin that interferes with the immune system's ability to function properly. Subsequently, major burns may result in immunosuppression.
- Generalized sepsis is a common and serious complication; the larger the wound, the greater the risk of infection.
- More severe burn states may result in the development of disseminated intravascular coagulation.

RENAL SYSTEM
- Hemoconcentration and decreased intravascular volumes cause decreased renal perfusion and decreased urinary output.
- Prolonged decreased renal perfusion leads to acute tubular necrosis and renal failure.

RESPIRATORY SYSTEM
- Neck burns or swelling from heat and smoke exposure or chemical injury to the mucosa of the respiratory tract can lead to respiratory distress.
- Restricted respiratory expansion from chest burns or eschar formation can lead to respiratory distress.
- Smoke inhalation or inhalation of other caustic substances results in pulmonary injury, such as bronchitis or respiratory distress.
- Hypoxia may result from a decreased amount of oxygen circulating through the blood that may be caused by inhalation of carbon monoxide, a by-product of combustion that displaces oxygen from hemoglobin molecules.

HISTORY
- Cause of the burn revealed
- Preexisting medical conditions

PHYSICAL FINDINGS
- Depth and size of the burn assessed
- Severity of the burn estimated—diagnosed as major, moderate, or minor based on affected body surface area and depth of injury
- Respiratory distress and cyanosis
- Edema
- Alteration in pulse rate, strength, and regularity
- Stridor, wheezing, crackles, and rhonchi
- S_3 or S_4
- Hypotension
- Soot marks on face

DIAGNOSTIC TEST RESULTS
- Arterial blood gas levels may show evidence of smoke inhalation, decreased alveolar function, and hypoxia.
- Complete blood count may show decreased hemoglobin level and hematocrit, if blood loss occurs.
- Abnormal electrolyte levels may result from fluid losses and shifts.
- Blood urea nitrogen level may increase with fluid losses.
- Glucose level in children may be decreased because of limited glycogen storage.
- Urinalysis may show myoglobinuria and hemoglobinuria.
- Carboxyhemoglobin level is increased.
- Electrocardiography shows myocardial ischemia, injury, or arrhythmias, especially in electrical burns.
- Fiber-optic bronchoscopy shows edema of the airways.

GENERAL
- Elimination of the burn source
- Airway, breathing, and circulation assessed and secured
- Prevention of hypoxia
- I.V. fluids through a large-bore I.V. line (see *Fluid replacement after a burn,* page 78)
- Adults: urine output of 30 to 50 ml/hour
- Child weighing less than 66 lb (30 kg): urine output of 1 ml/kg/hour
- Nasogastric tube and urinary catheter insertion
- Wound care

DIET
- Nothing by mouth until severity of burn established; then high-protein, high-calorie
- Increased hydration with high-calorie, high-protein drinks, not free water
- Total parenteral nutrition, if unable to take food by mouth

ACTIVITY
- With limitations based on extent and location of burn
- Physical therapy

MEDICATIONS
- Booster of tetanus toxoid
- Analgesics
- Antibiotics
- Antianxiolytics
- Osmotic diuretics

SURGERY
- Loose tissue and blister debridement
- Escharotomy
- Skin grafting

(continued)

NURSING DIAGNOSES

- Acute pain
- Anxiety
- Decreased cardiac output
- Deficient fluid volume
- Disturbed body image
- Hypothermia
- Imbalanced nutrition: Less than body requirements
- Impaired gas exchange
- Impaired physical mobility
- Impaired skin integrity
- Ineffective airway clearance
- Ineffective coping
- Ineffective protection
- Ineffective tissue perfusion: Peripheral
- Risk for infection
- Risk for posttraumatic stress disorder

EXPECTED OUTCOMES

The patient will:

- express feeling of increased comfort and decreased pain
- express feelings of decreased anxiety
- maintain adequate cardiac output
- maintain fluid volume within the acceptable range
- express positive feelings about self
- maintain normal body temperature
- maintain daily caloric requirements
- maintain adequate ventilation and oxygenation
- attain the highest degree of mobility possible within the confines of the injury
- exhibit improved or healed wounds or lesions that are clean, pink, and free of purulent drainage
- maintain a patent airway
- demonstrate effective coping mechanisms
- verbalize methods to prevent burns
- exhibit signs of adequate peripheral perfusion
- remain free from signs and symptoms of infection
- express feelings and fears about the traumatic event.

NURSING INTERVENTIONS

- Initiate aggressive burn treatment.
- Use strict sterile technique.
- Remove smoldering clothing.
- Remove constricting items.
- Monitor vital signs, intake and output, hydration and nutritional status, and respiratory status.
- Provide adequate hydration.
- Assess pain level, and provide analgesics, as ordered.
- Perform appropriate wound care.
- Weigh the patient daily.
- Encourage verbalization and provide emotional support.
- Observe for signs of infection and other complications.

PATIENT TEACHING

Be sure to cover:

- injury, diagnostic testing, and treatment
- wound care
- medication administration, dosage, and possible adverse effects
- developing a dietary plan
- signs and symptoms of complications
- available rehabilitation facilities, if appropriate
- available psychological counseling, if needed
- available resource and support services.

RESOURCES

Organizations

American Burn Association: *www.ameriburn.org*

National Center for Injury Prevention and Control: *www.cdc.gov/ncipc*

Selected references

Anwar, M.U., et al. "Smoking, Substance Abuse, Psychiatric History, and Burns: Trends in Adult Patients," *Journal of Burn Care & Rehabilitation* 26(6):493-501, November-December 2005.

Atlas of Pathophysiology, 2nd ed. Philadelphia: Lippincott Williams & Wilkins, 2005.

Burd, A., and Noronha, F. "What's New in Burns Trauma?" *Surgical Practice* 9(4):126-36, November 2005.

Cinat, M., and Carson, J. "Burns and Motor Vehicle Crashes," *Topics in Emergency Medicine* 28(1):56-67, January-March 2006.

DeSanti, L. "Pathophysiology and Current Management of Burn Injury," *Advances in Skin & Wound Care* 18(6):323-32, July-August 2005.

Smith, J., et al. "The Psychology of Burn Care," *Journal of Trauma Nursing* 13(3):105-106, July-September 2006.

Fluid replacement after a burn

To replace fluid in an adult with a burn, use one of the following formulas:

FIRST 24 HOURS

Evans

- 1 ml × patient's weight in kg × % total body surface area (TBSA) burn (0.9% normal saline solution)
- 1 ml × patient's weight in kg × % TBSA burn (colloid solution)

Brooke

- 1.5 ml × patient's weight in kg × % TBSA burn (lactated ringer's solution)
- 0.5 ml × patient's weight in kg × % TBSA burn (colloid solution)

Parkland

- 4 ml × patient's weight in kg × % TBSA burn (lactated Ringer's solution). Give one-half of volume in first 8 minutes; then infuse remainder over 16 minutes.

SECOND 24 HOURS

Evans

- 50% of first 24-hour replacement (0.9% normal saline solution)
- 2,000 ml (dextrose 5% in water [D_5W])

Brooke

- 50% to 75% of first 24-hour replacement (lactated Ringer's solution)
- 2,000 ml (D_5W)

Parkland

- 30% to 60% of calculated plasma volume (25% albumin)
- Volume to maintain desired urine output (D_5W)

Disorders affecting the management of burns

This chart highlights disorders that affect the management of burns.

DISORDER	SIGNS AND SYMPTOMS	DIAGNOSTIC TEST RESULTS	TREATMENT AND CARE
Burn shock (complication)	◆ Tachycardia ◆ Tachypnea ◆ Cyanosis ◆ Weak, rapid, thready pulse ◆ Cold, clammy skin ◆ Hypotension ◆ Reduced urinary output progressing to anuria ◆ Restlessness and irritability progressing to unconsciousness and absent reflexes ◆ Peripheral edema	◆ Potassium, serum lactate, and blood urea nitrogen levels are elevated. ◆ Urine specific gravity is greater than 1.020; urine osmolality is increased. ◆ Blood pH and partial pressure of arterial oxygen are decreased, and partial pressure of carbon dioxide is increased. ◆ Coagulation studies may detect disseminated intravascular coagulation (DIC).	◆ Institute and monitor continuous cardiac monitoring. ◆ Administer analgesics and antiarrhythmics. ◆ Administer blood replacement therapy. ◆ Initiate prompt and adequate fluid volume replacement therapy to restore intravascular volume and raise blood pressure. ◆ Administer supplemental oxygen. ◆ Monitor vital signs and signs and symptoms of deficient fluid volume, such as tachycardia, hypotension, weak peripheral pulses, dry mucous membranes, and decreased urine output (less than 0.5 ml/kg/hour). ◆ Monitor the patient carefully for signs of neurological impairment, such as confusion, memory loss, insomnia, lethargy, and combativeness. ◆ Monitor the patient for signs of impaired peristalsis, such as vomiting or fecal impaction. To prevent Curling's ulcers, initiate early enteral feedings and maintain gastric pH greater than 5 by administering antacids and histamine-2 receptor antagonists.
Compartment syndrome (complication)	◆ Increased pain at the affected part ◆ Decreased touch sensation at the affected part ◆ Increased weakness of the affected part ◆ Increased swelling and pallor ◆ Decreased pulses and capillary refill	◆ Creatinine kinase levels are increased because of muscle tissue injury or necrosis. ◆ Intracompartmental tissue pressures are increased. ◆ Arteriograms or venograms show blocked vessels with embolus, thrombus, or other vascular injury. ◆ Transcutaneous Doppler venous flow studies show impaired venous flow.	◆ Assist with procedures to relieve the constricting forces. An emergency fasciotomy may be necessary. ◆ Apply ice and elevate the affected extremity to no more than 5″ (12.7 cm) above heart level. ◆ Provide pain relief. Opioids may be necessary. ◆ Monitor neurovascular status closely to detect developing or worsening compartment syndrome. ◆ Administer I.V. mannitol (Osmitrol), a systemic diuretic, to reduce intracompartmental pressures.
Sepsis (complication)	◆ Labile temperature ◆ Tachycardia ◆ Tachypnea ◆ Hypotension ◆ Hyperglycemia ◆ Nausea and vomiting ◆ Lethargy and malaise	◆ Blood cultures as well as sputum, urine, and wound tissue cultures isolate the organism. ◆ Platelet count is decreased, and white blood cell count ranges from 15,000 to 30,000/mm^3, suggesting leukocytosis.	◆ Administer I.V. antibiotics to control the infection. Depending on the organism, a combination of antibiotics may be necessary. ◆ Monitor vital signs closely. ◆ Administer vasopressors. ◆ Monitor serum antibiotic levels. ◆ Provide meticulous burn wound and other care to prevent introducing microorganisms into the patient, who's typically immunocompromised. ◆ Apply topical antibiotics to the burn to prevent wound infection, that may develop into systemic sepsis.

Cardiac tamponade LIFE-THREATENING DISORDER

OVERVIEW

◆ Increase in intrapericardial pressure caused by fluid accumulation in the pericardial sac
◆ Impaired diastolic filling of the heart
◆ More common in males than in females
◆ Occurs acutely with 2% of penetrating chest traumas

CAUSES
◆ Acute myocardial infarction
◆ Cardiac catheterization
◆ Cardiac surgery
◆ Chronic renal failure
◆ Connective tissue disorders
◆ Drug reaction
◆ Effusion in cancer, bacterial infections, tuberculosis and, rarely, acute rheumatic fever
◆ Hemorrhage from nontraumatic cause
◆ Hypothyroidism
◆ Idiopathic (possibly)
◆ Trauma to the chest
◆ Viral, postirradiation, or idiopathic pericarditis

PATHOPHYSIOLOGY

◆ Typically, a coexisting disorder prompts fluid accumulation. If it accumulates rapidly around the heart, as little as 50 ml of fluid can create an emergency situation.
◆ Pericardial effusion associated with cancer may not produce immediate signs and symptoms because the fibrous wall of the pericardial sac can gradually stretch to accommodate as much as 1 to 2 L of fluid. (See *Disorders affecting management of cardiac tamponade,* page 83.)

CARDIOVASCULAR SYSTEM
◆ Pressure resulting from fluid accumulation in the pericardium decreases ventricular filling and cardiac output, resulting in cardiogenic shock and death, if left untreated. (See *Understanding cardiac tamponade.*)

UP CLOSE

Understanding cardiac tamponade

The pericardial sac, which surrounds and protects the heart, is composed of several layers. The fibrous pericardium is the tough outermost membrane; the inner membrane, called the serous membrane, consists of the visceral and parietal layers. The visceral layer clings to the heart and is also known as the epicardial layer of the heart. The parietal layer lies between the visceral layer and the fibrous pericardium. The pericardial space—between the visceral and parietal layers—contains 10 to 30 ml of pericardial fluid. This fluid lubricates the layers and minimizes friction when the heart contracts.

In cardiac tamponade, blood or fluid fills the pericardial space, compressing the heart chambers, increasing intracardiac pressure, and obstructing venous return. As blood flow into the ventricles falls, so does cardiac output. Without prompt treatment, low cardiac output can be fatal.

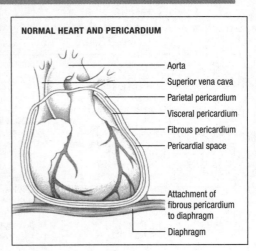

NORMAL HEART AND PERICARDIUM

- Aorta
- Superior vena cava
- Parietal pericardium
- Visceral pericardium
- Fibrous pericardium
- Pericardial space
- Attachment of fibrous pericardium to diaphragm
- Diaphragm

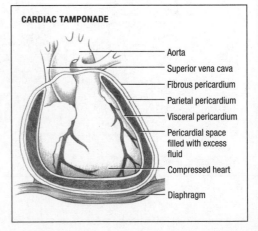

CARDIAC TAMPONADE

- Aorta
- Superior vena cava
- Fibrous pericardium
- Parietal pericardium
- Visceral pericardium
- Pericardial space filled with excess fluid
- Compressed heart
- Diaphragm

WARNING *Cardiac tamponade may cause a cardiac condition called pulseless electrical activity (PEA). With PEA, isolated electrical activity occurs sporadically without evidence of myocardial contraction. Unless the underlying cardiac tamponade is identified and treated quickly, PEA will result in death.*

GASTROINTESTINAL SYSTEM
◆ Cardiac tamponade alters systemic venous return secondary to increased compression of the right atrium. This results in increased volume in the right ventricle. Blood then accumulates in the venous circulation, causing hepatomegaly.

IMMUNE SYSTEM
◆ Exudative fluid accumulation may occur secondary to the inflammatory process that occurs in certain autoimmune disorders, such as systemic lupus erythematosus; infections, such as human immunodeficiency virus; or malignancy, such as cancer.

RESPIRATORY SYSTEM
◆ Large pleural effusions have been associated with cardiac tamponade. These effusions cause increased intrapleural pressure, which transmits to the pericardial space and impairs ventricular filling, causing the same physiologic outcome as cardiac tamponade.

ASSESSMENT

HISTORY
◆ Presence of one or more causes
◆ Dyspnea
◆ Shortness of breath
◆ Chest pain
◆ Syncope
◆ Palpitations

PHYSICAL FINDINGS
◆ Vary with volume of fluid and speed of fluid accumulation
◆ Diaphoresis
◆ Anxiety and restlessness
◆ Pallor or cyanosis
◆ Jugular vein distention
◆ Edema
◆ Rapid, weak pulses
◆ Hepatomegaly
◆ Decreased arterial blood pressure
◆ Increased central venous pressure
◆ Pulsus paradoxus
◆ Narrow pulse pressure
◆ Muffled heart sounds

DIAGNOSTIC TEST RESULTS
◆ Electrocardiography may show low voltage complexes in the precordial leads.
◆ Hemodynamic monitoring shows equalization of mean right atrial, right ventricular diastolic, pulmonary artery wedge, and left ventricular diastolic pressures.
◆ Echocardiography may show an echo-free space, indicating fluid accumulation in the pericardial sac.
◆ Chest X-rays show slightly widened mediastinum and enlargement of the cardiac silhouette.

TREATMENT

GENERAL
◆ Pericardiocentesis, if necessary

DIET
◆ As tolerated

ACTIVITY
◆ Bed rest until resolved

MEDICATIONS
◆ Oxygen
◆ Intravascular volume expansion
◆ Inotropic agents

SURGERY
◆ Pericardial window
◆ Subxiphoid pericardiotomy
◆ Complete pericardectomy
◆ Thoracotomy

(continued)

NURSING CONSIDERATIONS

NURSING DIAGNOSES

- Activity intolerance
- Acute pain
- Anxiety
- Decreased cardiac output
- Deficient fluid volume
- Impaired gas exchange
- Ineffective tissue perfusion: Cardiopulmonary
- Risk for infection

EXPECTED OUTCOMES

The patient will:

- maintain ability to perform activities of daily living to the fullest extent possible
- express feelings of increased comfort and decreased pain
- identify strategies to reduce anxiety
- maintain hemodynamic stability and adequate cardiac output
- maintain adequate fluid volume
- maintain adequate ventilation and oxygenation
- maintain adequate cardiopulmonary perfusion
- remain free from signs and symptoms of infection.

NURSING INTERVENTIONS

- Administer oxygen therapy, as needed.
- Assist with pericardiocentesis, if necessary.
- Monitor vital signs, intake and output, cardiac rhythm, hemodynamics, and arterial blood gas levels.
- Give prescribed drugs.
- Provide reassurance.
- Infuse I.V. solutions, as ordered.
- Maintain the chest drainage system, if used.
- Assess for signs and symptoms of increasing tamponade.
- Observe for complications.
- Prepare for surgery, if needed.

PATIENT TEACHING

Be sure to cover:

- disorder, diagnostic testing, and treatment
- medication administration, dosage, and possible adverse effects
- when to notify the practitioner
- preoperative and postoperative care
- emergency procedures.

RESOURCES

Organizations

American Heart Association: *www.americanheart.org*
National Heart, Lung, and Blood Institute: *www.nhlbi.nih.gov*

Selected references

Chen, I.C., et al. "Atrial Flutter with Cardiac Tamponade as Initial Presentation of Tuberculosis Pericarditis," *The American Journal of Emergency Medicine* 25(1):108-10, January 2007.

The Merck Manual of Diagnosis & Therapy, 18th ed. Whitehouse Station, N.J.: Merck & Co., Inc., 2006.

Sagrista-Sauleda, J., et al. "Low-Pressure Cardiac Tamponade: Clinical and Hemodynamic Profile," *Circulation* 114(9):945-52, August 2006.

Seferovic, P.M., et al. "Management Strategies in Pericardial Emergencies," *Herz* 31(9):891-900, December 2006.

Disorders affecting management of cardiac tamponade

This chart highlights disorders that affect the management of cardiac tamponade.

DISORDER	SIGNS AND SYMPTOMS	DIAGNOSTIC TEST RESULTS	TREATMENT AND CARE
End-stage renal disease (coexisting)	◆ Reduced urine output ◆ Hypotension or hypertension ◆ Pleural friction rub ◆ Altered level of consciousness	◆ Blood urea nitrogen (BUN) is elevated. ◆ Creatinine clearance and potassium levels are increased. ◆ Urine specific gravity, blood pH, bicarbonate level, hemoglobin, and hematocrit are decreased.	◆ Monitor intake and output; check weight daily. ◆ Monitor vital signs for signs of decreased cardiac output. ◆ Assess lungs for changes in breath sounds. ◆ Watch for signs of infection. ◆ Monitor serum laboratory results, including BUN, creatinine, and electrolyte levels.
Lung cancer (coexisting)	◆ Dyspnea ◆ Pleural friction rub ◆ Wheezing ◆ Decreased breath sounds ◆ Dilated chest and abdominal veins ◆ Pain	◆ Cytologic sputum analysis shows dense pulmonary malignancy. ◆ Liver function tests are abnormal, especially with metastasis. ◆ Chest X-ray shows advanced lesions. ◆ Contrast studies of the bronchial tree demonstrate the size and location as well as spread of the lesion. ◆ Computed tomography scan of the chest can detect malignant pleural effusion.	◆ Monitor respiratory status for dyspnea and changes in breath sounds. ◆ Administer oxygen. ◆ Assess the patient's pain level, and administer medications. ◆ Monitor chest X-ray for development of pleural effusion. ◆ Provide support for patients undergoing testing for metastatic disease. ◆ Check for pulsus paradoxus.
Myocardial infarction (MI) (coexisting)	◆ Severe, persistent chest pain ◆ Feeling of impending doom ◆ Fatigue ◆ Nausea and vomiting ◆ Shortness of breath ◆ Anxiety ◆ Muffled heart sounds ◆ Hypotension or hypertension	◆ Electrocardiogram (ECG) reveals ST-segment changes. ◆ Total creatine kinase (CK) and CK-MB isoenzyme levels are elevated over a 72-hour period. ◆ Myoglobin is elevated within 3 to 6 hours. ◆ Troponin level is elevated. ◆ Echocardiography shows ventricular-wall motion abnormalities. ◆ Multiple-gated acquisition scan or radionuclide ventriculography identifies acutely damaged muscle. ◆ Homocysteine and C-reactive protein levels are elevated.	◆ Assess the patient for specific type of pain, and monitor him for changes. ◆ Note cardiac rhythm and check peripheral pulses. ◆ Assess heart sounds for muffled tones, and auscultate for pericardial friction rub. ◆ Be alert for signs of decreased cardiac output, such as decreased blood pressure and dyspnea. ◆ Be prepared to administer an antiarrhythmic, to possibly assist with pacemaker insertion, or to assist with cardioversion to treat cardiac arrhythmias. ◆ Be prepared to administer thrombolytic therapy (streptokinase or recombinant tissue plasminogen) to preserve myocardial tissue. ◆ Percutaneous transluminal coronary angioplasty may be performed to restore blood flow to the heart muscle. ◆ Be prepared to administer other drugs, including antiplatelets (such as aspirin) to inhibit platelet aggregation; sublingual or I.V. nitrates (such as nitroglycerin) to relieve pain, increase cardiac output, and reduce myocardial workload; morphine for pain and sedation; and angiotensin-converting enzyme inhibitors to improve survival rate in large anterior-wall MI. ◆ Administer supplemental oxygen. ◆ Assist with pulmonary artery catheterization, used to detect left- or right-sided heart failure and to monitor the patient's response to treatment. ◆ Assess and record the severity of chest pain. ◆ Monitor vital signs frequently. ◆ Watch for signs and symptoms of fluid retention (crackles, cough, tachypnea, and edema). ◆ Carefully monitor daily weight, intake and output, and serum enzyme levels.

Cardiomyopathy

- Disease of the heart muscle fibers that occurs in three main forms: dilated (most common), hypertrophic, and restrictive (extremely rare) (see *Comparing cardiomyopathies*)
- Second most common direct cause of sudden death
- Approximately 5 to 8 Americans out of 100,000 with dilated cardiomyopathy

- Men and blacks at greatest risk for dilated form
- Prognosis for dilated cardiomyopathy usually poor because it goes undiagnosed until its in advanced stages
- Two types of hypertrophic cardiomyopathy: nonobstructive hypertrophic cardiomyopathy and hypertrophic obstructive cardiomyopathy (HOCM)
- Almost 50% of all sudden deaths in competitive athletes age 35 or younger caused by HOCM

- If severe, restrictive cardiomyopathy irreversible

CAUSES
Dilated cardiomyopathy
- Idiopathic (or primary) disease or associated with another condition, such as diabetes or thyroid disease
- Cardiotoxic effects of drugs or alcohol
- Chemotherapy
- Drug hypersensitivity
- Hypertension
- Ischemic heart disease

UP CLOSE

Comparing cardiomyopathies

Cardiomyopathies include various structural or functional abnormalities of the ventricles. They're grouped into three main pathophysiologic types—dilated, hypertrophic, and restrictive. These conditions may lead to heart failure by impairing myocardial structure and function.

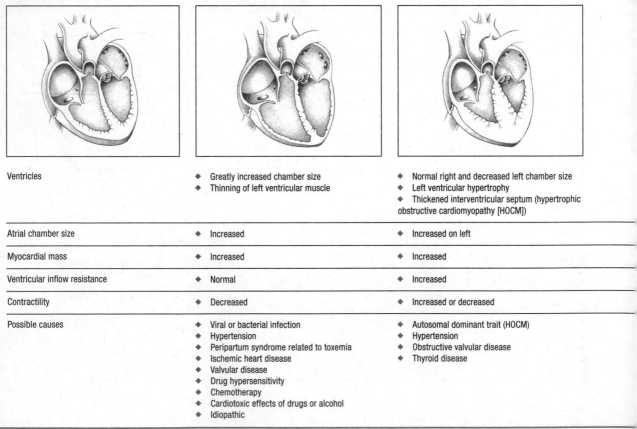

	NORMAL HEART	DILATED CARDIOMYOPATHY	HYPERTROPHIC CARDIOMYOPATHY
Ventricles		◆ Greatly increased chamber size ◆ Thinning of left ventricular muscle	◆ Normal right and decreased left chamber size ◆ Left ventricular hypertrophy ◆ Thickened interventricular septum (hypertrophic obstructive cardiomyopathy [HOCM])
Atrial chamber size		◆ Increased	◆ Increased on left
Myocardial mass		◆ Increased	◆ Increased
Ventricular inflow resistance		◆ Normal	◆ Increased
Contractility		◆ Decreased	◆ Increased or decreased
Possible causes		◆ Viral or bacterial infection ◆ Hypertension ◆ Peripartum syndrome related to toxemia ◆ Ischemic heart disease ◆ Valvular disease ◆ Drug hypersensitivity ◆ Chemotherapy ◆ Cardiotoxic effects of drugs or alcohol ◆ Idiopathic	◆ Autosomal dominant trait (HOCM) ◆ Hypertension ◆ Obstructive valvular disease ◆ Thyroid disease

- Peripartum syndrome related to preeclampsia and eclampsia
- Valvular disease
- Viral or bacterial infections

Hypertrophic cardiomyopathy
- Exact cause unknown
- Inherited
- Pressure overload hypertension
- Aortic valve stenosis
- Transmission by autosomal dominant trait (HOCM)

Restrictive cardiomyopathy
- Carcinoid heart disease

RESTRICTIVE CARDIOMYOPATHY

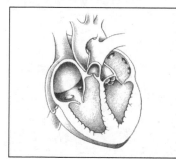

- Decreased ventricular chamber size
- Left ventricular hypertrophy

- Increased

- Normal

- Increased

- Decreased

- Amyloidosis
- Sarcoidosis
- Hemochromatosis
- Infiltrative neoplastic disease
- Collagen-vascular diseases
- Tumors

- Connective tissue disorder
- Heart transplant
- Idiopathic or associated with another condition (for example, amyloidosis or endomyocardial fibrosis)
- Mediastinal radiation

RISK FACTORS
- Coronary artery disease
- Myocardial infarction
- Diabetes
- Hypertension
- Pregnancy
- Viral infections
- Alcohol or illegal drug use

PATHOPHYSIOLOGY

- Cardiomyopathy results from extensively damaged myocardial muscle fibers.

CARDIOVASCULAR SYSTEM
Dilated cardiomyopathy
- When the renin-angiotensin system, which regulates cardiac output, can no longer do its job, the heart begins to fail. Left ventricular dilation occurs as venous return and systemic vascular resistance rise.
- Eventually, the atria dilate as more work is required to pump blood into the full ventricles, resulting in cardiomegaly.
- Blood pooling in the ventricles increases the risk of emboli. (See *Disorders affecting management of cardiomyopathy,* pages 88 and 89.)

Nonobstructive hypertrophic cardiomyopathy
- Unlike dilated cardiomyopathy, which affects systolic function, hypertrophic cardiomyopathy primarily affects diastolic function.
- The hypertrophied ventricle becomes stiff, noncompliant, and unable to relax during ventricular filling.
- Ventricular filling is reduced, and left ventricular filling pressure rises, causing a rise in left atrial and pulmonary venous pressures and leading to venous congestion and dyspnea. Ventricular filling time is further

---

reduced as a compensatory response to tachycardia, leading to low cardiac output.
- If papillary muscles (attached to the atrioventricular valves) become hypertrophied and don't close completely during contraction, mitral insufficiency occurs.

Hypertrophic obstructive cardiomyopathy
- The features of HOCM include asymmetrical left ventricular hypertrophy; hypertrophy of the intraventricular septum; rapid, forceful contractions of the left ventricle; impaired relaxation; and obstruction to left ventricular outflow.
- The forceful ejection of blood draws the anterior leaflet of the mitral valve to the intraventricular septum, which causes early closure of the outflow tract, decreasing ejection fraction.
- Intramural coronary arteries are abnormally small and may not be sufficient to supply the hypertrophied muscle with enough blood and oxygen to meet the increased needs of the hyperdynamic muscle.

Restrictive cardiomyopathy
- Stiffness of the ventricle is caused by left ventricular hypertrophy and endocardial fibrosis and thickening, which reduce the ability of the ventricle to relax and fill during diastole.
- The rigid myocardium fails to contract completely during systole, resulting in decreased cardiac output.

RESPIRATORY SYSTEM
Dilated cardiomyopathy
- Contractility in the left ventricle is reduced.
- Systolic function declines and stroke volume, ejection fraction, and cardiac output fall.
- End-diastolic volumes rise, resulting in pulmonary congestion.

RENAL SYSTEM
- The kidneys are stimulated to retain sodium and water to maintain cardiac output, resulting in vasoconstriction.

(continued)

HISTORY
◆ Onset of dilated or restrictive cardiomyopathy generally insidious
◆ Frequent exacerbations—regardless of the form
◆ Signs of left-sided heart failure

PHYSICAL FINDINGS
Dilated cardiomyopathy
◆ Shortness of breath
◆ Tachypnea
◆ Orthopnea
◆ Dyspnea on exertion
◆ Paroxysmal nocturnal dyspnea
◆ Fatigue
◆ Dry cough at night
◆ Peripheral edema
◆ Hepatomegaly
◆ Right-upper-quadrant pain (secondary to hepatic engorgement)
◆ Jugular vein distention
◆ Weight gain

◆ Peripheral cyanosis
◆ Tachycardia as a compensatory response to low cardiac output
◆ Pansystolic murmur
◆ Third (S_3) and fourth (S_4) heart sound gallop rhythms
◆ Irregular pulse, if atrial fibrillation exists
◆ Worsening renal function

Nonobstructive hypertropic cardiomyopathy
◆ Dyspnea
◆ Fatigue
◆ Angina
◆ Peripheral pulse with a characteristic double impulse (pulsus biferiens)
◆ Abrupt arterial pulse
◆ Irregular pulse, if atrial fibrillation exists

HOCM
◆ Systolic ejection murmur along the left sternal border and at the apex
◆ Angina

◆ Syncope
◆ Activity intolerance
◆ Abrupt arterial pulse
◆ Irregular pulse, if atrial fibrillation exists
◆ Displacement of point of maximum impulse inferiorly and laterally

Restrictive cardiomyopathy
◆ Fatigue
◆ Dyspnea, orthopnea
◆ Chest pain
◆ Edema
◆ Liver engorgement
◆ Peripheral cyanosis
◆ Pallor
◆ S_3 or S_4 gallop rhythms
◆ Jugular vein distention
◆ Systolic murmurs

DIAGNOSTIC TEST RESULTS
◆ Echocardiography may reveal asymmetry of the left ventricle and hypertrophy, obstruction of outflow of the left ventricle, decreased ejection frac-

---

Comparing diagnostic test results in cardiomyopathy

DIAGNOSTIC TEST	DILATED CARDIOMYOPATHY	HYPERTROPHIC CARDIOMYOPATHY	RESTRICTIVE CARDIOMYOPATHY
Electrocardiography	Biventricular hypertrophy, sinus tachycardia, atrial enlargement, atrial and ventricular arrhythmias, bundle-branch block, and ST-segment and T-wave abnormalities	Left ventricular hypertrophy, ST-segment and T-wave abnormalities, left anterior hemiblock, Q waves in precordial and inferior leads, ventricular arrhythmias and, possibly, atrial fibrillation	Low voltage, hypertrophy, atrioventricular conduction defects, and left-axis deviation
Echocardiography	Left ventricular thrombi, global hypokinesia, enlarged atria, left ventricular dilation and, possibly, valvular abnormalities, decreased ejection fraction, and possible pericardial effusion	Asymmetrical thickening of the left ventricular wall and intraventricular septum and left atrial dilation	Increased left ventricular muscle mass, normal or reduced left ventricular cavity size, and decreased systolic function; rules out constrictive pericarditis
Chest X-ray	Cardiomegaly, pulmonary congestion, pulmonary venous hypertension, and pleural or pericardial effusions	Cardiomegaly	Cardiomegaly, pericardial effusion, and pulmonary congestion
Cardiac catheterization	Elevated left atrial and left ventricular end-diastolic pressures, left ventricular enlargement, and mitral and tricuspid incompetence; may identify coronary artery disease as a cause	Elevated ventricular end-diastolic pressure and, possibly, mitral insufficiency, hyperdynamic systolic function, and aortic valve pressure gradient (if aortic valve is stenotic)	Reduced systolic function and myocardial infiltration; increased left ventricular end-diastolic pressure; rules out constrictive pericarditis
Radionuclide studies	Left ventricular dilation and hypokinesis, and reduced ejection fraction	Reduced left ventricular volume, increased muscle mass, and ischemia	Left ventricular hypertrophy with restricted ventricular filling and reduced ejection fraction

tion, endocardial thickening, and decreased cardiac output.

- Chest X-ray may reveal cardiomegaly associated with any of the cardiomyopathies.
- Cardiac catheterization with possible heart biopsy reveals endocardial fibrosis and thickening. It may also show decreased ejection fraction. (See *Comparing diagnostic test results in cardiomyopathy.*)

TREATMENT

GENERAL
- Treatment of underlying cause, if identifiable
- Cardioversion
- Symptomatic treatment

DIET
- Low-sodium, supplemented by vitamin therapy
- No alcohol, if cardiomyopathy caused by alcoholism

ACTIVITY
- Rest periods

MEDICATIONS
Dilated cardiomyopathy
- Cardiac glycosides
- Diuretics
- Angiotensin-converting enzyme (ACE) inhibitors
- Angiotensin receptor blockers
- Oxygen
- Anticoagulants
- Vasodilators
- Antiarrhythmics
- Beta-adrenergic blockers

Hypertrophic cardiomyopathy
- Beta-adrenergic blockers
- Calcium channel blockers
- Amiodarone, unless atrioventricular block exists
- Antibiotic prophylaxis

  WARNING *If propranolol is to be discontinued, don't stop the drug abruptly; doing so may cause rebound effects, resulting in myocardial infarction or sudden death.*

Restrictive cardiomyopathy
- Cardiac glycosides
- Diuretics
- Vasodilators
- ACE inhibitors
- Anticoagulants
- Corticosteroids

SURGERY
Dilated cardiomyopathy
- Permanent pacemaker (biventricular pacemaker for cardiac resynchronization therapy)
- Revascularization, such as coronary artery bypass graft surgery
- Valve repair or replacement
- Heart transplantation
- Possible cardiomyoplasty
- Implantable cardioverter-defibrillator (ICD)

Hypertrophic cardiomyopathy
- Ventricular myotomy or myectomy alone or combined with mitral valve replacement
- ICD
- Heart transplantation

Restrictive cardiomyopathy
- Permanent pacemaker
- Heart transplantation

NURSING CONSIDERATIONS

NURSING DIAGNOSES
- Activity intolerance
- Anxiety
- Decreased cardiac output
- Excess fluid volume
- Fatigue
- Hopelessness
- Impaired gas exchange
- Impaired physical mobility
- Ineffective breathing pattern
- Ineffective denial
- Ineffective role performance
- Ineffective tissue perfusion: Cardiopulmonary

EXPECTED OUTCOMES
The patient will:
- maintain ability to perform activities of daily living to the fullest extent possible
- verbalize strategies to reduce anxiety

- maintain adequate cardiac output and hemodynamic stability
- develop no complications of excess fluid volume
- express feelings of energy and decreased fatigue
- make decisions about his care, as appropriate
- maintain adequate ventilation and oxygenation
- maintain joint mobility and range of motion (ROM)
- maintain a respiratory rate within 5 breaths/minute of baseline
- recognize and accept limitations of chronic illness and the changes in lifestyle that are needed
- resume and maintain as many former roles as possible
- maintain adequate cardiopulmonary perfusion.

NURSING INTERVENTIONS
- Administer oxygen, as needed.
- Monitor vital signs, hemodynamics, intake and output, and daily weights.
- Assess for signs and symptoms of progressive heart failure.
- Alternate periods of rest with required activities of daily living.
- Provide active or passive ROM exercises.
- Consult with the dietitian to provide a low-sodium diet.
- Check serum potassium levels for hypokalemia, especially if therapy includes cardiac glycosides.
- Offer support and encourage the patient to express his feelings.
- Allow the patient and his family to express their fears and concerns and help them identify effective coping strategies.

PATIENT TEACHING

Be sure to cover:
- disorder, diagnostic testing, and treatment
- medication administration, dosage, and possible adverse effects
- need for antibiotic prophylaxis before dental work or surgery to prevent infective endocarditis

(continued)

- warnings against strenuous activity, which may precipitate syncope or sudden death
- need to avoid Valsalva's maneuver or sudden position changes
- how to contact local support groups and community cardiopulmonary resuscitation classes for the family.

RESOURCES

Organizations
Mayo Clinic: *www.mayoclinic.com*
National Heart, Lung, and Blood Institute: *www.nhlbi.nih.gov*

Selected references
Dakin, C., et al. "HAART to Heart: HIV Related Cardiomyopathy and Other Cardiovascular Complications," *AACN Advanced Critical Care* 17(1):18-29, January-March 2006.

Maisch, B., et al. "Management of Patients with Suspected (Peri)myocarditis and Inflammatory Dilated Cardiomyopathy," *Herz* 31(9):881-90, December 2006.

The Merck Manual of Diagnosis & Therapy, 18th ed. Whitehouse Station, N.J.: Merck & Co., Inc., 2006.

Towbin, J.A., et al. "Incidence, Causes, and Outcomes of Dilated Cardiomyopathy in Children," *JAMA* 296(15):1867-876, October, 2006.

Disorders affecting management of cardiomyopathy

This chart highlights disorders that affect the management of cardiomyopathy.

DISORDER	SIGNS AND SYMPTOMS	DIAGNOSTIC TEST RESULTS	TREATMENT AND CARE
Arrhythmias (complication)	• Irregularly irregular pulse rhythm with normal or abnormal heart rate • Radial pulse rate slower than apical pulse rate • Palpable peripheral pulse with stronger contractions • Evidence of decreased cardiac output, such as hypotension and light-headedness, with new-onset atrial fibrillation and a rapid ventricular rate	• Electrocardiography (ECG) shows atrial fibrillation (no clear P waves, irregularly irregular ventricular response, uneven baseline fibrillatory waves, and a wide variation in R-R intervals resulting in loss of atrial kick). Atrial fibrillation may be preceded by premature atrial contractions.	• Interventions aim to reduce the ventricular response rate to less than 100 beats/minute, establish anticoagulation, and restore and maintain a sinus rhythm. • Administer drug therapy to control the ventricular response. • If the patient is hemodynamically unstable, synchronized electrical cardioversion should be performed immediately. • A transesophageal echocardiogram may be obtained before cardioversion to rule out the presence of thrombi in the atria. • If drug therapy is used, monitor serum drug levels, and observe the patient for evidence of toxicity. • If the patient isn't on a cardiac monitor, be alert for an irregular pulse and differences in the radial and apical pulse rates. • Monitor the patient's peripheral and apical pulses; watch for evidence of decreased cardiac output and heart failure. • Tell the patient to report changes in pulse rate, dizziness, feeling faint, chest pain, and signs of heart failure, such as dyspnea and peripheral edema.
Heart failure (complication)	• Cough that produces pink, frothy sputum • Cyanosis of the lips and nail beds • Pale, cool, clammy skin • Diaphoresis • Jugular vein distention • Ascites • Pulsus alternans • Tachycardia • Hepatomegaly • Decreased pulse pressure • Third (S_3) and fourth (S_4) heart sounds • Moist, basilar crackles • Rhonchi • Expiratory wheezing • Decreased pulse oximetry • Peripheral edema • Decreased urinary output	• B-type natriuretic peptide immunoassay is elevated. • Chest X-ray shows increased pulmonary vascular markings, interstitial edema, or pleural effusions and cardiomegaly. • ECG reveals heart enlargement, ischemia, tachycardia, extrasystole, or atrial fibrillation. • Pulmonary artery pressure, pulmonary artery wedge pressure, and left ventricular end-diastolic pressure are elevated in the presence of left-sided heart failure; right atrial or central venous pressure is elevated in right-sided heart failure.	• Administer supplemental oxygen and mechanical ventilation if necessary. • Place the patient in Fowler's position. • Administer diuretics, inotropic drugs, vasodilators, angiotensin-converting enzyme inhibitors, angiotensin receptor blockers, cardiac glycosides, beta-adrenergic blockers, or electrolyte supplements. • Initiate cardiac monitoring. • Recurrent heart failure from valvular dysfunction may require surgery. • Maintain adequate cardiac output, and monitor hemodynamic stability. • Assess for deep vein thrombosis, and apply antiembolism stockings, as appropriate.

DISORDER	SIGNS AND SYMPTOMS	DIAGNOSTIC TEST RESULTS	TREATMENT AND CARE
Systemic or pulmonary embolization (complication)	◆ Dyspnea, which may be accompanied by anginal or pleuritic chest pain ◆ Tachycardia ◆ Productive cough ◆ Blood-tinged sputum ◆ Low-grade fever ◆ Pleural effusion ◆ Massive hemoptysis ◆ Chest splinting ◆ Leg edema ◆ Pleural friction rub ◆ Signs of circulatory collapse (weak, rapid pulse and hypotension) ◆ Signs of hypoxia (restlessness and anxiety) *With a large embolus* ◆ Cyanosis ◆ Syncope ◆ Jugular vein distention ◆ Right ventricular S_3 gallop ◆ Increased intensity of a pulmonic component of second heart sound ◆ Crackles	◆ Chest X-ray helps to rule out other pulmonary diseases; areas of atelectasis, elevated diaphragm and pleural effusion, prominent pulmonary artery and, occasionally, the characteristic wedge-shaped infiltrate suggesting pulmonary infarction or focal oligemia of blood vessels are apparent. ◆ Lung scan shows perfusion defects in areas beyond occluded vessels; however, it doesn't rule out microemboli. ◆ Pulmonary angiography (the most definitive test) reveals evidence of emboli. ◆ ECG may show right-axis deviation; right bundle-branch block; tall, peaked P waves; depression of ST segments and T-wave inversions (indicating right-sided heart strain); and supraventricular tachyarrhythmias in extensive pulmonary embolism. A pattern sometimes observed is S wave in lead I, Q wave in lead III, and inverted T wave in lead III. ◆ Arterial blood gas (ABG) analysis showing decreased partial pressure of arterial oxygen and partial pressure of arterial carbon dioxide are characteristic but don't always occur.	◆ Give supplemental oxygen. ◆ Check ABG levels if the patient develops worsening dyspnea. ◆ Be prepared to provide endotracheal intubation with assisted ventilation if breathing is severely compromised. ◆ Administer heparin through continuous drip. Monitor coagulation studies daily. Watch closely for nosebleed, petechiae, and other signs of abnormal bleeding; check stools for occult blood. Patients should be protected from trauma and injury; avoid I.M. injections, and maintain pressure over venipuncture sites for 5 minutes, or until bleeding stops, to reduce hematoma. ◆ After the patient is stable, encourage him to move about often and assist him with isometric and range-of-motion exercises. Check pedal pulses, temperature, and color of feet to detect venostasis. Never massage the patient's legs. ◆ Help the patient walk as soon as possible after surgery to prevent venostasis. ◆ Maintain adequate nutrition and fluid balance to promote healing. ◆ Incentive spirometry can assist in deep breathing. ◆ Warn the patient not to cross his legs; this promotes thrombus formation. ◆ To relieve anxiety, explain procedures and treatments. Encourage the patient's family to participate in his care. ◆ Most patients need treatment with an oral anticoagulant (warfarin [Coumadin]) for 3 to 6 months after a pulmonary embolism. Advise these patients to watch for signs of bleeding (bloody stools, blood in urine, and large ecchymoses), to take the prescribed medication exactly as ordered, not to change dosages without consulting their health care provider, and to avoid taking additional medications (including aspirin and vitamins). ◆ Stress the importance of follow-up laboratory tests to monitor anticoagulant therapy. ◆ Low-molecular-weight heparin may be given to prevent pulmonary embolism in high-risk patients.

Cerebral contusion

OVERVIEW

- Ecchymosis of brain tissue that results from head injury
- May occur at any age

CAUSES

- Acceleration-deceleration or coup-contrecoup injuries
- Falls
- Gunshot wounds
- Head trauma
- Motor vehicle accidents
- Stab wounds

RISK FACTORS

- Unsteady gait
- Participation in contact sports
- Anticoagulant therapy

PATHOPHYSIOLOGY

- Cerebral contusion causes brain tissue to bruise.
- Although major body systems can be affected because the brain functions as the control center, the most serious problems occur in the neurologic system.

NEUROLOGIC SYSTEM

- When injuries cause the brain to strike against bony prominences inside the skull (especially to the sphenoidal ridges), intracranial hemorrhage or hematoma can occur.
- The patient may suffer brain herniation (shifting of tissue from areas of high pressure to areas of lower pressure) as the tissue attempts to compensate for the increased pressure. This shifting, however, causes the blood supply to the shifted area to close off. (See *Disorders affecting management of cerebral contusion*, page 93.)
- Secondary effects, such as brain swelling, may accompany serious contusions, resulting in increased intracranial pressure (ICP) and herniation.

ASSESSMENT

HISTORY

- Head injury or motor vehicle accident
- Loss of consciousness
- Possible involuntary evacuation of bowel and bladder

PHYSICAL FINDINGS

- Unconscious patient who's pale and motionless, with altered vital signs
- Conscious patient who's drowsy or easily disturbed
- Scalp wound
- Headache
- Dizziness
- Vomiting
- Forgetfulness
- Hemiparesis
- Personality changes, such as restlessness or agitation

DIAGNOSTIC TEST RESULTS

- Computed tomography scan and magnetic resonance imaging show areas of injury.
- Electroencephalography and cerebral angiography help confirm diagnosis.

TREATMENT

GENERAL
- Maintenance of a patent airway
- Administration of I.V. fluids
- Minimization of environmental stimuli
- Safety measures

DIET
- Nothing by mouth until fully conscious

ACTIVITY
- Based on neurologic status
- Initially, bed rest, with head of bed raised to promote drainage
- Avoidance of contact sports

MEDICATIONS
- Oxygen, if needed
- Nonopioid analgesics
- Anticonvulsants
- Antibiotics
- Corticosteroids

SURGERY
- Craniotomy
- Suturing of scalp wounds

NURSING CONSIDERATIONS

NURSING DIAGNOSES
- Acute pain
- Anxiety
- Decreased intracranial adaptive capacity
- Disturbed sensory perception: Kinesthetic, tactile
- Impaired verbal communication
- Ineffective coping
- Risk for deficient fluid volume
- Risk for infection
- Risk for injury
- Risk for posttrauma syndrome

EXPECTED OUTCOMES
The patient will:
- express feelings of increased comfort and decreased pain
- identify measures to reduce anxiety
- maintain a stable neurologic state
- maintain optimal functioning within the limits of the kinesthetic and tactile impairment
- use language or an alternative form of communication to communicate needs
- use support systems to assist with coping
- maintain adequate fluid volume
- remain free from signs and symptoms of infection
- remain free from injury
- express feelings and fears about the traumatic event.

NURSING INTERVENTIONS
- Monitor neurologic status, especially for signs of increased ICP (See *What happens with increased ICP*, page 92.)
- Reorient the patient, as necessary.
- Give prescribed drugs (no aspirin).
- Protect from injury.
- Monitor vital signs (awaken patient every 2 hours during first 24 hours).
- Check for cerebrospinal fluid (CSF) leakage.

PATIENT TEACHING

Be sure to cover:
- injury, diagnostic testing, and treatment
- medication administration, dosage, and possible adverse effects
- need to avoid coughing, sneezing, or blowing the nose until after recovery
- observation for CSF drainage
- how the family can detect and report mental status changes
- importance of avoiding smoking and alcohol
- signs and symptoms of infection
- follow-up care with a neurologist, as indicated
- consultation with a social worker for further support and counseling, as needed.

RESOURCES
Organizations
American Academy of Neurology: *www.aan.com*
Brain Injury Society: *www.bisociety.org*
Head Injury Hotline: *www.headinjury.com*
Med Help International: *www.medhelp.org*

Selected references
Canobbio, M. *Mosby's Handbook of Patient Teaching*, 3rd ed. St. Louis: Mosby–Year Book, Inc., 2006.

Chamberlain, D.J. "The Experience of Surviving Traumatic Brain Injury," *Journal of Advanced Nursing* 54(4):407-17, May 2006.

Goldberg, L.D., and Dimeff, R.J. "Sideline Management of Sports-Related Concussions," *Sports Medicine and Arthroscopy Review* 14(4):199-205, December 2006.

(continued)

What happens with increased ICP

Intracranial pressure (ICP) is the pressure exerted within the intact skull by the intracranial volume—about 10% blood, 10% cerebrospinal fluid (CSF), and 80% brain tissue water. The rigid skull allows very little space for expansion of these substances. When ICP increases to pathologic levels, brain damage can result.

The brain compensates for increases in ICP by regulating the volumes of the three substances in the following ways:

◆ limiting blood flow to the head
◆ displacing CSF into the spinal canal
◆ increasing absorption or decreasing production of CSF—withdrawing water from brain tissue into the blood and excreting it through the kidneys.

When compensatory mechanisms become over-worked, small changes in volume lead to large changes in pressure.

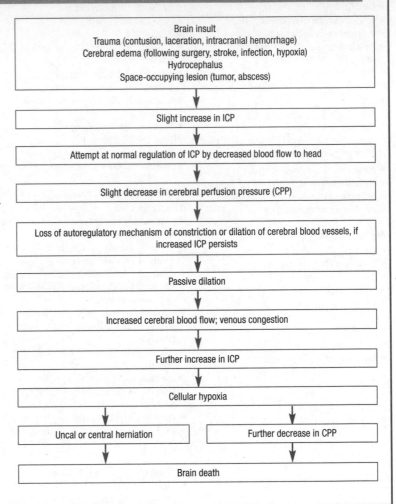

Brain insult
Trauma (contusion, laceration, intracranial hemorrhage)
Cerebral edema (following surgery, stroke, infection, hypoxia)
Hydrocephalus
Space-occupying lesion (tumor, abscess)

↓

Slight increase in ICP

↓

Attempt at normal regulation of ICP by decreased blood flow to head

↓

Slight decrease in cerebral perfusion pressure (CPP)

↓

Loss of autoregulatory mechanism of constriction or dilation of cerebral blood vessels, if increased ICP persists

↓

Passive dilation

↓

Increased cerebral blood flow; venous congestion

↓

Further increase in ICP

↓

Cellular hypoxia

↓   ↓

Uncal or central herniation   Further decrease in CPP

↓   ↓

Brain death

Disorders affecting management of cerebral contusion

This chart highlights disorders that affect the management of cerebral contusion.

DISORDER	SIGNS AND SYMPTOMS	DIAGNOSTIC TEST RESULTS	TREATMENT AND CARE
Brain herniation (complication)	*Intracerebral hemorrhage or hematoma* ♦ Nuchal rigidity ♦ Photophobia ♦ Nausea and vomiting ♦ Dizziness ♦ Seizures ♦ Decreased respiratory rate ♦ Progressive obtundation *Epidural hemorrhage or hematoma* ♦ Contralateral hemiparesis ♦ Progressively severe headache ♦ Ipsilateral pupillary dilation ♦ Signs of increased intracranial pressure (ICP) ♦ Decrease in pulse and respiratory rates ♦ Increase in systolic blood pressure *Epidural hematoma* ♦ Drowsiness and confusion ♦ Dilation of one or both pupils ♦ Hyperventilation ♦ Nuchal rigidity ♦ Bradycardia ♦ Decorticate or decerebrate posturing	♦ Computed tomography (CT) scan may reveal herniation.	♦ Check vital signs, level of consciousness, and pupil size every 15 minutes. ♦ Establish and maintain a patent airway. Intubation may be needed. ♦ Observe for cerebrospinal fluid (CSF) drainage from the patient's ears, nose, or mouth. If the patient's nose is draining CSF, wipe it—don't let him blow. If an ear is draining, cover it lightly with sterile gauze, but don't pack it. ♦ Take seizure precautions. ♦ Agitated behavior may be caused by hypoxia or increased ICP, so check for these symptoms. Speak in a calm voice, and touch the patient gently. Don't make any sudden, unexpected moves. ♦ Restrict total fluid intake to 1,200 to 1,500 ml/day to reduce fluid volume and intracellular swelling. ♦ A craniotomy may be necessary to locate and control bleeding and to aspirate blood. ♦ Epidural and subdural hematomas may be drained through burr holes in the skull. ♦ Administer I.V. mannitol, steroids, or diuretics to control decreased ICP.
Intracranial hemorrhage or hematoma (complication)	*Subacute or chronic subdural hemorrhage or hematoma* ♦ May not occur until days after the injury *Acute subdural hematoma* ♦ Loss of consciousness ♦ Weakness ♦ Paralysis	♦ CT scan may reveal a mass confirming a hematoma or hemorrhage. ♦ Skull X-ray may reveal a mass confirming a hematoma or hemorrhage. ♦ Arteriography may reveal altered blood flow in the area.	♦ Follow treatment and care for brain herniation.
Seizure (complication)	♦ Aura ♦ Loss of consciousness ♦ Dyspnea ♦ Fixed and dilated pupils ♦ Incontinence	♦ EEG slows abnormal wave patterns and the focus of the seizure activity. ♦ Magnetic resonance imaging may show pathologic changes. ♦ Brain mapping identifies seizure areas.	♦ Ensure patient safety; initiate seizure precautions. ♦ Monitor neurologic and respiratory status. ♦ Observe and document the seizure activity (body movement, respiratory pattern, duration of seizure, loss of consciousness, incontinence, and pupillary changes). ♦ Administer medications, as ordered. ♦ Monitor vital signs, intake and output, and laboratory values.

Chronic glomerulonephritis

OVERVIEW

- Slow, progressive disease that's characterized by inflammation of the glomeruli structure of the kidney, which results in sclerosis and scarring and may progress to renal failure
- Usually undetected until progressive phase begins
- By the time symptoms of proteinuria, granular tube casts, and hematuria develop, generally irreversible
- Third leading cause of end-stage renal disease in United States and leading cause internationally

CAUSES

- Focal glomerulosclerosis
- Goodpasture's syndrome
- Hemolytic uremic syndrome
- Membranoproliferative glomerulonephritis
- Membranous glomerulopathy
- Poststreptococcal glomerulonephritis
- Rapidly progressive glomerulonephritis
- Systemic lupus erythematosus

PATHOPHYSIOLOGY

- In nearly all types of glomerulonephritis, the epithelial layer of the glomerular membrane is disturbed, causing a loss of the negative charge.

RENAL SYSTEM

- Chronic glomerulonephritis progresses slowly—over a period of 20 to 30 years—leading to changes in the renal parenchyma.
- Kidney tissue atrophies, and the functional mass of nephrons decreases significantly, resulting in decreased glomerular filtration.
- The cortex of the parenchyma thins, but the calices and pelves remain normal.
- Renal biopsy of the kidney tissue in the late stages of glomerulonephritis shows hyalinization of the glomeruli, loss of tubules, and fibrosis of kidney tissue.
- The late stages of the disease produce symptoms related to uremia, which requires dialysis or renal transplantation.
- Glomerular injury causes proteinuria because of the increased permeability of the glomerular capillaries.
- Chronic glomerulonephritis eventually progresses to chronic renal failure.

CARDIOVASCULAR SYSTEM

- Hypertension results from the sclerosis of renal arterioles; severe hypertension may cause cardiac hypertrophy, leading to heart failure.
- Fluid overload may result from oliguria leading to peripheral edema and heart failure.
- Severe hyperkalemia can result in cardiac arrest and should be treated as a medical emergency.

ENDOCRINE AND METABOLIC SYSTEMS

- Renal failure leads to electrolyte, fluid, and acid-base imbalances.
- Proteinuria leads to serum protein loss.

GASTROINTESTINAL SYSTEM

- Accumulation of toxins results in nausea, vomiting, and anorexia.
- Coagulopathies increase the risk of GI bleeding.

IMMUNE AND HEMATOLOGIC SYSTEMS

- Renal failure compromises the immune system, leading to an increased risk of infection.
- Decreased erythropoiesis related to renal failure leads to anemia resulting in fatigue, malaise, and dyspnea.

INTEGUMENTARY SYSTEM

- The accumulation of waste products leads to dry skin, brittle hair, and pruritus.
- Hyperphosphatemia worsens pruritus and can cause the patient to scratch until the skin integrity is compromised.
- Coagulation abnormalities, such as prolonged clotting time, may cause ecchymoses or petechiae.
- Deposition of uremic toxins in the skin results in darkened or yellow skin tones.

MUSCULOSKELETAL SYSTEM

- Alterations in calcium and phosphorous balance lead to hypocalcemia, placing the patient at risk for pathological fractures.
- Hyperkalemia, a medical emergency, may result in muscle weakness. (See *Disorders affecting management of chronic glomerulonephritis*, page 97.)

NEUROLOGIC SYSTEM

- Nerve cells are affected by the accumulation of waste products leading to irritability, changes in mental status, peripheral neuropathies, ataxia, asterixis seizures and, if left untreated, coma.

RESPIRATORY SYSTEM

- Hypervolemia may result in fluid accumulation in the lungs leading to crackles, dyspnea, orthopnea, and pulmonary edema.
- Hyperventilation occurs as a result of metabolic acidosis.

HISTORY

- Decreased urine output
- Signs and symptoms of uremia: weakness, fatigue, weight loss, anorexia, pruritus, changes in sleep habits, and seizures
- History of infection

PHYSICAL FINDINGS

- Irritability, drowsiness, or confusion
- Altered level of consciousness
- Dry, pruritic skin
- Hematuria, petechiae, and ecchymosis
- Proteinuria
- In children, encephalopathy with seizures and local neurologic deficits
- In elderly patients, vague, nonspecific symptoms, such as nausea, fatigue, and arthralgia
- Altered urinary elimination (oliguria)
- Edema
- Tachycardia
- Bibasilar crackles
- Uremic breath odor
- Hypertension
- Anorexia, nausea, and vomiting

DIAGNOSTIC TEST RESULTS

- Urinalysis commonly reveals proteinuria; red blood cells and casts may be in the urine, indicating chronic renal disease processes.
- Creatinine clearance is reduced.
- Blood studies reveal elevated blood urea nitrogen and serum creatinine levels, low hemoglobin and hematocrit levels, platelet abnormalities, metabolic acidosis, and mild hypocalcemia, hyperphosphatemia, and hyperkalemia.
- Electrocardiography (ECG) may show arrhythmias due to electrolyte imbalances.

    WARNING *Hyperkalemia is a medical emergency. ECG changes consistent with hyperkalemia include a widening QRS segment, disappearing P waves, and tall, peaked T waves.*

- X-ray, I.V. urography, ultrasonography, or computed tomography reveals kidneys that are smaller than normal.
- Renal biopsy performed in the early stages (when proteinuria and hematuria are present) shows an increase in the number and types of cells infiltrating the glomerular tissue, deposition of immune complexes, and vessel sclerosis.

GENERAL

- Treatment of the primary disease
- Correction of electrolyte imbalance
- Blood transfusions
- Dialysis
- Plasmapheresis

DIET

- Fluid restriction
- Restriction of potassium, sodium, and phosphorus
- Adequate caloric intake and essential amino acids
- Possible restriction of protein

ACTIVITY

- As tolerated

MEDICATIONS

- Angiotensin-converting enzyme inhibitors
- Angiotensin II receptor blockers
- Beta-adrenergic blockers
- Calcium channel blockers
- Antibiotics
- Anticoagulants
- Diuretics
- Vasodilators
- Corticosteroids

SURGERY

- Kidney transplantation
- Dialysis access implantation

NURSING DIAGNOSES

- Acute pain
- Decreased cardiac output
- Excess fluid volume
- Fatigue
- Imbalanced nutrition: Less than body requirements
- Impaired physical mobility
- Ineffective health maintenance
- Ineffective role performance
- Risk for infection
- Risk for injury

EXPECTED OUTCOMES

The patient will:

- report increased comfort and decreased pain
- maintain hemodynamic stability
- maintain adequate fluid balance
- verbalize importance of balancing activity with adequate rest periods
- verbalize appropriate food choices
- maintain joint mobility and muscle strength
- identify risk factors that exacerbate the condition and modify lifestyle accordingly
- resume regular roles and responsibilities to the fullest extent possible
- remain free from signs or symptoms of infection
- remain free from injury.

NURSING INTERVENTIONS

- Monitor vital signs, intake and output, daily weight, and laboratory studies.
- Provide appropriate skin care and oral hygiene.
- Encourage the patient to express his feelings about the disorder, and provide emotional support.
- Give prescribed drugs.
- Assist the patient in locating a facility that will provide chronic hemodialysis or peritoneal dialysis training, if chronic renal failure develops.
- Observe for signs of renal failure.

(continued)

Be sure to cover:
◆ disorder, diagnostic testing, and treatment
◆ medication administration, dosage, and possible adverse effects
◆ how to assess for signs of increasing renal failure
◆ reporting signs of infection
◆ recording daily weight and reporting increase of 2 or more pounds in 1 week.

RESOURCES
Organizations
American Academy of Pediatrics: *www.aap.org*
American Association of Kidney Patients: *www.aakp.org*
Harvard University Consumer Health Information: *www.intelihealth.com*
National Institute of Diabetes & Digestive & Kidney Diseases: *www.niddk.nih.gov*

Selected references
Inaguma,. D., et al. "Effect of an Educational Program on the Predialysis Period for Patients with Chronic Renal Failure," *Clinical and Experimental Nephrology* 10(4):274-78, December 2006.

Javaid, B., and Quigg, R.J. "Treatment for Glomerulonephritis: Will We Ever Have Options Other than Steroids and Cytotoxics?" *Kidney International* 67(5):1692-703, May 2005.

Mitch, W., and Klahr, S. *Handbook of Nutrition & the Kidney,* 5th ed. Philadelphia: Lippincott Williams & Wilkins, 2005.

Disorders affecting management of chronic glomerulonephritis

This chart highlights disorders that affect the management of chronic glomerulonephritis.

DISORDER	SIGNS AND SYMPTOMS	DIAGNOSTIC TEST RESULTS	TREATMENT AND CARE
Heart failure (complication)	◆ Dyspnea ◆ Cyanosis of the lips and nail beds ◆ Pale, cool, clammy skin ◆ Diaphoresis ◆ Jugular vein distention ◆ Ascites ◆ Pulsus alternans ◆ Tachycardia ◆ Hepatomegaly ◆ Decreased pulse pressure ◆ Third (S_3) and fourth (S_4) heart sounds ◆ Moist, basilar crackles ◆ Rhonchi ◆ Expiratory wheezing ◆ Decreased pulse oximetry ◆ Peripheral edema ◆ Decreased urinary output	◆ B-type natriuretic peptide immunoassay is elevated. ◆ Chest X-ray shows increased pulmonary vascular markings, interstitial edema, or pleural effusions and cardiomegaly. ◆ Electrocardiogram (ECG) reveals heart enlargement or ischemia, tachycardia, extrasystole, or atrial fibrillation. ◆ Pulmonary artery pressure, pulmonary artery wedge pressure, and left ventricular end-diastolic pressure are elevated in the presence of left-sided heart failure; right atrial or central venous pressure is elevated in right-sided heart failure.	◆ Administer supplemental oxygen and mechanical ventilation, if needed. ◆ Place the patient in Fowler's position. ◆ Administer diuretics, inotropic drugs, vasodilators, angiotensin-converting enzyme inhibitors, angiotensin receptor blockers, cardiac glycosides, beta-adrenergic blockers, and electrolyte supplements. ◆ Initiate cardiac monitoring. ◆ Recurrent heart failure from valvular dysfunction may require surgery. ◆ A ventricular assist device may be needed. ◆ Maintain adequate cardiac output, and monitor hemodynamic stability. ◆ Assess for deep vein thrombosis, and apply antiembolism stockings, as appropriate.
Hyperkalemia (complication)	◆ Nausea ◆ Muscle weakness ◆ Paresthesia ◆ Diarrhea ◆ Abdominal cramps ◆ Irritability ◆ Hypotension ◆ Irregular heart rate ◆ Possible cardiac arrhythmias	◆ Serum potassium level is greater than 5 mEq/L. ◆ Arterial pH is decreased. ◆ ECG shows tall, peaked T waves, and possibly flattened P waves, prolonged PR intervals, widened QRS complexes, and depressed ST segments.	◆ Determine and remove the underlying cause, if possible. ◆ Administer a rapid infusion of 10% calcium gluconate to decrease myocardial irritability. ◆ Administer insulin and 10% to 50% glucose I.V. for severe hyperkalemia. ◆ Administer sodium polystyrene sulfonate orally or rectally using an enema for mild hyperkalemia. ◆ Initiate dialysis as a final treatment option, or if the hyperkalemia is related to renal failure. ◆ Discontinue medications that may cause hyperkalemia. ◆ Monitor cardiac rhythm and response to treatment. ◆ Implement a potassium-restricted diet.
Pericarditis (complication)	◆ Pericardial friction rub ◆ Sharp, sudden pain, usually starting over the sternum and radiating to the neck, shoulders, back, and arms ◆ Shallow, rapid respirations ◆ Mild fever ◆ Dyspnea, orthopnea, and tachycardia ◆ Muffled and distant heart sounds ◆ Pallor, clammy skin ◆ Hypotension, pulsus paradoxus ◆ Jugular vein distention	◆ ECG may reveal diffuse ST-segment elevation, downsloping PR segments and upright T waves, possibly diminished QRS complexes when pericardial effusion exists, and arrhythmias. ◆ Erythrocyte sedimentation rate is elevated. ◆ Echocardiogram may show an echo-free space between the ventricular wall and the pericardium and reduced pumping action of the heart. ◆ Chest X-ray may be normal with acute pericarditis. The cardiac silhouette may be enlarged with a water bottle shape caused by fluid accumulation, if pleural effusion is present.	◆ Maintain bed rest as long as fever and pain persist to reduce metabolic needs. ◆ Administer medications, such as nonsteroidal anti-inflammatory drugs (NSAIDs), to relieve pain and reduce inflammation; give corticosteroids if NSAIDs are ineffective. ◆ Prepare for pericardiocentesis or pericardectomy. ◆ Place the patient in an upright position to relieve dyspnea and chest pain. ◆ Administer supplemental oxygen, as indicated. ◆ Monitor vital signs and cardiovascular status for signs of cardiac compression or cardiac tamponade.

Chronic obstructive pulmonary disease

OVERVIEW

- Results from emphysema, chronic bronchitis, asthma, or any combination of these disorders
- Most common chronic lung disease, affecting about 17 million Americans, with rising prevalence
- Affects more males than females and more Whites than Blacks
- Tends to progressively worsen

CAUSES

- Cigarette smoking
- Genetic deficiency of alpha$_1$-antitrypsin
- Environmental pollution
- Organic or inorganic dusts and noxious gas exposure
- Possible genetic predisposition

PATHOPHYSIOLOGY

- There's usually more than one underlying respiratory condition coexisting; most commonly, bronchitis and emphysema occur together.

RESPIRATORY SYSTEM

- Smoking impairs ciliary action and macrophage functions, causing airway inflammation, increased mucus production, destruction of alveolar septae, and peribronchiolar fibrosis. Early inflammatory changes may reverse if the patient stops smoking before lung destruction becomes extensive.
- Mucus plugs and narrowed airways cause air trappings, as in asthma, chronic bronchitis, and emphysema.
- Alveoli hyperinflate on expiration.
- On inspiration, airways enlarge, allowing air to pass beyond the obstruction; on expiration, airways narrow and gas flow is prevented.

CARDIOVASCULAR SYSTEM

- Chronic hypoxemia and acidosis may result in constriction of the pulmonary vasculature, which eventually leads to increased pulmonary pressure and ventricular hypertrophy or cor pulmonale.

ASSESSMENT

HISTORY

- Smoking
- Shortness of breath
- Chronic cough
- Anorexia and weight loss
- Malaise
- Frequent respiratory tract infections

PHYSICAL FINDINGS

- Barrel chest
- Pursed-lip breathing
- Use of accessory muscles
- Cyanosis
- Productive cough
- Clubbed fingers and toes
- Tachypnea
- Decreased tactile fremitus
- Decreased chest expansion
- Hyperresonance
- Decreased breath sounds
- Crackles
- Inspiratory wheeze
- Prolonged expiratory phase with grunting respirations
- Distant heart sounds
- Severe respiratory failure (see *Disorders affecting management of COPD,* pages 100 and 101)

DIAGNOSTIC TEST RESULTS

- Arterial blood gas (ABG) analysis reveals decreased partial pressure of arterial oxygen and normal or increased partial pressure of arterial carbon dioxide.
- X-ray may show advanced emphysema, flattened diaphragm, reduced vascular markings at lung periphery, vertical heart, enlarged anteroposterior chest diameter, and large retrosternal airspace. During an asthma attack, there will be evidence of hyperinflation and air trapping. (See *Air trapping in COPD.*) In chronic bronchitis, there will be evidence of hyperinflation and increased bronchovascular markings.
- Pulmonary function studies show increased residual volume, total lung capacity, and compliance; and decreased vital capacity, diffusing capacity, and expiratory volumes.

UP CLOSE

Air trapping in COPD

In chronic obstructive pulmonary disease (COPD), mucus plugs and narrowed airways trap air (also called *ball-valving*). During inspiration, the airways enlarge and gas enters; on expiration, the airways narrow, and air can't escape. This process commonly occurs in asthma and chronic bronchitis.

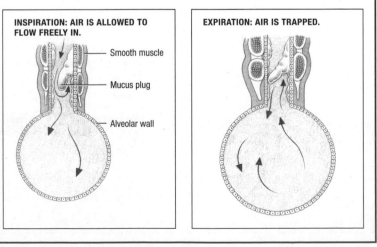

INSPIRATION: AIR IS ALLOWED TO FLOW FREELY IN.
— Smooth muscle
— Mucus plug
— Alveolar wall

EXPIRATION: AIR IS TRAPPED.

During an asthma attack, the forced expiratory volume will be decreased. In chronic bronchitis, the forced expiratory volume will be decreased, and the diffusing capacity will be normal.

- Electrocardiography may show arrhythmias consistent with hypoxemia.

TREATMENT

GENERAL

- Smoking cessation
- Chest physiotherapy
- Possible transtracheal catheterization
- Home oxygen therapy
- Mechanical ventilation (in acute exacerbations)
- Avoidance of air pollutants
- Ultrasonic or mechanical nebulizer treatments
- Chest tube insertion for pneumothorax

DIET

- Adequate hydration
- High-protein, high-calorie

ACTIVITY

- As tolerated

MEDICATIONS

- Bronchodilators
- Anticholinergics
- Mucolytics
- Corticosteroids
- Antibiotics
- Oxygen

SURGERY

- Tracheostomy, if ventilator dependent

NURSING CONSIDERATIONS

NURSING DIAGNOSES

- Activity intolerance
- Anxiety
- Fatigue
- Fear
- Impaired gas exchange
- Ineffective airway clearance
- Ineffective breathing pattern
- Interrupted family processes
- Risk for infection

EXPECTED OUTCOMES

The patient will:

- perform activities of daily living within the limitations of the disease
- identify strategies to reduce anxiety
- verbalize the importance of balancing activity with adequate rest periods
- discuss fears and concerns
- maintain adequate ventilation and oxygenation
- maintain a patent airway
- maintain an effective breathing pattern
- along with family members, identify and contact available support systems, as needed
- remain free from signs or symptoms of infection.

NURSING INTERVENTIONS

- Administer oxygen therapy, and monitor ABG results.
- Monitor vital signs, pulse oximetry, intake and output, and daily weight.
- Give prescribed drugs.
- Provide supportive care.
- Help the patient adjust to lifestyle changes necessitated by a chronic illness.
- Encourage the patient to express his fears and concerns.
- Perform chest physiotherapy.
- Provide a high-calorie, protein-rich diet in small, frequent meals.
- Encourage daily activity and diversional activities.
- Provide frequent rest periods.
- Observe for complications and deterioration of respiratory status.

PATIENT TEACHING

Be sure to cover:

- disorder, diagnostic testing, and treatment
- medication administration, dosage, and possible adverse effects
- when to notify the practitioner
- energy conservation techniques
- importance of receiving an influenza vaccine yearly
- avoidance of smoking and areas where smoking is permitted
- avoidance of crowds and people with known infections
- home oxygen therapy, if indicated
- coughing and deep breathing exercises
- need for a high-calorie, protein-rich diet
- adequate oral fluid intake
- avoidance of respiratory irritants
- signs and symptoms of respiratory failure and complications
- smoking cessation programs.

WARNING *Urge the patient to notify the practitioner if he experiences a sudden onset of worsening dyspnea or sharp pleuritic chest pain exacerbated by chest movement, breathing, or coughing. This could be signs of a pneumothorax.*

RESOURCES

Organizations

National Emphysema Foundation: *www.emphysemafoundation.org*
National Institute of Drug Abuse: *www.nida.nih.gov*
Tobacco Information and Prevention Source: *www.cdc.gov/tobacco*

Selected references

Bauldoff, G., and Diaz, P. "Improving Outcomes for COPD Patients," *The Nurse Practitioner* 31(8):26-43, August 2006.

Nettina, S.M. *Lippincott Manual of Nursing Practice,* 8th ed. Philadelphia: Lippincott Williams & Wilkins, 2006.

Pinkowish, M. "Critical Care: Differences in Men and Women with Oxygen Dependent COPD," *AJN* 106(12):72cc-72cc, December 2006.

Sandland, C.J., et al. "A Profile of Daily Activity in Chronic Obstructive Pulmonary Disease," *Journal of Cardiopulmonary Rehabilitation* 25(3):181-83, May-June 2005.

Tiukinhoy, S., and Rochester, C. "Impact of Pulmonary Rehabilitation on Psychosocial Morbidity in Patients with Severe Chronic Obstructive Pulmonary Disease," *Journal of Cardiopulmonary Rehabilitation* 26(4):246, July-August 2006.

(continued)

Disorders affecting management of COPD

This chart highlights disorders that affect the management of chronic obstructive pulmonary disease (COPD).

DISORDER	SIGNS AND SYMPTOMS	DIAGNOSTIC TEST RESULTS	TREATMENT AND CARE
Acute respiratory failure (complication)	◆ Increased respiratory rate ◆ Cyanosis ◆ Crackles ◆ Rhonchi ◆ Wheezing ◆ Diminished breath sounds ◆ Restlessness ◆ Confusion ◆ Loss of concentration ◆ Irritability ◆ Coma ◆ Tachycardia ◆ Increased cardiac output ◆ Increased blood pressure ◆ Cardiac arrhythmias	◆ Arterial blood gas (ABG) analysis shows deteriorating values and a pH below 7.35. ◆ Chest X-rays identify a pulmonary disease or condition. ◆ Electrocardiogram (ECG) may show ventricular arrhythmias or right ventricular hypertrophy. ◆ Pulse oximetry reveals decreasing arterial oxygen saturation. ◆ White blood cell (WBC) count detects underlying infection.	◆ Monitor the effects of oxygen therapy. ◆ Maintain a patent airway; prepare for endotracheal intubation, if indicated. ◆ For the intubated patient, suction, as needed, after hyperoxygenation. Observe for change in quantity, consistency, and color of sputum. ◆ Observe closely for respiratory arrest. ◆ Auscultate for chest sounds. ◆ Monitor ABG levels, and report changes immediately. ◆ Monitor serum electrolyte levels and correct imbalances. ◆ Monitor fluid balance by recording input and output or daily weight. ◆ Check the cardiac monitor for arrhythmias. ◆ Administer antibiotics, bronchodilators, corticosteroids, positive inotropic agents, vasopressors, or diuretics.
Cor pulmonale (complication)	◆ Progressive dyspnea worsening on exertion ◆ Tachypnea ◆ Orthopnea ◆ Edema ◆ Weakness ◆ Dependent edema ◆ Distended neck veins ◆ Enlarged, tender liver ◆ Tachycardia ◆ Hypotension ◆ Weak pulse	◆ Pulmonary artery pressure (PAP) shows increased right ventricular pressures. ◆ Echocardiography or angiography indicates right ventricular enlargement. ◆ Chest X-ray suggests right ventricular enlargement. ◆ ABG analysis shows a partial pressure of arterial oxygen of less than 70 mm Hg. ◆ ECG may show various arrhythmias. ◆ Pulmonary function tests are consistent with the underlying disorder.	◆ Provide meticulous respiratory care, including oxygen therapy, suctioning as needed, and deep-breathing and coughing exercises. ◆ Monitor ABG values and monitor for signs of respiratory failure (change in pulse rate; deep, labored respirations; and increased fatigue on exertion). ◆ Monitor fluid status carefully; limit fluid intake to 1,000 to 2,000 ml/day, and provide a low-sodium diet. ◆ Monitor serum potassium levels if the patient is receiving diuretics; low serum potassium levels can potentiate arrhythmias. ◆ Encourage bed rest. ◆ Administer digoxin, diazoxide, nitroprusside, hydralazine, angiotensin-converting enzyme inhibitors, calcium channel blockers, prostaglandins, heparin, or corticosteroids.
Heart failure (complication)	*Left-sided heart failure* ◆ Dyspnea ◆ Orthopnea ◆ Paroxysmal nocturnal dyspnea ◆ Fatigue ◆ Nonproductive cough ◆ Crackles ◆ Hemoptysis ◆ Tachycardia ◆ Third (S_3) and fourth (S_4) heart sounds ◆ Cool, pale skin ◆ Restlessness and confusion	◆ Chest X-rays may show pulmonary vascular markings, interstitial edema, or pleural effusion and cardiomegaly. ◆ ECG may indicate hypertrophy, ischemic changes, or infarction, and may reveal tachycardia and extrasystoles. ◆ Liver function tests are abnormal; blood urea nitrogen (BUN) and creatinine levels are elevated. ◆ Prothrombin time is prolonged. ◆ B-natriuretic peptide assay may be elevated. ◆ Echocardiography may reveal left ventricular hypertrophy, dilation, and abnormal contractility. ◆ PAP, pulmonary artery wedge pressure, and left ventricular end-diastolic pressure are elevated in the presence of left-sided heart failure; right atrial or central venous pressure is elevated in right-sided heart failure.	◆ Place patient in Fowler's position, and give supplemental oxygen. ◆ Weigh the patient daily. ◆ Check for peripheral edema. ◆ Administer diuretics, beta-adrenergic blockers, digoxin, inotropics (dobutamine or milrinone), nesiritide, nitrates, or morphine. ◆ Monitor intake and output, vital signs, and mental status. ◆ Auscultate for S_3 and crackles or rhonchi. ◆ Prepare the patient for coronary artery bypass surgery, angioplasty, or heart transplantation. ◆ Monitor BUN; creatinine; and serum potassium, sodium, chloride, and magnesium levels.

DISORDER	SIGNS AND SYMPTOMS	DIAGNOSTIC TEST RESULTS	TREATMENT AND CARE
Heart failure (complication) *(continued)*	*Right-sided heart failure* ◆ Jugular vein distention ◆ Positive hepatojugular reflex ◆ Right upper quadrant pain ◆ Anorexia ◆ Nausea ◆ Nocturia ◆ Weight gain ◆ Edema ◆ Ascites or anasarca	◆ Radionuclide ventriculography may reveal ejection fraction of less than 40% in diastolic dysfunction.	◆ Institute continuous cardiac monitoring to identify and treat arrhythmias promptly. ◆ Encourage lifestyle modifications or changes.
Hypertension (complication)	◆ Usually asymptomatic ◆ Elevated blood pressure readings on at least two consecutive occasions ◆ Occipital headache ◆ Epistaxis ◆ Bruits ◆ Dizziness ◆ Confusion ◆ Fatigue ◆ Blurry vision ◆ Nocturia ◆ Edema	◆ Serial blood pressure measurements reveal elevations of 140/90 mm Hg or greater on two or more separate occasions. ◆ Urinalysis may show protein, casts, red blood cells, or WBCs. ◆ BUN and serum creatinine levels are elevated, suggesting renal disease. ◆ Complete blood count may reveal polycythemia or anemia. ◆ Excretory urography may reveal renal atrophy. ◆ ECG may show left ventricular hypertrophy or ischemia. ◆ Chest X-rays may show cardiomegaly. ◆ Echocardiography may reveal left ventricular hypertrophy.	◆ Monitor the patient's blood pressure, his response to antihypertensive medications, and laboratory studies. ◆ Encourage lifestyle modifications or changes (such as a reduced-sodium diet). ◆ Monitor for complications of hypertension such as stroke, myocardial infarction, and renal disease. ◆ Administer thiazide diuretics, angiotensin-converting enzyme inhibitors, angiotensin receptor blockers, beta-adrenergic blockers, or calcium channel blockers.
Respiratory acidosis (complication)	◆ Restlessness ◆ Confusion ◆ Apprehension ◆ Somnolence ◆ Fine or flapping tremor ◆ Coma ◆ Headaches ◆ Dyspnea ◆ Tachypnea ◆ Papilledema ◆ Depressed reflexes ◆ Hypoxemia ◆ Tachycardia ◆ Hypertension or hypotension ◆ Atrial and ventricular arrhythmias	◆ ABG analysis reveals a partial pressure of arterial carbon dioxide greater than 45 mm Hg, a pH less than 7.35, normal HCO_3^- level in the acute stage, and elevated HCO_3^- in the chronic stage. ◆ Chest X-ray may reveal the pulmonary cause (for example, heart failure, pneumonia, COPD, or pneumothorax). ◆ Potassium level is greater than 5 mEq/L. ◆ Serum chloride is low.	◆ Be alert for critical changes in the patient's respiratory, central nervous system, and cardiovascular functions. Report changes in function, ABG levels, and electrolyte status immediately. ◆ Maintain adequate hydration. ◆ Maintain a patent airway, and provide mechanical ventilation if necessary. Perform tracheal suction regularly and chest physiotherapy, if ordered. Continuously monitor ventilator settings and respiratory status. ◆ Monitor patients with COPD and chronic carbon dioxide retention for signs of acidosis. ◆ Administer oxygen at low flow rates, as indicated. ◆ Monitor patients who receive opioids and sedatives carefully.

Chronic renal failure

OVERVIEW

- Progressive loss of renal function
- Usually asymptomatic until more than 75% of glomerular filtration is lost and worsening as renal function declines
- Fatal unless treated; to sustain life, may require maintenance dialysis or kidney transplantation
- Affects about 2 in 100,000 people
- May occur at any age but more common in adults
- Affects more males than females and more Blacks than Whites

CAUSES

- Chronic glomerular disease
- Chronic infections such as chronic pyelonephritis
- Collagen diseases such as systemic lupus erythematosus
- Congenital anomalies such as polycystic kidney disease
- Endocrine disease
- Nephrotoxic agents
- Obstructive processes such as calculi
- Vascular diseases

PATHOPHYSIOLOGY

- Nephron destruction eventually causes irreversible renal damage.
- Disease may progress through the following stages: reduced renal reserve, renal insufficiency, renal failure, and end-stage renal disease.

RENAL SYSTEM

- Oliguria occurs as a result of decreased glomerular filtration rate (GFR).
- Hyperkalemia occurs as a result of decreased GFR and metabolic acidosis.
- Hyperphosphatemia and hypocalcemia occur because the kidney can't excrete phosphorus.

CARDIOVASCULAR SYSTEM

- Hypertension and edema occur with fluid accumulation and hypervolemia.
- Fluid overload may cause pulmonary and peripheral edema, possibly leading to heart failure because of how these conditions increase the heart's workload. (See *Disorders affecting management of chronic renal failure*, page 105.)
- Acute pulmonary edema and hypertensive crisis may result from nephron loss and decreased kidney size, causing decreased blood flow to the kidneys.
- Arrhythmias and cardiac arrest may result from hyperkalemia.

ENDOCRINE AND METABOLIC SYSTEMS

- Metabolic acidosis occurs because the kidney can't excrete hydrogen ions and reabsorb sodium and bicarbonate.

GASTROINTESTINAL SYSTEM

- Nausea, vomiting, and anorexia occur with uremia.
- GI bleeding may occur with coagulation abnormalities and uremic gastric irritation.

IMMUNE AND HEMATOLOGIC SYSTEMS

- Anemia occurs because of decreased erythropoiesis, glomerular filtration of erythrocytes, or bleeding associated with platelet dysfunction.
- Infection and sepsis may occur because of decreased white blood cell–mediated immunity.
- A hypercoagulable state results from anticoagulant abnormalities, which leads to bleeding and clotting difficulties.

INTEGUMENTARY SYSTEM

- Accumulation of uremic toxins leads to dryness, pruritus, pallor, purpura, and (rarely) the deposition of the uremic toxins on the skin (uremic frost).

MUSCULOSKELETAL SYSTEM

- Muscle weakness may result from hyperkalemia.
- Pathological bone fractures may be caused by prolonged hypocalcemia.

NEUROLOGIC SYSTEM

- Altered mental status and peripheral neuropathies are related to the effects of uremic toxins on the highly sensitive nerve cells.
- Headache, drowsiness, irritability, and seizures result from central nervous system involvement and, without treatment, may progress to coma.

RESPIRATORY SYSTEM

- Tachypnea and labored breathing result from anemia, causing tissue hypoxia. Respiratory rate and effort also increase to compensate for metabolic acidosis.
- Fluid overload may lead to pulmonary congestion, impaired gas exchange, and ineffective breathing.

HISTORY

- Predisposing factors
- Dry mouth
- Fatigue
- Nausea
- Hiccups
- Muscle cramps
- Fasciculations, twitching
- Infertility, decreased libido
- Amenorrhea
- Impotence
- Pathologic fractures

PHYSICAL FINDINGS

- Decreased urine output
- Hypotension or hypertension
- Altered level of consciousness
- Peripheral edema
- Cardiac arrhythmias
- Bibasilar crackles
- Pleural friction rub
- Gum ulceration and bleeding
- Uremic fetor
- Abdominal pain on palpation
- Poor skin turgor
- Pale, yellowish bronze skin color
- Thin, brittle fingernails and dry, brittle hair
- Growth retardation (in children)

DIAGNOSTIC TEST RESULTS

- Blood urea nitrogen, serum creatinine, sodium, and potassium levels are elevated.
- Arterial blood gas values show decreased arterial pH and bicarbonate levels and evidence of metabolic acidosis.
- Hematocrit and hemoglobin level are low; red blood cell (RBC) survival time is decreased.
- Mild thrombocytopenia and platelet defects appear.
- Aldosterone secretion is increased.
- Blood glucose may show hyperglycemia.
- Blood chemistry may show elevated triglycerides.
- High-density lipoprotein levels are decreased.
- Urine specific gravity is fixed at 1.010.
- Urinalysis shows proteinuria, glycosuria, and urinary RBCs, leukocytes, casts, and crystals.
- Kidney-ureter-bladder radiography, excretory urography, nephrotomography, renal scan, and renal arteriography show reduced kidney size.
- Renal biopsy allows histologic identification of the underlying pathology.
- Electroencephalography shows changes suggesting metabolic encephalopathy.

GENERAL

- Hemodialysis or peritoneal dialysis

DIET

- Low-protein (with peritoneal dialysis, high protein), high-calorie, low-sodium, low-phosphorus, and low-potassium
- Fluid restriction

ACTIVITY

- As tolerated
- Rest periods when fatigued

MEDICATIONS

- Loop diuretics
- Cardiac glycosides
- Antihypertensives
- Antiemetics
- Iron and folate supplements
- Erythropoietin
- Antipruritics
- Supplementary vitamins and essential amino acids

SURGERY

- Creation of vascular access for dialysis
- Possible kidney transplantation

(continued)

NURSING CONSIDERATIONS

NURSING DIAGNOSES

- Acute pain
- Decreased cardiac output
- Disabled family coping
- Excess fluid volume
- Imbalanced nutrition: Less than body requirements
- Impaired gas exchange
- Impaired oral mucous membrane
- Impaired urinary elimination
- Ineffective coping
- Ineffective sexuality patterns
- Ineffective tissue perfusion: Renal
- Interrupted family processes
- Powerlessness
- Risk for infection
- Risk for injury

EXPECTED OUTCOMES

The patient (or family) will:

- report increased comfort and decreased pain
- maintain hemodynamic stability
- demonstrate adaptive coping behaviors
- remain free from fluid overload
- verbalize appropriate food choices according to the prescribed diet
- maintain adequate ventilation and oxygenation
- maintain intact oral mucous membranes
- demonstrate the ability to manage urinary elimination problems
- use support resources and exhibit adaptive coping behaviors
- resume sexual activity to the fullest extent possible
- remain free from fluid overload
- verbalize the effect the patient's condition has on the family unit
- verbalize feelings of control over condition and own well-being
- remain free from signs or symptoms of infection
- remain free from injury.

NURSING INTERVENTIONS

- Give prescribed drugs.
- Perform meticulous skin care.
- Encourage the patient to express feelings.
- Provide emotional support.
- Monitor renal function studies, vital signs, intake and output, and daily weight.
- Observe for signs and symptoms of fluid overload and bleeding.
- Assess dialysis access site for thrill and bruit and signs of infection.

PATIENT TEACHING

Be sure to cover:

- disorder, diagnostic testing, and treatment
- dietary changes
- fluid restrictions
- dialysis needs and site care, as appropriate
- importance of wearing or carrying medical identification
- follow-up care
- availability of resource and support services.

RESOURCES

Organizations

American Association of Kidney Patients: *www.aakp.org*
National Institute of Diabetes & Digestive & Kidney Diseases: *www.niddk.nih.gov*
National Kidney Foundation: *www.kidney.org*

Selected references.

Hamilton, R., and Hawley, S. "Quality of Life Outcomes Related to Anemia Management of Patients with Chronic Renal Failure," *Clinical Nurse Specialist* 20(3):139-43, May-June 2006.

Inaguma, D., et al. "Effect of an Educational Program on the Predialysis Period for Patients with Chronic Renal Failure," *Clinical and Experimental Nephrology* 10(4):274-78, December 2006.

Lederer, E., and Ouseph, R. "Chronic Kidney Disease," *American Journal of Kidney Diseases* 49(1):162-71, January 2007.

Lim, W.H., et al. "Renal Transplantation Reverses Functional Deficiencies in Circulating Dendritic Cell Subsets in Chronic Renal Failure Patients," *Transplantation* 81(2):160-68, January 2006.

Disorders affecting management of chronic renal failure

This chart highlights disorders that affect the management of chronic renal failure.

DISORDER	SIGNS AND SYMPTOMS	DIAGNOSTIC TEST RESULTS	TREATMENT AND CARE
Anemia (complication)	◆ Possibly asymptomatic early; signs and symptoms developing as anemia becomes more severe ◆ Dyspnea on exertion ◆ Fatigue ◆ Listlessness, inability to concentrate ◆ Pallor, irritability ◆ Tachycardia ◆ Brittle, thinning nails	◆ Total iron binding capacity is elevated and serum iron levels are decreased. ◆ Bone marrow aspiration reveals reduced iron stores and reduced production of red blood cell (RBC) precursors. ◆ Complete blood count reveals decreased hemoglobin and hematocrit and low mean corpuscular hemoglobin. ◆ RBC indices reveal decreased cells that are microcytic and hypochromic.	◆ Assess for decreased perfusion to vital organs, including heart and lungs; monitor for dyspnea, chest pain, and dizziness. ◆ Administer oxygen therapy to prevent hypoxemia. ◆ Monitor vital signs for changes. ◆ Administer iron replacement therapy. ◆ Administer blood products if anemia is severe. ◆ Allow for frequent rest periods. ◆ Monitor laboratory studies.
Hyperkalemia (complication)	◆ Nausea ◆ Muscle weakness ◆ Paresthesia ◆ Diarrhea ◆ Abdominal cramps ◆ Irritability ◆ Hypotension ◆ Irregular heart rate ◆ Possible cardiac arrhythmias	◆ Serum potassium level is greater than 5 mEq/L. ◆ Arterial pH is decreased. ◆ Electrocardiogram (ECG) shows tall peaked T waves, possibly flattened P waves, prolonged PR intervals, widened QRS complexes, and depressed ST segments.	◆ Administer a rapid infusion of 10% calcium gluconate to decrease myocardial irritability. ◆ Administer insulin and 10% to 50% glucose I.V. for severe hyperkalemia. ◆ Administer sodium polystyrene sulfate orally or rectally using an enema for mild hyperkalemia. ◆ Initiate dialysis as a final treatment option. ◆ Discontinue medications or I.V. fluids that may contribute to hyperkalemia. ◆ Monitor cardiac rhythm and potassium levels for response to treatment. ◆ Implement a potassium-restricted diet.
Pulmonary edema (complication)	◆ Restlessness and anxiety ◆ Rapid, labored breathing ◆ Intense, productive cough ◆ Frothy, blood-tinged sputum ◆ Mental status changes ◆ Jugular vein distention ◆ Wheezing ◆ Crackles ◆ Third heart sound (S_3) ◆ Tachycardia ◆ Hypotension ◆ Thready pulse ◆ Peripheral edema	◆ Chest X-ray shows diffuse haziness of the lung fields, cardiomegaly, and pleural effusion. ◆ Arterial blood gas (ABG) analysis shows hypoxemia, hypercapnia, or acidosis. ◆ Pulse oximetry may indicate decreased oxygenation of the blood. ◆ Hemodynamic readings may reveal increased pulmonary artery wedge pressures. ◆ ECG may show valvular disease and left ventricular hypokinesis or akinesis.	◆ Administer oxygen therapy, and be prepared to assist with endotracheal intubation and mechanical ventilation, if necessary. ◆ Closely monitor for changes in the patient's respiratory status. ◆ Institute energy conserving strategies. ◆ Implement fluid and sodium restriction. ◆ Administer diuretics, antiarrhythmics, preload and afterload reducing agents, bronchodilators, and vasopressors. ◆ Measure cardiac output, pulmonary artery pressures, and central venous pressure. ◆ Obtain daily weight. ◆ Monitor vital signs, pulse oximetry, and ABG values.

Cirrhosis

◆ Diffuse destruction and fibrotic regeneration of hepatic cells resulting in hepatic dysfunction
◆ Several types: Laënnec's; postnecrotic; biliary; idiopathic; Budd-Chiari syndrome (see *What happens in portal hypertension*), which involves epigastric pain, liver enlargement, and ascites caused by hepatic vein obstruction; and, rarely, cardiac cirrhosis, which results from right-sided heart failure.
◆ Tenth most common cause of death in the United States
◆ Most common among those ages 45 to 75
◆ Occurs in twice as many males as females

CAUSES

Laënnec's or micronodular cirrhosis
◆ Chronic alcoholism
◆ Malnutrition

Postnecrotic or macronodular cirrhosis
◆ Complication of viral hepatitis
◆ Possible after exposure to such liver toxins as arsenic, carbon tetrachloride, and phosphorus

Biliary cirrhosis
◆ Prolonged biliary tract obstruction or inflammation

Idiopathic cirrhosis (cryptogenic)
◆ Chronic inflammatory bowel disease
◆ Sarcoidosis

UP CLOSE

What happens in portal hypertension

Portal hypertension (elevated pressure in the portal vein) occurs when blood flow meets increased resistance. This common result of cirrhosis may also stem from mechanical obstruction and occlusion of the hepatic veins (Budd-Chiari syndrome).

As the pressure in the portal vein rises, blood backs up into the spleen and flows through collateral channels to the venous system, bypassing the liver. Thus, portal hypertension causes:
◆ splenomegaly with thrombocytopenia
◆ dilated collateral veins (esophageal varices, hemorrhoids, or prominent abdominal veins)
◆ ascites.

In many patients, the first sign of portal hypertension is bleeding esophageal varices (dilated tortuous veins in the submucosa of the lower esophagus).

Esophageal varices commonly cause massive hematemesis, requiring emergency care to control hemorrhage and prevent hypovolemic shock.

Superior vena cava
Right atrium
Azygos vein
Esophagus
Esophageal varices
Inferior vena cava
Hepatic vein
Enlarged spleen
Short gastric vein
Left gastric vein
Relative increase in hepatic artery flow
Portal vein pressure rising from 10 mm Hg to 20 mm Hg or more
Splenic vein

RISK FACTORS

- Alcoholism
- Toxins
- Biliary obstruction
- Hepatitis
- Metabolic disorders

PATHOPHYSIOLOGY

- Cirrhosis begins with hepatic scarring or fibrosis. The scar begins as an increase in extracellular matrix components—fibril-forming collagens, proteoglycans, fibronectin, and hyaluronic acid. The site of collagen deposition varies with the cause.
- Hepatocyte function is eventually impaired as the matrix changes. Fat-storing cells are believed to be the source of new matrix components.
- Contraction of these cells may also contribute to disruption of the lobular architecture and obstruction of blood or bile flow.
- Cellular changes producing bands of scar tissue also disrupt the lobular structure.

ENDOCRINE SYSTEM

- Testicular atrophy, menstrual irregularities, gynecomastia, and loss of chest and axillary hair result from decreased hormone metabolism.

HEMATOLOGIC SYSTEM

- Bleeding tendencies (nosebleeds, easy bruising, bleeding gums), splenomegaly, and anemia resulting from thrombocytopenia (secondary to splenomegaly and decreased vitamin K absorption) may develop.
- Portal hypertension may occur, which can result in enlarged superficial abdominal veins, hemorrhoids, and hemorrhage from esophageal varices. (See *Disorders affecting management of cirrhosis,* page 109.)

HEPATIC SYSTEM

- Jaundice results from decreased bilirubin metabolism.
- Hepatomegaly occurs secondary to liver scarring and portal hypertension.

- Ascites and edema of the legs result from portal hypertension and decreased plasma proteins.
- Hepatic encephalopathy may occur from ammonia toxicity.
- Hepatorenal syndrome results from advanced liver disease and subsequent renal failure.

INTEGUMENTARY SYSTEM

- Abnormal pigmentation, spider nevi, palmar erythema, and jaundice are related to impaired hepatic function.
- Severe pruritus develops secondary to jaundice from bilirubinemia.
- Extreme dryness and poor tissue turgor are related to malnutrition.

NEUROLOGIC SYSTEM

- Progressive signs or symptoms of hepatic encephalopathy, including lethargy, mental changes, slurred speech, asterixis, peripheral neuritis, paranoia, hallucinations, extreme obtundation, and coma may be secondary to urea conversion and consequent delivery of toxic ammonia to the brain.

RESPIRATORY SYSTEM

- Pleural effusion and limited thoracic expansion occur because of abdominal ascites.
- Interference with efficient gas exchange causes hypoxia.

ASSESSMENT

HISTORY

- Chronic alcoholism
- Malnutrition
- Viral hepatitis
- Exposure to liver toxins, such as arsenic and certain medications
- Prolonged biliary tract obstruction or inflammation

Early stage

- Vague signs and symptoms
- Abdominal pain
- Diarrhea, constipation
- Fatigue
- Nausea, vomiting
- Muscle cramps

Later stage

- Chronic dyspepsia
- Constipation
- Pruritus
- Weight loss
- Bleeding tendency, such as frequent nosebleeds, easy bruising, and bleeding gums
- Hepatic encephalopathy

PHYSICAL FINDINGS

- Telangiectasis on the cheeks
- Spider angiomas on the face, neck, arms, and trunk
- Gynecomastia
- Umbilical hernia
- Distended abdominal blood vessels
- Ascites
- Testicular atrophy
- Menstrual irregularities
- Palmar erythema
- Clubbed fingers
- Thigh and leg edema
- Ecchymosis
- Anemia
- Jaundice
- Palpable, large, firm liver with a sharp edge (early finding)
- Enlarged spleen
- Asterixis
- Slurred speech, paranoia, hallucinations

(continued)

DIAGNOSTIC TEST RESULTS

◆ Liver enzymes, such as alanine aminotransferase, aspartate aminotransferase, total serum bilirubin, and indirect bilirubin are elevated; total serum albumin and protein levels are decreased; prothrombin time is prolonged; hemoglobin, hematocrit, and serum electrolyte levels are decreased; vitamins A, C, and K are deficient.
◆ Urine levels of bilirubin and urobilinogen are increased; fecal urobilinogen levels are decreased.
◆ Ammonia levels are elevated.
◆ Abdominal X-rays show liver and spleen size and cysts or gas in the biliary tract or liver; liver calcification; and massive ascites.
◆ Computed tomography and liver scans determine liver size, identify liver masses, and visualize hepatic blood flow and obstruction.
◆ Radioisotope liver scans show liver size, blood flow, or obstruction.
◆ Liver biopsy, the definitive test for cirrhosis, reveals hepatic tissue destruction and fibrosis.
◆ Esophagogastroduodenoscopy reveals bleeding esophageal varices, stomach irritation or ulceration, and duodenal bleeding and irritation.

TREATMENT

GENERAL
◆ Removal or alleviation of underlying cause
◆ Paracentesis for ascites
◆ Esophageal balloon tamponade with bleeding varices
◆ Sclerotherapy with acute bleeding
◆ I.V. fluids
◆ Blood transfusion

DIET
◆ Restricted sodium consumption
◆ Restricted fluid intake
◆ Alcohol abstinence
◆ High-calorie

ACTIVITY
◆ Frequent rest periods, as needed

MEDICATIONS
◆ Vitamin and nutritional supplements
◆ Antacids
◆ Potassium-sparing diuretics
◆ Beta-adrenergic blockers and vasopressin
◆ Ammonia detoxicant
◆ Antiemetics

SURGERY
◆ Peritoneovenous shunt to divert ascites into venous circulation
◆ Portal-systemic shunts
◆ Liver transplantation

NURSING CONSIDERATIONS

NURSING DIAGNOSES
◆ Activity intolerance
◆ Excess fluid volume
◆ Hopelessness
◆ Imbalanced nutrition: Less than body requirements
◆ Risk for deficient fluid volume
◆ Risk for impaired skin integrity
◆ Risk for injury

EXPECTED OUTCOMES
The patient will:
◆ perform activities of daily living without fatigue or exhaustion
◆ maintain normal fluid volume and show no signs of circulatory overload
◆ participate in decisions about care
◆ maintain adequate caloric intake
◆ maintain an adequate fluid balance
◆ maintain skin integrity
◆ remain free from injury.

NURSING INTERVENTIONS
◆ Monitor vital signs and laboratory values.
◆ Give prescribed I.V. fluids and blood products.
◆ Give prescribed drugs.
◆ Encourage verbalization and provide support.
◆ Provide appropriate skin care.
◆ Assess hydration and nutritional status.
◆ Obtain daily abdominal girth measurements and daily weight.
◆ Observe for bleeding tendencies.
◆ Reposition every two hours, assess skin integrity, and provide skin care.

◆ Note any changes in mentation and behavior.

PATIENT TEACHING

Be sure to cover:
◆ disorder, diagnostic testing, and treatment
◆ medication administration, dosage, and possible adverse effects
◆ over-the-counter medications that may increase bleeding tendencies
◆ dietary modifications
◆ need to avoid infections and abstain from alcohol
◆ need to avoid sedatives and acetaminophen (hepatotoxic)
◆ need for high-calorie diet with small, frequent meals
◆ available alcohol cessation programs and support groups.

RESOURCES
Organizations
Alcoholics Anonymous: *www.alcoholics-anonymous.org*
American Liver Foundation: *www.liverfoundation.org*
Digestive Disease National Coalition: *www.ddnc.org*
National Institute of Diabetes & Digestive & Kidney Diseases: *www.niddk.nih.gov*

Selected references
Dangleben, D.A. "Impact of Cirrhosis on Outcomes in Trauma," *Journal of the American College of Surgeons* 203(6):908-13, December 2006.
Giouleme, O.I., et al. "Pathogenesis of Osteoporosis in Liver Cirrhosis," *Hepatogastroenterology* 53(72):938-43, November-December 2006.
Reshetnyak, V.I. "Concept on the Pathogenesis and Treatment of Primary Biliary Cirrhosis," *World Journal of Gastroenterology* 12(45):7250-262, December 2006.
Saner, F.H., et al. "Severe Neurological Events Following Liver Transplantation," *Archives of Medical Research* 38(1):75-79, January 2007.
Sargent, S., and Martin, W. "Renal Dysfunction in Liver Cirrhosis," *British Journal of Nursing* 15(1):12-16, January 2006.

Disorders affecting management of cirrhosis

This chart highlights disorders that affect the management of cirrhosis.

DISORDER	SIGNS AND SYMPTOMS	DIAGNOSTIC TEST RESULTS	TREATMENT AND CARE
Esophageal varices (complication)	◆ Massive hematemesis ◆ Tachycardia ◆ Tachypnea ◆ Hypotension ◆ Decreased pulses ◆ Dry mucous membranes ◆ Poor skin turgor ◆ Altered level of consciousness	◆ Endoscopy identifies ruptured varix as the bleeding site and excludes other potential sources in the upper GI tract. ◆ Complete blood count reveals decreased hemoglobin level; hematocrit; and red blood cell, white blood cell, and platelet counts. ◆ Coagulation studies reveal prolonged prothrombin time secondary to hepatocellular disease. ◆ Serum chemistry tests may reveal elevated blood urea nitrogen, sodium, total bilirubin and ammonia levels, and decreased serum albumin resulting from liver damage and elevated liver enzyme levels.	◆ Assess the patient for the extent of blood loss. ◆ Ensure a patent airway, and assess breathing and circulation. ◆ Monitor cardiac and respiratory status. ◆ Administer supplemental oxygen, and monitor its effects. ◆ Monitor oxygen saturation and arterial blood gas (ABG) levels. ◆ Prepare for endotracheal intubation, as indicated. ◆ Monitor vital signs continuously. ◆ Perform hemodynamic and cardiac monitoring. ◆ Administer fluid replacement and blood component therapy. ◆ Obtain serial hemoglobin level and hematocrit. ◆ Monitor input and output closely; assess all losses from the GI tract. ◆ Assist with balloon tamponade, as necessary, and maintain pressure; monitor for vomiting and respiratory distress closely. ◆ Prepare for surgery, as necessary. ◆ Provide emotional support. ◆ Administer sclerosing agents or vasopressin.
Portal hypertension (complication)	◆ Bleeding from esophageal varices ◆ Ascites ◆ Confusion	◆ Portal venous pressures exceed 10 mm Hg. ◆ Angiography helps to identify patency of the portal vein and development of collateral vessels. ◆ Platelet count is decreased. ◆ Hemoglobin and hematocrit (with bleeding) are decreased.	◆ Ensure a patent airway, and assess breathing and circulation. ◆ Administer supplemental oxygen, and monitor its effects. ◆ Monitor oxygen saturation and ABG levels. ◆ Assess the patient for the extent of blood loss. ◆ Monitor cardiac and respiratory status. ◆ Prepare the patient for surgery to insert a portosystemic shunt to decrease portal hypertension. ◆ Prepare for endotracheal intubation, as indicated. ◆ Monitor vital signs continuously. ◆ Perform hemodynamic and cardiac monitoring. ◆ Administer fluid replacement and blood component therapy. ◆ Obtain serial hemoglobin level and hematocrit. ◆ Monitor input and output; assess all losses from the GI tract.

Crohn's disease

OVERVIEW

- Inflammatory bowel disease that may affect any part of the GI tract but commonly involves the terminal ileum
- 50% of cases involving colon and small bowel; 33%, terminal ileum; 10% to 20%, only colon
- Extends through all layers of the intestinal wall; may involve regional lymph nodes and mesentery
- Occurs equally in males and females
- Occurs more commonly in Jewish people
- Onset usually before age 30

CAUSES

- Exact cause unknown
- Lymphatic obstruction and infection among contributing factors

RISK FACTORS

- History of allergies
- Immune disorders
- Genetic predisposition—10% to 20% of patients having one or more affected relatives; sometimes occurring in monozygotic twins
- Smoking
- Left-handedness
- Adult appendectomy
- Use of oral contraceptives, nonsteroidal anti-inflammatory drugs, and antibiotics

PATHOPHYSIOLOGY

- Crohn's disease involves slow, progressive inflammation of the bowel.
- Lymphatic obstruction is caused by enlarged lymph nodes.
- Edema, mucosal ulceration, fissures, and abscesses occur. (See *Disorders affecting management of Crohn's disease*, page 113.)

GASTROINTESTINAL SYSTEM

- Elevated patches of closely packed lymph follicles (Peyer's patches) develop in the small intestinal lining.
- Fibrosis occurs, thickening the bowel wall and causing stenosis.
- Inflamed bowel loops adhere to other diseased or normal loops.
- The diseased bowel becomes thicker, shorter, and narrower.
- Malabsorption of bile salts may occur, causing steatorrhea, fat-soluble vitamin deficiency, and gallstones.

RENAL SYSTEM

- Fat malabsorption occurs from loss of functional mucosal absorptive surface.
- Calcium is trapped and may cause increased oxalate excretion, which may cause renal calculi to form.

MUSCULOSKELETAL SYSTEM

- Ankylosing spondylitis, seronegative arthritis, and sacroiliitis occur as a result of the chronic inflammatory process.

ASSESSMENT

HISTORY

- Gradual onset of signs and symptoms, marked by periods of remission and exacerbation
- Fatigue and weakness
- Fever, flatulence, nausea
- Steady, colicky, or cramping abdominal pain that usually occurs in the right lower abdominal quadrant
- Diarrhea that may worsen after emotional upset or ingestion of poorly tolerated foods, such as milk, fatty foods, and spices
- Weight loss

PHYSICAL FINDINGS

- Possible soft or semiliquid stool, usually without gross blood
- Right lower abdominal quadrant tenderness or distention
- Possible abdominal mass, indicating adherent loops of bowel
- Hyperactive bowel sounds
- Bloody diarrhea
- Perianal and rectal abscesses

DIAGNOSTIC TEST RESULTS

- Occult blood in stools may be present.
- Hemoglobin (Hb) level and hematocrit may be decreased.
- White blood cell count and erythrocyte sedimentation rate may be increased.
- Serum potassium, calcium, magnesium, and Hb levels may be decreased.
- Hypoglobulinemia from intestinal protein loss may occur.
- Vitamin B_{12} and folate deficiency may occur.
- Small bowel X-rays may show irregular mucosa, ulceration, and stiffening.

- Barium enema reveals the string sign (segments of stricture separated by normal bowel) and may also show fissures and narrowing of the lumen.
- Sigmoidoscopy and colonoscopy show patchy areas of inflammation and may also reveal the characteristic coarse irregularity (cobblestone appearance) of the mucosal surface.
- Biopsy reveals granulomas in up to 50% of all specimens.

TREATMENT

GENERAL
- Stress reduction

DIET
- Avoidance of foods that worsen diarrhea
- Avoidance of raw fruits and vegetables if blockage occurs
- Adequate caloric and protein intake
- Parenteral nutrition, if necessary

ACTIVITY
- Reduced

MEDICATIONS
- Corticosteroids
- Immune modifiers
- Infliximab
- Sulfonamides
- Aminosalysilates
- Antibacterials and antiprotozoals
- Antispasmodics
- Antidiarrheals
- Opioids
- Vitamin supplements

SURGERY
- Indicated for acute intestinal obstruction
- Colectomy with ileostomy

NURSING CONSIDERATIONS

NURSING DIAGNOSES
- Acute pain
- Diarrhea
- Disturbed body image
- Imbalanced nutrition: Less than body requirements
- Ineffective coping
- Ineffective tissue perfusion: GI
- Risk for deficient fluid volume
- Risk for impaired skin integrity
- Risk for injury

EXPECTED OUTCOMES
The patient will:
- express feelings of increased comfort and decreased pain
- regain normal intestinal function
- express positive feelings about self
- maintain adequate caloric intake
- exhibit adequate coping mechanisms, and seek appropriate sources of support
- exhibit signs of adequate GI perfusion
- maintain normal fluid volume
- maintain skin integrity
- remain free from injury.

NURSING INTERVENTIONS
- Monitor vital signs; intake and output, including amount and characteristics of stool; daily weight; serum electrolytes and glucose; Hb; and stools for occult blood.
- Observe for signs of infection or obstruction and bleeding, especially with steroid use.
- Provide emotional support to the patient and his family.
- Provide meticulous skin care after each bowel movement.
- Schedule patient care to include rest periods throughout the day.
- Assist with dietary modification.
- Give prescribed iron supplements and blood transfusions.
- Give prescribed analgesics.
- Assess abdominal pain and distention.

(continued)

Be sure to cover:
- disorder, diagnostic testing, and treatment
- medication administration, dosage, and possible adverse effects
- importance of adequate rest
- how the patient can identify and reduce sources of stress
- prescribed dietary changes
- available smoking cessation programs
- contact information for enterostomal therapist and local support groups.

RESOURCES

Organizations

Crohn's and Colitis Foundation of America: *www.ccfa.org*

National Digestive Diseases Clearinghouse: *www.nddc.nih.gov*

United Ostomy Association, Inc.: *www.uoa.org*

Selected references

Dudley-Brown, S., and Bean, K. "Symptom Correlates in Inflammatory Bowel Disease," *Gastroenterology Nursing* 28(2):165, March-April 2005.

Fletcher, P.C., and Schneider, M.A. "Is There Any Food I Can Eat? Living with Inflammatory Bowel Disease and/or Irritable Bowel Syndrome," *Clinical Nurse Specialist* 20(5):241-47, September-October 2006.

Ghosh, S., et al. "Is Thiopurine Therapy in Ulcerative Colitis as Effective as in Crohn's Disease?" *Gut* 55(1):6-8, January 2006.

Kane, S. "Urogenital Complications of Crohn's Disease," *The American Journal of Gastroenterology* 101(Suppl 3):S640-43, December 2006.

Disorders affecting management of Crohn's disease

This chart highlights disorders that affect the management of Crohn's disease.

DISORDER	SIGNS AND SYMPTOMS	DIAGNOSTIC TEST RESULTS	TREATMENT AND CARE
Abdominal abscess (coexisting and complication)	◆ Persistent abdominal pain ◆ Focal tenderness ◆ Fever ◆ Prolonged ileus	◆ White blood cell (WBC) count is elevated. ◆ Liver function studies are abnormal. ◆ Blood cultures reveal bacteremia. ◆ Ultrasonography identifies abscess. ◆ Abdominal computed tomography scan identifies a fluid-filled extraluminal structure or air bubble and inflammatory edema in adjacent fat.	◆ Administer antibiotics, as prescribed. ◆ Monitor laboratory studies. ◆ Prepare the patient for surgery for drainage of abscess. ◆ Provide appropriate postoperative care and wound care.
Intestinal obstruction (complication)	◆ Diffuse abdominal discomfort ◆ Abdominal tenderness ◆ Rebound tenderness ◆ Abdominal distention ◆ Decreased bowel sounds (early) then absent bowel sounds	◆ Abdominal X-rays reveal the presence and location of intestinal gas or fluid; in small bowel obstruction, typical "step-ladder" pattern emerges. ◆ Barium enema reveals a distended air-filled colon or closed loop of sigmoid with extreme distention. ◆ WBC count is elevated.	◆ Insert a nasogastric tube, and monitor drainage. ◆ Monitor GI status. ◆ Don't allow the patient to take anything by mouth; administer fluids and parenteral nutrition until patient is able to resume diet. ◆ Provide analgesic for pain. ◆ Prepare the patient for surgery, if indicated.
Malnutrition (complication)	◆ Diarrhea ◆ Steatorrhea ◆ Flatulence and abdominal discomfort ◆ Nocturia ◆ Weakness and fatigue ◆ Edema ◆ Amenorrhea ◆ Glossitis ◆ Peripheral neuropathy ◆ Bruising ◆ Bone pain ◆ Skeletal deformities	◆ Stool specimen for fat reveals excretion of greater than 6 g of fat/day. ◆ D-xylose absorption test shows less than 20% of 25 g of D-xylose in the urine after 5 hours. ◆ Schilling test reveals deficiency of vitamin B_{12} absorption. ◆ Culture of duodenal and jejunal contents confirms bacterial overgrowth. ◆ GI barium studies show characteristic features of the small intestine. ◆ Small intestine biopsy reveals atrophy of the mucosal villi.	◆ Assess nutritional status; monitor daily calorie count and obtain daily weight. ◆ Evaluate the patient's tolerance to foods. ◆ Assess fluid status; administer fluid replacement. ◆ Administer dietary supplements and vitamins. ◆ Monitor laboratory values, especially electrolytes and coagulation studies. ◆ Assist with nutritional therapy, such as peripheral parenteral nutrition or total parenteral nutrition.

Cushing's syndrome

- Clinical manifestations of glucocorticoid excess, particularly cortisol
- May also reflect excess secretion of mineralocorticoids and androgens
- Classified as primary, secondary, or iatrogenic, depending on etiology
- Prognosis dependent on early diagnosis, identification of underlying cause, and effective treatment
- More common in females than in males and may occur at any age

CAUSES

- Corticotropin-producing tumor in another organ
- Cortisol-secreting adrenal tumor
- Excess production of corticotropin
- Pituitary microadenoma
- Prolonged exposure to elevated levels of endogenous or exogenous glucocorticoids

PATHOPHYSIOLOGY

- Cortisol excess results in anti-inflammatory effects and excess catabolism of protein and peripheral fat to support hepatic glucose production.
- The mechanism that triggers the secretion may be corticotropin dependent (elevated plasma corticotropin levels stimulate the adrenal cortex to produce excess cortisol), or corticotropin independent (excess cortisol is produced by the adrenal cortex or exogenously administered).
- Excess cortisol suppresses the hypothalamic-pituitary-adrenal axis.

CARDIOVASCULAR SYSTEM

- Sodium and secondary fluid retention leads to hypertension, possibly leading to heart failure and left ventricular hypertrophy.
- Capillary weakness may occur from protein loss, leading to bleeding and ecchymosis.

ENDOCRINE SYSTEM

- Diabetes mellitus develops because of cortisol-induced insulin resistance and increased gluconeogenesis in the liver. (See *Disorders affecting management of Cushing's syndrome,* pages 116 and 117.)

GASTROINTESTINAL SYSTEM

- Peptic ulcer may occur because of an increase in gastric secretions and pepsin production and a decrease in gastric mucus.

IMMUNOLOGIC SYSTEM

- The patient's susceptibility to infection is increased as a result of decreased lymphocyte production and suppressed antibody formation. Resistance to stress is decreased.

INTEGUMENTARY SYSTEM

- Decreased collagen and weakened tissues result in integumentary changes, such as increased body hair, purple striae, acne, facial plethora, and poor wound healing.

MUSCULOSKELETAL SYSTEM

- Muscle weakness caused by hypokalemia or loss of muscle mass from increased catabolism may occur.
- Pathologic fractures may occur because of decreased bone mineral ionization, osteopenia, osteoporosis, and skeletal growth retardation in children.

NEUROLOGIC SYSTEM

- The patient may have insomnia as a result of cortisol's role in neurotransmission.

RENAL AND UROLOGIC SYSTEMS

- Fluid retention occurs secondary to sodium restriction.
- Potassium excretion increases.
- Ureteral calculi result from increased bone demineralization associated with hypercalciuria.

HISTORY

- Use of synthetic steroids
- Fatigue
- Muscle weakness
- Sleep disturbances
- Polyuria
- Thirst
- Frequent infections (immunosuppression)
- Water retention
- Amenorrhea
- Decreased libido
- Irritability; emotional instability
- Symptoms resembling those of hyperglycemia
- Impotence
- Headache

PHYSICAL FINDINGS

- Thin hair
- Moon-shaped face
- Hirsutism
- Buffalo-hump–like back
- Thin extremities
- Muscle wasting and weakness
- Petechiae, ecchymoses, and purplish striae
- Delayed wound healing
- Swollen ankles
- Hypertension
- Central obesity
- Acne
- Osteopenic growth retardation in children

DIAGNOSTIC TEST RESULTS

- Salivary free cortisol is elevated.
- Corticotropin in adrenal disease is decreased and excess pituitary or ectopic secretion of corticotropin is increased.
- Blood chemistry may show hypernatremia, hypokalemia, hypocalcemia, and elevated blood glucose.
- Urinary free cortisol is elevated.
- Serum cortisol is elevated in the morning.
- Glycosuria is evident.
- Ultrasonography, computed tomography scan, and magnetic resonance imaging may show the location of a pituitary or adrenal tumor.

- A low-dose dexamethasone suppression test shows failure of plasma cortisol levels to be suppressed.

TREATMENT

GENERAL
- Management to restore hormone balance and reverse Cushing's syndrome, including radiation, drug therapy, or surgery

DIET
- High-protein, high-potassium, low-calorie, low-sodium

ACTIVITY
- As tolerated

MEDICATIONS
- Aminoglutethimide
- Antifungals
- Antihypertensives
- Diuretics
- Potassium supplements
- Antineoplastics, antihormonals
- Glucocorticoids

⚡ **WARNING** *Glucocorticoid administration on the morning of surgery can help prevent acute adrenal insufficiency during surgery. Cortisol therapy is essential during and after surgery to help the patient tolerate the physiologic stress caused by removal of the pituitary or adrenal glands.*

SURGERY
- Possible hypophysectomy or pituitary irradiation
- Bilateral adrenalectomy
- Excision of nonendocrine corticotropin-producing tumor, followed by drug therapy

NURSING CONSIDERATIONS

NURSING DIAGNOSES
- Activity intolerance
- Disturbed body image
- Excess fluid volume
- Impaired skin integrity
- Ineffective coping
- Risk for infection
- Risk for injury
- Sexual dysfunction

EXPECTED OUTCOMES
The patient will:
- perform activities of daily living as tolerated within the confines of the disorder
- express positive feelings about self
- maintain normal fluid volume
- maintain skin integrity
- demonstrate adaptive coping behaviors
- remain free from signs and symptoms of infection
- remain free from injury
- verbalize feelings related to sexual impairment.

NURSING INTERVENTIONS
- Monitor vital signs, intake and output, daily weights, and serum electrolyte results.
- Give prescribed drugs.
- Consult a dietitian.
- Use protective measures to reduce the risk of infection.
- Use meticulous hand-washing technique.
- Schedule adequate rest periods.
- Institute safety precautions.
- Provide meticulous skin care.
- Encourage verbalization of feelings.
- Offer emotional support.
- Help to develop effective coping strategies.

After transsphenoidal approach to hypophysectomy
- Keep the head of the bed elevated at least 30 degrees.
- Maintain nasal packing.
- Provide frequent mouth care.
- Avoid activities that increase intracranial pressure (ICP).
- Evaluate for cerebrospinal fluid leak.

After bilateral adrenalectomy and hypophysectomy
- Monitor neurologic and behavioral status.
- Administer medication for severe nausea, vomiting, and diarrhea.
- Assess bowel sounds.
- Observe for signs of increased ICP, diabetes insipidus, and hemorrhage and shock.

PATIENT TEACHING

Be sure to cover:
- disorder, diagnostic testing, and treatment
- medication administration, dosage, and possible adverse effects
- when to notify the practitioner
- need for lifelong steroid replacement
- need to wear medical identification bracelet
- prevention of infection
- signs and symptoms of adrenal crisis
- stress-reduction strategies
- follow-up care.

RESOURCES
Organizations
Addison and Cushing International Federation:
www.nvacp.nl/page.php?main=5
Cushing's Support and Research Foundation, Inc.: *www.csrf.net*
Endocrine Society: *www.endo-society.org*
National Adrenal Diseases Foundation: *www.medhelp.org/www/nadf.htm*

Selected references
Brown, R.L., and Weiss, R.E. "An Approach to the Evaluation and Treatment of Cushing's Disease," *Expert Review of Anticancer Therapy* Suppl 9:S37-46, September 2006.
Nettina, S.M. *Lippincott Manual of Nursing Practice*, 8th ed. Philadelphia: Lippincott Williams & Wilkins, 2006.
Salgado, L.R., et al. "Cushing's Disease Arising from a Clinically Nonfunctioning Pituitary Adenoma," *Endocrine Pathology* 17(2):191-99, Summer 2006.
Simmons Holcomb, S. "Hospital Nursing: Confronting Cushing's Syndrome," *Nursing* 35(9):32hn1-32hn6, September 2005.

(continued)

Disorders affecting management of Cushing's syndrome

This chart highlights disorders that affect the management of Cushing's syndrome.

DISORDER	SIGNS AND SYMPTOMS	DIAGNOSTIC TEST RESULTS	TREATMENT AND CARE
Diabetes insipidus (complication)	◆ Extreme polyuria—usually 4 to 6 L/day—may be up to 30 L/day ◆ Polydipsia, especially for cold drinks ◆ Nocturia ◆ Fatigue (in severe cases) ◆ Dehydration, characterized by weight loss, poor tissue turgor, dry mucous membranes, constipation, muscle weakness, dizziness, tachycardia, and hypotension	◆ Urinalysis reveals almost colorless urine of low osmolality (less than 200 mOsm/kg) and low specific gravity (less than 1.005). ◆ Water deprivation test demonstrates renal inability to concentrate urine (evidence of antidiuretic hormone deficiency). ◆ Vasopressin injection results in decreased urine output and increased urine specific gravity (with central diabetes insipidus).	◆ Administer thiazide diuretics to reduce urine volume by increasing mild salt depletion. ◆ Administer fluid replacement according to urine output; monitor intake and output. ◆ Monitor for signs and symptoms of hypovolemic shock; monitor vital signs and cardiovascular and respiratory systems. ◆ Measure urine specific gravity. ◆ Provide skin and mouth care. ◆ Monitor electrolyte values, and provide supplemental therapy, if indicated.
Diabetes mellitus (coexisting)	◆ Weight loss despite voracious hunger ◆ Weakness ◆ Vision changes ◆ Frequent skin and urinary tract infections ◆ Dry, itchy skin ◆ Poor skin turgor ◆ Dry mucous membranes ◆ Dehydration ◆ Decreased peripheral pulses ◆ Cool skin temperature ◆ Decreased reflexes ◆ Orthostatic hypotension ◆ Muscle wasting ◆ Loss of subcutaneous fat ◆ Fruity breath odor because of ketoacidosis	◆ Fasting plasma glucose is 126 mg/dl or greater on at least two occasions; a random blood glucose level is 200 mg/dl or greater. ◆ Blood glucose level is 200 mg/dl or greater 2 hours after ingesting 75 g of oral dextrose. ◆ Ophthalmologic examination may show diabetic retinopathy.	◆ Check blood glucose levels periodically because steroid replacement may necessitate adjustment of the insulin dosage. ◆ Keep a late-morning snack available in case the patient becomes hypoglycemic. ◆ Keep accurate records of vital signs, weight, fluid intake, urine output, and calorie intake. ◆ Monitor serum glucose and urine acetone levels. ◆ Monitor for acute complications of diabetic therapy, especially hypoglycemia (vagueness, slow cerebration, dizziness, weakness, pallor, tachycardia, diaphoresis, seizures, and coma); immediately give carbohydrates in the form of fruit juice, hard candy, honey or, if the patient is unconscious, glucagon or I.V. dextrose. ◆ Be alert for signs of hyperosmolar coma (polyuria, thirst, neurologic abnormalities, and stupor). This hyperglycemic crisis requires I.V. fluids and insulin replacement. ◆ Provide meticulous skin care, especially to the feet and legs. Treat all injuries, cuts, and blisters. ◆ Administer insulin replacement or oral antidiabetics. ◆ Observe for signs of urinary tract and vaginal infections. ◆ Encourage adequate fluid intake.
Hypertension (coexisting)	◆ Usually asymptomatic ◆ Elevated blood pressure readings on at least two consecutive occasions ◆ Occipital headache ◆ Epistaxis ◆ Bruits ◆ Dizziness ◆ Confusion ◆ Fatigue ◆ Blurry vision ◆ Nocturia ◆ Edema	◆ Serial blood pressure measurements reveal elevations of 140/90 mm Hg or greater on two or more separate occasions. ◆ Urinalysis may show protein, casts, red blood cells or white blood cells (WBCs). ◆ Blood urea nitrogen and serum creatinine levels are elevated. ◆ Complete blood count may reveal polycythemia or anemia. ◆ Excretory urography may reveal renal atrophy. ◆ Electrocardiography may show left ventricular hypertrophy or ischemia. ◆ Chest X-rays may show cardiomegaly. ◆ Echocardiography may reveal left ventricular hypertrophy.	◆ Monitor blood pressure, response to antihypertensive medication, and laboratory studies. ◆ Maintain a reduced-sodium diet. ◆ Monitor for complications of hypertension, such as signs of stroke or myocardial infarction. ◆ Administer thiazide diuretics, angiotensin-converting enzyme inhibitors, angiotensin receptor blockers, or calcium channel blockers.

DISORDER	SIGNS AND SYMPTOMS	DIAGNOSTIC TEST RESULTS	TREATMENT AND CARE
Osteoporosis (complication)	◆ Dowager's hump ◆ Back pain (thoracic and lumbar) ◆ Loss of height ◆ Unsteady gait ◆ Joint pain ◆ Weakness	◆ Dual photon or dual energy X-ray absorptiometry can detect bone loss. ◆ X-rays reveal characteristic degeneration in the lower vertebrae. ◆ Parathyroid levels may be elevated. ◆ Bone biopsy allows direct examination of changes in bone cells and the rate of bone turnover.	◆ Provide supportive devices such as a back brace. ◆ Encourage lifestyle modifications, such as weight loss, exercise program, and dietary modifications. ◆ Offer analgesics and heat for pain relief. ◆ Administer calcium and vitamin D supplements to stimulate bone formation. ◆ Give sodium fluoride to stimulate bone formation; give calcitonin to reduce bone resorption and slow the decline in bone mass.
Peptic ulcer (coexisting)	◆ Recent loss of weight or appetite ◆ Anorexia ◆ Feeling of fullness or distention ◆ Pain that may be worsened by eating or may be relieved by it ◆ Sharp, burning or gnawing, epigastric pain ◆ Hyperactive bowel sounds ◆ Possible epigastric tenderness in the midline and midway between the umbilicus and the xiphoid process ◆ Anemic pallor	◆ Barium swallow or upper GI and small-bowel series may reveal the presence of the ulcer. ◆ Upper GI endoscopy or esophagogastroduodenoscopy confirms the presence of an ulcer and permits cytologic studies and biopsy to rule out *Helicobacter pylori* or cancer. ◆ Laboratory analysis may disclose occult blood in stools. ◆ Immunoglobulin A anti-*H. pylori* test on a venous blood sample can be used to detect antibodies to *H. pylori*. ◆ Gastric secretory studies show hyperchlorhydria. ◆ Carbon 13 urea breath test results reflect activity of *H. pylori*.	◆ Support the patient emotionally, and offer reassurance. ◆ Administer antacids, antimicrobials, misoprostol, anticholinergics, histamine-2-blockers, or proton gastric pump inhibitors, and monitor the patient for the desired effects. Also watch for adverse reactions. Most medications should alleviate the patient's discomfort, so ask whether his pain is relieved. ◆ Provide six small meals or small hourly meals, as ordered. Advise the patient to eat slowly, chew thoroughly, and have small snacks between meals. ◆ Schedule the patient's care so that he can get plenty of rest.
Urinary calculi (complication)	◆ Pain that travels from the costovertebral angle to the flank and then to the suprapubic region and external genitalia (classic renal colic pain) ◆ Constant, dull pain and possible back pain (if calculi are in the renal pelvis and calyces) ◆ Severe abdominal pain ◆ Nausea and vomiting ◆ Fever and chills ◆ Hematuria ◆ Abdominal distention ◆ Anuria (rare)	◆ Kidney-ureter-bladder radiography reveals most renal calculi. ◆ Excretory urography helps confirm the diagnosis and determine the size and location of calculi. ◆ Kidney ultrasonography detects obstructive changes. ◆ Urine culture of a midstream specimen may indicate pyuria, a sign of urinary tract infection. ◆ A 24-hour urine collection reveals elevated calcium oxalate, phosphorus, and uric acid excretion levels. ◆ Calculus analysis shows mineral content.	◆ To aid diagnosis, maintain a 24- to 48-hour record of urine pH using nitrazine pH paper. Strain all urine through gauze or a tea strainer, and save all solid material recovered for analysis. ◆ To facilitate spontaneous passage of calculi, encourage the patient to walk, if possible. Also force fluids to maintain a urine output of 3 to 4 L/day (urine should be very dilute and colorless). ◆ If the patient can't drink the required amount of fluid, give supplemental I.V. fluids. ◆ Record intake and output and daily weight to assess fluid status and renal function. ◆ Medicate the patient for pain when he's passing a calculus. ◆ To help acidify urine, offer fruit juices, especially cranberry juice. *If the patient had calculi surgically removed* ◆ Anticipate that the patient will have an indwelling catheter or a nephrostomy tube. ◆ Unless one of his kidneys was removed, expect bloody drainage from the catheter. ◆ Check dressings regularly for bloody drainage. ◆ Immediately report excessive drainage or a rising pulse rate, which are symptoms of hemorrhage. ◆ Use sterile technique when changing dressings or providing catheter care. ◆ Watch for signs of infection, such as a rising temperature or chills. ◆ Administer antibiotics, meperidine, morphine, antimicrobials, or allopurinol.

Cystic fibrosis

OVERVIEW

- Chronic, progressive, inherited, incurable disease affecting exocrine (mucus-secreting) glands
- Transmitted as an autosomal recessive trait
- Genetic mutation that involves chloride transport across epithelial membranes (more than 100 specific mutations of the gene identified)
- Characterized by major aberrations in sweat gland, respiratory, and GI functions
- Causes of symptoms: increased viscosity of bronchial, pancreatic, and other mucous gland secretions and consequent destruction of glandular ducts (see *Disorders affecting management of cystic fibrosis*, pages 121 to 123.)
- Accounts for almost all cases of pancreatic enzyme deficiency in children
- Clinical effects apparent soon after birth or take years to develop
- Death typically from pneumonia, emphysema, or atelectasis
- Most common fatal genetic disease of white children
- 25% chance of transmission with each pregnancy when both parents are carriers of the recessive gene
- Incidence highest in people of northern European ancestry
- Less common in Blacks, Native Americans, and people of Asian ancestry
- Occurs equally in both sexes

CAUSES

- Autosomal recessive mutation of gene on chromosome 7q, which encodes a membrane-associated protein called the *cystic fibrosis transmembrane regulator (CFTR)*; exact function of CFTR unknown, but appears to help regulate chloride and sodium transport across epithelial membranes
- Abnormal coding found on as many as 350 CFTR alleles

PATHOPHYSIOLOGY

- Most cases arise from the mutation that affects the genetic coding for a single amino acid, causing CFTR to malfunction.
- CFTR resembles other transmembrane transport proteins, but it lacks the phenylalanine that's present in the protein produced by normal genes. This regulator interferes with cyclic adenosine monophosphate–regulated chloride channels and transport of other ions by preventing adenosine triphosphate from binding to the protein or by interfering with activation by protein kinase.
- The mutation affects volume-absorbing epithelia (in the airways and intestines), salt-absorbing epithelia (in sweat ducts), and volume-secretory epithelia (in the pancreas). Lack of phenylalanine leads to dehydration and, ultimately, to glandular duct obstruction.

RESPIRATORY SYSTEM

- Thick secretions and dehydration occur as a result of ionic imbalance.
- Chronic airway infections by *Staphylococcus aureus, Pseudomonas aeruginosa*, and *Pseudomonas cepacia* may develop, possibly due to abnormal airway surface fluids and failure of lung defenses.
- Accumulation of thick secretions in the bronchioles and alveoli results in dyspnea.
- Stimulation of the secretion-removal reflex produces a paroxysmal cough.
- Barrel chest, cyanosis, and clubbing of fingers and toes result from chronic hypoxia.
- Obstructed glandular ducts occur, leading to peribronchial thickening; this obstruction is due to increased viscosity of bronchial, pancreatic, and other mucous gland secretions.

CARDIOVASCULAR SYSTEM

- Fatal shock and arrhythmias may result from hyponatremia and hypochloremia from sodium lost in sweat.

- Pulmonary hypertension can result in cardiac dysfunction in adult cystic fibrosis patients with severe lung disease.
- Pulmonary hypertension and cor pulmonale in cystic fibrosis are thought to be related to progressive destruction of the lung parenchyma and pulmonary vasculature and to pulmonary vasoconstriction secondary to hypoxemia.

ENDOCRINE SYSTEM

- Retention of bicarbonate and water due to the absence of CFTR chloride channel in the pancreatic ductile epithelia limits membrane function and leads to retention of pancreatic enzymes, chronic cholecystitis and cholelithiasis, and the ultimate destruction of the pancreas.
- Diabetes, pancreatitis, and hepatic failure can develop because of the disease's effects on the intestines, pancreas, and liver.

GASTROINTESTINAL SYSTEM

- Obstruction of the small and large intestines results from inhibited secretion of chloride and water and excessive absorption of liquid.
- Biliary cirrhosis occurs because of retention of biliary secretions.
- Malnutrition and malabsorption of fat-soluble vitamins (A, D, E, and K) are caused by deficiencies of trypsin, amylase, and lipase from obstructed pancreatic ducts, preventing the conversion and absorption of fat and protein in the intestinal tract.

GENITOURINARY SYSTEM

- In males, a bilateral congenital absence of the vas deferens is accompanied by a lack of sperm in the semen.
- In females, secondary amenorrhea and increased mucus in the reproductive tracts block the passage of ova.

HISTORY

- Recurring bronchitis and pneumonia
- Nasal polyps and sinusitis
- Wheezing
- Dry, nonproductive cough
- Shortness of breath
- Abdominal distention, vomiting, constipation
- Frequent, bulky, foul-smelling, and pale stool with a high fat content
- Poor weight gain
- Poor growth
- Ravenous appetite
- Hematemesis

PHYSICAL FINDINGS

- Wheezy respirations
- Dry, nonproductive, paroxysmal cough
- Dyspnea
- Tachypnea
- Bibasilar crackles and hyperresonance
- Barrel chest
- Cyanosis, and clubbing of the fingers and toes
- Distended abdomen
- Thin extremities
- Sallow skin with poor turgor
- Delayed sexual development
- Neonatal jaundice
- Hepatomegaly
- Rectal prolapse
- Failure to thrive

DIAGNOSTIC TEST RESULTS

- Sweat tests using pilocarpine solution reveals sodium and chloride values.
- Stool specimen analysis shows absence of trypsin.
- Deoxyribonucleic acid testing shows presence of the delta F 508.
- Liver enzyme tests may show hepatic insufficiency.
- Serum albumin level is decreased.
- Serum electrolytes may show hypochloremia and hyponatremia.
- Arterial blood gas analysis shows hypoxemia.
- Chest X-rays may show early signs of lung obstruction.
- High-resolution chest computed tomography scan shows bronchial wall thickening, cystic lesions, and bronchiectasis.
- Pulmonary function tests show decreased vital capacity, elevated residual volume, and decreased forced expiratory volume in 1 second.

GENERAL

- Based on organ systems involved
- Chest physiotherapy, nebulization, and breathing exercises several times per day
- Postural drainage
- Gene therapy (experimental)
- Annual influenza vaccination

DIET

- Salt supplements
- High-fat, high-protein, high-calorie

ACTIVITY

- As tolerated

MEDICATIONS

- Dornase alfa, a pulmonary enzyme given by aerosol nebulizer
- Antibiotics
- Oxygen therapy, as needed
- Oral pancreatic enzymes
- Bronchodilators
- Prednisone
- Vitamin A, D, E, and K supplements

SURGERY

- Heart-lung transplantation

(continued)

NURSING DIAGNOSES

◆ Anxiety
◆ Delayed growth and development
◆ Disabled family coping
◆ Fear
◆ Imbalanced nutrition: Less than body requirements
◆ Impaired gas exchange
◆ Ineffective airway clearance
◆ Ineffective breathing pattern
◆ Ineffective coping

EXPECTED OUTCOMES

The patient (or his family) will:
◆ identify strategies to reduce anxiety
◆ achieve age-appropriate growth to the fullest extent possible
◆ express concerns about coping with the illness
◆ discuss fears and concerns
◆ consume adequate calories daily
◆ maintain adequate ventilation and oxygenation
◆ maintain a patent airway
◆ maintain an effective breathing pattern
◆ use a support system to assist with coping.

NURSING INTERVENTIONS

◆ Administer oxygen therapy, as needed.
◆ Monitor vital signs, pulse oximetry, intake and output, and daily weight.
◆ Assess hydration and respiratory status.
◆ Give prescribed drugs.
◆ Administer pancreatic enzymes with meals and snacks.
◆ Perform chest physiotherapy and postural drainage.
◆ Provide a well-balanced, high-protein, high-calorie diet; include adequate fats.
◆ Provide vitamin A, D, E, and K supplements, if indicated.
◆ Ensure adequate oral fluid intake.
◆ Provide exercise and activity periods.
◆ Encourage breathing exercises.
◆ Provide the young child with play periods.

◆ Enlist the help of the physical therapy department and play therapists, if available.
◆ Provide emotional support.
◆ Include family members in all phases of the child's care.

Be sure to cover:
◆ disorder, diagnostic testing, and treatment
◆ medication administration, dosage, and possible adverse effects
◆ when to notify the practitioner
◆ aerosol therapy
◆ chest physiotherapy
◆ signs and symptoms of infection
◆ complications
◆ available local support groups and resources.

RESOURCES

Organizations

American Academy of Pediatrics: *www.aap.org*
Cystic Fibrosis Foundation: *www.cff.org*
National Institute of Diabetes & Digestive & Kidney Diseases: *www.niddk.nih.gov*

Selected references

Christian, B., and D'Auria, J. "Building Life Skills for Children with Cystic Fibrosis; Effectiveness of an Intervention," *Nursing Research* 55(5):300-307, September-October 2006.

Connors, P., and Ulles, M. "The Physical, Psychological and Social Implications of Caring for the Pregnant Patient and Newborn with Cystic Fibrosis," *Journal of Perinatal and Neonatal Nursing* 19(4):301-15, October-December 2005.

Diseases, 4th ed. Philadelphia: Lippincott Williams & Wilkins, 2006.

Gayer, D., and Ganong, L. "Family Structure and Mothers' Caregiving of Children with Cystic Fibrosis," *Journal of Family Nursing* 12(4):390-412, November 2006.

Hink, H, and Schellhase, D. "Transitioning Families to Adult Cystic Fibrosis Care," *Journal for Specialists in Pediatric Nursing* 11(4):260-63, October 2006.

Disorders affecting management of cystic fibrosis

This chart highlights disorders that affect the management of cystic fibrosis.

DISORDER	SIGNS AND SYMPTOMS	DIAGNOSTIC TEST RESULTS	TREATMENT AND CARE
Acute respiratory failure (complication)	◆ Changes in respiratory rate (may be increased, decreased, or normal depending on the cause) ◆ Cyanosis ◆ Crackles ◆ Rhonchi ◆ Wheezing ◆ Diminished breath sounds ◆ Restlessness ◆ Confusion ◆ Loss of concentration ◆ Irritability ◆ Coma ◆ Tachycardia ◆ Increased cardiac output ◆ Elevated blood pressure ◆ Arrhythmias	◆ Arterial blood gas (ABG) analysis indicates respiratory failure by deteriorating values and a pH below 7.35. ◆ Chest X-rays identify pulmonary disease. ◆ Electrocardiogram (ECG) may show ventricular arrhythmias or right ventricular hypertrophy. ◆ Pulse oximetry reveals decreasing arterial oxygen saturation. ◆ White blood cell count detects underlying infection.	◆ Monitor the patient for effects of oxygen therapy. ◆ Maintain a patent airway; prepare for endotracheal intubation, if indicated. ◆ In the intubated patient, suction, as needed, after hyperoxygenation. Observe for change in quantity, consistency, and color of sputum. ◆ Observe closely for respiratory arrest. ◆ Auscultate for chest sounds. ◆ Monitor ABG levels, and report changes immediately. ◆ Monitor serum electrolyte levels, and correct imbalances. ◆ Monitor fluid balance by recording intake and output or daily weight. ◆ Check cardiac monitor for arrhythmias. ◆ Administer antibiotics, corticosteroids, bronchodilators, vasopressors, and diuretics.
Diabetes mellitus (complication)	◆ Weight loss despite voracious hunger ◆ Weakness ◆ Vision changes ◆ Frequent skin and urinary tract infections ◆ Dry, itchy skin ◆ Poor skin turgor ◆ Dry mucous membranes ◆ Dehydration ◆ Decreased peripheral pulses ◆ Cool skin ◆ Decreased reflexes ◆ Orthostatic hypotension ◆ Muscle wasting ◆ Loss of subcutaneous fat ◆ Fruity breath odor because of ketoacidosis	◆ Two-hour postprandial blood glucose is 200 mg/dl or greater. ◆ Fasting blood glucose is 126 mg/dl or higher after at least an 8-hour fast.	◆ Monitor the patient's blood glucose level. ◆ Watch for signs of diabetic neuropathy (numbness or pain in the hands and feet, footdrop, impotence, neurogenic bladder). ◆ Watch for signs of infection (increased temperature), signs of cardiac distress (chest pain, palpitations, dyspnea, confusion), changes in vision, peripheral numbness or tingling, constipation, anorexia, and blisters or skin openings (particularly on the feet). ◆ Monitor serum potassium levels when administering diuretics because thiazide and loop diuretics promote potassium excretion. ◆ Monitor intake and output, and watch for signs of dehydration. ◆ Review with the patient foods that are high and low in sodium and potassium. ◆ Administer oral antidiabetics and injectable insulin.
Heart failure (complication)	*Left-sided heart failure* ◆ Dyspnea ◆ Orthopnea ◆ Paroxysmal nocturnal dyspnea ◆ Fatigue ◆ Nonproductive cough ◆ Crackles ◆ Hemoptysis ◆ Tachycardia ◆ Third (S_3) and fourth (S_4) heart sounds ◆ Cool, pale skin ◆ Restlessness ◆ Confusion	◆ Chest X-rays may show pulmonary vascular markings, interstitial edema, or pleural effusion and cardiomegaly. ◆ ECG may indicate hypertrophy, ischemic changes, or infarction and may reveal tachycardia and extrasystoles. ◆ Liver function tests are abnormal. ◆ Blood urea nitrogen (BUN) and creatinine levels are elevated. ◆ Prothrombin time is prolonged.	◆ Place patient in Fowler's position and give supplemental oxygen. ◆ Administer angiotensin-converting inhibitors, digoxin, diuretics, beta-adrenergic blockers, inotropic agents, nesiritide, nitrates, and morphine. ◆ Weigh the patient daily. ◆ Check for peripheral edema.

(continued)

DISORDER	SIGNS AND SYMPTOMS	DIAGNOSTIC TEST RESULTS	TREATMENT AND CARE
Heart failure (complication) (continued)	*Right-sided heart failure* ◆ Jugular vein distention ◆ Positive hepatojugular reflex ◆ Right upper quadrant pain ◆ Anorexia, nausea ◆ Nocturia ◆ Weight gain ◆ Edema ◆ Ascites or anasarca	◆ B-natriuretic peptide assay may be elevated. ◆ Echocardiography may reveal left ventricular hypertrophy, dilation, and abnormal contractility. ◆ Pulmonary artery pressure, pulmonary artery wedge pressure, and left ventricular end-diastolic pressure are elevated in left-sided heart failure; right atrial or central venous pressure is elevated in right-sided heart failure. ◆ Radionuclide ventriculography may reveal ejection fraction less than 40% in diastolic dysfunction.	◆ Monitor intake and output, vital signs, and mental status. ◆ Auscultate for S_3 and crackles or rhonchi. ◆ Monitor BUN; creatinine; and serum potassium, sodium, chloride, and magnesium levels. ◆ Institute continuous cardiac monitoring to identify and treat arrhythmias promptly.
Liver failure (complication)	◆ Ascites ◆ Shortness of breath ◆ Right upper quadrant tenderness ◆ Jaundice ◆ Nausea and anorexia ◆ Fatigue and weight loss ◆ Pruritus ◆ Oliguria ◆ Splenomegaly ◆ Peripheral edema ◆ Varices ◆ Weight loss	◆ Liver function studies reveal elevated aspartate aminotransferase, alanine aminotransferase, alkaline phosphatase, and bilirubin levels. ◆ Blood studies reveal anemia, impaired red blood cell production, elevated bleeding and clotting times, low blood glucose levels, and increased serum ammonia levels. ◆ Urine osmolarity is increased. ◆ Liver scan may show filling defects.	◆ Provide meals low in protein and high in carbohydrates. ◆ Auscultate lung sounds for crackles, rhonchi, or stridor. Observe for any signs of airway obstruction including labored breathing, severe hoarseness, and dyspnea. ◆ Administer supplemental humidified oxygen. ◆ Monitor oxygen saturation with continuous pulse oximetry and serial ABG studies for evidence of hypoxemia and respiratory acidosis. ◆ Anticipate the need for endotracheal intubation and mechanical ventilation should the patient's respiratory status deteriorate. ◆ Administer I.V. fluid therapy. Obtain laboratory specimens to assess for drug, electrolytes, and glucose levels. Anticipate administering normal saline solution and vasopressors if the patient is hypotensive, or dextrose 5% in water if the patient is hypoglycemic. ◆ Maintain salt restriction, and administer potassium-sparing diuretics if the patient has ascites. ◆ For the patient who has a history of chronic alcohol abuse, use of dextrose solutions may precipitate Wernicke-Korsakoff syndrome, a thiamine deficiency with severe neurologic impairment. ◆ Place the patient in semi-Fowler's position to maximize chest expansion. Keep the patient as quiet and comfortable as possible to minimize oxygen demands. ◆ Monitor for encephalopathy; lactulose may provide palliative treatment.

DISORDER	SIGNS AND SYMPTOMS	DIAGNOSTIC TEST RESULTS	TREATMENT AND CARE
Malnutrition (complication)	◆ Generalized malnutrition ◆ Diarrhea ◆ Steatorrhea ◆ Flatulence and abdominal discomfort ◆ Nocturia ◆ Weakness and fatigue ◆ Edema ◆ Amenorrhea ◆ Anemia ◆ Glossitis ◆ Peripheral neuropathy ◆ Bruising ◆ Bone pain ◆ Skeletal deformities ◆ Fractures ◆ Tetany ◆ Paresthesia	◆ Stool specimen for fat reveals excretion of greater than 6 g of fat/day. ◆ D-xylose absorption test shows less than 20% of 25 g of D-xylose in the urine after 5 hours. ◆ Schilling test reveals deficiency of vitamin B_{12} absorption. ◆ Culture of duodenal and jejunal contents confirms bacterial overgrowth in the proximal bowel. ◆ GI barium studies show characteristic features of the small intestine. ◆ Small intestine biopsy reveals atrophy of the mucosal villi.	◆ Observe nutritional status and progress with daily calorie counts and weight checks. ◆ Evaluate the patient's tolerance to foods. ◆ Assess fluid status; record intake and output and the number of stools. ◆ Administer dietary supplements and vitamins. ◆ Assess for signs and symptoms of dehydration, such as dry skin and mucous membranes and poor skin turgor. ◆ Check serum electrolyte levels, and monitor coagulation studies. ◆ Assist with nutritional therapy, such as peripheral parenteral nutrition or total parenteral nutrition, and monitor for effects.

Decompression sickness LIFE-THREATENING DISORDER

OVERVIEW

◆ Involves a complex process called *dysbarism*, which results from changed barometric pressure
◆ Pressure increases as depth under the water increases—such as that experienced in free or assisted dives—which affects gases dissolved in the blood and areas of the body that have hollow spaces and viscous organs
◆ Incidence ranging from 4 per 100,000 to 15.4 per 100,000
◆ Classified as type I (mild), type II (serious), or as one that results in embolization

CAUSES

◆ Ascending from a dive too quickly
◆ Flying after diving

RISK FACTORS

◆ Inadequate decompression
◆ Surpassing no-decompression limits
◆ Increased depth and duration of dives
◆ Repeated dives
◆ Failure to take recommended safety stops during a dive
◆ Obesity
◆ Smoking
◆ Alcohol use
◆ Fatigue
◆ Age and gender (increased risk in males over age 42)
◆ Poor physical condition
◆ Dehydration
◆ Illness affecting lung or circulatory efficiency
◆ Previous musculoskeletal injury (scar tissue decreases diffusion)
◆ Cold water (vasoconstriction decreases nitrogen offloading)
◆ Heavy work (produces a vacuum effect in which tendon use causes gas pockets)
◆ Rough sea conditions
◆ Heated diving suits (can lead to dehydration)

PATHOPHYSIOLOGY

◆ The reduction in pressure that occurs during a too-rapid ascent at the end of a dive can release dissolved gases (in particular, nitrogen) from the tissues and blood, which form bubbles in the body, impacting organ systems.
◆ These bubbles can cause loss of cell function, mechanical compression, and stretching of the blood vessels and nerves and may also activate the blood coagulation system, releasing vasoactive substances, and act as emboli by blocking circulation. (See *Disorders affecting management of decompression sickness*, page 127.)

CARDIOVASCULAR SYSTEM

◆ Fluid shifts from the intravascular to extravascular spaces resulting in tachycardia and postural hypotension.
◆ Thrombi may form from activation of blood coagulation and release of vasoactive substances from cells lining the blood vessels.
◆ Bubble formation may result in a thrombus.
◆ Coronary artery embolization of gas bubbles can lead to myocardial infarction or arrhythmia.

NEUROLOGIC SYSTEM

◆ In deep water, nitrogen increasingly dissolves in the blood and, at higher partial pressures, it alters the electrical properties of cerebral cellular membranes, which causes an anesthetic effect (nitrogen narcosis).
◆ Alterations in reasoning, memory, response time, and problems, such as idea fixation, overconfidence, and calculation errors occur.
◆ Cerebral embolization of gas bubbles can result in stroke or seizures.

RESPIRATORY SYSTEM

◆ As the person ascends, lag occurs before saturated tissues release nitrogen back into the blood. Ascending too quickly causes dissolved nitrogen to return to a gaseous state while still in the blood or tissues, causing bubbles to form.
◆ Bubbles in the tissues cause local tissue dysfunction; if located in the blood, embolization results.
◆ Pulmonary overpressurization can cause large gas emboli to lodge in coronary, cerebral, and other systemic arterioles.

HISTORY

- One or more risk factors present
- Recent dive with symptoms occurring within 10 to 20 minutes after resurfacing
- Headache, dizziness, and profound anxiousness initially; later, more dramatic symptoms, including unresponsiveness, shock, and seizures

PHYSICAL FINDINGS

Type I decompression sickness

- Mild pains that resolve within 10 minutes of onset (niggles)
- Pruritus (skin bends)
- Skin rash (mottling or marbling of the skin, or a papular or plaquelike rash)
- Orange-peel skin (rarely)
- Pitting edema
- Anorexia, nausea
- Excessive fatigue
- Dull, deep, throbbing, toothache-type pain in a joint, tendon, or tissue (the bends)
- Limited limb movement with crunching sound when joint moved

Type II decompression sickness

- Symptoms mimicking spinal cord trauma (lower back pain progressing to paresis, paralysis, paresthesia, loss of sphincter control, girdle pain, or lower trunk pain)
- Headaches or vision disturbances
- Dizziness
- Tunnel vision
- Changes in mental status
- Nausea, vomiting, vertigo, nystagmus, tinnitus, and partial deafness
- Burning substernal discomfort on inspiration, nonproductive coughing that can become paroxysmal, and severe respiratory distress
- Subcutaneous emphysema
- Signs and symptoms of hypovolemic shock or arterial gas embolization
- Depending on where the gas emboli travel, possible signs and symptoms of myocardial infarction, stroke, and seizures

DIAGNOSTIC TEST RESULTS

- No specific diagnostic tests exist for decompression sickness; however, hyperbaric oxygen therapy may be useful in differential diagnosis.
- Laboratory studies, including blood glucose, electrolytes, oxygen saturation, ethanol level, and carboxyhemoglobin, can help determine the cause of mental status changes or shock.
- Chest X-ray may identify injury to the lungs and chest and show evidence of pneumothorax, pneumomediastinum, subcutaneous emphysema, pneumocranium, alveolar hemorrhage, and decreased pulmonary blood flow.
- Magnetic resonance imaging may reveal spinal lesions or localized decompression sickness injury.
- Electrocardiography determines cardiac status and identifies possible cardiac arrhythmias.

GENERAL

- Establishment of airway, breathing, and circulation; cardiopulmonary resuscitation, if indicated
- Hyperbaric oxygen therapy

DIET

- Oral fluids, as tolerated

ACTIVITY

- Minimal activity until decompressed

MEDICATIONS

- 100% oxygen therapy
- Aspirin
- Corticosteroids
- Over-the-counter pain relievers

WARNING *Don't administer opioids because they further depress the respiratory system.*

(continued)

NURSING CONSIDERATIONS

NURSING DIAGNOSES
- Anxiety
- Deficient fluid volume
- Fear
- Impaired gas exchange
- Ineffective breathing pattern

EXPECTED OUTCOMES
The patient will:
- express reduced levels of anxiety
- achieve and maintain adequate fluid volumes
- use support systems to assist with coping
- maintain adequate ventilation and oxygenation
- demonstrate effective breathing pattern.

NURSING INTERVENTIONS
- Monitor airway, breathing, and circulation.
- During recompression, advise the patient to alternate breathing oxygen for 5 minutes with breathing air for 5 minutes.
- Administer fluids or encourage oral fluid intake.
- Assess neurologic, cardiovascular, and respiratory status.
- Assist with transport to hyperbaric facility.

PATIENT TEACHING

Be sure to cover:
- disorder, diagnostic testing, and treatment
- medication administration, dosage, and possible adverse effects
- hyperbaric treatment
- need for diver education
- importance of follow-up care and clearance before diving again.

RESOURCES
Organizations
The Divers Alert Network (DAN): *www.diversalertnetwork.org*

Selected references
Holck, P., and Hunter, R. "NIHSS Applied to Cerebral Neurological Dive Injuries as a Tool for Dive Injury Severity Stratification," *Undersea & Hyperbaric Medicine* 33(4):271-80, July-August 2006.

McMullin, A.M. "Scuba Diving: What You and Your Patients Need to Know," *Cleveland Clinic Journal of Medicine* 73(8):711-16, August 2006.

Schipke, J., et al. "Decompression Sickness Following Breath-Hold Diving," *Research in Sports Medicine* 14(3):163-78, July-September 2006.

Strategies for Managing Multisystem Disorders. Philadelphia: Lippincott Williams & Wilkins, 2006.

Disorders affecting management of decompression sickness

This chart highlights disorders that affect the management of decompression sickness.

DISORDER	SIGNS AND SYMPTOMS	DIAGNOSTIC TEST RESULTS	TREATMENT AND CARE
Avascular necrosis (complication)	◆ Pain in extremity ◆ Decreased circulation distally ◆ Edema ◆ Warmth to site	◆ X-rays, computed tomography (CT) scan, and magnetic resonance imaging (MRI) may help differentiate diagnosis of avascular necrosis.	◆ Monitor extremities for adequate circulation, but handle extremity gently to avoid further trauma. ◆ Prepare the patient for surgery to alleviate condition. ◆ Monitor effects of antibiotics; also monitor for sepsis.
Dehydration (coexisting)	◆ Tachycardia ◆ Dry mucous membranes ◆ Poor skin turgor ◆ Decreased blood pressure ◆ Decreased urine output ◆ Lethargy ◆ Delayed capillary refill	◆ Urine specific gravity is elevated. ◆ Blood urea nitrogen (BUN) and creatinine are elevated. ◆ Completed blood count reveals elevated hematocrit.	◆ Encourage small amounts of oral fluids. ◆ Administer I.V. fluids. ◆ Administer electrolyte solutions, oral or I.V., to correct imbalances. ◆ Monitor vital signs, including central and peripheral pulses and capillary refill approximately every 15 minutes. ◆ Monitor neurologic status for increasing lethargy or seizures.
Intravascular volume depletion (complication)	◆ Shock (tachycardia, tachypnea, hypotension, decreased urine output)	◆ Elevated potassium, serum lactate, and BUN levels may be present in hypovolemic shock. ◆ Urine specific gravity is greater than 1.020; urine osmolality is increased. ◆ Blood pH and partial pressure of arterial oxygen is decreased; partial pressure of arterial carbon dioxide is increased.	◆ Ensure a patent airway and adequate circulation. Begin cardiopulmonary resuscitation (CPR). ◆ Monitor for signs of shock (tachycardia, hypotension, decreased pulmonary artery and central venous pressures, decreased urine output). ◆ Maintain I.V. therapy, and monitor effect of fluid bolus. ◆ Monitor electrolyte status and effects of electrolyte replacements. ◆ If the patient is awake and alert, rehydrate orally. ◆ Administer oxygen and monitor pulse oximetry.
Massive venous air embolism (complication)	◆ If in an extremity: decreased peripheral circulation, pain, discoloration ◆ If pulmonary or cardiac: shortness of breath, chest pain, tachycardia, tachypnea, respiratory distress ◆ If in cerebral circulation: signs of stroke (change in mental status, facial drooping, weakness of one side of the body)	◆ Chest X-ray, CT scan, and MRI may show evidence of air embolism. ◆ Arterial blood gas analysis may show decreased partial pressure of arterial oxygen, increased carbon dioxide level, and respiratory acidosis.	◆ Ensure a patent airway and adequate circulation. Begin CPR. ◆ Monitor for respiratory distress (dyspnea, shortness of breath, decreasing oxygen saturations). ◆ Monitor for signs of cardiovascular collapse (hypotension, tachycardia, diaphoresis, diminished pulse). ◆ Administer oxygen, and monitor the patient closely for its effects. ◆ Monitor the patient's neurologic status. ◆ Maintain patency of I.V. lines
Vascular occlusion (complication)	*Peripheral occlusion* ◆ Pain ◆ Pulselessness ◆ Pallor ◆ Paresthesia to extremity *Cardiac occlusion* ◆ Signs of myocardial infarction (chest pain, diaphoresis, shortness of breath) *Neurologic occlusion* ◆ Signs of stroke (change in mental status, facial drooping, weakness on one side of the body)	◆ Cardiac enzymes may reveal elevated CK-MB and troponin levels. ◆ A venogram may detect the specific site of occlusion.	◆ Monitor for signs of myocardial infarction, arrhythmias, stroke, and peripheral vascular occlusion. ◆ Maintain patency of I.V. lines. ◆ Monitor intake and output. ◆ Administer antiarrhythmics, and monitor the patient for their effects. ◆ Monitor the patient for changes in pulses and peripheral circulation. ◆ Administer oxygen and monitor pulse oximetry. ◆ Monitor effects of thrombolytics.

Diabetes mellitus

OVERVIEW

- Chronic disease of absolute or relative insulin deficiency or resistance
- Characterized by disturbances in carbohydrate, protein, and fat metabolism
- Two primary forms of diabetes mellitus (DM):
- Type 1: characterized by absolute insulin insufficiency; usually occurs before age 30, although it may occur at any age
- Type 2: characterized by insulin resistance with varying degrees of insulin secretory defects; usually occurs in obese adults after age 30, although it may be seen in obese North American youths of African-American, Native American, or Hispanic descent
- Affects about 8% of the population of the United States
- About one-third of patients with DM undiagnosed
- Incidence of type 2 diabetes increasing with age
- More common in males than in females

CAUSES

- Autoimmune disease (type 1)
- Genetic factors

RISK FACTORS

- Viral infections (type 1)
- Obesity (type 2)
- Physiologic or emotional stress
- Sedentary lifestyle (type 2)
- Pregnancy
- Medications, such as thiazide diuretics, adrenal corticosteroids, and hormonal contraceptives

PATHOPHYSIOLOGY

- In persons genetically susceptible to type 1 diabetes, a triggering event, possibly a viral infection, causes production of autoantibodies against the beta cells of the pancreas.
- The resultant destruction of the beta cells leads to a decline in and ultimate lack of insulin secretion.
- Insulin deficiency leads to hyperglycemia, enhanced lipolysis (decomposition of fat), and protein catabolism. These characteristics occur when more than 90% of the beta cells have been destroyed.
- Type 2 diabetes mellitus is caused by one or more of the following factors: impaired insulin secretion, inappropriate hepatic glucose production, or peripheral insulin receptor insensitivity.
- Insulin deficiency compromises the body tissues' access to essential nutrients for fuel and storage. (See *Disorders affecting management of diabetes mellitus,* pages 131 to 133.)

CARDIOVASCULAR SYSTEM

- Arterial thrombosis may develop due to persistent activated thrombogenic pathways and impaired fibrinolysis.

GASTROINTESTINAL SYSTEM

- Autonomic neuropathy leads to abdominal discomfort and pain, causing gastroparesis and constipation.
- Nausea, diarrhea, or constipation may develop due to dehydration, electrolyte imbalances, or autonomic neuropathy.

METABOLIC SYSTEM

- Impaired or absent insulin function prevents normal metabolism of carbohydrates, fats, and proteins, leading to weight loss.
- Muscle cramps, irritability, and emotional lability result from electrolyte imbalances.

NEUROLOGIC SYSTEM

- Low intracellular glucose levels may result in headaches, fatigue, lethargy, reduced energy levels, and impaired school and work performance.
- Vision changes, such as blurring, occur due to glucose-induced swelling.
- Numbness and tingling occur due to neural tissue damage.

RENAL SYSTEM

- Polyuria and polydipsia occur because of high serum osmolality caused by high serum glucose levels.

ASSESSMENT

HISTORY
- Polydipsia
- Polyuria, nocturia
- Polyphagia
- Dry mucous membranes
- Poor skin turgor
- Weight loss
- Weakness, fatigue
- Vision changes
- Frequent skin and urinary tract infections
- Dry, itchy skin
- Sexual problems
- Numbness or pain in the hands or feet
- Postprandial feeling of nausea or fullness
- Nocturnal diarrhea

Type 1
- Rapidly developing symptoms

Type 2
- Vague, long-standing symptoms that develop gradually
- Family history of DM
- Pregnancy
- Severe viral infection
- Other endocrine diseases
- Recent stress or trauma
- Use of drugs that increase blood glucose levels

PHYSICAL FINDINGS
- Retinopathy or cataract formation
- Skin changes, especially on the legs and feet
- Muscle wasting and loss of subcutaneous fat (type 1)
- Obesity, particularly in the abdominal area (type 2)
- Poor skin turgor
- Dry mucous membranes
- Decreased peripheral pulses
- Cool skin temperature
- Diminished deep tendon reflexes
- Orthostatic hypotension
- Characteristic "fruity" breath odor in ketoacidosis
- Signs and symptoms of hypovolemia and shock in severe ketoacidosis and hyperosmolar hyperglycemic state

DIAGNOSTIC TEST RESULTS
- Fasting plasma glucose level is greater than or equal to 126 mg/dl on at least two occasions.
- Random blood glucose level is greater than or equal to 200 mg/dl.
- Two-hour postprandial blood glucose level is greater than or equal to 200 mg/dl.
- Glycosylated hemoglobin (Hb A_{1C}) is increased.
- Urinalysis may show acetone or glucose.
- Ophthalmologic examination may show diabetic retinopathy.

TREATMENT

GENERAL
- American Diabetes Association recommendations to reach target glucose, Hb A_{1C} lipid, and blood pressure levels
- Tight glycemic control for prevention of complications
- Self-monitoring of capillary glucose levels

DIET
- Modest caloric restriction for weight loss or maintenance

ACTIVITY
- Regular aerobic exercise

MEDICATIONS
- Exogenous insulin (type 1 or possibly type 2)
- Oral antihyperglycemic drugs (type 2)

SURGERY
- Pancreas transplantation

(continued)

NURSING DIAGNOSES

◆ Deficient fluid volume
◆ Disabled family coping
◆ Disturbed sensory perception: Tactile, visual
◆ Imbalanced nutrition: Less than body requirements
◆ Imbalanced nutrition: More than body requirements
◆ Impaired skin integrity
◆ Impaired urinary elimination
◆ Ineffective coping
◆ Ineffective tissue perfusion: Cardiopulmonary, peripheral, renal
◆ Risk for infection
◆ Risk for injury
◆ Sexual dysfunction

EXPECTED OUTCOMES

The patient will:
◆ maintain adequate fluid balance
◆ develop adequate coping mechanisms and support systems
◆ maintain optimal functioning within the confines of the tactile and visual impairment
◆ maintain daily calorie requirements
◆ maintain weight within an acceptable range
◆ maintain skin integrity
◆ have balanced intake and output
◆ demonstrate adaptive coping behaviors
◆ exhibit signs of adequate cardiopulmonary, peripheral, and renal perfusion
◆ remain free from signs and symptoms of infection
◆ remain free from injury
◆ discuss feelings about sexual impairment.

NURSING INTERVENTIONS

◆ Give prescribed drugs.
◆ Give rapidly absorbed carbohydrates for hypoglycemia or, if the patient is unconscious, glucagon or I.V. dextrose, as ordered.
◆ Administer I.V. fluids and insulin replacement for hyperglycemic crisis, as ordered.
◆ Provide meticulous skin care, especially to the feet and legs.

◆ Treat all injuries, cuts, and blisters immediately.
◆ Avoid constricting hose, slippers, or bed linens.
◆ Encourage adequate fluid intake.
◆ Encourage verbalization of feelings.
◆ Offer emotional support.
◆ Help patient to develop effective coping strategies.
◆ Monitor vital signs, intake and output, daily weight.
◆ Monitor serum glucose, urine acetone, and electrolytes.
◆ Assess renal and cardiovascular status facility policy and clinical status.
◆ Observe for signs and symptoms of:
– hypoglycemia
– hyperglycemia
– hyperosmolar coma
– urinary tract and vaginal infections
– diabetic neuropathy.

Be sure to cover:
◆ disorder, diagnostic testing, and treatment
◆ medication administration, dosage, and possible adverse effects
◆ when to notify the practitioner
◆ prescribed meal plan
◆ prescribed exercise program
◆ signs and symptoms of:
– infection
– hypoglycemia
– hyperglycemia
– diabetic neuropathy
◆ self-monitoring of blood glucose
◆ complications of hyperglycemia
◆ foot care
◆ annual regular ophthalmologic examinations
◆ safety precautions
◆ management of diabetes during illness
◆ available resource and support services.

RESOURCES

Organizations

American Diabetes Association: *www.diabetes.org*
Juvenile Diabetes Research Foundation International: *www.jdf.org*
National Institute of Diabetes, Digestive, and Kidney Diseases: *www.niddk.nih.gov*

Selected references

Delmas, L. "Best Practices in the Assessment and Management of Diabetic Foot Ulcers," *Rehabilitation Nursing* 31(6):228-34, November-December 2006.
Gallegos, E.C., et al. "Metabolic Control of Adults with Type 2 Diabetes Mellitus through Education and Counseling," *Journal of Nursing Scholarship* 38(4):344-51, 2006.
Miller, C. "Using Standards of Care to Drive Evidence-Based Clinical Practice and Outcomes for Diabetes Mellitus," *Home Healthcare Nurse* 24(5):307-12, May 2006.
Wien, M. "A Review of Macronutrient Considerations for Persons with Prediabetes," *Topics in Clinical Nutrition* 21(2):64-75, April-June 2006.

Disorders affecting management of diabetes mellitus

This chart highlights disorders that affect the management of diabetes mellitus.

DISORDER	SIGNS AND SYMPTOMS	DIAGNOSTIC TEST RESULTS	TREATMENT AND CARE
Coronary artery disease (complication)	◆ Angina or feeling of burning, squeezing, or tightness in the chest that may radiate to the left arm, neck, jaw, or shoulder blade ◆ Nausea and vomiting ◆ Cool extremities and pallor ◆ Diaphoresis ◆ Xanthelasma (fat deposits on the eyelids)	◆ Electrocardiogram (ECG) may be normal between anginal episodes. During angina, it may show ischemic changes (T-wave inversion, ST-segment depression, arrhythmias). ◆ Computed tomography may identify calcium deposits in coronary arteries. ◆ Stress testing may detect ST-segment changes during exercise or pharmacologic stress. ◆ Coronary angiography reveals location and degree of stenosis, obstruction, and collateral circulation. ◆ Intravascular ultrasound may define coronary anatomy and luminal narrowing. ◆ Myocardial perfusion imaging detects ischemic areas as cold spots. ◆ Stress echocardiography shows abnormal wall motion in ischemic areas. ◆ Rest perfusion imaging rules out myocardial infarction.	◆ During anginal attacks, monitor the patient's blood pressure and heart rate. Obtain an ECG during the episode and before administering nitroglycerin or other nitrates. Record duration of pain, amount of medication required to relieve it, and accompanying symptoms. ◆ Keep nitroglycerine available for immediate use. Instruct the patient to call immediately whenever he feels chest, arm, or neck pain. ◆ Before cardiac catheterization, explain the procedure and reinforce learning of the procedure. ◆ After catheterization, review recommended treatment. Check distal pulses, and monitor catheter site for bleeding. To counter diuretic effect of the dye, make sure the patient drinks plenty of fluids. Assess potassium levels. ◆ If the patient is scheduled for surgery, explain the procedure and reinforce teaching. ◆ Administer nitrates, beta-adrenergic blockers, calcium channel blockers, antiplatelets, antilipemics, and antihypertensives. ◆ After surgery, monitor blood pressure, intake and output, breath sounds, chest tube drainage, and ECG. Monitor for arrhythmias. Give vigorous chest physiotherapy. ◆ Before discharge, stress the need to follow the prescribed drug regimen, exercise program, and diet.
Diabetic ketoacidosis (complication)	◆ Acetone breath ◆ Dehydration ◆ Weak and rapid pulse ◆ Kussmaul's respirations	◆ Blood glucose level is slightly above normal. ◆ Serum ketone level is elevated. ◆ Serum potassium is normal or elevated initially and then drops. ◆ Urine glucose is positive; urine acetone is high. ◆ Serum phosphorus, magnesium, and chloride are decreased. ◆ Serum osmolality is slightly elevated, ranging from 300 to 350 mOsm/L. ◆ Hematocrit is slightly elevated. ◆ Arterial blood gas (ABG) analysis reveals metabolic acidosis. ◆ ECG shows arrhythmias.	◆ Assess level of consciousness (LOC) and maintain airway patency. ◆ Monitor vital signs at least every 15 minutes initially and then hourly, as indicated; monitor hemodynamic status. ◆ Institute continuous cardiac monitoring and treat arrhythmias. ◆ Administer I.V. replacement therapy with normal saline to correct fluid deficit; dextrose may be added to prevent hypoglycemia. ◆ Administer regular insulin I.V., as ordered; monitor blood glucose levels and serum electrolyte levels frequently. ◆ Anticipate potassium replacement after insulin therapy is initiated; replace electrolytes, as needed. ◆ If the patient is comatose, obtunded, or vomiting, insert a nasogastric (NG) tube to suction. ◆ Monitor the patient for signs of complications, such as infection, diabetic neuropathy, and hypoglycemia. ◆ Perform teaching regarding treatment regimen for diabetes; enlist the assistance of a diabetes educator and nutritionist, as needed.

(continued)

DISORDER	SIGNS AND SYMPTOMS	DIAGNOSTIC TEST RESULTS	TREATMENT AND CARE
Hyperosmolar hyperglycemic nonketotic syndrome (complication)	◆ Polyuria ◆ Thirst ◆ Neurologic abnormalities ◆ Stupor	◆ Blood glucose is markedly elevated above normal, usually greater than 800 mg/dl. ◆ Urine acetone is negative; serum ketones are negative. ◆ Urine glucose is positive. ◆ Serum osmolality is elevated, usually above 350 mOsm/L. ◆ Serum electrolyte levels reveal hypokalemia, hypophosphatemia, hypomagnesemia, and hypochloremia. ◆ Serum creatinine and blood urea nitrogen (BUN) are elevated. ◆ Hematocrit is slightly elevated.	◆ Assess LOC and maintain a patent airway. ◆ Monitor vital signs at least every 15 minutes initially and then hourly, as indicated; monitor hemodynamic status. ◆ Institute continuous cardiac monitoring, and treat arrhythmias. ◆ Administer I.V. replacement therapy with isotonic or half-normal saline to correct fluid deficit. ◆ Administer regular insulin I.V.; monitor blood glucose levels and serum electrolyte levels frequently. ◆ Replace electrolytes, as necessary, according to laboratory studies. ◆ If the patient is comatose, obtunded, or vomiting, insert an NG tube to suction. ◆ Assess peripheral circulation. ◆ Perform range-of-motion exercises every 2 hours; use intermittent pneumatic sequential compression devices. ◆ Assess for hypoglycemia, diabetic neuropathy, or signs of infection. ◆ Consult a dietitian to plan a recommended diet; enlist assistance of a diabetes educator.
Hypertension (complication)	◆ Usually asymptomatic ◆ Elevated blood pressure readings on at least two consecutive occasions ◆ Occipital headache ◆ Epistaxis ◆ Bruits ◆ Dizziness, confusion, fatigue ◆ Blurry vision ◆ Nocturia ◆ Edema	◆ Serial blood pressure measurements reveal elevations of 140/90 mm Hg or greater on two or more separate occasions. ◆ Urinalysis may show protein, casts, red blood cells, or white blood cells. ◆ BUN and serum creatinine are elevated. ◆ Complete blood count may reveal polycythemia or anemia. ◆ Excretory urography may reveal renal atrophy. ◆ ECG may show left ventricular hypertrophy or ischemia. ◆ Chest X-rays may show cardiomegaly. ◆ Echocardiography may reveal left ventricular hypertrophy.	◆ Monitor blood pressure, the patient's response to antihypertensives, and laboratory studies. ◆ Encourage a reduced-sodium diet. ◆ Monitor for complications of hypertension, such as signs of stroke or myocardial infarction and renal disease. ◆ Administer thiazide diuretics, angiotensin-converting enzyme inhibitors, angiotensin receptor blockers, beta-adrenergic blockers, and calcium channel blockers.
Hypoglycemia (complication)	◆ Decreased LOC ◆ Shakiness ◆ Sweating ◆ Numbness and tingling of extremities ◆ Hunger ◆ Irritability, anxiety	◆ Blood glucose level is less than normal.	◆ Monitor blood glucose level. ◆ Administer dextrose 50% I.V. if the patient is unable to eat or drink. ◆ Give the patient juice and carbohydrates (such as crackers) if the patient is awake and alert. ◆ Assess for the cause of hypoglycemia (such as extreme exercise, taking antidiabetic medication without eating, or illness).

DISORDER	SIGNS AND SYMPTOMS	DIAGNOSTIC TEST RESULTS	TREATMENT AND CARE
Pneumonia (complication)	◆ Coughing, sputum production ◆ Pleuritic chest pain ◆ Shaking chills and fever ◆ Possible crackles	◆ Chest X-ray shows infiltrates. ◆ Sputum smear shows acute inflammatory cells. ◆ Positive blood cultures in patients with infiltrates suggest sepsis. ◆ Transtracheal aspirate of secretions or bronchoscopy are positive for organisms.	◆ Maintain a patent airway and adequate oxygenation. Measure ABG levels. ◆ Teach the patient to deep breathe and cough effectively. ◆ Assist with endotracheal intubation or tracheostomy, as necessary; suction to remove secretions. ◆ Obtain sputum specimens, as directed, and monitor for results; administer antibiotics, as needed, and record the patient's response to treatment. ◆ Maintain hydration and treat fever; fluid and electrolyte replacement may be necessary. ◆ Maintain adequate nutrition; supplemental oral feedings or parenteral nutrition may be needed; monitor intake and output. ◆ Dispose of secretions properly. ◆ Administer appropriate antibiotics.
Retinopathy (complication)	◆ Progressive blindness or loss of vision	◆ Indirect ophthalmoscopy shows retinal changes, such as microaneurysms, retinal hemorrhages, edema, venous dilation exudates, and vitreous hemorrhage. ◆ Fluorescein angiography shows leakage of fluorescein from new blood vessels and differentiates between microaneurysms and true hemorrhages. ◆ History reveals long-standing diabetes and decreased vision.	◆ Carefully control blood glucose levels, and monitor levels closely. ◆ If the patient complains of sudden, unilateral vision loss, arrange for immediate ophthalmologic evaluation. ◆ Monitor blood pressure. ◆ Encourage the patient to comply with the prescribed regimen for treating diabetes. ◆ Assist with laser photocoagulation, which cauterizes the leaking blood vessels and eliminates the cause of the edema, as needed.
Wound infection (complication	◆ Wound that doesn't heal properly ◆ Foul discharge and inflammation at wound site ◆ Fever	◆ Culture confirms wound infection.	◆ Administer appropriate antibiotics, and monitor the patient for their effects. ◆ Maintain hydration and treat fever; fluid and electrolyte replacement may be necessary. ◆ Maintain adequate nutrition; supplemental oral feedings or parenteral nutrition may be needed; monitor intake and output. ◆ Perform dressing changes, and look for signs of healing; debridement may be necessary.

◣ Disseminated intravascular coagulation LIFE-THREATENING DISORDER

OVERVIEW

- Syndrome of activated coagulation characterized by bleeding or thrombosis
- Complicates diseases and conditions that accelerate clotting, causing occlusion of small blood vessels, organ necrosis, depletion of circulating clotting factors and platelets, and activation of the fibrinolytic system
- Mortality rate greater than 50%
- Also known as *DIC, consumption coagulopathy,* and *defibrination syndrome*

CAUSES

- Disorders that produce necrosis, such as extensive burns and trauma
- Infection, sepsis
- Neoplastic disease
- Obstetric complications
- Other disorders, such as heat stroke, shock, incompatible blood transfusion, drug reactions, cardiac arrest, surgery necessitating cardiopulmonary bypass, acute respiratory distress syndrome, diabetic ketoacidosis, pulmonary embolism, and sickle cell anemia

PATHOPHYSIOLOGY

- Typical accelerated clotting results in generalized activation of prothrombin and a consequent excess of thrombin. (See *Three mechanisms of DIC.*)
- Excess thrombin converts fibrinogen to fibrin, producing fibrin clots in the microcirculation.
- This process consumes exorbitant amounts of coagulation factors (especially platelets, factor V, prothrombin, fibrinogen, and factor VIII), causing thrombocytopenia, deficiencies in factors V and VIII, hypoprothrombinemia, and hypofibrinogenemia.
- Circulating thrombin activates the fibrinolytic system, which lyses fibrin clots into fibrinogen degradation products (FDPs).
- The hemorrhage that occurs may be due largely to the anticoagulant activity of FDPs and depletion of plasma coagulation factors. (See *Disorders affecting management of DIC,* page 137.)

NEUROLOGIC SYSTEM

- Cerebral hemorrhage may occur and result in neurologic dysfunction due to decreased perfusion and increased intracerebral pressure.

CARDIOVASCULAR SYSTEM

- Fibrin deposition in small and midsize vessels may lead to ischemia and necrosis and cause clinical dysfunction of that particular organ due to decreased perfusion.
- Pain may occur in a specific area of ischemia, such as chest pain or limb pain.
- Hypovolemic shock may result from uncontrolled hemorrhage.

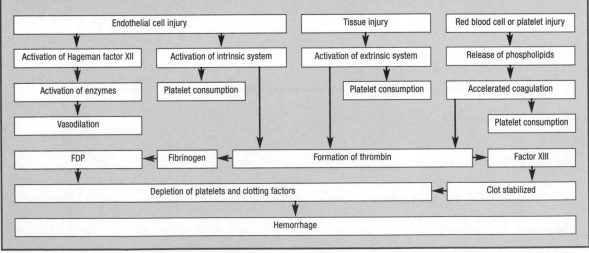

Three mechanisms of DIC

However disseminated intravascular coagulation (DIC) begins, accelerated clotting (characteristic of DIC) usually results in excess thrombin, which in turn causes fibrinolysis with excess fibrin formation and fibrin degradation products (FDP), activation of fibrin-stabilizing factor (factor XIII), consumption of platelet and clotting factors, and, eventually, hemorrhage.

RESPIRATORY SYSTEM

◆ Microemboli may cause obstruction of pulmonary vessels, resulting in pulmonary emboli.
◆ Hemorrhage may cause decreased circulating oxygen, resulting in respiratory failure.

RENAL SYSTEM

◆ Disruption of adequate perfusion of kidneys may cause acute renal failure.

HISTORY

◆ Abnormal bleeding without a history of a serious hemorrhagic disorder; bleeding that may occur at all bodily orifices
◆ Possible presence of one of the causes of DIC
◆ Possible signs of bleeding into the skin, such as cutaneous oozing, petechiae, ecchymoses, and hematomas
◆ Possible bleeding from surgical or invasive procedure sites, such as incisions or venipuncture sites
◆ Possible nausea and vomiting; severe muscle, back, and abdominal pain; chest pain; hemoptysis; epistaxis; seizures; and oliguria
◆ Possible GI bleeding, hematuria

PHYSICAL FINDINGS

◆ Petechiae
◆ Acrocyanosis
◆ Dyspnea, tachypnea
◆ Mental status changes, including confusion

DIAGNOSTIC TEST RESULTS

◆ Serum platelet count is decreased (less than 150,000/ml).
◆ Serum fibrinogen level is decreased (less than 170 mg/dl).
◆ Prothrombin time is prolonged (more than 19 seconds).
◆ Partial thromboplastin time is prolonged (more than 40 seconds).
◆ FDPs are increased (commonly greater than 45 mcg/ml, or positive at less than 1:100 dilution).
◆ Result of D-dimer test (specific fibrinogen test for DIC) is positive at less than 1:8 dilution.
◆ Blood clotting factors V and VIII are diminished.
◆ Complete blood count shows hemoglobin levels less than 10 g/dl.
◆ Blood urea nitrogen level is elevated (greater than 25 mg/dl), and serum creatinine levels are elevated (greater than 1.3 mg/dl).

GENERAL

◆ Treatment of the underlying condition
◆ Possibly, supportive care alone if the patient isn't actively bleeding

DIET

◆ No restrictions

ACTIVITY

◆ As tolerated

MEDICATIONS
For active bleeding

◆ Administration of blood, fresh frozen plasma, platelets, or packed red blood cells
◆ Cryoprecipitate
◆ Antithrombin III
◆ Fluid replacement

(continued)

NURSING DIAGNOSES

♦ Acute pain
♦ Anxiety
♦ Fatigue
♦ Fear
♦ Impaired gas exchange
♦ Impaired physical mobility
♦ Impaired tissue integrity
♦ Ineffective tissue perfusion: Cerebral, GI, renal
♦ Risk for deficient fluid volume
♦ Risk for injury

EXPECTED OUTCOMES

The patient will:

♦ express feelings of increased comfort and decreased pain
♦ verbalize strategies to reduce anxiety level
♦ express feelings of energy and decreased fatigue
♦ use available support systems to assist in coping with fears
♦ maintain adequate ventilation and oxygenation
♦ perform activities of daily living with the maximum level of mobility and independence
♦ have reduced redness, swelling, and pain at the site of impaired tissue
♦ maintain a blood pressure high enough to maintain cerebral, GI, and renal perfusion pressure but low enough to prevent intracranial bleeding and cerebral swelling
♦ maintain fluid balance
♦ remain free from injury.

NURSING INTERVENTIONS

♦ Provide emotional support.
♦ Provide adequate rest periods.
♦ Give prescribed analgesics, as necessary.
♦ Reposition the patient every 2 hours, and provide meticulous skin care.
♦ Give prescribed oxygen therapy.

⚡ **WARNING** *To prevent clots from dislodging and causing fresh bleeding, don't vigorously rub the affected areas when bathing.*

♦ Protect the patient from injury.

♦ If bleeding occurs, use pressure and topical hemostatic agents to control bleeding.
♦ Limit venipunctures whenever possible.
♦ Watch for transfusion reactions and signs of fluid overload.
♦ Measure the amount of blood lost, weigh dressings and linen, and record drainage.
♦ Weigh the patient daily, particularly with renal involvement.
♦ Monitor vital signs, pulse oximetry, and results of serial blood studies.
♦ Observe for signs of shock.
♦ Monitor intake and output, especially when administering blood products.

Be sure to cover (with the patient and his family):

♦ disorder, diagnostic testing, and treatment
♦ medication administration, dosage, and possible adverse effects
♦ signs and symptoms of bleeding
♦ follow-up care.

RESOURCES

Organizations

American Heart Association: *www.americanheart.org*
Mayo Clinic: *www.mayoclinic.com*

Selected references

Kasper, D.L., et al., eds. *Harrison's Principles of Internal Medicine,* 16th ed. New York: McGraw-Hill Book Co., 2005.

Nguyen, T.C., and Carcillo, J.A. "Bench-to-Bedside: Thrombocytopenia-Associated Multiple Organ Failure: A Newly Appreciated Syndrome in the Critically Ill," *Critical Care* 10(6):235, November 2006.

Weidermann, C.J., and Kaneider, N.C. "A Systematic Review of Antithrombin Concentrate Use in Patients with Disseminated Intravascular Coagulation of Severe Sepsis," *Blood Coagulation & Fibrinolysis* 17(7):521-26, October 2006.

Disorders affecting management of DIC

This chart highlights disorders that affect the management of disseminated intravascular coagulation (DIC).

DISORDER	SIGNS AND SYMPTOMS	DIAGNOSTIC TEST RESULTS	TREATMENT AND CARE
Deep vein thrombophlebitis (complication)	◆ Homans' sign elicited ◆ Severe pain in affected extremity ◆ Fever, chills ◆ Malaise ◆ Swelling and cyanosis of the affected extremity ◆ Affected area possibly warm to touch	◆ Doppler ultrasonography identifies reduced blood flow to the area of the thrombus and any obstruction to venous blood flow. ◆ Plethysmography shows decreased circulation distal to the affected area. ◆ Plebography (also called *venography*) shows filling defects and diverted blood flow and usually confirms the diagnosis.	◆ Administer anticoagulants and monitor for adverse effects, such as bleeding, dark tarry stools, and coffee-ground vomitus. ◆ Assess pulses, skin color, and temperature of the affected extremity. ◆ Measure and record the circumference of the affected extremity. ◆ Perform range-of-motion exercises with the unaffected extremities and turn the patient every 2 hours. ◆ Apply warm soaks to improve circulation and relieve pain and inflammation. ◆ Assess for signs of pulmonary emboli.
Hypovolemic shock (complication)	◆ Pallor ◆ Decreased level of consciousness (LOC) ◆ Hypotension ◆ Tachycardia ◆ Cool, clammy skin ◆ Urine output less than 25 ml/hr	◆ Central venous pressure, pulmonary wedge pressure, and cardiac output are decreased. ◆ Hematocrit, hemoglobin, and red blood cell and platelet counts are low. ◆ Serum potassium, sodium, lactic dehydrogenase, blood urea nitrogen, and creatinine are elevated. ◆ Urine specific gravity is increased. ◆ Arterial blood gas (ABG) analysis shows respiratory acidosis.	◆ Assess extent of fluid loss. ◆ Administer fluid and blood replacement. ◆ Administer supplemental oxygen. ◆ Monitor vital signs and intake and output. ◆ Monitor respiratory status and pulse oximetry. ◆ Assist with endotracheal intubation, if necessary. ◆ Prepare the patient for surgery to control bleeding.
Sepsis (complication)	◆ Agitation ◆ Anxiety ◆ Altered LOC ◆ Tachycardia ◆ Hypotension ◆ Rapid, shallow respirations ◆ Fever ◆ Urine output less than 25 ml/hr	◆ Blood cultures are positive for the infecting organism. ◆ Complete blood count reveals whether anemia, neutropenia, and thrombocytopenia are present. ◆ ABG studies show metabolic acidosis. ◆ Blood urea nitrogen and creatinine levels are increased. ◆ Electrocardiography shows ST-segment depression, inverted T waves, and arrhythmias.	◆ Identify and treat underlying cause of sepsis. ◆ Monitor vital signs frequently. ◆ Administer antibiotics. ◆ Administer I.V. fluids to replace intravascular volume. ◆ Administer vasopressors if fluid resuscitation doesn't maintain blood pressure. ◆ Assess respiratory status. ◆ Prepare for intubation and mechanical ventilation, if needed.

Drug overdose LIFE-THREATENING DISORDER

OVERVIEW

- Results from ingestion of a drug through inhalation, injection, or direct absorption through the skin and mucous membranes
- May also occur as a result of impaired drug clearance, creating toxic drug levels
- Most commonly involves ingestion of more than recommended amount of prescription or over-the-counter medications
- Also referred to as *drug poisoning* or *drug toxicity*

CAUSES
- Accidental ingestion
- Intentional ingestion

RISK FACTORS
- Age
- Inadequate knowledge of medication
- Polypharmacy
- Drug addiction
- Depression
- Organ dysfunction, causing impaired drug clearance

PATHOPHYSIOLOGY

- The effects of drug overdose depend on:
- type of substance ingested
- amount of substance ingested
- patient's tolerance to the toxin
- number of toxins ingested
- time between ingestion and treatment.
- Changes produced by a drug overdose commonly result from an exaggeration of the drug's normal therapeutic and adverse effects.
- Synergistic effects occur when a drug combination produces a response that's greater than the response that would occur if the drugs were taken alone.
- Antagonistic effects occur when the combined response of a drug combination is less than the response produced by either drug alone.
- Some toxins, such as acetaminophen and ethylene glycol, have organ-

specific toxic effects. (See *Understanding specific drug toxicities.* Also see *Disorders affecting management of a drug overdose,* pages 142 and 143.)

CARDIOVASCULAR SYSTEM
- Hypotension and arrhythmias occur after ingestion of beta-adrenergic blockers and calcium channel blockers.

NERVOUS SYSTEM
- Depressed level of consciousness (LOC) typically occurs after ingestion of sedatives and opioids.

RESPIRATORY SYSTEM
- Hypoventilation typically occurs after ingestion of sedatives and opioids.

ASSESSMENT

HISTORY
- One or more risk factors present
- Evidence of ingestion of drugs

PHYSICAL FINDINGS
- Dilated pupils
- Tremors or seizures
- Possible coma or posturing neurologically
- Rapid respirations, Kussmaul's respirations, or no respirations
- Hypotension
- Cardiac arrhythmia or cardiac arrest
- Diaphoretic, pink-tinged, or cyanotic skin
- Dry mouth, diarrhea, nausea, vomiting, or hematemesis (see *Assessing drug overdose,* pages 140 and 141)

DIAGNOSTIC TEST RESULTS
- Toxicologic studies of the mouth, vomitus, urine, stool, blood, or the victim's hands or clothing confirm the diagnosis.
- Drug screens identify the toxin and amount. If possible, the family or patient should bring the container of the ingested substance to the facility for a comparable study.

- Abdominal X-rays may reveal iron pills or other radiopaque substances such as calcium, enteric-coated aspirin, and phenothiazine.
- Arterial blood gas levels aid in ruling out hypoxia, hypercapnia, and metabolic acidosis as the cause of the patient's altered LOC.
- Blood glucose level aids in ruling out hypoglycemia as the cause of the patient's altered LOC.
- Electrocardiography reveals ischemia, arrhythmias, and widened QRS complexes associated with cyclic antidepressant therapy.
- Serum electrolyte levels reveal high anion gap (associated with methanol, ethylene glycol, iron, and salicylate toxicity); low anion gap (associated with lithium toxicity); hyperkalemia (associated with ethylene glycol and methanol toxicity); hypokalemia (associated with loop diuretics and salicylate toxicity); and hypocalcemia (associated with ethylene glycol toxicity).
- Complete blood count may reveal leukocytosis secondary to ethylene glycol toxicity.
- Coagulation studies may reveal prolonged coagulation times suggesting warfarin toxicity.

TREATMENT

GENERAL
- Emergency resuscitation; support for the patient's airway, breathing, and circulation
- Gastric lavage for patients who have ingested a potentially lethal amount of drug or toxin and present within 1 hour of ingestion
- Dialysis, if indicated
- Psychiatric evaluation and intervention, if appropriate

DIET
- Nothing by mouth if LOC altered

ACTIVITY
- Based on effects of overdose

MEDICATIONS

- Administration of an antidote, if available
- Activated charcoal
- Cathartics, such as sorbitol, magnesium citrate, or magnesium sulfate
- Diuretic

NURSING CONSIDERATIONS

NURSING DIAGNOSES

- Decreased cardiac output
- Ineffective airway clearance
- Ineffective breathing pattern
- Risk for aspiration
- Risk for injury
- Risk for suicide

EXPECTED OUTCOMES

The patient will:
- maintain adequate cardiac output

UP CLOSE

Understanding specific drug toxicities

ACETAMINOPHEN

Acetaminophen, the active ingredient in many over-the-counter analgesics and antipyretics, is the most commonly reported pharmaceutical ingestion in adults and children. The drug is rapidly absorbed and metabolized in the liver. Normally, a small amount of acetaminophen (less than 5%) is metabolized to a toxic intermediate metabolite, N-acetyl-para-benzoquinoneimine (NAPQI), which is further metabolized by glutathione to nontoxic products.

NAPQI is a powerful oxidizing agent that leads to cell death by bonding to cellular proteins. After an acute single toxic dose (7.5 g in an adult), the glutathione is used up and can't regenerate fast enough to detoxify all of the intermediate metabolite. Consequently, NAPQI builds up, causing liver damage. Evidence of liver damage may not be apparent until 24 to 36 hours after ingestion.

ALCOHOL

All alcohol, including ethanol, ethylene glycol, methanol, and isopropanol, is rapidly absorbed from the GI tract and metabolized by the liver enzyme alcohol dehydrogenase. Isopropanol and methanol also are easily absorbed through the skin and mucous membranes and can result in toxicity. Ethylene glycol and methanol are the most toxic alcohols. Ethylene glycol commonly is found in antifreeze and cleaning solutions; methanol is found in windshield washer fluid and solvents. Both are minimally toxic before metabolism, but in addition to their inebriating effects, have specific organ toxicity once metabolized. Both alcohols are metabolized in the liver, and blood levels above 20 mg/dl are considered toxic for both.

Metabolism of ethylene glycol produces glycolaldehyde, glycolic acid, glyoxylic acid, and oxalic acid. Symptoms result from the direct effects of these toxins and progress through three stages. Symptoms in stage I (first 12 hours) include altered mental status, seizures, and severe anion-gap metabolic acidosis. Cardiac toxicity occurs in stage II (12 to 36 hours). Stage III, renal failure, the hallmark of ethylene glycol toxicity, occurs at 36 to 48 hours.

Metabolism of methanol produces formaldehyde and formic acid. Folic acid is required for further metabolism to nontoxic products. Symptoms of methanol toxicity appear 12 to 24 hours after ingestion and result primarily from the effects of formic acid. Formic acid damages the optic nerve. Hemorrhages also have been found in a portion of the basal ganglia called the *putamen*. Symptoms include severe anion-gap metabolic acidosis caused by acid production, hypotension, visual changes that can progress to blindness, coma, and sudden respiratory arrest.

COCAINE

Cocaine blocks the reuptake of norepinephrine, epinephrine, and dopamine, causing excesses at the postsynaptic receptor sites. This leads to central and peripheral adrenergic stimulation and to a generalized vasoconstriction that affects multiple organs. These effects may include hypertension, hyperthermia, tachycardia, excited delirium, and seizures. Hyperthermia can cause rhabdomyolysis and later renal failure. Direct effects on the heart include increased myocardial oxygen consumption, coronary artery spasm, ischemia, myocardial infarction, depressed myocardial contractility, acute heart failure, sudden death from arrhythmias, and dilated cardiomyopathy. Recent studies have shown that cocaine increases platelet aggregation and thrombus formation. I.V. drug users are also at risk for endocarditis.

CYCLIC ANTIDEPRESSANTS

Cyclic antidepressants are responsible for almost half of all overdose-related adult admissions to critical care units and are the leading cause of overdose-related deaths in emergency departments. Cyclic drugs include the older tricyclics, such as amitriptyline and nortriptyline, and such newer agents as maprotiline (Ludiomil). These drugs are rapidly absorbed from the GI tract, although absorption may be delayed in large overdoses because of anticholinergic adverse effects. They're metabolized in the liver.

In an overdose, the enzymes responsible for metabolism become saturated, and some of the drug and its metabolites are secreted into the bile and gastric fluid to be reabsorbed later. Toxicity results from central and peripheral blockage of norepinephrine reuptake, anticholinergic effects, and quinidine-like effects on the heart. Central nervous system (CNS) effects may include initial agitation followed rapidly by lethargy, coma, and seizures. Anticholinergic effects include tachycardia, mydriasis, dry and flushed skin, hypoactive bowel sounds, and urine retention. Cardiovascular effects include hypotension, arrhythmias, and quinidine-like changes on the electrocardiogram with widening of the QRS complex.

ORGANOPHOSPHATES AND CARBAMATES

Organophosphates and carbamates are commonly found in pesticides and account for 80% of pesticide-related hospital admissions. They are highly lipid-soluble and easily absorbed through skin and mucous membranes. The primary mechanism of toxicity is cholinesterase inhibition, which leads to excess acetylcholine at muscarinic, nicotinic, and CNS receptors. The effects of excessive acetylcholine include increased salivation and lacrimation, muscle fasciculations and weakness, constricted pupils, decreased level of consciousness, and seizures. Bradycardia is typically present, but tachycardia has also been reported.

(continued)

Assessing drug overdose

DRUG	ASSESSMENT FINDINGS
Acetaminophen	◆ Plasma levels greater than 300 mcg/ml 4 hours after ingestion; 50 mcg/ml 12 hours after ingestion (suggestive of hepatoxicity) ◆ Nausea, vomiting, diaphoresis, and anorexia 12 to 24 hours after ingestion ◆ Cyanosis ◆ Anemia ◆ Jaundice ◆ Skin eruptions ◆ Fever ◆ Emesis ◆ Delirium ◆ Methemoglobinemia progressing to central nervous system (CNS) depression, coma, vascular collapse, seizures, and death
Amphetamines, cocaine	◆ Abdominal cramps ◆ Aggressiveness ◆ Arrhythmias ◆ Confusion ◆ Diarrhea ◆ Fatigue ◆ Hallucinations ◆ Hyperreflexia ◆ Nausea, vomiting ◆ Restlessness ◆ Seizures ◆ Tachypnea ◆ Tremor ◆ Coma ◆ Death
Anticholinergics	◆ Blurred vision ◆ Decreased or absent bowel sounds ◆ Dilated, nonreactive pupils ◆ Dry mucous membranes ◆ Dysphagia ◆ Flushed, hot, dry skin ◆ Hypertension ◆ Hyperthermia ◆ Increased respiratory rate ◆ Tachycardia ◆ Urine retention
Anticoagulants	◆ Hematuria ◆ Internal or external bleeding ◆ Skin necrosis
Antihistamines	◆ Drowsiness ◆ Moderate anticholinergic symptoms (selected histamine-1 antagonists) ◆ Respiratory depression ◆ Seizures ◆ Coma

DRUG	ASSESSMENT FINDINGS
Barbiturates	◆ Areflexia ◆ Confusion ◆ Pulmonary edema ◆ Respiratory depression ◆ Slurred speech ◆ Sustained nystagmus ◆ Somnolence ◆ Unsteady gait ◆ Coma
Benzodiazepines	◆ Bradycardia ◆ Confusion ◆ Dyspnea ◆ Hypoactive reflexes ◆ Hypotension ◆ Impaired coordination ◆ Labored breathing ◆ Slurred speech ◆ Somnolence
CNS depressants	◆ Absent pupillary reflexes ◆ Apnea ◆ Dilated pupils ◆ Hypotension ◆ Hypothermia followed by fever ◆ Inadequate ventilation ◆ Loss of deep tendon reflexes ◆ Tonic muscle spasms ◆ Coma
Iron supplements	◆ GI irritation with epigastric pain, nausea, vomiting ◆ Diarrhea (initially green, then tarry, then progressing to melena) ◆ Hematemesis ◆ Metabolic acidosis ◆ Hepatic dysfunction ◆ Renal failure ◆ Bleeding diathesis ◆ Circulatory failure ◆ Coma ◆ Death
Nonsteroidal anti-inflammatory drugs	◆ Abdominal pain ◆ Apnea ◆ Cyanosis ◆ Dizziness ◆ Drowsiness ◆ Headache ◆ Nausea, vomiting ◆ Nystagmus ◆ Paresthesia ◆ Sweating

DRUG	ASSESSMENT FINDINGS
Opioids	◆ Respiratory depression with or without CNS depression and miosis ◆ Hypotension ◆ Bradycardia ◆ Hypothermia ◆ Shock ◆ Cardiopulmonary arrest ◆ Circulatory collapse ◆ Pulmonary edema ◆ Seizures
Phenothiazines	◆ Abnormal involuntary muscle movements ◆ Agitation ◆ Arrhythmias ◆ Autonomic nervous system dysfunction ◆ Deep, unarousable sleep ◆ Extrapyramidal symptoms ◆ Hypotension ◆ Hypothermia or hyperthermia ◆ Seizures

DRUG	ASSESSMENT FINDINGS
Salicylates	◆ Hyperpnea ◆ Metabolic acidosis ◆ Respiratory alkalosis ◆ Tachypnea
Tricyclic antidepressants	◆ CNS stimulation (first 12 hours after ingestion) – Agitation – Confusion – Constipation, ileus – Dry mucous membranes – Hallucinations – Hyperthermia – Irritation – Parkinsonism – Pupillary dilation – Seizures – Urine retention ◆ CNS depression – Cardiac irregularities – Cyanosis – Decreased or absent reflexes – Hypotension – Hypothermia – Sedation

◆ maintain a patent airway
◆ exhibit an effective breathing pattern
◆ show no signs or symptoms of aspiration
◆ remain free from injury
◆ not express or exhibit suicidal ideation.

NURSING INTERVENTIONS

◆ Administer medications, as prescribed.
◆ Monitor respiratory, cardiovascular, and neurologic status.
◆ Initiate resuscitative measures, if indicated.
◆ Initiate surveillance measures, if suicidal intention is suspected.
◆ Provide support and encourage verbalization of feelings.

PATIENT TEACHING

Be sure to cover:
◆ causes of drug overdose
◆ medication administration, dosage, and possible adverse effects
◆ safety measures to avoid reccurence
◆ available support services, if indicated.

RESOURCES
Organizations
American Association of Poison Control Centers: *www.aapcc.org*

Selected references
Branagan, O., and Grogan, L. "Providing Health Education on Accidental Drug Overdose," *Nursing Times* 102(6):32-33, February 2006.
Captain, C. "Is Your Patient a Suicide Risk?" *Nursing* 36(8):43-47, August 2006.
Forti, R.J., and Adam, H.M. "Opiate Overdose," *Pediatrics in Review* 28(1):35-36, January 2007.

Hickman, M., et al. "London Audit of Drug-Related Overdose Deaths: Characteristics and Typology, and Implications for Prevention and Monitoring," *Addiction* 102(2):317-23, February 2007.

(continued)

Disorders affecting management of a drug overdose

This chart highlights disorders that affect the management of a drug overdose.

DISORDER	SIGNS AND SYMPTOMS	DIAGNOSTIC TEST RESULTS	TREATMENT AND CARE
Arrhythmias (complication)	◆ May be asymptomatic ◆ Dizziness, hypotension, syncope ◆ Weakness ◆ Cool, clammy skin ◆ Altered level of consciousness (LOC) ◆ Reduced urine output ◆ Shortness of breath ◆ Chest pain	◆ Electrocardiography (ECG) detects arrhythmias and ischemia and infarction that may result in arrhythmias. ◆ Laboratory testing may reveal electrolyte abnormalities, acid-base abnormalities, or drug toxicities that may cause arrhythmias. ◆ Holter monitoring, event monitoring, and loop recording can detect arrhythmias and effectiveness of drug therapy during a patient's daily activities. ◆ Exercise testing may detect exercise-induced arrhythmias. ◆ Electrophysiologic testing identifies the mechanism of an arrhythmia and the location of accessory pathways; it also assesses the effectiveness of antiarrhythmics, radiofrequency ablation, and implanted cardioverter-defibrillators.	◆ When life-threatening arrhythmias develop, rapidly assess LOC, respirations, and pulse rate. ◆ Initiate cardiopulmonary resuscitation, if indicated. ◆ Evaluate cardiac output resulting from arrhythmias. ◆ If the patient develops heart block, prepare for cardiac pacing. ◆ Administer antiarrhythmics, as ordered, and prepare to assist with medical procedures, if indicated. ◆ Assess intake and output every hour; insert an indwelling urinary catheter, as indicated, to ensure accurate urine measurement. ◆ Document arrhythmias in a monitored patient, and assess for possible causes and effects. ◆ If the patient's pulse is abnormally rapid, slow, or irregular, watch for signs of hypoperfusion, such as hypotension and diminished urine output. ◆ Monitor the patient for predisposing factors, such as fluid and electrolyte imbalance or possible drug toxicity.
Liver failure (complication)	◆ Ascites, shortness of breath ◆ Right upper quadrant tenderness ◆ Jaundice ◆ Nausea and anorexia ◆ Fatigue and weight loss ◆ Pruritus ◆ Oliguria ◆ Splenomegaly ◆ Peripheral edema ◆ Varices ◆ Bleeding tendencies ◆ Petechia ◆ Amenorrhea ◆ Gynecomastia	◆ Liver function studies reveal elevated levels of aspartate aminotransferase, alanine aminotransferase, alkaline phosphatase, and bilirubin. ◆ Blood studies reveal anemia, impaired red blood cell production, elevated bleeding and clotting times, low blood glucose levels, and increased serum ammonia levels. ◆ Urine osmolarity is increased. ◆ Liver scan may show filling defects.	◆ Auscultate lung sounds for crackles, rhonchi, or stridor. Observe for signs of respiratory distress, including labored breathing and dyspnea. ◆ Administer supplemental humidified oxygen. ◆ Administer lactulose, potassium-sparing diuretics, and potassium supplements. ◆ Monitor oxygen saturation for evidence of hypoxemia with continuous pulse oximetry and serial arterial blood gas (ABG) studies. Anticipate the need for endotracheal intubation and mechanical ventilation if patient's respiratory status deteriorates. ◆ Monitor ABG studies for increasing partial pressure of arterial carbon dioxide and decreasing pH (respiratory acidosis). ◆ Administer I.V. fluid therapy. Obtain laboratory specimens to assess for drug, electrolytes, and glucose levels. Anticipate administering normal saline solution and vasopressors if the patient is hypotensive and administering dextrose 5% in water if the patient is hypoglycemic. ◆ For the patient who has a history of chronic alcohol abuse, use of dextrose solutions may precipitate Wernicke-Korsakoff syndrome, a thiamine deficiency with severe neurologic impairment. ◆ Place the patient in semi-Fowler's position to maximize chest expansion. Keep the patient as quiet and comfortable as possible to minimize oxygen demands. ◆ Monitor for encephalopathy; lactulose may provide palliative treatment.

DISORDER	SIGNS AND SYMPTOMS	DIAGNOSTIC TEST RESULTS	TREATMENT AND CARE
Renal failure (complication)	◆ Oliguria (early) ◆ Metabolic acidosis ◆ Nausea, vomiting ◆ Dry mucous membranes ◆ Headache ◆ Confusion ◆ Seizures ◆ Drowsiness ◆ Irritability ◆ Dry, pruritic skin ◆ Uremic breath odor ◆ Hypotension (early) ◆ Hypertension with arrhythmias (later) ◆ Systemic edema ◆ Pulmonary edema ◆ Kussmaul's respirations ◆ Tachycardia ◆ Bibasilar crackles ◆ Altered LOC	◆ Blood urea nitrogen, serum creatinine, and potassium levels are elevated. ◆ Bicarbonate level, hematocrit, hemoglobin, and pH are decreased. ◆ Urine studies show casts, cellular debris, and decreased specific gravity; in glomerular diseases, proteinuria and urine osmolality close to serum osmolality are present; urine sodium level is less than 20 mEq/L if oliguria results from decreased perfusion and more than 40 mEq/L if the cause is intrarenal. ◆ Creatinine clearance test measures glomerular filtration rate and reflects the number of remaining functioning nephrons. ◆ ECG shows tall, peaked T waves; widening QRS; and disappearing P waves if hyperkalemia is present. ◆ Ultrasonography, abdominal and kidney-ureter-bladder X-rays, excretory urography, renal scan, retrograde pyelography, computerized tomography, and nephrotomography reveal abnormalities of the urinary tract.	◆ Administer hypertonic glucose, insulin, diuretics, and sodium bicarbonate. ◆ Measure intake and output, including body fluids, nasogastric output, and diarrhea. Weigh the patient daily. ◆ Measure hemoglobin and hematocrit; replace blood components. ◆ Monitor vital signs; check and report for signs of pericarditis (pleuritic chest pain, tachycardia, pericardial friction rub), inadequate renal perfusion (hypotension), and acidosis. ◆ Maintain proper electrolyte balance. Monitor potassium levels and monitor for hyperkalemia (malaise, anorexia, paresthesia, muscle weakness) and ECG changes. ◆ If patient receives hypertonic glucose and insulin infusions, monitor potassium and glucose levels. If giving sodium polystyrene sulfonate rectally, make sure patient doesn't retain it and become constipated to prevent bowel perforation. ◆ Maintain nutritional status with a high-calorie, low-protein, low-sodium, low-potassium diet and vitamin supplements. ◆ Monitor the patient carefully during peritoneal dialysis. ◆ If patient requires hemodialysis, monitor vascular access site carefully, and assess patient and laboratory studies carefully.

Electric shock

- Electric current that passes through body
- Physical damage dependent on the intensity of current, resistance of the tissues it passes through, type of current, and frequency and duration of current flow
- Classified as lightning, low-voltage (less than 600 V), and high-voltage (greater than 600 V)
- Causes more than 500 deaths annually
- More common in males ages 20 to 40

CAUSES

- Accidental contact with an exposed part of an electrical appliance or wiring
- Flash of electric arcs from high-voltage power lines or machines
- Lightning

PATHOPHYSIOLOGY

- Electrical energy results in altered cell membrane resting potential, causing depolarization in muscles and nerves.
- Electric shock alters normal electrical activity of the heart and brain.
- Electric shock resulting from a high-frequency current generates more heat in tissues than a low-frequency current, resulting in burns and local tissue coagulation and necrosis.
- Muscle tetany is elicited.
- Tissue destruction and coagulative necrosis occurs.

CARDIOVASCULAR SYSTEM

- If it passes through the heart, even the smallest electric current may induce ventricular fibrillation (or another arrhythmia) that progresses to fibrillation or myocardial infarction. (See *Disorders affecting management of electric shock,* pages 146 and 147.)

INTEGUMENTARY SYSTEM

- Electric shock from a high-frequency current usually causes burns, local tissue coagulation, and necrosis.
- Low-frequency currents can cause serious burns if the contact with the current is concentrated in a small area (for example, if a toddler bites into an electric cord).

MUSCULOSKELETAL SYSTEM

- Cell membrane resting potential is altered, causing depolarization in muscles. Muscle tetany can occur.
- Contusions, fractures, and other injuries can result from violent muscle contractions, falls, or being thrown during the shock.

NEUROLOGIC SYSTEM

- Cell membrane resting potential is altered, causing depolarization in nerves. Numbness, tingling, or sensorimotor deficits can occur.

RENAL SYSTEM

- Electrical current causes coagulation necrosis and tissue ischemia, which liberates myoglobin and hemoglobin, which then precipitate in the renal tubules, causing tubular necrosis and renal shutdown.

RESPIRATORY SYSTEM

- Respiratory paralysis occurs because of the electric current's direct effect on the respiratory nerve center or because of prolonged contraction of respiratory muscles.
- After momentary shock, hyperventilation may follow initial muscle contraction.

ASSESSMENT

HISTORY
◆ Exposure to electricity or lightning
◆ Loss of consciousness
◆ Muscle pain
◆ Fatigue
◆ Headache
◆ Nervous irritability

PHYSICAL FINDINGS
◆ Determined by voltage exposure
◆ Burns
◆ Local tissue coagulation
◆ Entrance and exit injuries
◆ Cyanosis
◆ Apnea
◆ Markedly decreased blood pressure
◆ Cold skin
◆ Unconsciousness
◆ Numbness or tingling or sensorimotor deficits

DIAGNOSTIC TEST RESULTS
◆ Urinalysis shows evidence of myoglobin.
◆ Computed tomography or magnetic resonance imaging may rule out intracranial bleeding or contusion of the brain if the patient is unresponsive or unconscious.
◆ Chest X-rays reveal internal damage such as fractures or dislocations.
◆ Electrocardiogram (ECG) reveals cardiac arrhythmias.

TREATMENT

GENERAL
◆ Separation of victim from current source
◆ Stabilization of cervical spine
◆ Emergency measures
◆ Treatment of acid-base imbalance
◆ Vigorous fluid replacement

DIET
◆ No restrictions if swallowing ability intact

ACTIVITY
◆ Based on outcome of interventions

MEDICATIONS
◆ Osmotic diuretics
◆ Tetanus prophylaxis

NURSING CONSIDERATIONS

NURSING DIAGNOSES
◆ Acute pain
◆ Anxiety
◆ Decreased cardiac output
◆ Impaired skin integrity
◆ Impaired spontaneous ventilation
◆ Ineffective tissue perfusion: Cardiopulmonary
◆ Risk for injury
◆ Risk for posttrauma syndrome

EXPECTED OUTCOMES
The patient will:
◆ express feelings of increased comfort and decreased pain
◆ express feelings of decreased anxiety
◆ maintain cardiac output
◆ regain skin integrity
◆ maintain adequate ventilation either spontaneously or with assisted ventilation
◆ exhibit signs of adequate cardiopulmonary perfusion
◆ verbalize methods to prevent future injury from electric shock
◆ express feelings and fears about the traumatic event.

NURSING INTERVENTIONS
◆ Separate the victim from the current source while maintaining personal safety.
◆ Provide emergency treatment.
◆ Give rapid I.V. fluid infusion.
◆ Obtain a 12-lead ECG.
◆ Give prescribed drugs.
◆ Monitor cardiac rhythm, intake and output, and neurologic status.
◆ Observe for sensorimotor deficits and changes in peripheral neurovascular status.

(continued)

Be sure to cover:
◆ injury, diagnostic testing, and treatment
◆ how to avoid electrical hazards at home and at work
◆ electrical safety regarding children.

RESOURCES
Organizations
Harborview Injury Prevention and Research Center: *www.depts.washington.edu/hiprc*
National Center for Injury Prevention and Control: *www.cdc.gov/ncipc*

Selected references
Diseases, 4th ed. Philadelphia: Lippincott Williams & Wilkins, 2006.
Hendler, N. "Overlooked Diagnoses in Chronic Pain: Analysis of Survivors of Electric Shock and Lightning Strike," *Journal of Occupational & Environmental Medicine* 47(8):796-805, August 2005.
Rivera, J., et al. "Severe Stunned Myocardium after Lightning Strike," *Critical Care Medicine* 35(1):280-85, January 2007.
Wick, R., et al. "Fatal Electrocution in Adults: A 30-Year Study," *Medicine, Science and the Law* 46(2):166-72, April 2006.

Disorders affecting management of electric shock

This chart highlights disorders that affect the management of electric shock.

DISORDER	SIGNS AND SYMPTOMS	DIAGNOSTIC TEST RESULTS	TREATMENT AND CARE
Atrial fibrillation (complication)	◆ Irregularly irregular pulse rhythm with normal or abnormal heart rate ◆ Radial pulse rate slower than apical pulse rate ◆ Palpable peripheral pulse with stronger contractions ◆ Evidence of decreased cardiac output, such as hypotension and light-headedness, with new-onset atrial fibrillation and a rapid ventricular rate	◆ Electrocardiography reveals no clear P waves, irregularly irregular ventricular response, and uneven baseline fibrillatory waves; wide variation in R-R intervals results in loss of atrial kick. Atrial fibrillation may be preceded by premature atrial contractions.	◆ Interventions aim to reduce the ventricular response rate to less than 100 beats/minute, establish anticoagulation, and restore and maintain a sinus rhythm. ◆ Treatment typically includes drug therapy (calcium channel blockers, beta-adrenergic blockers, antiarrhythmics, cardiac glycosides, anticoagulants) to control the ventricular response or a combination of electrical cardioversion and drug therapy. If drug therapy is used, monitor serum drug levels, and observe the patient for evidence of toxicity. ◆ If the patient is hemodynamically unstable, synchronized electrical cardioversion should be performed right away. It's most successful if done within 48 hours after onset of atrial fibrillation. ◆ A transesophageal echocardiogram may be obtained before cardioversion to rule out the presence of thrombi in the atria. ◆ Tell the patient to report changes in pulse rate, dizziness, feeling faint, chest pain, and signs of heart failure, such as dyspnea and peripheral edema. ◆ If the patient isn't on a cardiac monitor, be alert for an irregular pulse and differences in the radial and apical pulse rates. ◆ Monitor the patient's peripheral and apical pulses; watch for evidence of decreased cardiac output and heart failure.

DISORDER	SIGNS AND SYMPTOMS	DIAGNOSTIC TEST RESULTS	TREATMENT AND CARE
Burn shock (complication)	◆ Tachycardia ◆ Tachypnea ◆ Cyanosis ◆ Weak, rapid, thready pulse ◆ Cold, clammy skin ◆ Hypotension ◆ Reduced urinary output progressing to anuria ◆ Restlessness and irritability progressing to unconsciousness and absent reflexes ◆ Peripheral edema	◆ Potassium, serum lactate, and blood urea nitrogen levels are elevated. ◆ Urine specific gravity is greater than 1.020; urine osmolality is increased. ◆ Blood pH and partial pressure of arterial oxygen are decreased, and partial pressure of carbon dioxide is increased. ◆ Coagulation studies may detect disseminated intravascular coagulation.	◆ Monitor cardiac rhythm. ◆ Administer analgesics and antiarrhythmics. ◆ Initiate and maintain I.V. fluid replacement therapy. ◆ Administer blood replacement therapy. ◆ Administer supplemental oxygen. ◆ Monitor vital signs, including central and peripheral pulses and capillary refill, approximately every 15 minutes. ◆ Monitor the patient for signs of deficient fluid volume, such as tachycardia, hypotension, weak peripheral pulses, dry mucous membranes, and decreased urine output. ◆ Monitor the patient carefully for signs of neurological impairment, such as confusion, memory loss, insomnia, lethargy, and combativeness. ◆ Monitor the patient for signs of impaired peristalsis, such as vomiting or fecal impaction.
Heart failure (complication)	◆ Cough that produces pink, frothy sputum ◆ Cyanosis of the lips and nail beds ◆ Pale, cool, clammy skin ◆ Diaphoresis ◆ Jugular vein distention ◆ Ascites ◆ Pulsus alternans ◆ Tachycardia ◆ Hepatomegaly ◆ Decreased pulse pressure ◆ Third (S_3) and fourth (S_4) heart sounds ◆ Moist, basilar crackles ◆ Rhonchi ◆ Expiratory wheezing ◆ Decreased pulse oximetry ◆ Peripheral edema ◆ Decreased urinary output	◆ B-type natriuretic peptide immunoassay is elevated. ◆ Chest X-ray shows increased pulmonary vascular markings, interstitial edema, or pleural effusions and cardiomegaly. ◆ Electrocardiography reveals heart enlargement or ischemia, tachycardia, extrasystole, or atrial fibrillation. ◆ Pulmonary artery pressure, pulmonary artery wedge pressure, and left ventricular end-diastolic pressure are elevated in left-sided heart failure; right atrial or central venous pressure is elevated in right-sided heart failure.	◆ Limit fluid and sodium intake to decrease preload. ◆ Monitor the patient for signs of embolization (hematuria, pleuritic chest pain, left-upper-quadrant pain). ◆ Monitor oxygenation status, auscultate lung fields, and evaluate arterial blood gas studies. ◆ Monitor urine output. ◆ Administer supplemental oxygen and mechanical ventilation. ◆ Place the patient in Fowler's position. ◆ Administer diuretics, inotropic drugs, vasodilators, angiotensin-converting enzyme inhibitors, angiotensin receptor blockers, cardiac glycosides, beta-adrenergic blockers, and electrolyte supplements. ◆ Initiate cardiac monitoring. ◆ Recurrent heart failure from valvular dysfunction may require surgery. ◆ A ventricular assist device may be needed. ◆ Maintain adequate cardiac output, and monitor hemodynamic stability. ◆ Assess for deep vein thrombosis, and apply antiembolism stockings.

Emphysema

- Chronic lung disease characterized by permanent enlargement of air spaces distal to the terminal bronchioles and by exertional dyspnea
- One of several diseases usually labeled collectively as chronic obstructive pulmonary disease or chronic obstructive lung disease
- Most common cause of death from respiratory disease in the United States
- More prevalent in males than in females
- Affects about 2 million Americans
- Affects 1 in 3,000 neonates

CAUSES

- Cigarette smoking
- Genetic deficiency of alpha$_1$-antitrypsin

PATHOPHYSIOLOGY

- Recurrent inflammation associated with the release of proteolytic enzymes from lung cells causes abnormal, irreversible enlargement of the air spaces distal to the terminal bronchioles.
- The alveolar septa are initially destroyed, eliminating a portion of the capillary bed and increasing air volume in the acinus.
- This breakdown leaves the alveoli unable to recoil normally after expanding and results in bronchiolar collapse on expiration. The damaged or destroyed alveolar walls can't support the airways to keep them open.
- The amount of air that can be expired passively is diminished, thus trapping air in the lungs and leading to overdistension.
- Hyperinflation of the alveoli produces bullae (air spaces) adjacent to the pleura (blebs). Septal destruction also decreases airway calibration.
- Part of each inspiration is trapped because of increased residual volume and decreased calibration. (See *What happens in emphysema.*)

CARDIOVASCULAR SYSTEM

- Pulmonary hypertension causes cor pulmonale as the heart's workload increases and the right ventricle hypertrophies to force blood through the lungs. As this compensatory mechanism fails, the right ventricle dilates. (See *Disorders affecting management of emphysema,* pages 150 and 151.)
- As blood viscosity increases due to prolonged hypoxia, pulmonary hypertension increases, and heart failure can occur.

HEMATOLOGIC SYSTEM

- Hypoxia causes the bone marrow to produce more red blood cells (RBCs), and blood viscosity increases, aggravating pulmonary hypertension.

ASSESSMENT

HISTORY

- Smoking
- Shortness of breath
- Chronic cough
- Anorexia and weight loss
- Malaise

UP CLOSE

What happens in emphysema

In normal, healthy breathing, air moves in and out of the lungs to meet metabolic needs. A change in airway size compromises the lungs' ability to circulate sufficient air.

In a patient with emphysema, recurrent pulmonary inflammation damages and eventually destroys the alveolar walls, creating large air spaces. This breakdown leaves the alveoli unable to recoil normally after expanding and results in bronchiolar collapse on expiration. This traps air within the lungs.

Associated pulmonary capillary destruction usually allows a patient with severe emphysema to match ventilation to perfusion and thus avoid cyanosis.

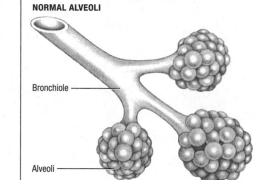

NORMAL ALVEOLI

Bronchiole

Alveoli

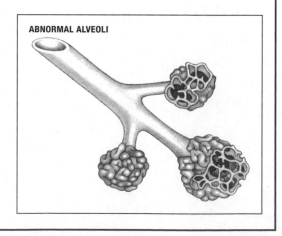

ABNORMAL ALVEOLI

PHYSICAL FINDINGS

- Barrel chest
- Pursed-lip breathing
- Use of accessory muscles
- Cyanosis
- Clubbed fingers and toes
- Tachypnea
- Decreased tactile fremitus
- Decreased chest expansion
- Hyperresonance
- Decreased breath sounds
- Crackles
- Inspiratory wheeze
- Prolonged expiratory phase with grunting respirations
- Distant heart sounds

DIAGNOSTIC TEST RESULTS

- Arterial blood gas analysis shows decreased partial pressure of oxygen; partial pressure of carbon dioxide is normal until late in the disease and then it's increased.
- RBC count shows an increased hemoglobin level late in the disease then it's increased.
- Chest X-ray may show:
- flattened diaphragm
- reduced vascular markings at the lung periphery
- overaeration of the lungs
- vertical heart
- enlarged anteroposterior chest diameter
- large retrosternal air space.
- Pulmonary function tests typically show:
- increased residual volume and total lung capacity
- reduced diffusing capacity
- increased inspiratory flow.
- Electrocardiography may show tall, symmetrical P waves in leads II, III, and aV_F; a vertical QRS axis; and signs of right ventricular hypertrophy late in the disease.

TREATMENT

GENERAL

- Chest physiotherapy
- Possible transtracheal catheterization and home oxygen therapy
- Mechanical ventilation (in acute exacerbations)

DIET

- Adequate hydration
- High-protein, high-calorie

ACTIVITY

- As tolerated

MEDICATIONS

- Bronchodilators
- Anticholinergics
- Mucolytics
- Corticosteroids
- Antibiotics
- Oxygen

SURGERY

- Chest tube insertion for pneumothorax

NURSING CONSIDERATIONS

NURSING DIAGNOSES

- Anxiety
- Fatigue
- Fear
- Impaired gas exchange
- Ineffective airway clearance
- Ineffective breathing pattern
- Interrupted family processes
- Risk for infection

EXPECTED OUTCOMES

The patient will:

- identify strategies to reduce anxiety
- verbalize the importance of balancing activity with adequate rest periods
- discuss fears and concerns
- maintain adequate ventilation and oxygenation
- maintain a patent airway
- maintain effective breathing pattern

- along with family members, identify and contact available support systems, as needed
- remain free from signs or symptoms of infection.

NURSING INTERVENTIONS

- Give prescribed drugs.
- Provide supportive care.
- Help the patient adjust to lifestyle changes necessitated by a chronic illness.
- Encourage the patient to express his fears and concerns.
- Perform chest physiotherapy.
- Provide a high-calorie, protein-rich diet.
- Give small, frequent meals.
- Encourage daily activity and diversional activities.
- Provide frequent rest periods.
- Monitor vital signs, intake and output, and daily weight.
- Observe for complications.
- Assess respiratory status per facility policy and clinical status.
- Monitor activity tolerance.

PATIENT TEACHING

Be sure to cover:

- disorder, diagnostic testing, and treatment
- medication administration, dosage, and possible adverse effects
- when to notify the practitioner
- energy conservation techniques
- importance of receiving influenza and pneumonia vaccines yearly
- avoidance of smoking and areas where smoking is permitted
- avoidance of crowds and people with known infections
- home oxygen therapy, if indicated
- transtracheal catheter care, if needed
- coughing and deep-breathing exercises
- proper use of handheld inhalers
- need for a high-calorie, protein-rich diet
- adequate oral fluid intake
- avoidance of respiratory irritants
- signs and symptoms of pneumothorax

(continued)

WARNING *Urge the patient to notify the practitioner if he experiences a sudden onset of worsening dyspnea or sharp pleuritic chest pain exacerbated by chest movement, breathing, or coughing.*

◆ available smoking-cessation programs.

RESOURCES
Organizations
National Emphysema Foundation: *www.emphysemafoundation.org*
National Institute of Drug Abuse: *www.nida.nih.gov*
Tobacco Information and Prevention Source: *www.cdc.gov/tobacco*

Selected references
Bauldoff, G., and Diaz, P. "Improving Outcomes for COPD Patients," *The Nurse Practitioner* 31(8):26-43, August 2006.
Nettina, S.M. *Lippincott Manual of Nursing Practice*, 8th ed. Philadelphia: Lippincott Williams & Wilkins, 2006.
Teramots, S., and Ishii, I. "Aging, the Aging Lung, and Senile Emphysema are Different," *American Journal of Respiratory Critical Care Medicine* 175(2):197-98, January 2007.

Disorders affecting management of emphysema

This chart highlights disorders that affect the management of emphysema.

DISORDER	SIGNS AND SYMPTOMS	DIAGNOSTIC TEST RESULTS	TREATMENT AND CARE
Cor pulmonale (complication)	◆ Progressive dyspnea worsening on exertion ◆ Tachypnea ◆ Orthopnea ◆ Edema ◆ Weakness ◆ Dependent edema ◆ Jugular vein distention ◆ Enlarged tender liver ◆ Tachycardia ◆ Hypotension ◆ Weak pulse	◆ Pulmonary artery pressures show increased right ventricular pressures. ◆ Echocardiography or angiography indicates right ventricular enlargement. ◆ Chest X-ray suggests right ventricular enlargement. ◆ Arterial blood gas (ABG) analysis shows partial pressure of arterial oxygen (Pao_2) of less than 70 mm Hg. ◆ Electrocardiography may show various arrhythmias. ◆ Pulmonary function tests are consistent with underlying disorder.	◆ Provide meticulous respiratory care, including oxygen therapy; suctioning, as needed; and deep-breathing and coughing exercises. ◆ Monitor ABG values and monitor for signs of respiratory failure (change in pulse rate, deep labored respiration's, and increased fatigue on exertion). ◆ Monitor fluid status carefully; limit fluid intake to 1,000 to 2,000 ml/day, and provide a low sodium diet. ◆ Monitor serum potassium levels if patient is receiving diuretics; low serum potassium levels can potentiate arrhythmias. ◆ Administer digoxin, antibiotics, vasodilators, and oxygen.
Peptic ulcer disease (complication)	◆ Pallor ◆ Epigastric tenderness ◆ Hyperactive bowel sounds *Gastric ulcer* ◆ Recent weight or appetite loss ◆ Nausea or vomiting ◆ Pain triggered or worsened by eating *Duodenal ulcer* ◆ Pain relieved by eating; may occur 1½ hours to 3 hours after food intake ◆ Pain that awakens the patient from sleep ◆ Weight gain	◆ Barium swallow or upper GI and small-bowel series may reveal the presence of the ulcer. ◆ Upper GI endoscopy or esophagogastroduodenoscopy confirms the presence of an ulcer and permits cytologic studies and biopsy to rule out *Helicobacter pylori* or cancer. ◆ Upper GI tract X-rays reveal mucosal abnormalities. ◆ Laboratory analysis may disclose occult blood in stools. ◆ Immunoglobulin A anti-*H. pylori* test on a venous blood sample can be used to detect *H. pylori* antibodies. ◆ Serologic testing may disclose clinical signs of infection such as an elevated white blood cell (WBC) count. ◆ Gastric secretory studies show hyperchlorhydria. ◆ Carbon 13 urea breath test results reflect activity of *H. pylori*.	◆ Support the patient emotionally, and offer reassurance. ◆ Administer proton pump inhibitors, histamine-2-receptor agonists, gastric acid pump inhibitors, sedatives, anticholinergics (with duodenal ulcers), and prostaglandin analogs. ◆ Provide six small meals or small hourly meals, as ordered. Advise the patient to eat slowly, chew thoroughly, and have small snacks between meals. ◆ Schedule the patient's care so that he can get plenty of rest. ◆ Teach the patient about peptic ulcer disease, and help him to recognize its signs and symptoms. ◆ Explain scheduled diagnostic tests and prescribed therapies. ◆ Review symptoms associated with complications, and urge him to notify the physician if any occur. ◆ Emphasize the importance of complying with treatment, even after his symptoms are relieved.

DISORDER	SIGNS AND SYMPTOMS	DIAGNOSTIC TEST RESULTS	TREATMENT AND CARE
Respiratory failure (complication)	◆ Cyanosis of the oral mucosa, lips, and nail beds ◆ Yawning and use of accessory muscles ◆ Pursed-lip breathing ◆ Nasal flaring ◆ Ashen complexion ◆ Cold, clammy skin ◆ Rapid breathing ◆ Asymmetrical chest movement ◆ Decreased tactile fremitus over an obstructed bronchi or pleural effusion ◆ Increased tactile fremitus over consolidated lung tissue ◆ Hyperresonance ◆ Wheezing (in asthma) ◆ Diminished or absent breath sounds ◆ Rhonchi (in bronchitis) ◆ Crackles (in pulmonary edema)	◆ ABG analysis indicates respiratory failure by deteriorating values (typically Pao_2 less than 60 mm Hg and partial pressure of arterial carbon dioxide greater than 45 mm Hg) and a pH below 7.35. ◆ Chest X-ray identifies pulmonary diseases or conditions, such as emphysema, atelectasis, lesions, pneumothorax, infiltrates, and effusions. ◆ Electrocardiography may show arrhythmias, which are commonly found with cor pulmonale and myocardial hypoxia. ◆ Pulse oximetry reveals a decreasing arterial oxygen saturation; a mixed venous oxygen saturation level of less than 50% indicates impaired tissue oxygenation. ◆ Complete blood count may reveal an elevated WBC count, which helps detect an underlying infection as the cause. ◆ Abnormally low hemoglobin and hematocrit levels signal blood loss, indicating a decreased oxygen-carrying capacity. ◆ Serum electrolyte levels may reveal hypokalemia resulting from compensatory hyperventilation, the body's attempt to correct acidosis, or hypochloremia if the patient develops metabolic alkalosis. ◆ Blood cultures, sputum culture, and Gram stain may identify pathogens.	◆ To reverse hypoxemia, administer oxygen at appropriate concentrations to maintain Pao_2 at a minimum pressure range of 50 to 60 mm Hg. The patient with chronic obstructive pulmonary disease usually requires only small amounts of supplemental oxygen. Watch for a positive response, such as improved breathing, color, and ABG values. ◆ Maintain a patent airway. If the patient retains carbon dioxide, encourage him to cough and breathe deeply with pursed lips. If he's alert, have him use an incentive spirometer. ◆ If the patient is intubated and lethargic, reposition him every 1 to 2 hours. Use postural drainage and percussion and vibration to help clear secretions. ◆ Observe the patient closely for respiratory arrest. Auscultate for chest sounds. Monitor ABG values, and report any changes immediately. Notify the physician of decreased oxygen saturation levels detected by pulse oximetry. ◆ Watch for treatment complications, especially oxygen toxicity and acute respiratory distress syndrome. ◆ Frequently monitor vital signs. Note and report an increasing pulse rate, increasing or decreasing respiratory rate, decreasing blood pressure, or febrile state. ◆ Monitor and record serum electrolyte levels carefully. Take appropriate steps to correct imbalances. Monitor fluid balance by recording the patient's intake and output and daily weight. ◆ Check the cardiac monitor for arrhythmias. ◆ Perform oral hygiene measures frequently. ◆ Position the patient for comfort and optimal gas exchange. ◆ Maintain the patient in a normothermic state to reduce the body's demand for oxygen. ◆ Schedule patient care activities to maximize the patient's energy level and provide needed rest.

Endocarditis

OVERVIEW

OVERVIEW

- Infection of the endocardium, heart valves, or cardiac prosthesis
- Three types: native valve (acute and subacute) endocarditis, prosthetic valve (early and late) endocarditis, and endocarditis related to I.V. drug abuse (usually involving the tricuspid valve)
- Mitral valve most commonly involved valve
- Up to 40% of affected patients having no underlying heart disease
- More common in males than in females
- Usually affects patients older than age 50
- Uncommon in children
- Rheumatic valvular disease occurring in about 25% of all cases
- Drug abusers with endocarditis commonly young males

CAUSES
Native valve endocarditis
- Alpha-hemolytic *Streptococcus* or enterococci (subacute form)
- Group B hemolytic *Streptococcus*
- *Staphylococcus aureus*

Prosthetic valve
- Alpha-hemolytic *Streptococcus*, enterococci, and *Staphylococcus* (late; 60 days or more after implant)
- *Staphylococcus*, gram-negative bacilli, and *Candida* (early; within 60 days after implant)
- Related to I.V. drug abuse

PATHOPHYSIOLOGY

- Fibrin and platelets cluster on valve tissue and engulf circulating bacteria or fungi. (See *Degenerative changes in endocarditis.*)
- This produces friable verrucous vegetation which, in turn, may cover the valve surfaces, causing deformities and destruction of valvular tissue. The vegetation may also extend to the chordae tendineae, causing them to rupture, leading to valvular insufficiency. (See *Disorders affecting management of endocarditis,* pages 154 and 155.)
- Vegetative growth on the heart valves, endocardial lining of a heart chamber, or the endothelium of a blood vessel may embolize to the spleen, kidneys, central nervous system, and lungs.

CARDIOVASCULAR SYSTEM
- Infective endocarditis can occur as a consequence of nonbacterial thrombotic endocarditis, which results from turbulence or trauma to the endothelial surface of the heart.
- The bacteria invade the vegetative lesions, leading to infective endocarditis.
- Atrial fibrillation can result as the cardiac muscle is destroyed (through progressive local tissue trauma and destruction).

MUSCULOSKELETAL SYSTEM
- Immune response to the infection and systemic infection can result in septic arthritis.

Degenerative changes in endocarditis

This illustration shows typical vegetations on the endocardium produced by fibrin and platelet deposits on infection sites.

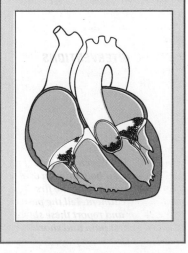

RENAL SYSTEM
- Fragments of lesions in the valves and endocardium can form emboli and travel in the bloodstream to the renal system where they may form renal infarctions and abscesses, resulting in glomerulonephritis.

ASSESSMENT

HISTORY
- Predisposing condition such as heart failure
- Nonspecific symptoms, such as weakness, fatigue, weight loss, anorexia, arthralgia, night sweats, and intermittent fever that may recur for weeks
- Dyspnea and chest pain (common with I.V. drug abusers)

PHYSICAL FINDINGS
- Petechiae on the skin (especially common on the upper anterior trunk) and on the buccal, pharyngeal, or conjunctival mucosa
- Splinter hemorrhages under the nails
- Clubbing of the fingers in patients with long-standing disease
- Heart murmur in all patients except those with early acute endocarditis and I.V. drug users with tricuspid valve infection
- Osler's nodes
- Roth's spots
- Janeway lesions
- Murmur that changes suddenly or a new murmur that develops in the presence of fever (classic physical sign)
- Splenomegaly in long-standing disease
- Dyspnea, tachycardia, and bibasilar crackles possible with left-sided heart failure
- Splenic infarction causing pain in the upper left quadrant, radiating to the left shoulder, and abdominal rigidity
- Renal infarction causing hematuria, pyuria, flank pain, and decreased urine output
- Cerebral infarction causing hemiparesis, aphasia, and other neurologic deficits

- Pulmonary infarction causing cough, pleuritic pain, pleural friction rub, dyspnea, and hemoptysis
- Peripheral vascular occlusion causing numbness and tingling in arm, leg, finger, or toe or signs of impending peripheral gangrene

DIAGNOSTIC TEST RESULTS
- Three or more blood cultures during a 24- to 48-hour period identify the causative organism (in up to 90% of patients).
- White blood cell count and differential is normal or elevated.
- Complete blood count and anemia panel show normocytic, normochromic anemia in subacute native valve endocarditis.
- Erythrocyte sedimentation rate and serum creatinine levels are elevated.
- Serum rheumatoid factor is positive in about 50% of all patients with endocarditis longer than 6 weeks.
- Urinalysis shows proteinuria and microscopic hematuria.
- Echocardiography may identify valvular damage in up to 80% of patients with native valve endocarditis.
- Electrocardiography may show atrial fibrillation and other arrhythmias that accompany valvular disease.

TREATMENT

GENERAL
- Prompt therapy that continues for several weeks
- Selection of anti-infective drug based on type of infecting organism and sensitivity studies
- With negative blood cultures (10% to 20% of subacute cases), possible I.V. antibiotic therapy (usually for 4 to 6 weeks) against probable infecting organism

DIET
- Sufficient fluid intake

ACTIVITY
- Bed rest

MEDICATIONS
- Aspirin
- Antibiotics

SURGERY
- With severe valvular damage, especially aortic insufficiency or infection of a cardiac prosthesis, possible corrective surgery if refractory heart failure develops or if an infected prosthetic valve must be replaced

NURSING CONSIDERATIONS

NURSING DIAGNOSES
- Activity intolerance
- Decreased cardiac output
- Deficient diversional activity
- Impaired gas exchange
- Impaired physical mobility
- Ineffective role performance
- Risk for infection

EXPECTED OUTCOMES
The patient will:
- carry out activities of daily living without weakness or fatigue
- maintain hemodynamic stability with adequate cardiac output
- express interest in using leisure time meaningfully
- maintain adequate ventilation and oxygenation
- maintain joint mobility and muscle strength
- express feelings about diminished capacity to perform usual roles
- remain free from further signs or symptoms of infection.

NURSING INTERVENTIONS
- Stress the importance of bed rest.
- Provide a bedside commode.
- Allow patient to express concerns.
- Obtain a history of allergies.
- Administer antibiotics in a timely manner.
- Administer oxygen.

   WARNING *Watch for signs of pulmonary embolization, a common occurrence during the first 3 months of treatment. Tell the patient to watch for and report these signs, which are chest pain and shortness of breath.*

- Monitor renal status.
- Perform frequent cardiovascular status assessments.
- Monitor vital signs and arterial blood gas analysis values.

PATIENT TEACHING

Be sure to cover:
- disorder, diagnostic testing, and treatment
- anti-infectives the patient needs to continue taking
- need to watch closely for fever, anorexia, and other signs of relapse about 2 weeks after treatment stops
- need for prophylactic antibiotics before dental work and some surgical procedures
- proper dental hygiene and avoiding flossing the teeth
- how to recognize symptoms of endocarditis and to notify the practitioner immediately if such symptoms occur
- available drug rehabilitation programs and support services, if appropriate.

RESOURCES
Organizations
American Heart Association: *www.americanheart.org*
Mayo Clinic: *www.mayoclinic.com*
National Heart, Lung and Blood Institute: *www.nhlbi.nih.gov/nhlbi/cardio*

Selected references
David, T.E., et al. "Surgical Treatment of Infective Endocarditis: A Continued Challenge," *Journal of Thoracic Cardiovascular Surgery* 133(1):144-49, January 2007.
Fink, A. "Endocarditis After Valve Replacement Surgery," *AJN* 106(2):40-51, February 2006.
Habib, G. "Management of Infective Endocarditis," *Heart* 92(1):124-30, January 2006.
The Merck Manual of Diagnosis & Therapy, 18th ed. Whitehouse Station, N.J.: Merck & Co., Inc., 2006.

(continued)

Disorders affecting management of endocarditis

This chart highlights disorders that affect the management of endocarditis.

DISORDER	SIGNS AND SYMPTOMS	DIAGNOSTIC TEST RESULTS	TREATMENT AND CARE
Atrial fibrillation (complication)	◆ Irregularly irregular pulse rhythm with normal or abnormal heart rate ◆ Radial pulse rate slower than apical pulse rate ◆ Palpable peripheral pulse with the stronger contractions ◆ Evidence of decreased cardiac output, such as hypotension and light-headedness, with new-onset atrial fibrillation and a rapid ventricular rate	◆ Electrocardiography shows no clear P waves, irregularly irregular ventricular response, and uneven baseline fibrillatory waves; wide variation in R-R intervals results in loss of atrial kick. ◆ Atrial fibrillation may be preceded by premature atrial contractions.	◆ Interventions aim to reduce the ventricular response rate to less than 100 beats/minute, to establish anticoagulation, and to restore and maintain a sinus rhythm. ◆ Treatment typically includes drug therapy to control the ventricular response or a combination of electrical cardioversion and drug therapy. ◆ If the patient is hemodynamically unstable, synchronized electrical cardioversion should be performed right away. ◆ A transesophageal echocardiogram may be obtained before cardioversion to rule out the presence of thrombi in the atria. ◆ If drug therapy is used, monitor serum drug levels, and observe the patient for evidence of toxicity. ◆ Tell the patient to report changes in pulse rate, dizziness, feeling faint, chest pain, and signs of heart failure, such as dyspnea and peripheral edema. ◆ If the patient isn't on a cardiac monitor, be alert for an irregular pulse and differences in the radial and apical pulse rates. ◆ Monitor the patient's peripheral and apical pulses; watch for evidence of decreased cardiac output and heart failure.
Heart failure (complication)	◆ Cough that produces pink, frothy sputum ◆ Cyanosis of the lips and nail beds ◆ Pale, cool, clammy skin ◆ Diaphoresis ◆ Jugular vein distention ◆ Ascites ◆ Pulsus alternans ◆ Tachycardia ◆ Hepatomegaly ◆ Decreased pulse pressure ◆ Third (S_3) and fourth (S_4) heart sounds ◆ Moist, basilar crackles ◆ Rhonchi ◆ Expiratory wheezing ◆ Decreased pulse oximetry ◆ Peripheral edema ◆ Decreased urinary output	◆ Cardiac output is decreased. ◆ B-type natriuretic peptide immunoassay is elevated. ◆ Chest X-ray shows increased pulmonary vascular markings, interstitial edema, or pleural effusions and cardiomegaly. ◆ Electrocardiography reveals heart enlargement or ischemia, tachycardia, extrasystole, or atrial fibrillation. ◆ Pulmonary artery pressure, pulmonary artery wedge pressure (PAWP), and left ventricular end-diastolic pressure are elevated in the presence of left-sided heart failure; right atrial or central venous pressure is elevated in right-sided heart failure.	◆ Limit fluid and sodium intake to decrease preload. ◆ Monitor for signs of embolization (hematuria, pleuritic chest pain, left upper quadrant pain). ◆ Monitor oxygenation status, auscultate lung fields, and evaluate arterial blood gas (ABG) studies. ◆ Monitor urine output. ◆ Administer supplemental oxygen and mechanical ventilation. ◆ Place the patient in Fowler's position. ◆ Administer diuretics, inotropic drugs, vasodilators, angiotensin-converting enzyme inhibitors, angiotensin-receptor blockers, cardiac glycosides, beta-adrenergic blockers, and electrolyte supplements. ◆ Initiate cardiac monitoring. ◆ Recurrent heart failure from valvular dysfunction may require surgery. ◆ A ventricular assist device may be needed. ◆ Maintain adequate cardiac output ,and monitor hemodynamic stability. ◆ Assess for deep vein thrombosis, and apply antiembolism stockings.

DISORDER	SIGNS AND SYMPTOMS	DIAGNOSTIC TEST RESULTS	TREATMENT AND CARE
Septic arthritis (complication)	◆ Abrupt single swollen joint with pain on active or passive movement ◆ Low-grade fever	◆ Synovial fluid analysis may reveal an elevated leukocyte count. ◆ Gram stain of synovial fluid may reveal the infecting organism. ◆ X-rays reveal the inflamed synovial tissue and accompanying fluid in the joint as well as a symmetric soft-tissue swelling around the involved joint. ◆ Magnetic resonance imaging reveals inflammatory changes and fluid.	◆ Practice strict sterile technique for all procedures. Wash hands carefully before and after giving care. Dispose of soiled linens and dressings properly. Prevent contact between immunosuppressed patients and infected patients. ◆ Watch for signs of joint inflammation (heat, redness, swelling, pain, or drainage). Monitor vital signs and fever pattern. Remember that corticosteroids mask signs of infection. ◆ Check splints or traction regularly. Keep the joint in proper alignment, but avoid prolonged immobilization. Start passive range-of-motion exercises immediately, and progress to active exercises as soon as the patient can move the affected joint and put weight on it. ◆ Monitor pain levels and medicate accordingly, especially before exercise, remembering that the pain of septic arthritis is easy to underestimate. Administer analgesics and opioids for acute pain and heat or ice packs for moderate pain. ◆ Warn the patient before the first aspiration that it will be painful. Carefully evaluate the patient's condition after joint aspiration.
Valvular insufficiency (complication)	◆ Orthopnea ◆ Dyspnea ◆ Fatigue ◆ Angina ◆ Palpitations ◆ Peripheral edema ◆ Jugular vein distention ◆ Hepatomegaly ◆ Tachycardia ◆ Crackles ◆ Pulmonary edema ◆ Murmurs	◆ Catheterization may show mitral insufficiency with increased left ventricular end-diastolic volume and pressure, and increased atrial pressure and PAWP. ◆ X-rays may show left atrial and ventricular enlargement and pulmonary venous congestion. ◆ Echocardiography shows abnormal valve leaflet motion and left atrial enlargement. ◆ Electrocardiography may show left atrial and ventricular hypertrophy, sinus tachycardia, and atrial fibrillation.	◆ Watch for signs of heart failure or pulmonary edema. ◆ Monitor for adverse effects of drug therapy. ◆ Teach the patient about diet restrictions, medications, and the importance of consistent follow-up care. ◆ Monitor vital signs, ABG studies, input and output, daily weight, blood chemistries, chest X-rays, and pulmonary artery readings. ◆ Therapies vary with the severity of symptoms.
Valvular stenosis (complication)	◆ Dyspnea ◆ Orthopnea ◆ Palpitations ◆ Peripheral edema ◆ Jugular vein distention ◆ Ascites ◆ Crackles ◆ Cardiac arrhythmias ◆ Murmurs	◆ PAWP is increased. ◆ Severe pulmonary hypertension is present. ◆ X-rays may reveal left atrial and ventricular enlargement, enlarged pulmonary arteries, and mitral valve calcification. ◆ Echocardiography may show a thickened mitral valve. ◆ Electrocardiography may show left atrial hypertrophy, atrial fibrillation, right ventricular hypertrophy, and right axis deviation.	◆ Watch for signs of heart failure or pulmonary edema. ◆ Monitor for adverse effects of drug therapy. ◆ Teach the patient about diet restrictions, medications, and the importance of consistent follow-up care. ◆ Monitor vital signs, ABG studies, input and output, daily weight, blood chemistries, chest X-rays, and pulmonary artery readings. ◆ Therapies vary with the severity of symptoms.

Esophageal varices

OVERVIEW

- Dilated, torturous veins in the submucosa of the lower esophagus resulting from portal hypertension (elevated pressure in the portal vein)
- May result in sudden and massive bleeding
- Accounts for approximately 10% of cases of upper GI bleeding
- 70% chance of experiencing additional bleeding episodes with one-third ending in death

CAUSES
- Cirrhosis
- Mechanical obstruction
- Occlusion of the hepatic veins (Budd-Chiari syndrome)

PATHOPHYSIOLOGY

- As pressure in the portal vein rises, blood backs up into the spleen and flows through collateral channels to the venous system, bypassing the liver.
- Splenomegaly; thrombocytopenia; dilated, collateral veins in the esophagus, abdomen, and rectum (hemorrhoids); and ascites may occur.

GASTROINTESTINAL SYSTEM
- The collateral circulation located in the submucosa of the lower esophagus and upper stomach results from communication between the portal vein and the gastric coronary vein.
- Increased blood flow and higher pressure resulting from the opening of these collaterals cause the submucosa veins near the esophagogastric junction to become dilated and protrude into the lumen.

CARDIOVASCULAR SYSTEM
- Hemorrhage from bleeding varices may cause circulatory collapse.

RESPIRATORY SYSTEM
- Impaired gas exchange may occur because of the possibility of aspiration pneumonitis. (*See Disorders affecting management of esophageal varices,* pages 158 and 159.)

ASSESSMENT

HISTORY
- History of excessive use of alcohol
- History of cirrhosis
- Mechanical irritation, straining on defecation, or rigorous coughing preceding the bleeding episode

PHYSICAL FINDINGS
- Massive hematemesis
- Varied level of consciousness depending on the degree of bleeding
- Tachycardia
- Tachypnea
- Hypotension
- Weak peripheral pulses
- Pale skin
- Circumoral pallor
- Dry mucous membranes
- Poor skin turgor
- Jaundice
- Splenomegaly
- Diminished urine output

DIAGNOSTIC TEST RESULTS

◆ Endoscopy identifies the ruptured varix as the bleeding site and excludes other potential sources in the upper GI tract.
◆ Complete blood count reveals decreased hemoglobin levels, hematocrit, and red blood cell count; white blood cell and platelet counts are decreased initially due to splenomegaly.
◆ Coagulation studies reveal prolonged prothrombin time secondary to hepatocellular disease.
◆ Serum chemistry tests may reveal elevated blood urea nitrogen, sodium, total bilirubin, and ammonia levels; decreased serum albumin due to liver damage; and elevated liver enzyme levels.
◆ Angiography helps to identify patency of the portal vein and development of collateral vessels.

GENERAL

◆ Esophagastric inflatable balloon
◆ Nasogastric (NG) tube
◆ Endoscopic therapy (sclerotherapy or ligation of varices)
◆ Blood products

DIET

◆ Nothing by mouth during bleeding episodes or prior to endoscopic therapy or surgery

ACTIVITY

◆ Bed rest during bleeding episodes

MEDICATIONS

◆ Beta-adrenergic blockers
◆ Antisecretory agents (somatostatin)
◆ Vasoconstrictors (vasopressin)
◆ Vasodilators

WARNING *Vasopressin may cause adverse reactions such as hypothermia, myocardial and GI tract ischemia, and acute renal failure; therefore, it should be used with caution. Propranolol may cause decreased pulse and blood pressures, which may impair the patient's cardiovascular response to hemorrhage.*

SURGERY

◆ Transjugular intrahepatic portosystemic shunt
◆ Portal systemic shunting
◆ Percutaneous transhepatic embolization

NURSING DIAGNOSES

◆ Anxiety
◆ Decreased cardiac output
◆ Deficient fluid volume
◆ Imbalanced nutrition: Less than body requirements
◆ Risk for aspiration

EXPECTED OUTCOMES

The patient will:
◆ express feelings of decreased anxiety
◆ maintain adequate cardiac output
◆ maintain fluid volume within normal limits
◆ maintain weight and nutritional status
◆ not aspirate.

NURSING INTERVENTIONS

◆ Monitor amount of bleeding, vital signs, and laboratory values.
◆ Administer fluid and blood products, as ordered.
◆ Administer prescribed medications.
◆ Monitor for signs and symptoms of aspiration.
◆ Maintain NG tube patency, and assess characteristics of drainage.
◆ Prepare for surgery, as indicated.
◆ Provide support and encourage verbalization of feelings.

(continued)

Be sure to cover:
- disorder, diagnostic testing, and treatment
- medication administration, dosage, and possible adverse effects
- preoperative and postoperative care
- need for lifestyle changes, if appropriate
- available support services, if indicated.

RESOURCES
Organizations
Alcoholics Anonymous: *www.alcoholics-anonymous.org*
American Liver Foundation: *www.liver-foundation.org*
Digestive Disease National Coalition: *www.ddnc.org*
Selected references
Kovalak, M., et al. "Endoscopic Screening for Varices in Cirrotic Patients; Data from a National Endoscopic Data-base," *Gastrointestinal Endoscopy* 65(1):82-88, January 2007.
Longacre, A., and Garcia-Tsao, G. "A Commonsense Approach to Esophageal Varices," *Clinics in Liver Disease* 10(3):613-25, August 2006.
Triantos, C., and Burroughs, A. "Prevention of the Development of Varices and First Portal Hypertensive Bleeding Episode," *Best Practice and Research in Clinical Gastroenterology* 21(1):31-42, 2007.

Disorders affecting management of esophageal varices

This chart highlights disorders that affect the management of esophageal varices.

DISORDER	SIGNS AND SYMPTOMS	DIAGNOSTIC TEST RESULTS	TREATMENT AND CARE
Aspiration pneumonia (complication)	• Fever • Chills • Sweats • Pleuritic chest pain • Cough • Sputum production • Hemoptysis • Dyspnea • Headache • Fatigue • Bronchial breath sounds over areas of consolidation • Crackles • Increased tactile fremitus • Unequal chest wall expansion	• Chest X-rays reveal infiltrates, confirming the diagnosis. • Sputum specimen for Gram stain and culture and sensitivity tests shows acute inflammatory cells. • White blood cell count indicates leukocytosis in bacterial pneumonia and a normal or low count in viral or mycoplasmal pneumonia. • Blood cultures reflect bacteremia and help to determine the causative organism. • Arterial blood gas (ABG) levels vary depending on the severity of pneumonia and the underlying lung state. • Bronchoscopy or transtracheal aspiration allows the collection of material for culture. Pleural fluid culture may also be obtained. • Pulse oximetry may show a reduced level of arterial oxygen saturation.	• Maintain a patent airway and adequate oxygenation. Measure the patient's ABG levels, especially if he's hypoxic. Administer supplemental oxygen if his partial pressure of arterial oxygen falls below 55 mm Hg. If he has an underlying chronic lung disease, give oxygen cautiously. • With severe pneumonia that requires endotracheal (ET) intubation or a tracheostomy with or without mechanical ventilation, provide thorough respiratory care and suction often, using sterile technique, to remove secretions. • Obtain sputum specimens, as needed. Use suction if the patient can't produce a specimen. Collect the specimens in a sterile container, and deliver them promptly to the microbiology laboratory. • Administer antibiotics and pain medication. Administer I.V. fluids and electrolyte replacement, if needed, for fever and dehydration. • Provide a high-calorie, high-protein diet of soft foods to offset the calories the patient uses to fight the infection. If necessary, supplement oral feedings with nasogastric (NG) tube feedings or parenteral nutrition. • To prevent aspiration during NG tube feedings, elevate the patient's head, check the tube position, and administer the feeding slowly. Don't give large volumes at one time because this can cause vomiting. • If the patient has an ET tube, inflate the tube cuff before feeding. Keep his head elevated after feeding. • Monitor the patient's fluid intake and output. • To control the spread of infection, dispose of secretions properly. Tell the patient to sneeze and cough into a disposable tissue, and tape a waxed bag to the side of the bed for used tissues. • Provide a quiet, calm environment, with frequent rest periods. Make sure the patient has diversionary activities appropriate to his age. • Listen to the patient's fears and concerns, and remain with him during periods of severe stress and anxiety. Encourage him to identify actions and care measures that promote comfort and relaxation. • Whenever possible, include the patient in decisions about his care. • Include family members in all phases of the patient's care, and encourage them to visit.

DISORDER	SIGNS AND SYMPTOMS	DIAGNOSTIC TEST RESULTS	TREATMENT AND CARE
Esophageal rupture (complication)	◆ Severe vomiting or retching ◆ Acute, severe chest or epigastric pain ◆ Subcutaneous emphysema ◆ Dysphagia ◆ Dysphonia ◆ Dyspnea ◆ Tachycardia ◆ Raspy, crunching sound heard over the precordium with each heartbeat ◆ Reduced breath sounds on side of perforation	◆ Chest X-ray may show mediastinal air, pleural effusion, free air under the diaphragm, pneumothorax, and hydropneumothorax. ◆ Lateral neck X-ray reveals air in fascial planes. ◆ Esophagram identifies perforation. ◆ Computed tomography scan with contrast reveals perforation. ◆ Esophagoscopy visualizes perforation.	◆ Assess respiratory and circulatory status; maintain a patent airway. ◆ Restrict anything by mouth; insert NG tube to aspirate gastric contents. ◆ Assess pain level; administer analgesics, as ordered, and evaluate effect. ◆ Administer antibiotics and antiemetics, as ordered. ◆ Prepare the patient for surgery; provide preoperative and postoperative teaching and care. ◆ Monitor for signs and symptoms of complications such as sepsis.
Hypovolemic shock (complication)	◆ Pallor ◆ Decreased level of consciousness ◆ Hypotension ◆ Tachycardia ◆ Cool, clammy skin ◆ Urine output less than 25 ml/hour	◆ Central venous pressure, pulmonary wedge pressure, and cardiac output are decreased. ◆ Hematocrit, hemoglobin, and red blood cell and platelet counts are low. ◆ Serum potassium, sodium, lactate dehydrogenase, blood urea nitrogen, and creatinine are elevated. ◆ Urine specific gravity is increased. ◆ Arterial blood gas analysis shows respiratory acidosis.	◆ Assess extent of fluid loss. ◆ Administer fluid and blood replacement. ◆ Administer supplemental oxygen. ◆ Monitor vital signs and intake and output. ◆ Monitor respiratory status and pulse oximetry. ◆ Assist with ET intubation, if necessary. ◆ Prepare the patient for surgery to control bleeding.

Fibromyalgia syndrome

OVERVIEW

- Diffuse pain syndrome that's observed in up to 15% of patients seen in general rheumatology practice and 5% of general medicine clinics
- Affects 90% more females than males
- May occur at almost any age, but incidence peaks between ages 20 and 60
- Formerly known as *fibrositis*
- Also called *FMS*

CAUSES

- Exact cause unknown
- May be multifactorial and influenced by stress, physical conditioning, abnormal sleep patterns, and neuroendocrine, psychiatric, or hormonal factors
- May be primary disorder or associated with underlying disease such as infection

PATHOPHYSIOLOGY

- Altered processing of nociceptive stimuli in the central nervous system (CNS) causes the perception of pain even with non-nociceptive stimuli.
- The disorder may be the result of abnormalities in pronociception and antinociception pathways.
- Several theories describe FMS:
- Blood flow to the muscle is decreased (due to poor muscle aerobic conditioning, rather than other physiologic abnormalities).
- Blood flow in the thalamus and caudate nucleus is decreased, leading to a lowered pain threshold.
- Endocrine dysfunction—such as abnormal pituitary-adrenal axis responses or abnormal levels of the neurotransmitter serotonin in brain centers—affects pain and sleep.
- The functioning of other pain-processing pathways is abnormal. (See *Disorders affecting management of fibromyalgia,* page 163.)

MUSCULOSKELETAL SYSTEM

- Diffuse pain in the neck, shoulder, and lower limbs affects ability to participate in vigorous activities or exercise.
- Activities of daily living may be difficult to accomplish due to fatigue and pain.

NEUROLOGIC SYSTEM

- Disturbed sleep patterns result in impaired cognitive thinking, labile emotions, and fatigue.
- Central sensitization caused by physical injury causes disruption of pain sensation and pain control.
- Depression frequently occurs due to difficulty in diagnosing cause of pain and fatigue.

ASSESSMENT

HISTORY

- Diffuse, dull, aching pain across neck and shoulders and in lower back and proximal limbs
- Pain that's typically worse in the morning, sometimes with stiffness; can be exacerbated by stress, lack of sleep, weather changes, and inactivity
- Sleep disturbances with frequent arousal and fragmented sleep or frequent waking throughout night (patient unaware of arousals)
- Possible reports of irritable bowel syndrome, tension headaches, puffy hands, and paresthesia

PHYSICAL FINDINGS

- Tender points elicited by applying a moderate amount of pressure to a specific location. (See *Tender points of fibromyalgia.*)

DIAGNOSTIC TEST RESULTS

- Diagnostic testing in FMS not associated with an underlying disease is generally negative for significant abnormalities.

TREATMENT

GENERAL
◆ Massage therapy
◆ Ultrasound treatments

DIET
◆ Well-balanced diet; weight reduction, if appropriate

ACTIVITY
◆ Regular, low-impact aerobic exercise program such as water aerobics
◆ Pre-exercise and postexercise stretching to minimize injury

MEDICATIONS
◆ Skeletal muscle relaxants (amitriptyline, nortriptyline, or cyclobenzaprine)
◆ Tricyclic antidepressants and serotonin reuptake inhibitors
◆ Anxiolytics
◆ Anticonvulsants (useful with chronic pain states)
◆ Nonsteroidal anti-inflammatory drugs
◆ Magnesium supplements
◆ Steroid or lidocaine injections
◆ Pramipexole (Mirapex), a dopamine agonist (possibly helpful in some patients)

Tender points of fibromyalgia

The patient with fibromyalgia syndrome may complain of specific areas of tenderness, which are shown in the illustrations below.

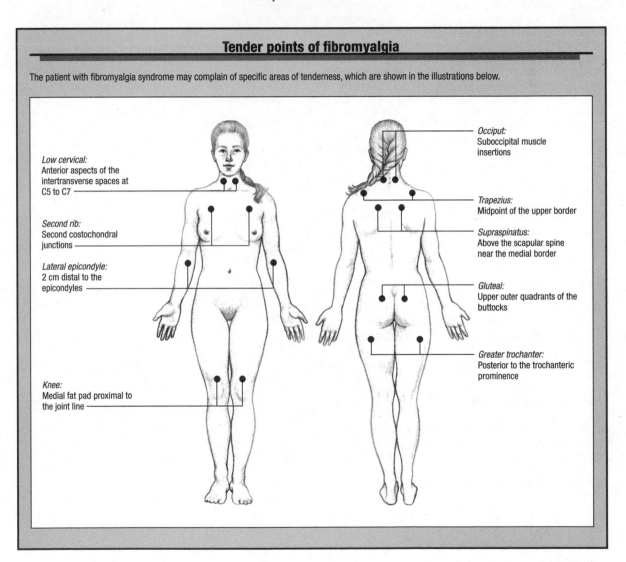

Low cervical:
Anterior aspects of the intertransverse spaces at C5 to C7

Second rib:
Second costochondral junctions

Lateral epicondyle:
2 cm distal to the epicondyles

Knee:
Medial fat pad proximal to the joint line

Occiput:
Suboccipital muscle insertions

Trapezius:
Midpoint of the upper border

Supraspinatus:
Above the scapular spine near the medial border

Gluteal:
Upper outer quadrants of the buttocks

Greater trochanter:
Posterior to the trochanteric prominence

(continued)

NURSING CONSIDERATIONS

NURSING DIAGNOSES
- Activity intolerance
- Chronic pain
- Disturbed sleep pattern
- Energy field disturbance
- Fatigue
- Hopelessness
- Impaired physical mobility
- Ineffective coping
- Ineffective health maintenance
- Ineffective role performance
- Powerlessness

EXPECTED OUTCOMES
The patient will:
- verbalize the importance of balancing activity, as tolerated, with rest
- express feelings of increased comfort and decreased pain
- express feelings of being well rested or will appear well rested
- express an increased sense of well-being
- verbalize feelings of increased energy
- make decisions on own behalf
- attain the highest degree of mobility possible within the confines of the disease
- demonstrate effective coping behaviors
- continue to receive treatments that help promote relaxation and inner well-being
- recognize limitations imposed by the illness and express feelings about these limitations
- express feelings of control over the pain.

NURSING INTERVENTIONS
- Give prescribed drugs.
- Provide emotional support.
- Encourage the patient to perform regular stretching exercises safely and effectively.
- Provide reassurance that FMS can be treated.
- Assess for sensory disturbances.
- Assess level of pain and effects of medication.
- Observe for signs of fatigue and depression.

PATIENT TEACHING

Be sure to cover:
- disorder, diagnostic testing, and treatment
- medication administration, dosage, and possible adverse effects
- importance of exercise in maintaining muscle conditioning, improving energy and, possibly, improving sleep quality
- avoidance of decongestants and caffeine before bedtime
- available support services, if appropriate.

RESOURCES
Organizations
American Fibromyalgia Syndrome Association, Inc.: *www.afsafund.org*
Arthritis Foundation: *www.arthritis.org*

Selected references
Hughes, L. "Physical and Psychological Variables That Influence Pain in Patients with Fibromyalgia," *Orthopaedic Nursing* 25(3):112-19, March-April 2006.

Nelson, P., and Tucker, S. "Developing an Intervention to Alter Castrophizing in Persons with Fibromyalgia," *Orthopaedic Nursing* 25(3):205-14, May-June 2006.

Prins, M.A., et al. "Sexual Functioning of Women with Fibromyalgia," *Clinical and Experimental Rheumatology* 24(5):555-61, September-October 2006.

Stuifbergen, A.K., et al. "Illness Perceptions and Related Outcomes Among Women with Fibromyalgia Syndrome," *Womens Health* 16(6):353-60, November-December 2006.

Disorders affecting management of fibromyalgia

This chart highlights disorders that affect the management of fibromyalgia.

DISORDER	SIGNS AND SYMPTOMS	DIAGNOSTIC TEST RESULTS	TREATMENT AND CARE
Chronic fatigue syndrome (coexisting)	◆ Myalgia ◆ Cognitive dysfunction ◆ Unrefreshing sleep ◆ Sore throat ◆ Tender cervical or axillary nodes ◆ Multiple joint pain without swelling ◆ Headaches ◆ Postexertional malaise lasting 24 hours or longer	◆ Lymphocyte differential may reveal reduced natural killer cell cytotoxicity, abnormal $CD4^+$:$CD8^+$ T-cell ratios, and mild lymphocytosis. ◆ Immunoglobulin profile may show decreased immunoglobulin subclasses. ◆ Immune complex profile may reveal circulating immune complexes. ◆ Antimicrosomal antibody testing may reveal increased levels of antimicrosomal antibodies.	◆ Provide emotional support. ◆ Begin a graded exercise program. ◆ Monitor response to treatment. ◆ Administer medications and observe for adverse effects. ◆ Monitor for signs and symptoms of complications.
Depression (complication or coexisting)	◆ Difficulty sleeping ◆ Difficulty concentrating or thinking clearly ◆ Profound loss of pleasure in all activities ◆ Change in eating patterns ◆ Agitation ◆ Psychomotor retardation ◆ Recent weight loss or gain ◆ Use of prescription, nonprescription, over-the-counter, or illegal drugs	◆ Psychiatric evaluation identifies symptoms meeting *DSM-IV-TR* criteria for major depression. ◆ Toxicology screening suggests drug use. ◆ Beck Depression Inventory shows the onset, severity, duration, and progression of depressive symptoms.	◆ Encourage participation in activities of daily living. ◆ Encourage verbalization of feelings. ◆ Encourage interaction with others. ◆ Administer medications and observe for adverse effects. ◆ Provide a structured routine. ◆ Identify support systems and encourage participation and interaction. ◆ Assess for suicidal ideation, and provide surveillance, if appropriate.
Substance dependence (complication)	◆ Substance often taken in larger amounts or for a longer time than the patient intended ◆ Persistent desire or one or more unsuccessful efforts to cut down or control substance use ◆ Excessive time devoted to activities necessary to obtain the substance ◆ Frequent intoxication or withdrawal symptoms when expected to fulfill major obligations at work, school, or home or when substance use is physically hazardous ◆ Impaired social, occupational, or recreational activities ◆ Continued substance use despite the recognition of a persistent or recurrent social, psychological, or physical problem that's caused or exacerbated by the use of the substance ◆ Marked tolerance ◆ Characteristic withdrawal symptoms ◆ Substance commonly taken to relieve or avoid withdrawal symptoms	◆ Serum or urine drug screen reveals the substance. ◆ Serum protein electrophoresis shows elevated serum globulin levels. ◆ Serum glucose measurement shows hypoglycemia. ◆ Complete blood count (CBC) shows leukocytosis. ◆ Liver function is abnormal. ◆ CBC shows elevated mean corpuscular hemoglobin levels. ◆ Uric acid levels are elevated. ◆ Blood urea nitrogen levels are decreased. ◆ Mental status examination findings fit *DSM-IV-TR* criteria for substance abuse.	◆ Maintain a quiet, safe environment. ◆ Institute seizure precautions. ◆ Set limits for dealing with demanding, manipulative behavior. ◆ Monitor vital signs, and observe behavior for suicide ideation. ◆ Observe for signs of complications. ◆ Evaluate nutritional status and provide appropriate diet. ◆ Administer medications and observe effects.

Gaucher's disease

OVERVIEW

◆ Most common lysosomal storage disease
◆ Occurs in three forms: type I (adult), type II (infantile), and type III (juvenile)
◆ Type II possibly fatal within 9 months of onset, usually from pulmonary involvement (see *Types of Gaucher's disease*)

CAUSES

◆ Autosomal recessive gene inheritance
◆ More than 100 mutations of the gene identified; however, mutation appearing is unrelated to the manifestations presented or the prognosis

PATHOPHYSIOLOGY

◆ The faulty gene is located on the long arm (designated as "q") of chromosome 1 in region 21 (1q21).
◆ Abnormal gene encoding leads to a deficiency in the enzyme glucocerebrosidase, which plays a major role in phagocytosis, breaking down dead cells and cellular debris.
◆ This deficiency causes an abnormal accumulation of glucocerebrosides in reticuloendothelial cells and in the storage compartments (lysosomes) of certain body cells.
◆ Lucosylceramide is an intermediate metabolite that forms from the breakdown of aging leukocytes. This metabolite, along with other fats and carbohydrates that aren't broken down, builds up in the monocytes and macrophages of the liver, spleen, bones, and bone marrow.
◆ These now enlarged cells are called Gaucher cells and can affect any organ in the body. (See *Disorders affecting management of Gaucher's disease*, page 167.)

HEMATOLOGIC SYSTEM

◆ Gaucher cells infiltrate the spleen, leading to splenomegaly and hypersplenism, which results in overfiltering of circulating blood cells, possibly leading to anemia, leukopenia, and thrombocytopenia.

◆ Fibrosis occurs, which affects red blood cell production, leading to anemia.
◆ Blood cell production is compromised by infiltration of the Gaucher cells in the bone marrow.

MUSCULOSKELETAL SYSTEM

◆ Infiltration of osteocytes can lead to musculoskeletal abnormalities.
◆ Remodeling of the distal femur and proximal tibia fails, producing a funnel-like, cylindrical-shaped bone instead of the typical flared shape.
◆ Diffuse and localized bone loss occurs along with cortical thinning and loss of coarse cancellous bone. Bone loss is most severe in the axial skeleton.
◆ Osteonecrosis occurs, most commonly affecting the femoral head or proximal humerus (although it may also affect the long bones), leading to pathologic fractures and bone pain.

NEUROLOGIC SYSTEM

◆ Enzyme deficiency can result in Gaucher cells developing within the cells of the central nervous system.
◆ Motor and sensory nerve dysfunction can occur leading to seizures, hypertonicity, spasticity, hyperreflexia, and cognitive dysfunction.

Types of Gaucher's disease

Gaucher's disease can be classified as one of three types—classification is based on the age of onset and the degree of neurologic involvement.

Type I Gaucher's disease is the most common form of all lysosomal disorders. It occurs primarily in the Ashkenazi Jewish population. Although most cases are diagnosed in adulthood, some cases are diagnosed in infancy; others aren't diagnosed until age 70 or older. The disease initially presents as painless splenomegaly. Bone involvement may be so severe that the patient is confined to a wheelchair.

Type II Gaucher's disease is a rare form. Onset usually occurs by age 3 months. The disease initially presents as hepatosplenomegaly. Trismus, strabismus, and backward flexion of the neck develop within a few months. The disease involves rapid neurologic deterioration. Most patients die before age 1.

Type III is also rare and combines features of type I and type II. Splenomegaly and bone marrow damage occur along with neurologic manifestations. Onset occurs at an older age and progresses at a slower rate than with type II disease.

HISTORY

Type I

- Severe episodic pain in the legs, arms, and back
- Pathologic fractures
- Vertebral compression
- Easy bruising and bleeding, anemia and, rarely, pancytopenia

Type II

- Motor dysfunction and spasticity
- Dysphagia
- Easy bruising and bleeding
- Seizures

Type III

- Seizures

PHYSICAL FINDINGS

Type I

- Collapsed hip joints
- Fever
- Abdominal distention (from hypotonicity of the large bowel)
- Hepatosplenomegaly
- Respiratory problems (pneumonia or, rarely, cor pulmonale)
- Yellow pallor and brown-yellow pigmentation on the face and legs (in older patients)

Type II

- Strabismus
- Muscle hypertonicity
- Retroflexion of the head
- Neck rigidity
- Laryngeal stridor
- Hyperreflexia
- Respiratory distress

Type III

- Hypertonicity
- Strabismus
- Poor coordination and mental ability

DIAGNOSTIC TEST RESULTS

- Direct assay of glucocerebrosidase activity, which can be performed on venous blood, confirms the diagnosis.
- Bone marrow aspiration shows Gaucher cells.
- Distal femur radiography shows flask-shaped bone.
- Magnetic resonance imaging of the skeleton, including femurs, shows infiltration of bone marrow and bone changes.
- Laboratory tests reveal increased serum acid phosphatase levels and decreased platelets and serum iron levels.
- EEG is abnormal after infancy in type III disease.

GENERAL

- Supportive care
- Genetic counseling
- Blood transfusions

DIET

- Well-balanced diet high in iron

ACTIVITY

- As tolerated

MEDICATIONS

- Enzyme replacement therapy
- Vitamins, including supplemental iron or liver extract
- Analgesics

SURGERY

- Partial or total splenectomy to combat hypersplenism or mechanical obstruction due to splenomegaly
- Bone marrow transplantation

(continued)

NURSING CONSIDERATIONS

NURSING DIAGNOSES
- Acute pain
- Fatigue
- Impaired gas exchange
- Impaired parenting
- Risk for injury

EXPECTED OUTCOMES
The patient will:
- express increased comfort and decreased pain
- demonstrate increased energy
- maintain adequate ventilation and oxygenation
- participate in child's care
- remain free from injury.

NURSING INTERVENTIONS
- Monitor respiratory status.
- Assist with ambulation and turn carefully to prevent injury.
- Encourage coughing and deep breathing every 2 hours and use of incentive spirometer every hour.
- Observe for signs and symptoms of bleeding; administer blood products, as ordered.
- Assess pain level; administer analgesics, as ordered, and evaluate effect.

PATIENT TEACHING

Be sure to cover:
- disorder, diagnostic testing, and treatment
- medication administration, dosage, and possible adverse effects
- preoperative and postoperative care, if appropriate
- safety measures
- signs and symptoms of complications.

RESOURCES
Organizations
National Gaucher Foundation: *www.gaucherdisease.org*
National Institute of Neurological Disorders and Stroke: *www.ninds.nih.gov*

Selected references
Costello, R., et al. "Gaucher Disease and Multiple Myeloma," *Leukemia & Lymphoma* 47(7):1365-368, July 2006.
Masood, Y., and Ali, A.S. "Enzyme Replacement Therapy in a Child with Gaucher Disease," *Journal of the College of Physicians and Surgeons-Pakistan* 16(12):786-88, December 2006.
Strategies for Managing Multisystem Disorders. Philadelphia: Lippincott Williams & Wilkins, 2006.

Disorders affecting management of Gaucher's disease

This chart highlights disorders that affect the management of Gaucher's disease.

DISORDER	SIGNS AND SYMPTOMS	DIAGNOSTIC TEST RESULTS	TREATMENT AND CARE
Anemia (complication)	◆ Possibly asymptomatic early; signs and symptoms developing as anemia becomes more severe ◆ Dyspnea on exertion and fatigue ◆ Listlessness, inability to concentrate ◆ Pallor, irritability ◆ Tachycardia ◆ Brittle, thinning nails	◆ Total iron binding capacity is elevated and serum iron levels are decreased (early on). ◆ Bone marrow aspiration reveals reduced iron stores and reduced production of red blood cell (RBC) precursors. ◆ Complete blood count reveals decreased hemoglobin and hematocrit and low mean corpuscular hemoglobin. ◆ RBC indices reveal decreased cells that are microcytic and hypochromic.	◆ Assess for decreased perfusion to vital organs, including heart and lungs; monitor for dyspnea, chest pain, and dizziness. ◆ Administer oxygen therapy to prevent hypoxemia. ◆ Frequently monitor vital signs for changes. ◆ Administer iron replacement therapy. ◆ Prepare to administer blood component therapy, such as packed RBCs, if anemia is severe. ◆ Allow for frequent rest periods.
Pathological fractures (complication)	◆ Increased pain with movement ◆ Inability to intentionally move body part ◆ Possible tingling sensation distal to fracture site ◆ Soft tissue edema ◆ Obvious deformity or shortening of limb ◆ Possible discoloration over fracture site ◆ Warmth, crepitus on palpation ◆ Numbness and coolness distal to site of fracture (indicative of possible nerve and vessel damage)	◆ Anteroposterior and lateral X-rays identify site of fracture, which displays as a break in the continuity of the bone. ◆ Computed tomography or magnetic resonance imaging (MRI) indicates fracture site. ◆ Angiography reveals possible vascular injury due to fracture.	◆ Prepare for immobilization of fracture site with a splint, cast, or traction. ◆ Perform neurovascular assessment every 1 to 2 hours to detect changes in circulation or sensation. ◆ Administer analgesics for pain control. ◆ Increase fluid intake and maintain diet. ◆ Elevate the fractured extremity; for a fractured hip, keep the patient flat with the foot of the bed elevated 25 degrees and legs abducted. ◆ Provide active and passive range-of-motion exercises for unaffected limbs. ◆ Encourage coughing, deep breathing, and incentive spirometry. ◆ Assess vital signs frequently, watching for signs and symptoms of pulmonary or fat embolism, such as dyspnea, tachypnea, tachycardia, hemoptysis, chest pain, and crackles.
Seizure (complications)	◆ Aura ◆ Loss of consciousness ◆ Dyspnea ◆ Fixed, dilated pupils ◆ Incontinence	◆ EEG slows abnormal wave patterns and the focus of the seizure activity. ◆ MRI may show pathologic changes. ◆ Brain mapping identifies seizure areas.	◆ Ensure patient safety; initiate seizure precautions. ◆ Monitor neurologic and respiratory status. ◆ Observe and document the seizure activity (body movement, respiratory pattern, duration of seizure, loss of consciousness, incontinence, and papillary changes). ◆ Administer medications. ◆ Monitor vital signs, intake and output, and laboratory values.
Thrombocytopenia (complication)	◆ Sudden onset of petechiae and ecchymosis or bleeding into mucous membranes ◆ Malaise, fatigue ◆ Blood-filled bullae in the mouth	◆ Platelet count is diminished to less than 100,000/µl. ◆ Bleeding time is prolonged. ◆ Prothrombin and partial thromboplastin times are normal. ◆ Bone marrow study may show ineffective platelet production.	◆ Administer blood products, as ordered; monitor laboratory results. ◆ Administer corticosteroids and monitor blood glucose levels. ◆ Protect from injury and monitor for signs of bleeding. ◆ Provide emotional support. ◆ Observe for signs and symptoms of complications.

Graft-versus-host disease

OVERVIEW

- Organ or graft donor's lymphocytes that recognize the *recipient's* cells as antigenetically different and attempt to destroy them
- May be acute or chronic:
- acute form: occurs within the first 100 days after a transplant
- chronic: occurs after the first 100 days of a transplant and involves an autoimmune response that affects multiple organs
- Less than one-half of recipients with histocompatibility identical to the donor developing graft-versus-host disease (GVHD); incidence increasing to greater than 60% when there is one antigen mismatch
- Highest mortality rates when development of chronic GVHD immediately follows acute GVHD

CAUSES

- Usually develops after a patient with impaired immune function—from congenital immunodeficiency, radiation treatment, or immunosuppressant therapy—receives a bone marrow transplant from an incompatible donor, following solid organ transplants, or from the transfusion of a blood product containing viable lymphocytes
- Maternal-fetal blood transfusions and intrauterine transfusions

PATHOPHYSIOLOGY

- Foreign or graft cells launch an attack against the host cells, which are incapable of rejecting them.
- Three criteria exist, including:
- immunologically competent cells in the graft
- graft recognition of the host as foreign
- inability of the host to react to the graft.
- The process begins when graft cells become sensitized to the recipient's class II antigens.
- Although the exact mechanism by which this occurs remains unclear, biopsy of active GVHD lesions usually reveals infiltration by mononuclear cells, eosinophils, and phagocytic and histiocytic cells.

GASTROINTESTINAL SYSTEM

- Severe diarrhea, severe abdominal pain, GI bleeding, and malabsorption occur as cell loss from the bowel progresses.
- Mild jaundice with elevated liver enzymes and possibly hepatic coma may result from liver damage. (See *Disorders affecting management of GVHD*, pages 170 and 171.)

IMMUNE SYSTEM

- Infections (mostly bacterial and fungal) due to granulocytopenia are an issue immediately after transplantation. Later, interstitial pneumonitis predominates.
- Because the patient is already immunocompromised from a graft or organ transplant, sepsis can occur.

INTEGUMENTARY SYSTEM

- A pruritic maculopapular rash may develop on palms and soles 10 to 30 days after transplant, possibly progressing to generalized erythema with bullous formation and desquamation.

ASSESSMENT

HISTORY

- Skin changes that resemble scleroderma, which can ultimately lead to ulcerations, joint contractures, and impaired esophageal motility

PHYSICAL FINDINGS

- Skin rash
- Severe diarrhea
- Jaundice
- Abdominal cramps
- GI bleeding

DIAGNOSTIC TEST RESULTS

- No single test or combination of tests proves definitive.
- Tissue biopsy usually reveals immunocompetent T cells along with the extent of lymphocytic infiltration and tissue damage.
- Repeat biopsies detect early histologic changes characteristic of rejection, determine the degree of change from previous biopsies, and monitor the course and success of treatment.
- Liver function studies reveal elevated levels of bilirubin, serum alkaline phosphatase, alanine aminotransferase, and aspartate aminotransferase.

TREATMENT

GENERAL
◆ Initial interventions focusing on prevention
◆ Depletion of donor marrow of T cells and radiating blood products before administration to prevent T-cell replication

DIET
◆ Restriction based on organ system affected

ACTIVITY
◆ As tolerated

MEDICATIONS
◆ Immunosuppressants (methotrexate)
◆ Corticosteroids (prednisone)
◆ Antithymocyte globulin, cyclosporine, cyclophosphamide, or tacrolimus

NURSING CONSIDERATIONS

NURSING DIAGNOSES
◆ Activity intolerance
◆ Disturbed body image
◆ Fatigue
◆ Hopelessness
◆ Hyperthermia
◆ Imbalanced nutrition: Less than body requirements
◆ Impaired skin integrity
◆ Impaired tissue integrity
◆ Ineffective coping
◆ Ineffective health maintenance
◆ Ineffective tissue perfusion: Cardiopulmonary, renal
◆ Interrupted family processes
◆ Powerlessness
◆ Risk for deficient fluid volume
◆ Risk for infection
◆ Social isolation

EXPECTED OUTCOMES
The patient will:
◆ verbalize the importance of balancing activity, as tolerated, with rest
◆ express feelings related to a changed body image
◆ express feelings of increased energy
◆ make decisions on own behalf
◆ maintain a normal body temperature
◆ exhibit no signs of malnutrition
◆ exhibit normal healing of wounds and lesions
◆ experience decreased areas of redness, swelling, and inflammation
◆ use support systems to assist with coping
◆ perform health maintenance activities according to the level of his ability
◆ maintain adequate cardiopulmonary and renal perfusion
◆ voice feelings about the condition and how it's affected the family
◆ express feelings of control over his well-being
◆ maintain a normal fluid balance
◆ remain free from signs and symptoms of infection
◆ maintain social interaction to the extent possible.

NURSING INTERVENTIONS
◆ Give prescribed immunosuppressants.
◆ Give prescribed antirejection therapies.
◆ Give prescribed antibiotics for infection.
◆ Monitor vital signs and function of the transplanted organ.
◆ Observe for signs and symptoms of infection and rejection.

(continued)

RESOURCES
Organizations
Centers for Disease Control and Prevention: *www.cdc.gov*
National Institutes of Health: *www.nih.gov*

Selected references
Diseases, 4th ed. Philadelphia: Lippincott Williams & Wilkins, 2006.
Shlomchik, W., et al. "Transplantation's Greatest Challenges: Advances in Chronic Graft-Versus-Host Disease," *Biology of Blood and Bone Marrow Transplant* 13(Suppl 1):2-10, January 2007.
Smith, D.M., and Kresie, L.A. "Preventing Transfusion-Associated Graft-Versus-Host Disease," *Transfusion* 47(1):173-74, January 2007.

Disorders affecting management of GVHD

This chart highlights disorders that affect the management of graft-versus-host disease (GVHD).

DISORDER	SIGNS AND SYMPTOMS	DIAGNOSTIC TEST RESULTS	TREATMENT AND CARE
Hypokalemia (complication)	◆ Abdominal cramps, nausea, vomiting ◆ Muscle weakness ◆ Irritability, malaise, confusion ◆ Paresthesia and progression to paralysis ◆ Decreased cardiac output and possible cardiac arrest at any point ◆ Respiratory paralysis ◆ Metabolic alkalosis ◆ Characteristic electrocardiogram (ECG) changes ◆ Orthostatic hypotension ◆ Irregular heart rate ◆ Decreased bowel sounds ◆ Speech changes	◆ Serum potassium level is below 3.5 mEq/L. ◆ Bicarbonate (HCO_3^-) levels and pH are elevated. ◆ Serum glucose levels are slightly elevated. ◆ ECG changes show a flattened T wave, a depressed ST segment, and a characteristic U wave.	◆ Be prepared to administer I.V. potassium chloride with an infusion pump (never as a bolus) to prevent cardiac arrhythmias and cardiac arrest. Infusion rates are generally 10 mEq/hour, but should not exceed 40 to 60 mEq/hour. ◆ Provide continuous cardiac monitoring during I.V. potassium chloride infusions, and report irregularities immediately, as well as toxic reactions. ◆ Assess the I.V. site for signs and symptoms of infiltration, phlebitis, or tissue necrosis. Advise the patient that I.V. potassium chloride administration can lead to burning at the infusion site. ◆ Monitor vital signs, ECG tracing, heart rate and rhythm, and respiratory status. ◆ Monitor serum potassium levels, intake and output, and signs of metabolic alkalosis. ◆ Provide a safe environment, and assess the patient's risk for injury. ◆ Assess for constipation and gastric distention, but avoid the use of laxatives because of the potassium losses associated with these medications. ◆ Avoid crushing slow-release potassium supplements. ◆ After the potassium has returned to a normal level, the patient may need further dietary counseling and prescription of a sustained-release oral potassium supplement. ◆ A patient taking a diuretic should be changed to a potassium-sparing diuretic to prevent excessive loss of potassium in the urine.

DISORDER	SIGNS AND SYMPTOMS	DIAGNOSTIC TEST RESULTS	TREATMENT AND CARE
Septic shock (complication)	Hyperdynamic phase ◆ Pink, flushed skin ◆ Agitation ◆ Anxiety ◆ Irritability ◆ Shortened attention span ◆ Rapid, shallow respirations ◆ Urine output below normal ◆ Rapid, full, bounding pulse ◆ Warm, dry skin ◆ Normal or slightly elevated blood pressure Hypodynamic phase ◆ Pale and possibly cyanotic skin (peripheral areas may be mottled) ◆ Decreased level of consciousness (obtundation and coma may be present) ◆ Possible rapid, shallow respirations ◆ Urine output less than 25 ml/hour or absent ◆ Weak, thready, and rapid pulse or absent pulse; may be irregular if arrhythmias are present ◆ Cold, clammy skin ◆ Hypotension, usually with a systolic pressure below 90 mm Hg or 50 to 80 mm Hg below the patient's previous level ◆ Crackles or rhonchi if pulmonary congestion is present	◆ Blood cultures are positive for the offending organism. ◆ Complete blood count shows the presence or absence of anemia and leukopenia, severe or absent neutropenia, and (usually) the presence of thrombocytopenia. ◆ Blood urea nitrogen and creatinine levels are increased, and creatinine clearance is decreased. ◆ Prothrombin time and partial thromboplastin time are abnormal. ◆ ECG shows ST-depression, inverted T waves, and arrhythmias resembling myocardial infarction. ◆ Serum lactate dehydrogenase levels are elevated with metabolic acidosis. ◆ Urine studies show increased specific gravity (more than 1.020) and osmolality and decreased sodium. ◆ Arterial blood gas analysis demonstrates elevated blood pH and partial pressure of arterial oxygen (Pao_2) and decreased partial pressure of arterial carbon dioxide ($Paco_2$) with respiratory alkalosis in early stages. As shock progresses, metabolic acidosis develops with hypoxemia indicated by decreased $Paco_2$, as well as decreasing Pao_2, HCO_3^-, and pH levels.	◆ Remove I.V., intra-arterial, or urinary drainage catheters, and send them to the laboratory to culture for the presence of the causative organism. New catheters can be reinserted in the intensive care unit. ◆ Start an I.V. infusion with normal saline solution or lactated Ringer's solution, using a large-bore (14G to 18G) catheter, which allows easier administration for subsequent blood transfusions. (*Caution:* Don't start I.V. infusions in the legs of a shock patient who has suffered abdominal trauma because infused fluid may escape through the ruptured vessel into the abdomen.) ◆ Record the patient's blood pressure, pulse and respiratory rates, and peripheral pulses every 1 to 5 minutes until he's stabilized. Record hemodynamic pressure readings every 15 minutes. Monitor cardiac rhythm continuously. Systolic blood pressure less than 80 mm Hg usually results in inadequate coronary artery blood flow, cardiac ischemia, arrhythmias, and further complications of low cardiac output. When blood pressure drops below 80 mm Hg, increase the oxygen flow rate, and notify the physician immediately. ◆ A progressive drop in blood pressure accompanied by a thready pulse generally signals inadequate cardiac output from reduced intravascular volume. Notify the physician and increase the infusion rate. ◆ Administer appropriate antimicrobial drugs I.V. to achieve effective blood levels rapidly. ◆ Measure hourly urine output. If output is less than 30 ml/hour in adults, increase the fluid infusion rate, but watch for signs of fluid overload, such as an increase in pulmonary artery wedge pressure. Notify the physician if urine output doesn't improve. A diuretic may be ordered to increase renal blood flow and urine output. ◆ Draw an arterial blood sample to measure blood gas levels. Administer oxygen by face mask or airway to ensure adequate tissue oxygenation. Adjust the oxygen flow rate to a higher or lower level, as blood gas measurements indicate. ◆ Provide emotional support to the patient and family members. ◆ Document the occurrence of a nosocomial infection, and report it to the infection-control nurse. Investigating all hospital-acquired infections can help identify their sources and prevent future infections.

Guillain-Barré syndrome

OVERVIEW

♦ Form of polyneuritis
♦ Acute, rapidly progressive, and potentially fatal
♦ Four variations: ascending, descending, Miller-Fischer variant and pure motor (see *Types of Guillain-Barré syndrome*)
♦ Three phases:
– Acute: beginning from first symptom, ending in 1 to 3 weeks
– Plateau: lasting several days to 2 weeks
– Recovery: coincides with remyelination and axonal process regrowth; extends over 4 to 6 months and may take up to 2 to 3 years; recovery possibly not complete
♦ Occurs equally in both sexes, typically between ages 30 and 50

CAUSES
♦ Exact cause unknown

RISK FACTORS
♦ Surgery
♦ Rabies or swine influenza vaccination
♦ Viral illness
♦ Hodgkin's or some other malignant disease
♦ Lupus erythematosus

PATHOPHYSIOLOGY

♦ Segmented demyelination of peripheral nerves occurs, preventing normal transmission of electrical impulses.
♦ Sensorimotor nerve roots are affected; autonomic nerve transmission may also be affected. (See *Understanding sensorimotor nerve degeneration.*)
♦ Although the primary pathophysiologic mechanism involves the nervous system, the overall effects of the disorder can affect multiple systems. (See *Disorders affecting management of Guillain-Barré syndrome*, pages 174 and 175.)

NEUROLOGIC SYSTEM
♦ The myelin sheath, which covers the nerve axons and conducts electrical impulses along the nerve pathways, degenerates.
♦ With degeneration comes inflammation, swelling, and patchy demyelination.
♦ As myelin is destroyed, the nodes of Ranvier, located at the junctures of the myelin sheaths, widen. This widening delays and impairs impulse transmission along the dorsal and ventral nerve roots, which affects sensory function, leading to tingling and numbness; and motor function, leading to muscle weakness, immobility, and paralysis.
♦ Other neurologic problems include sensory loss, loss of position sense, and diminished or absent deep tendon reflexes.

CARDIOVASCULAR SYSTEM
♦ Autonomic nervous system functioning may be affected, possibly leading to cardiac arrhythmias, tachycardia, bradycardia, hypertension, and postural hypotension.
♦ Vascular effects, primarily due to immobility from impaired motor function in conjunction with muscle weakness and paralysis, may lead to deep vein thrombosis.

GASTROINTESTINAL SYSTEM
♦ Swallowing may be impaired due to impaired cranial nerve function.
♦ Abdominal muscles are weakened because of nervous system dysfunction.
♦ Autonomic nervous system dysfunction can lead to decreased peristalsis, resulting in constipation. Bowel sphincter control may also be affected.

INTEGUMENTARY SYSTEM
♦ Immobility secondary to motor and sensory nerve dysfunction increases the risk of skin breakdown.

MUSCULOSKELETAL SYSTEM
♦ Effects on the musculoskeletal system are directly related to the impaired motor function from ventral nerve root involvement.
♦ Impaired motor function leads to weakened muscles.
♦ Paralysis leads to a significant decrease in mobility. Joint pain and contractures may occur.

RESPIRATORY SYSTEM
♦ Paralysis of the internal and external intercostal muscles leads to a reduction in functional breathing.
♦ Vagus nerve paralysis causes a loss of the protective mechanisms that respond to brachial irritation and foreign bodies and a diminished or absent gag reflex.

Types of Guillain-Barré syndrome

Four variations of Guillain-Barré syndrome have been identified: ascending, descending, Miller-Fischer variant, and pure motor. These classifications reflect the degree of peripheral nerve involvement.

In ascending Guillain-Barré syndrome, the most common form, weakness and numbness begin in the legs and progress upward to the trunk, arms, and cranial nerves. Symmetrical motor deficits range from paresis to quadriplegia. Sensory deficits involve mild numbness that's more severe in the toes. Reflexes are absent or diminished.

In descending Guillain-Barré syndrome, initial weakness of the cranial nerves, such as facial, glossopharyngeal, vagus, and hypoglossal nerves, progresses downward. Sensory deficits more commonly occur in the hands than in the feet. Reflexes are absent or diminished.

In Miller-Fisher variant Guillain-Barré syndrome, a rare form, ophthalmoplegia, areflexia, and pronounced ataxia occur, with no sensory loss.

In pure motor Guillain-Barré syndrome, a mild form, manifestations are similar to those of the ascending form, except that sensory deficits are absent.

- Immobility due to impaired motor function can lead to retained secretions, atelectasis, and pneumonia.

URINARY SYSTEM

- Motor and sensory nerve dysfunction may lead to impaired bladder muscle tone and sphincter muscle function, possibly affecting urinary elimination.
- Autonomic nervous system dysfunction can lead to urine retention and loss of urinary sphincter control.

ASSESSMENT

HISTORY

- Minor febrile illness 1 to 4 weeks before current symptoms
- Paresthesia in the legs
- Progression of symptoms to arms, trunk and, finally, the face
- Stiffness and pain in the calves

PHYSICAL FINDINGS

- Muscle weakness (major neurologic sign)
- Sensory loss, usually in the legs (spreads to arms)
- Difficulty talking, chewing, and swallowing
- Paralysis of the ocular, facial, and oropharyngeal muscles
- Loss of position sense
- Diminished or absent deep tendon reflexes

DIAGNOSTIC TEST RESULTS

- Cerebrospinal fluid (CSF) analysis may show a normal white blood cell count, an elevated protein count and, in severe disease, increased CSF pressure.
- Electromyography may demonstrate repeated firing of the same motor unit instead of widespread sectional stimulation.
- Nerve conduction studies show marked slowing of nerve conduction velocities.

TREATMENT

GENERAL

- Supportive measures
- Emotional support
- Maintenance of skin integrity
- Possible endotracheal (ET) intubation or tracheotomy
- Fluid volume replacement
- Plasmapheresis
- Possible tube feedings with ET intubation

DIET

- Adequate caloric intake

ACTIVITY

- Exercise program to prevent contractures

MEDICATIONS

- I.V. beta-adrenergic blockers
- Parasympatholytics
- I.V. immune globulin

SURGERY

- Possible tracheostomy
- Possible gastrostomy or jejunotomy feeding tube insertion

UP CLOSE

Understanding sensorimotor nerve degeneration

Guillain-Barré syndrome attacks the peripheral nerves so that they can't transmit messages to the brain correctly. Following is a synthesis of what goes wrong.

The myelin sheath degenerates for unknown reasons. This sheath covers the nerve axons and conducts electrical impulses along the nerve pathways. Degeneration brings inflammation, swelling, and patchy demyelination. As the disorder destroys myelin, the nodes of Ranvier (at the junction of the myelin sheaths) widen, which delays and impairs impulse transmission along the dorsal and anterior nerve roots.

Because the dorsal nerve roots handle sensory function, the patient may experience tingling and numbness. Similarly, because the anterior nerve roots are responsible for motor function, impairment causes varying weakness, immobility, and paralysis.

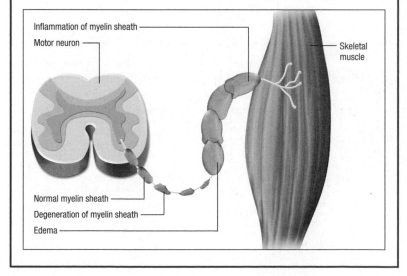

Inflammation of myelin sheath
Motor neuron
Skeletal muscle
Normal myelin sheath
Degeneration of myelin sheath
Edema

(continued)

NURSING CONSIDERATIONS

NURSING DIAGNOSES
- Anxiety
- Fear
- Imbalanced nutrition: Less than body requirements
- Impaired gas exchange
- Impaired physical mobility
- Impaired urinary elimination
- Impaired verbal communication
- Ineffective breathing pattern

EXPECTED OUTCOMES
The patient will:
- identify strategies to reduce anxiety
- express fears and concerns
- maintain required daily caloric intake
- maintain adequate ventilation and oxygenation
- maintain joint mobility and range of motion (ROM)
- establish routine urinary elimination patterns
- develop alternate means of expressing self
- maintain effective breathing pattern.

NURSING INTERVENTIONS
- Establish a means of communication before intubation is required, if possible.
- Reposition the patient every 2 hours, and assess skin integrity.
- Encourage coughing and deep-breathing exercises.
- Provide meticulous skin care.
- Provide passive ROM exercises.
- In case of facial paralysis, provide eye and mouth care.
- Provide emotional support.
- Give prescribed drugs.
- Monitor vital signs, arterial blood gas measurements, and pulse oximetry.
- Assess respiratory status and level of consciousness.
- Observe for signs of thrombophlebitis, urine retention, and response to medications.

PATIENT TEACHING

Be sure to cover:
- disorder, diagnostic testing, and treatment
- effective means of communication
- appropriate home care plan
- medication administration, dosage, and possible adverse effects
- physical and occupational and speech therapy, if indicated
- local support services, if indicated.

RESOURCES
Organizations
Guillain-Barré Syndrome Foundation, International: *www.gbsfi.com*
National Institutes of Health: *www.nih.gov*

Selected references
Ali, M.I., et al. "Mechanical Ventilation in Patients with Guillain-Barré Syndrome," *Respiratory Care* 51(12):1403-407, December 2006.
Atkinson, S.B., et al. "The Challenges of Managing and Treating Guillian-Barré Syndrome During the Acute Phase," *Dimensions in Critical Care Nursing* 25(6):256-63, November-December 2006.
Bernsen, R.A., et al. "The Effects of Guillian-Barré Syndrome on the Close Relatives of Patients During the First Year," *Journal of the Neurological Sciences* 244(1-2):69-75, May 2006.
Diseases, 4th ed. Philadelphia: Lippincott Williams & Wilkins, 2006.

Disorders affecting management of Guillain-Barré syndrome

This chart highlights disorders that affect the management of Guillain-Barré syndrome.

DISORDER	SIGNS AND SYMPTOMS	DIAGNOSTIC TEST RESULTS	TREATMENT AND CARE
Cardiac arrhythmias (complication)	- Palpitations - Chest pain - Dizziness - Weakness, fatigue - Irregular heart rhythm - Hypotension - Syncope - Altered level of consciousness (LOC) - Diaphoresis - Pallor - Cold clammy skin	- 12-lead electrocardiogram (ECG) identifies specific waveform changes associated with the arrhythmia. - Laboratory testing reveals electrolyte abnormalities, hypoxemia, or acid-base abnormalities. - Electrophysiologic testing identifies the mechanism of an arrhythmia and the location of accessory pathways.	- Evaluate the patient's ECG regularly for arrhythmia, and assess hemodynamic parameters, as indicated. Document arrhythmias and notify the physician immediately. - If the patient's pulse rate is abnormally rapid, slow, or irregular, watch for signs of hypoperfusion, such as hypotension and diminished urine output. - Administer antiarrhythmics and monitor for adverse effects. - If a life-threatening arrhythmia develops, rapidly assess the patient's LOC, pulse and respiratory rates, and hemodynamic parameters. Be alert for trends. Monitor EGG continuously. Be prepared to initiate cardiopulmonary resuscitation or cardioversion, if indicated. - Prepare for possible insertion of temporary pacemaker or implantable cardioverter-defibrillator, if indicated.

DISORDER	SIGNS AND SYMPTOMS	DIAGNOSTIC TEST RESULTS	TREATMENT AND CARE
Deep vein thrombosis (complication)	◆ Severe pain ◆ Fever ◆ Chills ◆ Malaise ◆ Swelling and cyanosis of the affected extremity ◆ Affected area possibly warm to the touch ◆ Positive Homans' sign (pain on dorsiflexion of the foot; false positives are common)	◆ Doppler ultrasonography identifies reduced blood flow to a specific area and any obstruction to venous flow, particularly in iliofemoral deep vein thrombophlebitis. ◆ Plethysmography shows decreased circulation distal to the affected area. ◆ Phlebography (also called *venography)* shows filling defects and diverted blood flow and usually confirms diagnosis.	◆ Administer anticoagulants and monitor for adverse effects, such as bleeding; dark, tarry stools; coffee-ground vomitus; and ecchymoses. ◆ Assess pulses, skin color, and temperature of affected extremity, and compare these findings with those of the unaffected extremity. ◆ Measure and record the circumference of the affected arm or leg daily. Compare this with the circumference of the other arm or leg. ◆ Maintain bed rest; use pillows for elevating the leg, placing them to support the entire length of the affected extremity and to prevent possible compression of the popliteal space. ◆ Perform range-of-motion exercises with unaffected extremities, and turn the patient every 2 hours. ◆ Apply warm soaks to improve circulation to the affected area and to relieve pain and inflammation. Give analgesics to relieve pain. ◆ Assess for signs of pulmonary emboli, such as crackles, dyspnea, hemoptysis, sudden changes in mental status, restlessness, and hypotension.
Respiratory failure (complication)	◆ Diminished chest movement ◆ Restlessness, irritability, confusion ◆ Decreasing LOC ◆ Pallor, possible cyanosis ◆ Tachypnea, tachycardia (strong and rapid initially, but thready and irregular in later stages) ◆ Cold, clammy skin and frank diaphoresis, especially around the forehead and face ◆ Diminished breath sounds; possible adventitious breath sounds ◆ Possible cardiac arrhythmias	◆ Arterial blood gas (ABG) analysis shows a low partial pressure of arterial oxygen (usually less than 70 mm Hg), partial pressure of arterial carbon dioxide greater than 45 mm Hg, and a normal bicarbonate level, indicating early respiratory failure. ◆ Serial vital capacity is less than 800 ml. ◆ ECG may show arrhythmias. ◆ Pulse oximetry reveals a decreased oxygen saturation level. Mixed venous oxygen saturation levels less than 50% indicate impaired tissue oxygenation.	◆ Institute oxygen therapy immediately to optimize oxygenation of pulmonary blood. ◆ Prepare for endotracheal (ET) intubation and mechanical ventilation; anticipate the need for high-frequency or pressure ventilation to force airways open. ◆ Administer bronchodilators to open airways, corticosteroids to reduce inflammation, continuous I.V. solutions of positive inotropic agents to increase cardiac output, vasopressors to induce vasoconstriction to maintain blood pressure, and diuretics to reduce fluid overload and edema. ◆ Assess the patient's respiratory status at least every 2 hours, or more often, as indicated. Observe for a positive response to oxygen therapy, such as improved breathing, color, and oximetry and ABG values. ◆ Position the patient for optimal breathing effort. ◆ Maintain a normothermic environment to reduce the patient's oxygen demand. ◆ Monitor vital signs, heart rhythm, and fluid intake and output. ◆ If intubated, auscultate the lungs to check for accidental intubation of the esophagus or the mainstem bronchus. Be alert for aspiration, broken teeth, nosebleeds, and vagal reflexes causing bradycardia, arrhythmias, and hypotension. ◆ Perform suctioning using strict aseptic technique when intubated. ◆ Monitor oximetry and capnography values to detect important indicators of changes in the patient's condition. ◆ Note the amount and quality of lung secretions and look for changes in the patient's status. ◆ Check cuff pressure on the ET tube to prevent erosion from an overinflated cuff. ◆ Implement measures to prevent nasal tissue necrosis. Position and maintain the nasotracheal tube midline in the nostrils, and reposition daily. Tape the tube securely but use skin protection measures and nonirritating tape to prevent skin breakdown. ◆ Provide a means of communication for patients who are intubated and alert.

Haemophilus influenzae infection

OVERVIEW

- Infection that most commonly attacks the respiratory system
- Common cause of epiglottiditis, laryngotracheobronchitis, pneumonia, bronchiolitis, otitis media, and meningitis
- Infrequent cause of bacterial endocarditis, conjunctivitis, facial cellulitis, septic arthritis, and osteomyelitis
- Incidence 10 times higher in Native Americans, possibly due to exposure, socioeconomic conditions, and genetic differences in immune responses
- *H. influenzae* type B (Hib) infection: predominantly affects children at a rate of 3% to 5%; lower incidence when a vaccine is administered at ages 2, 4, 6, and 15 months
- *H. influenzae* epiglottiditis: most common in children between ages 3 and 7, but can occur at any age
- Meningitis due to Hib: higher incidence in Black children than in White children

CAUSES

- *H. influenzae*, a gram-negative, pleomorphic aerobic bacillus

PATHOPHYSIOLOGY

- An antigenic response occurs with the invasion of bacteria.
- Systemic disease results from the invasion and hematogenous spread to distant sites, including the bones, joints, meninges. (See *Disorders affecting management of* Haemophilus influenzae *infection*, page 179.)

RESPIRATORY SYSTEM

- Bacteria is transmitted through direct contact or inhalation of infected airborne droplets.
- Colonization of the bacteria in the nasopharynx can cause sinusitis and epiglottiditis. With epiglottiditis, swelling and cellulitis of the epiglottis and supraglottic tissues causes the epiglottis to curl posteriorly and inferiorly, causing airway obstruction.
- Bacteria that disseminate into lung tissue cause bronchitis or pneumonia.
- Colonization in the lower respiratory tract with coexisting cystic fibrosis or chronic obstructive pulmonary disease can cause exacerbation of the disease.

CARDIOVASCULAR SYSTEM

- Bacterial infection of the heart muscle or valves results in pericarditis or endocarditis.
- If the infection is left untreated, sepsis may occur, causing circulatory compromise.

NEUROLOGIC SYSTEM

- Contaminated nasopharynx can cause transmission of bacteria into the pia-arachnoid space, with progression to adjacent tissues, causing meningeal inflammation and infection.

NEUROSENSORY SYSTEM

- Otitis media occurs when bacteria reach the middle ear through the eustachian tube.
- Orbital cellulitis occurs when buccal and periorbital regions are infected, resulting in sinusitis.

ASSESSMENT

HISTORY

- Possible report of recent viral infection
- Malaise
- Fatigue
- Fever

PHYSICAL FINDINGS

Epiglottiditis

- Restlessness and irritability
- Use of accessory muscles, inspiratory retractions, and stridor
- Sitting up, leaning forward with mouth open, tongue protruding, and nostrils flaring
- Expiratory rhonchi; diminishing breath sounds as the condition worsens
- Pharyngeal mucosa that may look reddened (rarely, with soft yellow exudate)
- Epiglottis that appears cherry-red with considerable edema
- Severe pain that makes swallowing difficult or impossible

Pneumonia

- Shaking chills
- Tachypnea
- Productive cough
- Impaired or asymmetrical chest movement caused by pleuritic pain
- Dullness over areas of lung consolidation

Meningitis

- Altered level of consciousness
- Seizures and coma as disease progresses
- Positive Brudzinski's and Kernig's signs
- Exaggerated and symmetrical deep tendon reflexes
- Nuchal rigidity
- Opisthotonos

DIAGNOSTIC TEST RESULTS

- Isolation of the organism in blood culture confirms infection.
- Hib meningitis is detected in cerebrospinal fluid cultures.

TREATMENT

GENERAL
◆ Airway maintenance (critical in epiglottiditis)

DIET
◆ Based on respiratory status (possible need for small, frequent meals)
◆ Nothing by mouth if unable to swallow adequately

ACTIVITY
◆ As tolerated

MEDICATIONS
◆ Antibiotics: cefotaxime (Claforan), ceftriaxone (Rocephin), amoxicillin and clavulanic acid (Augmentin)
◆ Glucocorticoids; dexamethasone (Decadron)

NURSING CONSIDERATIONS

NURSING DIAGNOSES
◆ Acute pain
◆ Anxiety
◆ Deficient fluid volume
◆ Imbalanced nutrition: Less than body requirements
◆ Impaired gas exchange
◆ Ineffective airway clearance
◆ Ineffective breathing pattern
◆ Risk for aspiration
◆ Risk for infection

EXPECTED OUTCOMES
The patient will:
◆ express feelings of increased comfort and decreased pain
◆ verbalize feelings of anxiety and fear
◆ attain and maintain normal fluid and electrolyte balance
◆ maintain nutritional health through oral intake of I.V. fluids
◆ maintain adequate ventilation and oxygenation
◆ maintain a patent airway
◆ maintain effective breathing pattern and not have adventitious breath sounds
◆ not aspirate
◆ remain free from signs and symptoms of infection.

NURSING INTERVENTIONS
◆ Maintain respiratory isolation.
◆ Maintain adequate respiratory function through cool humidification; oxygen, as needed; and croup or face tents.
◆ Keep emergency resuscitation equipment readily available.
◆ Suction, as needed.
◆ Give prescribed drugs.
◆ Maintain adequate nutrition and elimination.
◆ Monitor pulse oximetry and arterial blood gas results.

◆ Note complete blood count for signs of bone marrow depression when therapy includes ampicillin or chloramphenicol.
◆ Monitor vital signs and intake and output.
◆ Assess respiratory and neurologic status.

(continued)

Be sure to cover:
- ◆ disorder, diagnostic testing, and treatment
- ◆ medication administration, dosage, and possible adverse effects
- ◆ using a room humidifier or breathing moist air from a shower or bath, as necessary, for home treatment of a respiratory infection
- ◆ coughing and deep-breathing exercises to clear secretions
- ◆ disposal of secretions and use of proper hand-washing technique
- ◆ vaccinations to prevent future infections.

RESOURCES

Organizations

Centers for Disease Control and Prevention: *www.cdc.gov*

Harvard University Consumer Health Information: *www.intelihealth.com*

National Health Information Center: *www.health.gov/nhic/*

National Library of Medicine: *www.nlm.nih.gov*

Selected references

Heininger, U., and Zuberbuhler, M. "Immunization Rates and Timely Administration in Pre-school and School-Aged Children," *European Journal of Pediatrics* 165(2):124-29, February 2006.

Kasper, D.L., et al., eds. *Harrison's Principles of Internal Medicine,* 16th ed. New York: McGraw-Hill Book Co., 2005.

Sheff, B. "*Haemophilus Influenzae* Type B (Hib)," *Nursing* 36(1):31, January 2006.

Disorders affecting management of *Haemophilus influenzae* infection

This chart highlights disorders that affect the management of *Haemophilus influenzae*.

DISORDER	SIGNS AND SYMPTOMS	DIAGNOSTIC TEST RESULTS	TREATMENT AND CARE
Epiglottiditis (complication)	◆ Red, inflamed throat ◆ Fever ◆ Cyanosis ◆ Stridor ◆ Drooling ◆ Pale or cyanotic skin ◆ Restlessness or irritability ◆ Nasal flaring ◆ Use of accessory muscles for breathing	◆ Arterial blood gas analysis may show hypoxia. ◆ Lateral neck X-rays show an enlarged epiglottis and distended hypopharynx. ◆ Direct laryngoscopy shows swollen, beefy red epiglottis.	◆ Administer prescribed medications. ◆ Place the patient in a sitting position, and utilize a cool mist tent to administer oxygen, if possible. ◆ Encourage parents to remain with their child to decrease anxiety and provide comfort. ◆ Ensure adequate fluid intake. ◆ Minimize external stimuli.
Meningitis (complication)	◆ Nuchal rigidity ◆ Fever ◆ Photophobia ◆ Confusion ◆ Seizures ◆ Meningismus ◆ Rigors ◆ Profuse diaphoresis ◆ Kernig's and Brudzinski's signs ◆ Cranial nerve palsies	◆ White blood cell count is elevated. ◆ Blood cultures are positive in bacterial meningitis. ◆ Coagglutination test reveals the causative agent. ◆ Chest X-ray reveals a coexisting pneumonia. ◆ Lumbar puncture and cerebrospinal fluid analysis reveals increased levels of protein, positive Gram stain, positive culture, and decreased levels of glucose.	◆ Maintain standard precautions and respiratory isolation for 24 hours. ◆ Administer oxygen therapy. ◆ Assess neurologic status. ◆ Monitor vital signs and pulse oximetry readings. ◆ Administer prescribed medications. ◆ Observe for signs and symptoms of complications. ◆ Provide skin and mouth care.
Pneumonia (complication)	◆ Elevated temperature ◆ Cough with purulent, yellow, or bloody sputum ◆ Dyspnea ◆ Crackles ◆ Decreased breath sounds ◆ Pleuritic pain ◆ Chills ◆ Malaise ◆ Tachypnea	◆ Chest X-ray shows infiltrates. ◆ Sputum smear reveals acute inflammatory cells and causative organism.	◆ Administer antimicrobial therapy according to the causative organism. ◆ Provide oxygen therapy; assist with endotracheal intubation, if necessary. ◆ Administer analgesics, as needed. ◆ Provide a high-calorie diet, adequate fluid intake, and rest periods, as needed. ◆ Monitor vital signs and pulse oximetry readings.

Heart failure LIFE-THREATENING DISORDER

OVERVIEW

- Fluid buildup in the heart that affects cardiac output and oxygenation
- Usually occurs from a damaged left or right ventricle
- May result secondarily from left-sided heart failure
- Affects 1% of people older than age 50 and 10% of people older than age 80

CAUSES

- Anemia
- Arrhythmias
- Atherosclerosis with myocardial infarction
- Constrictive pericarditis
- Emotional stress
- Hypertension
- Increased salt or water intake
- Infections
- Mitral or aortic insufficiency
- Mitral stenosis secondary to rheumatic heart disease, constrictive pericarditis, or atrial fibrillation (see *Causes of heart failure*)
- Myocarditis
- Pregnancy
- Pulmonary embolism
- Thyrotoxicosis
- Ventricular and atrial septal defect

PATHOPHYSIOLOGY

LEFT-SIDED HEART FAILURE

- The pumping ability of the left ventricle fails, and cardiac output falls. (See *Classifying heart failure.*)
- Blood backs up into the right atrium and lungs, causing pulmonary congestion.

RIGHT-SIDED HEART FAILURE

- Ineffective contractile function of the right ventricle leads to blood backing up into the right atrium and the peripheral circulation, which results in peripheral edema and engorgement of the kidneys and other organs.
- Pump failure usually occurs in a damaged left ventricle (left-sided heart failure) but may occur in the right ventricle (right-sided heart failure) as a primary disorder or secondary to left-sided heart failure. Sometimes, left- and right-sided heart failure develop simultaneously. (See *What happens in heart failure,* pages 182 and 183.)

CARDIOVASCULAR SYSTEM

- Fluid buildup in the heart results in compromised cardiac output, pulmonary congestion, and diminished oxygenation.
- Ventricular hypertrophy develops with chronic occurrence, leading to increased conduction time and arrhythmias. (See *Disorders affecting management of heart failure,* page 185.)

GASTROINTESTINAL SYSTEM

- Congestion of the peripheral tissues leads to GI tract congestion and anorexia, GI distress, and weight loss.
- Liver failure can occur as a result of blood backing up into the peripheral circulation and subsequent engorgement of organs.

RENAL SYSTEM

- With right-sided heart failure, blood backs up into the right atrium and the peripheral circulation. The patient gains weight and develops peripheral edema and engorgement of the kidney and other organs.

RESPIRATORY SYSTEM

- As blood backs up into the right atrium, blood backs into the lungs, causing pulmonary congestion.

Causes of heart failure

CAUSE	EXAMPLES
Abnormal cardiac muscle function	◆ Myocardial infarction ◆ Cardiomyopathy
Abnormal left ventricular volume	◆ Valvular insufficiency ◆ High-output states: – chronic anemia – arteriovenous fistula – thyrotoxicosis – pregnancy – septicemia – beriberi – infusion of large volume of I.V. fluids in a short time period
Abnormal left ventricular pressure	◆ Hypertension ◆ Pulmonary hypertension ◆ Chronic obstructive pulmonary disease ◆ Aortic or pulmonic valve stenosis
Abnormal left ventricular filling	◆ Mitral valve stenosis ◆ Tricuspid valve stenosis ◆ Atrial myxoma ◆ Constrictive pericarditis ◆ Atrial fibrillation ◆ Impaired ventricular relaxation: – hypertension – myocardial hibernation – myocardial stunning

HISTORY

- Disorder or condition that can precipitate heart failure
- Dyspnea or paroxysmal nocturnal dyspnea
- Peripheral edema
- Fatigue
- Weakness
- Insomnia
- Anorexia
- Nausea
- Sense of abdominal fullness (particularly in right-sided heart failure)
- Substance abuse

PHYSICAL FINDINGS

- Cough that produces pink, frothy sputum
- Cyanosis of the lips and nail beds
- Pale, cool, clammy skin
- Diaphoresis
- Jugular vein distention
- Ascites
- Tachycardia
- Pulsus alternans
- Hepatomegaly and, possibly, splenomegaly
- Decreased pulse pressure
- S_3 and S_4 heart sounds
- Moist, bibasilar crackles, rhonchi, and expiratory wheezing
- Decreased pulse oximetry
- Peripheral edema
- Decreased urinary output

DIAGNOSTIC TEST RESULTS

- B-type natriuretic peptide immunoassay is elevated—the higher the elevation, the more severe the failure.
- Chest X-rays show increased pulmonary vascular markings, interstitial edema, or pleural effusion and cardiomegaly.
- Electrocardiography may reflect heart strain, enlargement, or ischemia. It may also reveal atrial enlargement, tachycardia, extrasystole, or atrial fibrillation.
- Pulmonary artery pressure monitoring may show elevated pulmonary artery and pulmonary artery wedge pressures, left ventricular end-diastolic pressure in left-sided heart failure, and elevated right atrial or central venous pressure in right-sided heart failure.

TREATMENT

GENERAL

- Antiembolism stockings
- Elevation of lower extremities

DIET

- Sodium restriction
- Fluid restriction
- Calorie restriction, if indicated
- Low-fat, if indicated

ACTIVITY

- As tolerated (walking encouraged)

MEDICATIONS

- Diuretics
- Oxygen
- Inotropic drugs
- Vasodilators
- Angiotensin-converting enzyme inhibitors
- Angiotensin receptor blockers
- Cardiac glycosides
- Diuretics
- Potassium supplements
- Beta-adrenergic blockers
- Anticoagulants

SURGERY

- Surgical replacement for valvular dysfunction with recurrent acute heart failure
- Heart transplantation
- Ventricular assist device
- Stent placement

Classifying heart failure

Heart failure is classified according to its pathophysiology. It may be right- or left-sided, systolic or diastolic, and acute or chronic.

RIGHT-SIDED OR LEFT-SIDED

Right-sided heart failure is the result of ineffective right ventricular contraction. It may be caused by an acute right ventricular infarction or pulmonary embolus. However, the most common cause is profound backward flow due to left-sided heart failure.

Left-sided heart failure is the result of ineffective left ventricular contraction. It may lead to pulmonary congestion or pulmonary edema and decreased cardiac output. Left ventricular myocardial infarction, hypertension, and aortic and mitral valve stenosis or regurgitation are common causes. As the decreased pumping ability of the left ventricle persists, fluid accumulates, backing up into the left atrium and then into the lungs. If this worsens, pulmonary edema and right-sided heart failure may also result.

SYSTOLIC OR DIASTOLIC

In patients with systolic heart failure, the left ventricle can't pump enough blood out to the systemic circulation during systole, and the ejection fraction falls. Consequently, blood backs up into the pulmonary circulation, pressure rises in the pulmonary venous system, and cardiac output falls.

In patients with diastolic heart failure, the left ventricle can't relax and fill properly during diastole, and the stroke volume falls. Therefore, larger ventricular volumes are needed to maintain cardiac output.

ACUTE OR CHRONIC

Acute refers to the timing of the onset of symptoms and whether compensatory mechanisms kick in. Typically, fluid status is normal or low, and sodium and water retention don't occur.

In patients with chronic heart failure, signs and symptoms have been present for some time, compensatory mechanisms have taken effect, and fluid volume overload persists. Drug therapy, diet changes, and activity restrictions usually help control symptoms.

(Text continues on page 184.)

What happens in heart failure

These step-by-step illustrations show what happens when myocardial damage leads to heart failure.

LEFT-SIDED HEART FAILURE

Increased workload and end-diastolic volume enlarge the left ventricle. Because of the lack of oxygen, however, the ventricle enlarges with stretched tissue rather than functional tissue. The patient may experience increased heart rate, pallor and cool tingling in the extremities, decreased cardiac output, and arrhythmias.

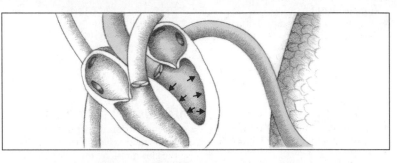

Diminished left ventricular function allows blood to pool in the ventricle and the atrium and eventually back up into the pulmonary veins and capillaries. The patient may experience dyspnea on exertion, confusion, dizziness, postural hypotension, decreased peripheral pulses and pulse pressure, cyanosis, and an S_3 gallop.

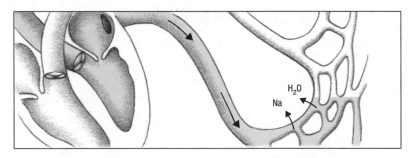

As the pulmonary circulation becomes engorged, rising capillary pressure pushes sodium (Na) and water (H_2O) into the interstitial space, causing pulmonary edema. Note coughing, subclavian retractions, crackles, tachypnea, elevated pulmonary artery pressure, diminished pulmonary compliance, and increased partial pressure of carbon dioxide.

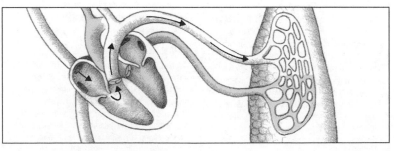

When the patient lies down, fluid in the extremities moves into systemic circulation. Because the left ventricle can't handle the increased venous return, fluid pools in the pulmonary circulation, worsening pulmonary edema. You may note decreased breath sounds, dullness on percussion, crackles, and orthopnea.

The right ventricle may now become stressed because it's pumping against greater pulmonary vascular resistance and left ventricular pressure. When this occurs, the patient's symptoms worsen.

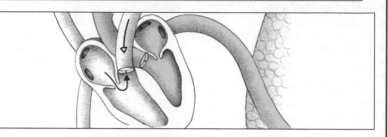

RIGHT-SIDED HEART FAILURE

The stressed right ventricle hypertrophies with the formation of stretched tissue. Increasing conduction time and deviation of the heart from its normal axis can cause arrhythmias. If the patient doesn't already have left-sided heart failure, he may experience increased heart rate, cool skin, cyanosis, decreased cardiac output, palpitations, and dyspnea.

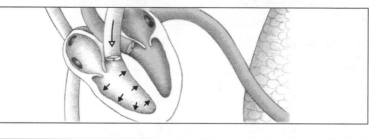

Blood pools in the right ventricle and right atrium. The backed-up blood causes pressure and congestion in the vena cava and systemic circulation. The patient has elevated central venous pressure, jugular vein distention, and hepatojugular reflux.

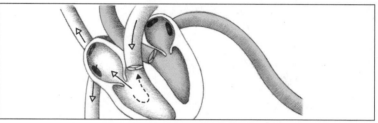

Backed-up blood also distends the visceral veins, especially the hepatic vein. As the liver and spleen become engorged, their function is impaired. The patient may develop anorexia, nausea, abdominal pain, palpable liver and spleen, weakness, and dyspnea secondary to abdominal distention.

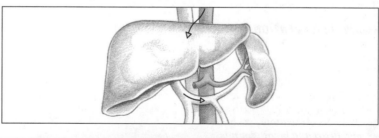

Increasing capillary pressure forces excess fluid from the capillaries into the interstitial space. This causes tissue edema, especially in the lower extremities and abdomen. The patient may experience weight gain, pitting edema, and nocturia.

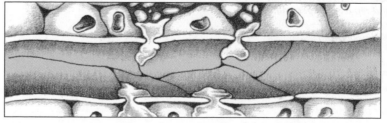

NURSING DIAGNOSES

◆ Activity intolerance
◆ Decreased cardiac output
◆ Excess fluid volume
◆ Fatigue
◆ Imbalanced nutrition: Less than body requirements
◆ Impaired gas exchange
◆ Ineffective airway clearance
◆ Ineffective breathing pattern
◆ Ineffective tissue perfusion: Cardiopulmonary

EXPECTED OUTCOMES

The patient will:
◆ carry out activities of daily living without excess fatigue or decreased energy
◆ maintain adequate cardiac output
◆ remain free from complications of fluid volume excess
◆ verbalize the importance of balancing activity with rest periods
◆ maintain adequate nutrition and hydration
◆ maintain adequate ventilation and oxygenation
◆ maintain a patent airway
◆ maintain an effective breathing pattern
◆ maintain hemodynamic stability.

NURSING INTERVENTIONS

◆ Place the patient in Fowler's position, and give supplemental oxygen.
◆ Provide continuous cardiac monitoring in acute and advanced stages.
◆ Assess respiratory status according to facility policy and clinical status.
● **WARNING** *Auscultate for abnormal heart and breath sounds, and report changes immediately.*
◆ Monitor intake and output, vital signs, and pulse oximetry.
◆ Assist the patient with range-of-motion exercises.
◆ Apply antiembolism stockings.
◆ Check for calf pain and tenderness.

◆ Monitor daily weight for peripheral edema and other signs and symptoms of fluid overload.
◆ Evaluate response to treatment.
◆ Assess for peripheral edema.
◆ Monitor blood urea nitrogen and serum creatinine, potassium, sodium, chloride, and magnesium levels.

Be sure to cover:
◆ disorder, diagnostic testing, and treatment
◆ medication administration, dosage, and possible adverse effects
◆ signs and symptoms of worsening heart failure
◆ when to notify the practitioner
◆ importance of follow-up care
◆ need to avoid high-sodium foods
◆ need to avoid fatigue
◆ instructions about fluid restrictions
◆ need to weigh himself every morning at the same time (before eating, after urinating); to keep record of weight; and to report weekly weight gain of 3 to 5 lb (1.5 to 2.5 kg)
◆ importance of smoking cessation, if appropriate
◆ weight reduction, as needed
◆ local support services.

RESOURCES

Organizations

American Heart Association: *www.americanheart.org*
Heart Failure Online: *www.heartfailure.org*

Selected references

Barnes, S., et al. "Characteristics and Views of Family Carers of Older People with Heart Failure," *International Journal of Palliative Nursing* 12(8):380-89, August 2006.

Inglis, S.C., et al. "Extending the Horizon in Chronic Heart Failure; Effects of Multidisciplinary Home-Based Intervention Relative to Usual Care," *Circulation* 114(23):2566-573, December 2006.

McCauley, K.M., et al. "Advanced Practice Nurse Strategies to Improve Outcomes and Reduce Cost in Elders with Heart Failure," *Disease Management* 9(5): 302-10, October 2006.

Quinn, C. "Low-Technology Heart Failure Care in Home Health; Improving Patient Outcomes," *Home Healthcare Nurse* 24(8):533-40, September 2006.

Disorders affecting management of heart failure

This chart highlights disorders that affect the management of heart failure.

DISORDER	SIGNS AND SYMPTOMS	DIAGNOSTIC TEST RESULTS	TREATMENT AND CARE
Pulmonary edema (complication)	◆ Restlessness and anxiety ◆ Rapid, labored breathing ◆ Intense, productive cough ◆ Frothy, bloody sputum ◆ Mental status changes ◆ Jugular vein distention ◆ Wheezing ◆ Crackles ◆ Third heart sound (S_3) ◆ Tachycardia ◆ Hypotension ◆ Thready pulse ◆ Peripheral edema ◆ Hepatomegaly	◆ Arterial blood gas (ABG) analysis shows hypoxemia, hypercapnia, or acidosis. ◆ Chest X-ray shows diffuse haziness of the lung fields, cardiomegaly, and pleural effusion. ◆ Pulse oximetry may reveal decreased oxygenation of the blood. ◆ Pulmonary artery catheterization may reveal increased pulmonary artery wedge pressures. ◆ Electrocardiogram (ECG) may show valvular disease and left ventricular hypokinesis or akinesis.	◆ Identify and attempt to correct or manage the underlying disease. ◆ Closely monitor for changes in the patient's respiratory status. ◆ Institute energy conservation strategies; plan activities as dictated by respiratory ability. ◆ Provide supplemental oxygen and mechanical ventilation, if indicated. ◆ Implement fluid and sodium restriction. ◆ Monitor intake and output. ◆ Implement cardiac monitoring. ◆ Administer antiarrhythmics, diuretics, preload and afterload reducing agents, bronchodilators, and vasopressors. ◆ Maintain adequate cardiac output. ◆ Weigh the patient daily. ◆ Monitor pulse oximetry, ABG, and hemodynamic values.
Renal failure (complication)	◆ Oliguria (initially) ◆ Azotemia ◆ Electrolyte imbalance ◆ Metabolic acidosis ◆ Anorexia, nausea, and vomiting ◆ Diarrhea or constipation ◆ Dry mucous membranes ◆ Headache ◆ Confusion ◆ Seizures ◆ Drowsiness ◆ Irritability ◆ Coma ◆ Dry skin ◆ Pruritus ◆ Pallor ◆ Purpura ◆ Uremic frost ◆ Hypotension (early) ◆ Hypertension with arrhythmias (later) ◆ Fluid overload ◆ Heart failure ◆ Systemic edema ◆ Anemia ◆ Altered clotting mechanisms ◆ Pulmonary edema ◆ Kussmaul's respirations	◆ Blood urea nitrogen, serum creatinine, and potassium levels are elevated. ◆ Bicarbonate level, hematocrit, hemoglobin, and pH are decreased. ◆ Urine studies show casts, cellular debris, decreased specific gravity; in glomerular diseases proteinuria and urine osmolality close to serum osmolality; urine sodium level is less than 20 mEq/L if oliguria results from decreased perfusion, and more than 40 mEq/L if the cause is intrarenal. ◆ Creatinine clearance tests reveal the number of remaining functioning nephrons. ◆ ECG shows tall, peaked T waves; widening QRS; and disappearing P waves if hyperkalemia is present. ◆ Ultrasonography, abdominal and kidney-ureter-bladder X-rays, excretory urography, renal scan, retrograde pyelography, computed tomography, and nephrotomography reveal abnormalities of the urinary tract.	◆ Measure input and output, including body fluids, nasogastric output, and diarrhea. Weigh the patient daily. ◆ Measure hemoglobin and hematocrit and replace blood components. ◆ Monitor vital signs; check and report for signs of pericarditis (pleuritic chest pain, tachycardia, pericardial friction rub), inadequate renal perfusion (hypotension), and acidosis. ◆ Maintain proper electrolyte balance. Monitor potassium levels and monitor the patient for hyperkalemia (malaise, anorexia, paresthesia, or muscle weakness) and ECG changes. ◆ Administer diuretics. ◆ If the patient receives hypertonic glucose and insulin infusions, monitor potassium and glucose levels. If giving sodium polystyrene sulfonate rectally, make sure the patient doesn't retain it and become constipated (to prevent bowel perforation). ◆ Maintain nutritional status with a high-calorie, low-protein, low-sodium, and low-potassium diet and vitamin supplements. ◆ Monitor the patient carefully during peritoneal dialysis. ◆ If the patient requires hemodialysis, monitor the venous access site carefully, and assess the patient and laboratory work carefully.

Heat syndrome LIFE-THREATENING DISORDER

OVERVIEW

- Occurs in two forms:
- Heat exhaustion—acute heat injury with hyperthermia caused by dehydration
- Heat stroke—extreme hyperthermia with thermoregulatory failure
- Affects males and females equally
- Increased incidence among older patients and neonates during excessively hot summer days

CAUSES

- Dehydration
- Drugs, such as phenothiazines, anticholinergics, and amphetamines
- Endocrine disorders
- Excessive clothing
- Excessive physical activity
- Heart disease
- Hot environment without ventilation
- Illness
- Infection (fever)
- Lack of acclimatization
- Neurologic disorder
- Sudden discontinuation of Parkinson's disease medications

RISK FACTORS

- Age
- Alcohol use
- Obesity
- Poor physical condition
- Salt and water depletion
- Socioeconomic status

PATHOPHYSIOLOGY

- Normal regulation of temperature is through evaporation (30% of body's heat loss) or vasodilation. When heat is generated or gained by the body faster than it can dissipate, the thermoregulatory mechanism is stressed and eventually fails.
- This causes hyperthermia to accelerate.
- Cerebral edema and cerebrovascular congestion occur.
- Cerebral perfusion pressure increases, and cerebral perfusion decreases.
- Tissue damage occurs when temperature exceeds 107.6° F (42° C), resulting in tissue necrosis, organ dysfunction, and failure. (See *Disorders affecting management of heat syndrome*, page 189.)

CARDIOVASCULAR SYSTEM

- Inadequate dissipation of heat results in elevated body temperature. Blood is redistributed to the periphery, electrolytes are lost through diaphoresis, intravascular volume diminishes, and cardiac output becomes inadequate.
- Cardiovascular collapse may occur.

NEUROVASCULAR SYSTEM

- Extreme body temperature results in decreased cerebral tissue perfusion, causing a change in sensorium, altered mental status, and seizures. If continued, the elevated temperature causes tissue necrosis, causing damage to cells. Cerebral edema and herniation may also occur.

RESPIRATORY SYSTEM

- Initially, heat stroke may cause tachypnea and hyperventilation due to central nervous system (CNS) stimulation.
- Prolonged elevated body temperature may cause hypoxia and acidosis, resulting in respiratory failure.

MUSCULOSKELETAL SYSTEM

- Heat stroke may cause muscle tenderness and cramping, followed by rhabdomyolysis.

RENAL SYSTEM

- Hypovolemia, diminished cardiac output, and myoglobinuria (as a result of rhabdomyolysis) may cause acute renal failure.

HISTORY

Heat exhaustion

- Prolonged activity in a very warm or hot environment
- Muscle cramps
- Nausea and vomiting
- Thirst
- Weakness
- Headache
- Fatigue
- Sweating
- Tachycardia

Heat stroke

- Same signs as heat exhaustion
- Exposure to high temperature and humidity without air circulation
- Blurred vision
- Confusion
- Hallucinations
- Decreased muscle coordination
- Syncope

PHYSICAL FINDINGS

Heat exhaustion

- Rectal temperature greater than 100° F (37.8° C)
- Pale skin
- Thready, rapid pulse
- Cool, moist skin
- Decreased blood pressure
- Irritability
- Syncope
- Impaired judgment
- Hyperventilation

Heat stroke

- Rectal temperature of at least 104° F (40° C)
- Red, diaphoretic, hot skin in early stages
- Gray, dry, hot skin in later stages
- Tachycardia
- Slightly elevated blood pressure in early stages
- Decreased blood pressure in later stages
- Tachypnea
- Decreased level of consciousness
- Signs of CNS dysfunction
- Altered mental status
- Hyperpnea
- Cheyne-Stokes respirations
- Anhidrosis (late sign)

DIAGNOSTIC TEST RESULTS

- Serum electrolytes are elevated, which may show hyponatremia and hypokalemia.
- Arterial blood gas levels may indicate respiratory alkalosis.
- Complete blood count may reveal leukocytosis and thrombocytopenia.
- Coagulation studies may show increased bleeding and clotting times.
- Urinalysis may show concentrated urine and proteinuria with tubular casts and myoglobinuria.
- Blood urea nitrogen may be elevated.
- Serum calcium level may be decreased.
- Serum phosphorus level may be decreased.
- Myoglobinuria may indicate rhabdomyolosis.

GENERAL

Heat exhaustion

- Cool environment
- Oral or I.V. fluid administration

Heat stroke

- Lowering the body temperature as rapidly as possible
- Evaporation, hypothermia blankets, and ice packs to the groin, axillae, and neck
- Supportive respiratory and cardiovascular measures

DIET

- Increased hydration; cool liquids only
- Avoidance of caffeine and alcohol

ACTIVITY

- Rest periods, as needed

(continued)

NURSING CONSIDERATIONS

NURSING DIAGNOSES
◆ Decreased cardiac output
◆ Deficient fluid volume
◆ Hyperthermia
◆ Impaired gas exchange
◆ Impaired home maintenance

EXPECTED OUTCOMES
The patient will:
◆ exhibit signs of adequate cardiac output
◆ express understanding of the need to maintain adequate fluid intake
◆ maintain a normal body temperature
◆ maintain adequate ventilation and oxygenation
◆ express understanding of how to prevent recurrent episodes of hyperthermia.

NURSING INTERVENTIONS
◆ Perform rapid cooling procedures.
◆ Provide supportive measures.
◆ Provide adequate fluid intake.
◆ Give prescribed drugs.
◆ Monitor vital signs, pulse oximetry, cardiac rhythm, intake and output, and myoglobin test results.
◆ Observe for signs of complications.

PATIENT TEACHING

Be sure to cover:
◆ disorder, diagnostic testing, and treatment
◆ how to avoid reexposure to high temperatures
◆ need to maintain adequate fluid intake
◆ need to wear loose clothing in hot weather
◆ activity limitation in hot weather.
◆ local support services, if indicated.

RESOURCES
Organizations
National Center for Injury Prevention and Control: *www.cdc.gov/ncipc*
National Institutes of Health: *www.nih.gov*

Selected references
Brueckmann, M., et al. "Beyond Sepsis: Activated Protein C and Heat Stroke," *Critical Care Medicine* 34(7):2020-2021, July 2006.
Kim, S.Y., et al. "A Case of Multiple Organ Failure Due to Heat Stroke Following a Warm Bath," *Korean Journal of Internal Medicine* 21(3):210-12, September 2006.
Thompson, H.J., et al. "Intensive Care Unit Management of Fever Following Traumatic Brain Injury," *Intensive Critical Care Nurse* 23(2):91-96, April 2007.

Disorders affecting management of heat syndrome

This chart highlights disorders that affect the management of heat syndrome.

DISORDER	SIGNS AND SYMPTOMS	DIAGNOSTIC TEST RESULTS	TREATMENT AND CARE
Acute respiratory failure (complication)	◆ Tachypnea ◆ Cyanosis ◆ Crackles, rhonchi, wheezing ◆ Diminished breath sounds ◆ Restlessness ◆ Altered mental status ◆ Tachycardia ◆ Increased cardiac output ◆ Increased blood pressure ◆ Cardiac arrhythmias	◆ Arterial blood gas (ABG) values show deteriorating values and a pH below 7.35. ◆ Chest X-ray shows pulmonary disease or condition. ◆ Electrocardiogram may show cardiac arrhythmia or right ventricular hypertrophy. ◆ Pulse oximetry shows decreasing arterial oxygen saturation.	◆ Administer oxygen therapy and monitor respiratory status; assist with endotracheal intubation and mechanical ventilation, if necessary. ◆ Assess breath sounds and note changes. ◆ Monitor ABG values and pulse oximetry. ◆ Monitor vital signs and intake and output. ◆ Monitor cardiac rhythm for arrhythmias. ◆ Administer antibiotics, bronchodilators, corticosteroids, positive inotropic agents, diuretics, vasopressors, or antiarrhythmics.
Dehydration (complication)	◆ Tachycardia ◆ Dry mucous membranes ◆ Poor skin turgor ◆ Decreased blood pressure ◆ Decreased urine output ◆ Lethargy ◆ Delayed capillary refill	◆ Urine specific gravity is elevated. ◆ Blood urea nitrogen and creatinine are elevated. ◆ Complete blood count reveals elevated hematocrit.	◆ Encourage small amounts of oral fluids. ◆ Administer I.V. fluids. ◆ Administer electrolyte solutions—oral or I.V.—to correct imbalances. ◆ Monitor vital signs, including central and peripheral pulses and capillary refill, approximately every 15 minutes. ◆ Monitor neurologic status for increasing lethargy or seizures.
Seizure (complication)	◆ Aura ◆ Loss of consciousness ◆ Dyspnea ◆ Fixed and dilated pupils ◆ Incontinence	◆ EEG shows abnormal wave patterns and the focus of the seizure activity. ◆ Magnetic resonance imaging may show pathologic changes. ◆ Brain mapping identifies seizure areas.	◆ Observe and record the seizure activity and duration. ◆ Assess postictal state. ◆ Protect the patient from injury. ◆ Assess neurologic and respiratory status. ◆ Administer medications. ◆ Monitor and record vital signs, intake and output, neurovital signs, and laboratory studies.

Hepatic failure

- Dysfunctional liver cells possible end result of any liver disease
- Prognosis generally poor
- Liver transplant only cure

CAUSES

- Nonviral hepatitis
- Viral hepatitis
- Cirrhosis
- Liver cancer

PATHOPHYSIOLOGY

- Complex syndrome involving impairment of multiple organs and body functions ensues. (See *Disorders affecting management of hepatic failure*, pages 192 and 193.)

NEUROLOGIC SYSTEM

- Hepatic encephalopathy develops when the liver can no longer detoxify the blood. Liver dysfunction and collateral vessels that shunt blood around the liver to the systemic circulation permit toxins absorbed from the GI tract to circulate freely to the brain. The normal liver transforms ammonia to urea, which the kidneys excrete. When the liver fails, ammonia blood levels rise and circulate to the brain.
- Short-chain fatty acids, serotonin, tryptophan, and false neurotransmitters may accumulate in the blood and contribute to hepatic encephalopathy.

RENAL SYSTEM

- Accumulation of vasoactive substances or a compensatory response to portal hypertension and the pooling of blood in the splenic circulation may lead to decreased glomerular filtration, oliguria, and hepatorenal syndrome (renal failure concurrent with liver disease; the kidneys appear normal but abruptly cease functioning).
- Hepatorenal syndrome causes expanded blood volume, accumulation

of hydrogen ions, and electrolyte disturbances.

ASSESSMENT

HISTORY
Prodromal stage (Grade I)
- Slight personality changes, such as agitation, belligerence, disorientation, or forgetfulness
- Trouble concentrating or thinking clearly
- Fatigue or drowsiness, slurred speech

Impending stage (Grade II)
- Confused and disoriented as to time, place, and person
- Ability to write becoming more difficult and illegible

Stuporous stage (Grade III)
- Marked mental confusion; commonly noisy and abusive (when aroused)

Comatose stage (Grade IV)
- Obtunded with no asterixis
- Possible seizures (usually uncommon)
- Progression to coma and death

PHYSICAL FINDINGS
- Jaundice
- Nausea and anorexia
- Abdominal pain or tenderness
- Fatigue and weight loss
- Pruritus
- Oliguria
- Splenomegaly
- Ascites
- Peripheral edema
- Esophageal varices
- Bleeding tendencies
- Petechiae

Prodromal stage (Grade I) hepatic encephalopathy
- Slurred speech
- Slight tremor

Impending stage (Grade II) hepatic encephalopathy
- Asterixis (liver flap, flapping tremor)
- Lethargy
- Aberrant behavior
- Apraxia

Stuporous stage (Grade III) hepatic encephalopathy
- Marked mental confusion
- Drowsiness
- Stupor
- Hyperventilation
- Muscle twitching
- Asterixis

Comatose stage (Grade IV) hepatic encephalopathy
- Fetor hepaticus (musty odor of breath and urine)
- Seizures
- Hyperactive reflexes
- Coma

DIAGNOSTIC TEST RESULTS
- Liver function tests reveal elevated levels of aspartate aminotransferase, alanine aminotransferase, alkaline phosphatase, and bilirubin.
- Blood studies reveal anemia, impaired red blood cell production, elevated bleeding and clotting times, low platelet levels, low blood glucose levels, low albumin, decreased blood urea nitrogen, and increased serum ammonia levels.
- Serum electrolyte studies commonly reveal hyponatremia and hypokalemia in patients with ascites.
- Urinalysis reveals increased urobilinogen, bilirubin, and osmolarity.
- Electroencephalogram is typically abnormal with hepatic encephalopathy, but the changes are nonspecific.

TREATMENT

GENERAL
- Airway and ventilation maintenance
- Eliminating the underlying cause

DIET
- High-calorie, protein-restricted, and possibly moderately sodium-restricted diet
- Possible enteral or parenteral nutritional therapy

ACTIVITY
- Bed rest
- Physical therapy
- Passive range-of-motion exercises

MEDICATIONS
- Lactulose
- Neomycin
- Potassium supplements
- Salt-poor albumin

SURGERY
- Possible liver transplantation

NURSING CONSIDERATIONS

NURSING DIAGNOSES
- Activity intolerance
- Anxiety
- Fear
- Imbalanced nutrition: Less than body requirements
- Ineffective breathing pattern
- Risk for aspiration
- Risk for impaired skin integrity
- Risk for infection
- Risk for injury

EXPECTED OUTCOMES
The patient will:
- perform activities of daily living within the confines of the disease process
- identify strategies to reduce anxiety
- discuss fears and concerns
- achieve adequate caloric and nutritional intake
- maintain adequate ventilation and oxygenation
- not experience aspiration
- maintain skin integrity
- remain free from signs and symptoms of infection
- remain free from injury.

NURSING INTERVENTIONS
- Provide rest periods during the day.
- Provide appropriate skin care.
- Give prescribed drugs and note effects.
- Assess hydration and nutritional status.
- Monitor daily weight and intake and output.
- Obtain daily abdominal girth measurements and daily weight.
- Observe for signs of complications.
- Provide emotional support to patient and family.

PATIENT TEACHING

Be sure to cover:
- disorder, diagnostic testing, and treatment
- medication administration, dosage, and possible adverse effects
- support services and end-of life care, if appropriate.

RESOURCES
Organizations
Alcoholics Anonymous:
   www.alcoholics-anonymous.org
American Liver Foundation:
   www.liverfoundation.org
Digestive Disease National Coalition:
   www.ddnc.org
National Digestive Diseases Information Clearinghouse:
   www.niddk.nih.gov/health/digest/nddic.htm

Selected references
Otsuka, Y., et al. "Postresection Hepatic Failure: Successful Treatment with Liver Transplantation," *Liver Transplantation* 13(5):672-79, May 2007.
Sargent, S., and Wainwright, S.P. "Quality of Life Following Emergency Liver Transplantation for Acute Liver Failure," *Nursing in Critical Care* 11(4):168-76, July-August 2006.
Wright, G., and Jalan, R. "Management of Hepatic Encephalopathy in Patients with Cirrhosis," *Best Practice & Research-Clinical Gastroenterology* 21(1):95-110, January 2007.

(continued)

Disorders affecting management of hepatic failure

This chart highlights disorders that affect the management of hepatic failure.

DISORDER	SIGNS AND SYMPTOMS	DIAGNOSTIC TEST RESULTS	TREATMENT AND CARE
GI hemorrhage (complication)	◆ Anxiety ◆ Agitation ◆ Confusion ◆ Tachycardia ◆ Hypotension ◆ Oliguria ◆ Diaphoresis ◆ Pallor ◆ Cool, clammy skin ◆ Hematochezia ◆ Hematemesis ◆ Melena	◆ Upper GI endoscopy reveals the source of bleeding, such as an ulcer, esophageal varices, or Mallory-Weiss tear. ◆ Colonoscopy reveals the source of bleeding, such as polyps. ◆ Complete blood count reveals a decrease in hemoglobin level and hematocrit (usually 6 to 8 hours after the initial symptoms) and the amount of blood lost (hematocrit may be normal initially, but then drops dramatically), increased reticulocyte and platelet levels, and decreased red blood cell count. ◆ Arterial blood gas (ABG) studies reveal low pH and bicarbonate levels, indicating lactic acidosis from massive hemorrhage and possible hypoxemia. ◆ A 12-lead electrocardiogram (ECG) may reveal evidence of cardiac ischemia secondary to hypoperfusion. ◆ Abdominal X-ray may indicate air under the diaphragm, suggesting ulcer perforation. ◆ Angiography may aid in visualizing the site of bleeding.	◆ Assess the patient for the amount of blood lost and begin fluid resuscitation. ◆ Obtain a type and cross match for blood component therapy. ◆ Ensure a patent airway, and assess breathing and circulation. Monitor cardiac and respiratory status closely, at least every 15 minutes or more, depending on the patient's condition. ◆ Administer supplemental oxygen. Monitor oxygen saturation and serial ABG levels for evidence of hypoxemia. Anticipate endotracheal intubation and mechanical ventilation should the patient's respiratory status deteriorate. Keep the patient in semi-Fowler's position to maximize chest expansion. Keep the patient as quiet and as comfortable as possible to minimize oxygen demands. ◆ Monitor vital signs continuously for changes indicating hypovolemic shock. Observe skin color and check capillary refill. Notify the physician if capillary refill is greater than 2 seconds. ◆ Assist with insertion of central venous or pulmonary artery catheter to evaluate hemodynamic status. Monitor hemodynamic parameters including central venous pressure, pulmonary artery wedge pressure, cardiac output, and cardiac index every 15 minutes to evaluate the patient's status and response to treatment. ◆ Assess level of consciousness (LOC) approximately every 30 minutes until the patient stabilizes, and then every 2 to 4 hours, as indicated by the patient's status. ◆ Obtain serial hemoglobin and hematocrit; notify the physician of hematocrit below the prescribed parameter. ◆ Monitor intake and output closely, including all losses from the GI tract. Insert an indwelling urinary catheter, and assess urine output hourly. Check stools and gastric drainage for occult blood. ◆ Provide emotional support and reassurance appropriately in the wake of massive GI bleeding. ◆ Administer histamine-2 receptor agonists and other agents, such as sucralfate, misoprostol, and omeprazole (a protein-pump inhibitor). ◆ Prepare the patient for endoscopic or surgical repair of bleeding sites. ◆ Assist with gastric intubation and gastric pH monitoring.

DISORDER	SIGNS AND SYMPTOMS	DIAGNOSTIC TEST RESULTS	TREATMENT AND CARE
Renal failure (complication)	◆ Oliguria (early) ◆ Electrolyte imbalance ◆ Metabolic acidosis ◆ Nausea, vomiting ◆ Dry mucous membranes ◆ Headache ◆ Confusion ◆ Seizures ◆ Drowsiness ◆ Irritability ◆ Dry, pruritic skin ◆ Uremic breath odor ◆ Hypotension (early) ◆ Hypertension with arrhythmias (later) ◆ Systemic edema ◆ Pulmonary edema ◆ Kussmaul's respirations ◆ Tachycardia ◆ Bibasilar crackles ◆ Altered LOC	◆ Blood urea nitrogen, serum creatinine, and potassium levels are elevated. ◆ Bicarbonate level, hematocrit, hemoglobin, and pH are decreased. ◆ Urine studies show casts, cellular debris, and decreased specific gravity; in glomerular diseases, proteinuria and urine osmolality are close to serum osmolality; urine sodium level is less than 20 mEq/L if oliguria results from decreased perfusion, and more than 40 mEq/L if the cause is intrarenal. ◆ Creatinine clearance tests reveal the number of remaining functioning nephrons. ◆ ECG shows tall, peaked T waves; widening QRS; and disappearing P waves if hyperkalemia is present. ◆ Ultrasonography, abdominal and kidney-ureter-bladder X-rays, excretory urography, renal scan, retrograde pyelography, computerized tomography, and nephrotomography reveal abnormalities of the urinary tract.	◆ Measure intake and output including body fluids, nasogastric output, and diarrhea; weigh the patient daily. ◆ Measure hemoglobin and hematocrit, and replace blood components, as ordered. ◆ Monitor vital signs. ◆ Check for and report signs of pericarditis (pleuritic chest pain, tachycardia, pericardial friction rub), inadequate renal perfusion (hypotension), and acidosis. ◆ Maintain proper electrolyte balance. Monitor for hyperkalemia (malaise, anorexia, paresthesia or muscle weakness) and ECG changes. ◆ If the patient receives hypertonic glucose and insulin infusions, monitor potassium and glucose levels. If giving sodium polystyrene sulfonate rectally, make sure the patient doesn't retain it and become constipated; doing so prevents bowel perforation. ◆ Maintain the patient's nutritional status with a high-calorie, low-protein, low-sodium, low-potassium diet and vitamin supplements. ◆ Monitor the patient carefully during peritoneal dialysis. ◆ If the patient requires hemodialysis, monitor the venous access site carefully; assess the patient and laboratory work carefully. ◆ Administer diuretics.

Hepatitis, viral

OVERVIEW

- Infection and inflammation of the liver caused by a virus
- Six types recognized—A, B, C, D, E, and G—and a seventh suspected
- Marked by hepatic cell destruction, necrosis, and autolysis, leading to anorexia, jaundice, and hepatomegaly
- Recovery possible in most patients because hepatic cells eventually regenerate with little or no residual damage
- Complications more likely with old age and serious underlying disorders
- Prognosis poor if edema and hepatic encephalopathy develop
- Hepatitis A occurring in nationwide epidemics
- Hepatitis B occurring predominantly in people ages 20 to 49
- About 1.25 million Americans chronically infected with hepatitis B
- About 3.9 million Americans chronically infected with hepatitis C

CAUSES
- Infection with one of the six major forms of viral hepatitis

Type A
- Transmittal by the fecal-oral or parenteral route
- Ingestion of contaminated food, milk, or water

Type B
- Transmittal by contact with contaminated human blood, secretions, and stool

Type C
- Transmittal primarily through needles shared by I.V. drug users or those used in tattooing, through blood transfusions, or through sharing nose paraphernalia used for sniffing cocaine

Type D
- Found only in patients with an acute or a chronic episode of hepatitis B

Type E
- Transmittal by parenteral route and commonly water-borne

Type G
- Thought to be blood-borne, with transmission similar to that of hepatitis B and C

PATHOPHYSIOLOGY

- Hepatic damage is usually similar in all types of viral hepatitis; however, varying degrees of cell injury and necrosis can occur. (See *Disorders affecting management of viral hepatitis,* pages 196 and 197.)
- On entering the body, the virus causes hepatocyte injury and cell death, either by directly killing the cells or by activating inflammatory and immune reactions, which, in turn, injure or destroy hepatocytes by lysing the infected or neighboring cells.
- Later, direct antibody attack against viral antigens causes further destruction of the infected cells.
- Edema and swelling of the interstitium lead to collapse of capillaries and decreased blood flow, tissue hypoxia, and scarring and fibrosis.

NEUROLOGIC SYSTEM
- Hepatic encephalopathy develops when the liver can no longer detoxify the blood. Liver dysfunction and collateral vessels that shunt blood around the liver to the systemic circulation permit toxins absorbed from the GI tract to circulate freely to the brain. The normal liver transforms ammonia to urea, which the kidneys then excrete. When the liver fails, ammonia blood levels rise and circulate to the brain, causing encephalopathic damage.
- Short-chain fatty acids, serotonin, tryptophan, and false neurotransmitters may accumulate in the blood and contribute to hepatic encephalopathy. (See *Recognizing asterixis.*)

RENAL SYSTEM
- Accumulation of vasoactive substances or a compensatory response to portal hypertension and the pooling of blood in the splenic circulation may lead to decreased glomerular filtration, oliguria, and hepatorenal syndrome (renal failure concurrent with liver disease; the kidneys appear normal but abruptly cease functioning).
- Hepatorenal syndrome causes expanded blood volume, accumulation of hydrogen ions, and electrolyte disturbances.

ASSESSMENT

HISTORY
- No signs or symptoms in 50% to 60% of people with hepatitis B
- No signs or symptoms in 80% of people with hepatitis C
- Revelation of a source of transmission

Prodromal stage
- Patient easily fatigued, with generalized malaise
- Anorexia, mild weight loss
- Depression
- Headache, photophobia
- Weakness
- Arthralgia, myalgia (hepatitis B)
- Nausea or vomiting
- Changes in the senses of taste and smell

Recognizing asterixis

With asterixis, the patient's wrists and fingers are observed to "flap" because there is a brief, rapid relaxation of dorsiflexion of the wrist.

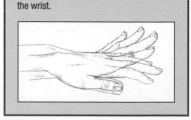

Clinical jaundice stage

- Pruritus
- Abdominal pain or tenderness
- Indigestion
- Anorexia
- Possible jaundice of sclerae, mucous membranes, and skin

Posticteric stage

- Most symptoms decreasing or subsiding

PHYSICAL FINDINGS
Prodromal stage

- Fever (100° to 102° F [37.8° to 38.9° C])
- Dark urine
- Clay-colored stools

Clinical jaundice stage

- Rashes, erythematous patches, or hives
- Abdominal tenderness in the right upper quadrant
- Enlarged and tender liver
- Splenomegaly
- Cervical adenopathy

Posticteric stage

- Decrease in liver enlargement

DIAGNOSTIC TEST FINDINGS

- With suspected viral hepatitis, routine hepatitis profile identifies antibodies specific to the causative virus, establishing the type of hepatitis:
- Type A: Detection of an antibody to hepatitis A confirms the diagnosis.
- Type B: The presence of hepatitis B surface antigens and hepatitis B antibodies confirms the diagnosis.
- Type C: The diagnosis depends on serologic testing for the specific antibody one or more months after the onset of acute illness; until then, diagnosis is principally established by obtaining negative test results for hepatitis types A, B, and D.
- Type D: Detection of intrahepatic delta antigens or immunoglobulin (Ig) M antidelta antigens in acute disease (or IgM and IgG in chronic disease) establishes the diagnosis.
- Type E: Detection of hepatitis E antigens support the diagnosis.
- Type G: Detection of hepatitis G ribonucleic acid supports the diagno-

sis (serologic assays are being developed).
- Additional findings from liver function studies support the diagnosis:
- Serum aspartate aminotransferase and serum alanine aminotransferase levels are increased in the prodromal stage of acute viral hepatitis.
- Serum alkaline phosphatase levels are slightly increased.
- Serum bilirubin level is elevated; level may stay elevated late in the disease, especially with severe disease.
- Prothrombin time is prolonged (more than 3 seconds longer than normal), indicating severe liver damage.
- White blood cell counts commonly reveal transient neutropenia and lymphopenia, followed by lymphocytosis.
- Liver biopsy may show chronic hepatitis.

TREATMENT

GENERAL
For hepatitis C

- Aimed at clearing hepatitis C from the body, stopping or slowing hepatic damage, and relieving symptoms
- Parenteral feeding, if appropriate

DIET

- Small, high-calorie, high-protein meals (reduced protein intake if signs of precoma—lethargy, confusion, mental changes—develop)
- Avoidance of alcohol

ACTIVITY

- Frequent rest periods, as needed
- Avoidance of contact sports and strenuous activity

MEDICATIONS

- Standard immunoglobulin
- Vaccine
- Alfa-2b interferon (hepatitis B and C)
- Antiemetics
- Cholestyramine (Questran)
- Lamivudine (Epivir) (hepatitis B)
- Ribavirin (Virazole) (hepatitis C)

SURGERY

- Possible liver transplant (hepatitis C)

NURSING CONSIDERATIONS

NURSING DIAGNOSES

- Activity intolerance
- Anxiety
- Fear
- Imbalanced nutrition: Less than body requirements
- Risk for infection
- Risk for injury

EXPECTED OUTCOMES
The patient will:

- perform activities of daily living within the confines of the disease process
- identify strategies to reduce anxiety
- discuss fears and concerns
- achieve adequate caloric and nutritional intake
- remain free from signs and symptoms of infection
- remain free from injury.

NURSING INTERVENTIONS

- Observe standard precautions to prevent transmission of the disease.
- Provide rest periods during the day.
- Give prescribed drugs.
- Encourage oral fluid intake.
- Assess hydration and nutritional status.
- Monitor daily weight and intake and output.
- Evaluate stool for color, consistency, amount, and frequency.
- Observe for signs of complications.

PATIENT TEACHING

Be sure to cover:

- disorder, diagnostic testing, and treatment
- medication administration, dosage, and possible adverse effects
- measures to prevent the spread of disease
- importance of rest and a proper diet
- need to abstain from alcohol

(continued)

- need to avoid over-the-counter medications, unless approved by the practitioner
- need for follow-up care
- support services, such as Alcoholics Anonymous, if indicated.

RESOURCES
Organizations
Alcoholics Anonymous:
www.alcoholics-anonymous.org
American Liver Foundation:
www.liver-foundation.org
Digestive Disease National Coalition:
www.ddnc.org

National Digestive Diseases Information Clearinghouse:
www.niddk.nih.gov/health/digest/nddic.htm

Selected references
Sheppard, K., and Hubbert, A. "The Patient Experience of Treatment of Hepatitis C," *Gastroenterology Nursing* 29(4):309-15, July-August 2006.
Stonsifer, E., et al. "Hepatitis in Primary Care: What NPs Can Do to Save Lives," *Nurse Practitioner* 31(6):53,55, June 2006.

Tierney, L., et al. *Current Medical Diagnosis and Treatment 2006.* New York: McGraw-Hill Book Co., 2006.
Vos, D., et al. "Needlestick Injury and Accidental Exposure to Blood: The Need for Improving the Hepatitis B Vaccination Grade Among Health Care Workers Outside the Hospital," *American Journal of Infection Control* 34(9):610-12, November 2006.

Disorders affecting management of viral hepatitis

This chart highlights disorders that affect the management of viral hepatitis.

DISORDER	SIGNS AND SYMPTOMS	DIAGNOSTIC TEST RESULTS	TREATMENT AND CARE
Esophageal varices (complication)	• Ascites • GI bleeding • Confusion • Forgetfulness • Jaundice	• Platelet levels are decreased. • White blood cell count is decreased. • Ammonia levels are elevated. • Endoscopy reveals esophageal varices.	• Monitor neurologic status. • Assist with paracentesis. • Monitor intake and output. • Monitor laboratory values. • Administer medications, as ordered. • Initiate aspiration precautions, if patient is lethargic, or administer enteral feedings. • Provide skin care and assess skin integrity.
Hepatic encephalopathy (complication)	• Jaundice • Nausea and anorexia • Abdominal pain or tenderness • Fatigue and weight loss • Pruritus • Oliguria • Splenomegaly • Ascites • Peripheral edema • Esophageal varices • Bleeding tendencies • Petechiae *Prodromal stage (Grade I)* • Personality changes such as agitation, belligerence, disorientation, and forgetfulness • Fatigue • Drowsiness • Slurred or slow speech • Slight tremor *Impending stage (Grade II)* • Confusion • Disoriented to time, place, and person • Asterixis (liver flap, flapping tremor)	• Liver function tests reveal elevated levels of aspartate aminotransferase, alanine aminotransferase, alkaline phosphatase, and bilirubin. • Blood studies reveal anemia, impaired red blood cell (RBC) production, elevated bleeding and clotting times, low platelet levels, low blood glucose levels, low albumin, decreased blood urea nitrogen (BUN), and increased serum ammonia levels. • Serum electrolyte studies commonly reveal hyponatremia and hypokalemia in patients with ascites. • Urinalysis reveals increased urobilinogen, bilirubin, and osmolarity. • EEG is typically abnormal with hepatic encephalopathy, but the changes are nonspecific.	• Frequently assess and record the patient's level of consciousness (LOC). Continually orient him to place and time. Remember to keep a daily record of the patient's handwriting to monitor the progression of neurologic involvement. • Promote rest, comfort, and a quiet atmosphere. • Monitor intake, output, and fluid and electrolyte balance. Check the patient's weight, and measure abdominal girth daily. Watch for and immediately report signs of anemia (decreased hemoglobin), alkalosis (increased serum bicarbonate), GI bleeding (melena, hematemesis), and infection. Monitor the patient's serum ammonia level. • Administer lactulose, neomycin, potassium supplements, and salt-poor albumin. Monitor the patient for the desired effects, and watch for adverse reactions. • Provide a low-protein diet, with carbohydrates supplying most of the calories. Provide good mouth care. Provide parenteral nutrition to the semicomatose or comatose patient. • Use appropriate safety measures to protect the patient from injury. Avoid physical restraints, if possible. • Provide emotional support for the patient's family during the terminal stage of encephalopathy.

DISORDER	SIGNS AND SYMPTOMS	DIAGNOSTIC TEST RESULTS	TREATMENT AND CARE
Hepatic encephalopathy (complication) *(continued)*	*Stuporous stage (Grade III)* ◆ Marked mental confusion ◆ Drowsiness ◆ Stupor ◆ Hyperventilation ◆ Muscle twitching ◆ Asterixis *Comatose stage (Grade IV)* ◆ Fetor hepaticus (musty odor of breath and urine) ◆ Seizures ◆ Hyperactive reflexes ◆ Coma		
Portal hypertension (complication)	◆ Massive hematemesis ◆ Varied LOC depending on degree of hepatic failure ◆ Tachycardia ◆ Hypotension ◆ Weak peripheral pulses ◆ Jaundice ◆ Splenomegaly ◆ Decreased urine output	◆ Endoscopy reveals bleeding site. ◆ Complete blood count reveals decreased hemoglobin levels, hematocrit, and RBC count. ◆ Coagulation studies reveal prolonged prothrombin time. ◆ BUN, sodium, total bilirubin, and ammonia levels may be elevated. ◆ Serum albumin may be decreased. ◆ Angiography identifies patency of portal vein and development of collateral vessels.	◆ Maintain nasogastric tamponade. ◆ Monitor amount of bleeding and laboratory studies. ◆ Monitor vital signs and pulse oximetry readings. ◆ Administer medications, I.V. fluids, and blood products. ◆ Initiate and maintain aspiration precautions. ◆ Observe for signs of complications. ◆ Identify and encourage beneficial lifestyle changes.
Renal failure (complication)	◆ Altered urinary elimination (oliguria or anuria) ◆ Irritability, drowsiness, or confusion ◆ Altered LOC ◆ Dry, pruritic skin ◆ Infection related to an altered immune status ◆ Hematuria, petechiae, and ecchymosis related to bleeding abnormalities ◆ Fatigue, dyspnea, and malaise related to anemia ◆ Anorexia, nausea, and vomiting ◆ Edema related to fluid retention ◆ Tachycardia ◆ Bibasilar crackles ◆ Uremic breath odor ◆ Hypertension or hypotension depending on the stage of acute renal failure ◆ Dry mucous membranes	◆ Blood studies show elevated BUN, serum creatinine, and potassium levels. Bicarbonate level, hematocrit, hemoglobin, and acid pH are decreased. ◆ Urine studies show casts, cellular debris, and decreased specific gravity. *In glomerular disease* ◆ Urine studies show proteinuria and a urine osmolality close to the serum osmolality. ◆ A creatinine clearance test reveals the number of functioning nephrons and measures the glomerular filtration rate. ◆ An electrocardiogram shows tall, peaked T waves; widening QRS complex; and disappearing P waves if hyperkalemia is present. ◆ Ultrasonography, abdominal and kidney-ureter-bladder X-rays, excretory urography, renal scan, retrograde pyelography, computerized tomography, and nephrotomography reveal abnormalities of the urinary tract.	◆ Measure and record intake and output. ◆ Follow standard precautions. ◆ Weigh the patient and measure his abdominal girth daily. ◆ Assess hematocrit and hemoglobin levels, and replace blood components. ◆ Monitor vital signs. Watch for and report signs of pericarditis (pleuritic chest pain, tachycardia, and pericardial friction rub), inadequate renal perfusion (hypotension), and acidosis. ◆ Maintain proper electrolyte balance. Strictly monitor potassium levels. Watch for symptoms of hyperkalemia. ◆ If the patient receives hypertonic glucose and insulin infusions, monitor potassium and glucose levels. If sodium polystyrene sulfonate is administered rectally, make sure the patient doesn't retain it and become constipated. This can lead to bowel perforation. ◆ Provide a diet high in calories and low in protein, sodium, and potassium, with vitamin supplements. ◆ Encourage frequent coughing and deep breathing; perform passive range-of-motion exercises. ◆ Test all stools for occult blood. ◆ Provide meticulous perineal care. ◆ Anticipate the need for peritoneal dialysis or hemodialysis. ◆ Administer medications after hemodialysis is completed. Many medications are removed from the blood during treatment. ◆ Administer diuretics.

Hodgkin's lymphoma

OVERVIEW

- Neoplastic disorder characterized by painless, progressive enlargement of lymph nodes, spleen, and other lymphoid tissue
- With appropriate treatment, 5-year survival rate about 90%
- Occurs in all races, but is slightly more common in whites
- Most common in people ages 15 to 38, except in Japan where it occurs exclusively in people older than age 50
- Incidence higher in males than in females

CAUSES
- Exact cause unknown

RISK FACTORS
- Genetic
- Viral
- Environmental

PATHOPHYSIOLOGY

- Enlarged lymphoid tissue results from proliferation of lymphocytes, histiocytes, eosinophils, and Reed-Sternberg cells. (See *Recognizing Reed-Sternberg cells.*)
- Untreated Hodgkin's lymphoma follows a variable but relentlessly progressive and ultimately fatal course. (See *Disorders affecting management of Hodgkin's lymphoma*, page 201.)

CARDIOVASCULAR SYSTEM
- Mediastinal mass causes chest pain and compromised cardiac circulation.

NEUROLOGIC SYSTEM
- Paraneoplastic syndromes cause central nervous system symptoms, such as neuropathy or cerebellar degeneration.

RESPIRATORY SYSTEM
- Chest mass may cause respiratory compromise.
- Immunodeficiency may cause increased risk of respiratory infection and development of pleural effusions.
- Treatment with radiation therapy and chemotherapy decreases immune status and increases risk for pulmonary infection.

ASSESSMENT

HISTORY
- Painless swelling of one of the cervical, axillary, or inguinal lymph nodes
- Persistent fever and night sweats
- Weight loss despite an adequate diet, with resulting fatigue and malaise
- Increasing susceptibility to infection

PHYSICAL FINDINGS
- Edema of the face and neck and jaundice
- Enlarged, rubbery lymph nodes in the neck (nodes enlarge during periods of fever and then revert to normal size)

DIAGNOSTIC TEST RESULTS
- Hematologic tests show mild to severe normocytic, normochromic anemia in 50% of patients; elevated, normal, or reduced white blood cell count and differential; and any combination of neutrophilia, lymphocytopenia, monocytosis, and eosinophilia.
- Serum alkaline phosphatase levels are elevated, indicating liver or bone involvement.
- Tests must first rule out other disorders that enlarge the lymph nodes.
- Lymph node biopsy confirms the presence of Reed-Sternberg cells, abnormal histiocyte proliferation, and

Recognizing Reed-Sternberg cells

The illustration at right shows Reed-Sternberg cells. Note the large, distinct nucleoli.

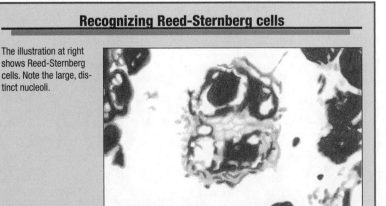

nodular fibrosis and necrosis. A lymph node biopsy is also used to determine lymph node and organ involvement.

- Staging laparotomy is necessary for patients younger than age 55 and for those without obvious stage III or IV disease, lymphocyte predominance subtype histology, or medical contraindications.

GENERAL

- For patient with stage I or II disease, radiation therapy alone
- For patient with stage III disease, radiation therapy and chemotherapy
- For patient with stage IV disease, chemotherapy alone (or chemotherapy and radiation therapy to involved sites), sometimes inducing complete remission
- Autologous bone marrow transplantation or autologous peripheral blood sternal transfusions and immunotherapy

DIET

- Well-balanced, high-calorie, high-protein

ACTIVITY

- Frequent rest periods

MEDICATIONS

- Chemotherapy
- Antiemetics
- Sedatives
- Antidiarrheals

NURSING DIAGNOSES

- Acute pain
- Anxiety
- Fatigue
- Fear
- Imbalanced nutrition: Less than body requirements
- Impaired oral mucous membranes
- Impaired skin integrity
- Ineffective coping
- Risk for infection

EXPECTED OUTCOMES

The patient will:

- express feelings of increased comfort and decreased pain
- verbalize feelings of decreased anxiety
- express feelings of increased energy
- express fears and concerns relating to diagnosis and condition
- maintain weight within an acceptable range
- exhibit intact mucous membranes
- demonstrate adequate skin integrity
- demonstrate effective coping mechanisms
- remain free from signs and symptoms of infection.

NURSING INTERVENTIONS

- Provide a well-balanced, high-calorie, high-protein diet.
- Provide frequent rest periods.
- Give prescribed drugs.
- Provide emotional support.
- Observe for complications of treatment.
- Evaluate pain management.
- Monitor lymph node enlargement and temperature.
- Note level of fatigue.
- Monitor daily weight and response to treatment.

(continued)

Be sure to cover:
◆ disorder, diagnostic testing, and treatment
◆ medication administration, dosage, and possible adverse effects
◆ signs and symptoms of infection
◆ importance of maintaining good nutrition
◆ pacing of activities to counteract therapy-induced fatigue
◆ importance of good oral hygiene
◆ avoidance of crowds and people with known infection
◆ importance of checking the lymph nodes
◆ available resource and support services.

RESOURCES
Organizations
American Cancer Society:
www.cancer.org
Guide to Internet Resources for Cancer:
www.cancerindex.org
National Cancer Institute:
www.cancer.gov

Selected references
Atlas of Pathophysiology, 2nd ed. Philadelphia: Lippincott Williams & Wilkins, 2005.

Kuppers, R., et al. "Advances in Biology, Diagnostics, and Treatment of Hodgkin's Disease," *Biology of Blood and Marrow Transplantation* 12(1 Suppl 1):66-76, January 2006.

Miyoshi, I., et al. "Cutaneous Involvement in Hodgkin's Disease," *Internal Medicine* 46(2):73-74, January 2007.

Ng, A., and Mauch, P. "The Impact of Treatment on the Risk of Second Malignancy After Hodgkin's Disease," *Annuals of Oncology* 17(12):1727-729, December 2006.

Disorders affecting management of Hodgkin's lymphoma

This chart highlights disorders that affect the management of Hodgkin's lymphoma.

DISORDER	SIGNS AND SYMPTOMS	DIAGNOSTIC TEST RESULTS	TREATMENT AND CARE
Coronary artery disease (complication)	◆ Angina or feeling of burning, squeezing, or tightness in the chest that may radiate to the left arm, neck, jaw, or shoulder blade ◆ Nausea and vomiting ◆ Cool extremities and pallor ◆ Diaphoresis ◆ Xanthelasma (fat deposits on the eyelids)	◆ Electrocardiogram (ECG) may be normal between anginal episodes. During angina attack, it may show ischemic changes ◆ Computed tomography scan may identify calcium deposits in coronary arteries. ◆ Stress testing may detect ST-segment changes. ◆ Coronary angiography reveals location and degree of stenosis, obstruction, and collateral circulation. ◆ Intravascular ultrasound may define anatomy and luminal narrowing. ◆ Myocardial perfusion imaging detects ischemic areas as cold spots. ◆ Stress echocardiography shows abnormal wall motion in ischemic areas. ◆ Rest perfusion imaging rules out myocardial infarction.	◆ During anginal attack, monitor the patient's vital signs and obtain an ECG. ◆ Administer nitrates, as ordered, and evaluate effect. ◆ Prepare for diagnostic studies, and monitor for complications when complete. ◆ Administer medications, as ordered. ◆ Provide emotional support. ◆ Provide teaching regarding appropriate lifestyle changes.
Pericarditis (complication)	◆ Pericardial friction rub ◆ Sharp, sudden pain, usually starting over the sternum and radiating to the neck, shoulders, back, and arms ◆ Shallow, rapid respirations ◆ Mild fever ◆ Dyspnea, orthopnea, and tachycardia ◆ Muffled and distant heart sounds ◆ Pale, clammy skin ◆ Hypotension, pulsus paradoxus ◆ Jugular vein distention	◆ ECG may reveal diffuse ST-segment elevation, downsloping PR segments and upright T waves, possible diminished QRS complexes when pericardial effusion exists, and arrhythmias. ◆ Erythrocyte sedimentation rate is elevated. ◆ Echocardiogram may show an echo-free space between the ventricular wall and the pericardium and reduced pumping action of the heart. ◆ Chest X-rays may be normal with acute pericarditis. The cardiac silhouette may be enlarged with a water bottle shape caused by fluid accumulation, if pleural effusion is present.	◆ Maintain bed rest as long as fever and pain persist to reduce metabolic needs. ◆ Administer medications, such as nonsteroidal anti-inflammatory (NSAIDs) drugs, to relieve pain and reduce inflammation; give corticosteroids if NSAIDs are ineffective. ◆ Prepare for pericardiocentesis or pericardectomy. ◆ Place the patient in an upright position to relieve dyspnea and chest pain. ◆ Administer supplemental oxygen, as indicated. ◆ Monitor vital signs and cardiovascular status for signs of cardiac tamponade.
Sepsis (complication)	◆ Agitation ◆ Anxiety ◆ Altered level of consciousness ◆ Tachycardia ◆ Hypotension ◆ Rapid, shallow respirations ◆ Fever ◆ Urine output less than 25 ml/hr	◆ Blood cultures are positive for the infecting organism. ◆ Complete blood count reveals whether anemia, neutropenia, and thrombocytopenia are present. ◆ Arterial blood gas studies show metabolic acidosis. ◆ Blood urea nitrogen and creatinine levels are increased. ◆ ECG shows ST-segment depression, inverted T waves, and arrhythmias.	◆ Identify and treat underlying cause of sepsis. ◆ Monitor vital signs frequently. ◆ Administer antibiotics. ◆ Administer I.V. fluids to replace intravascular volume. ◆ Administer vasopressors if fluid resuscitation doesn't maintain blood pressure. ◆ Assess respiratory status. ◆ Prepare for intubation and mechanical ventilation, if needed.

Hyperaldosteronism

- Hypersecretion of the mineralocorticoid aldosterone by the adrenal cortex
- Causes excessive reabsorption of sodium and water and excessive renal excretion of potassium
- May be primary (uncommon) or secondary
- Three times more common in females than in males
- Most common between ages 30 and 50

CAUSES

- Bartter's syndrome
- Benign aldosterone-producing adrenal adenoma (in 70% of patients)
- Bilateral adrenocortical hyperplasia (in children) or carcinoma (rarely)
- Conditions that produce a sodium deficit (Wilms' tumor)
- Conditions that reduce renal blood flow and extracellular fluid volume (renal artery stenosis)
- Heart failure
- Hepatic cirrhosis with ascites
- Nephrotic syndrome

PRIMARY HYPERALDOSTERONISM (CONN'S SYNDROME)

- Chronic excessive secretion of aldosterone is independent of the renin-angiotensin system and suppresses plasma renin activity.
- This aldosterone excess enhances sodium and water reabsorption and potassium loss by the kidneys, which leads to mild hypernatremia, hypokalemia, and increased extracellular fluid volume.

WARNING *Excessive ingestion of English black licorice or licorice-like substances can produce a syndrome similar to primary hyperaldosteronism because of the mineralocorticoid action of glycyrrhizic acid.*

SECONDARY HYPERALDOSTERONISM

- An extra-adrenal abnormality stimulates the adrenal gland to increase aldosterone production.

CARDIOVASCULAR SYSTEM

- Expansion of intravascular fluid volume results in volume-dependent hypertension and increased cardiac output. (See *Disorders affecting management of hyperaldosteronism*, page 205.)
- Hypokalemia may cause cardiac arrhythmias.

RESPIRATORY SYSTEM

- Development of metabolic alkalosis can result in hypoventilation and respiratory compromise.

MUSCULOSKELETAL SYSTEM

- Excessive potassium loss causes muscular weakness and tetany.

HISTORY

- Vision disturbances
- Nocturnal polyuria
- Polydipsia
- Fatigue
- Headaches
- Hypokalemia

PHYSICAL FINDINGS

- Muscle weakness
- Intermittent, flaccid paralysis
- Paresthesia
- High blood pressure
- Abdominal distention

DIAGNOSTIC TEST RESULTS

- Serum potassium levels are persistently low.
- Low plasma renin level that fails to increase appropriately during volume depletion (upright posture, sodium depletion) and high plasma aldosterone level that fails to decrease during volume expansion by salt loading confirm primary hyperaldosteronism in a hypertensive patient without edema.
- Serum bicarbonate level is elevated.
- Urine aldosterone levels are markedly increased.
- Plasma aldosterone levels are increased.
- Plasma renin levels (secondary) are increased.
- Suppression test distinguishes between primary and secondary hyperaldosteronism.
- Chest X-rays show left ventricular hypertrophy from chronic hypertension.
- Adrenal angiography or computed tomography scan localize the tumor.
- Electrocardiography may show signs of hypokalemia (ST-segment depression and U waves).

GENERAL
◆ Treatment of underlying cause (secondary)

DIET
◆ Low-sodium, high-potassium

MEDICATIONS
◆ Aldosterone antagonists
◆ Potassium-sparing diuretics (primary)
◆ Potassium supplements

SURGERY
◆ Unilateral adrenalectomy (primary)

NURSING DIAGNOSES
◆ Acute pain
◆ Decreased cardiac output
◆ Excess fluid volume
◆ Impaired physical mobility
◆ Impaired urinary elimination
◆ Ineffective coping
◆ Ineffective tissue perfusion: Cardiopulmonary

EXPECTED OUTCOMES
The patient will:
◆ express feelings of increased comfort and decreased pain
◆ maintain adequate cardiac output
◆ show no signs of circulatory overload
◆ maintain joint range of motion and muscle strength
◆ maintain a normal urine output
◆ demonstrate adaptive coping behaviors
◆ maintain hemodynamic stability.

NURSING INTERVENTIONS
◆ Watch for signs of tetany (muscle twitching, Trousseau's sign, Chvostek's sign).
◆ Give potassium replacement, and keep I.V. calcium gluconate available.
◆ After adrenalectomy, watch for weakness, hyponatremia, rising serum potassium levels, and signs of adrenal hypofunction, especially hypotension.
◆ Monitor intake and output, vital signs, weight, and serum electrolyte levels.
◆ Observe for cardiac arrhythmias.

(continued)

Be sure to cover:
◆ disorder, diagnostic testing, and treatment
◆ adverse effects of spironolactone, including hyperkalemia, impotence, and gynecomastia, if appropriate
◆ dietary restrictions
◆ how to take blood pressure measurements
◆ importance of wearing medical identification jewelry while taking steroid hormone replacement therapy.

RESOURCES
Organizations
Endocrine Society: *www.endo-society.org*
The Merck Manuals Online Medical Library: *www.merck.com/mmhe*
National Adrenal Diseases Foundation: *www.medhelp.org/www/nadf.htm*
National Institute of Diabetes & Digestive & Kidney Diseases: *www.niddk.nih.gov*
National Library of Medicine: *www.nlm.nih.gov*

Selected references
Al-Aloul, B., et al. "Atrial Fibrillation Associated with Hypokalemia Due to Primary Hyperaldosteronism (Conn's syndrome)," *Pacing and Clinical Electrophysiology* 29(11):1303-305, November 2006.
Calhoun, D. "Aldosterone and Cardiovascular Disease: Smoke and Fire," *Circulation* 114(24):2572-574, December 2006.
Williams, J.S., et al. "Prevalence of Primary Hyperaldosteronism in Mild to Moderate Hypertension Without Hypokalemia," *Journal of Human Hypertension* 20(2):129-36, February 2006.

Disorders affecting management of hyperaldosteronism

This chart highlights disorders that affect the management of hyperaldosteronism.

DISORDER	SIGNS AND SYMPTOMS	DIAGNOSTIC TEST RESULTS	TREATMENT AND CARE
Hypertension (complication)	◆ Usually asymptomatic ◆ Elevated blood pressure readings on at least two consecutive occasions ◆ Occipital headache ◆ Epistaxis ◆ Bruits ◆ Dizziness ◆ Confusion ◆ Fatigue ◆ Blurred vision ◆ Nocturia ◆ Peripheral edema	◆ Serial blood pressure measurements reveal elevations of 140/90 mm Hg on at least two or more separate occasions. ◆ Urinalysis may show protein, casts, red blood cells, or white blood cells. ◆ Blood urea nitrogen and creatinine levels are elevated, suggesting renal disease. ◆ Complete blood count may reveal polycythemia or anemia. ◆ Excretory urography may reveal renal atrophy. ◆ Electrocardiogram (ECG) may show left ventricular hypertrophy or ischemia. ◆ Chest X-rays may show cardiomegaly. ◆ Echocardiogram may reveal left ventricular hypertrophy.	◆ Monitor blood pressure readings and laboratory studies. ◆ Identify and encourage lifestyle modifications. ◆ Monitor for complications, such as stroke, myocardial infarction, and renal disease. ◆ Administer medications, as ordered, and monitor response.
Hypokalemia (complication)	◆ Dizziness ◆ Hypotension ◆ Arrhythmias ◆ Cardiac arrest ◆ Nausea, vomiting ◆ Anorexia ◆ Diarrhea ◆ Decreased peristalsis ◆ Abdominal distention ◆ Muscle weakness ◆ Fatigue ◆ Leg cramps	◆ Serum potassium is less than 3.5 mEq/L. ◆ Arterial blood gas (ABG) analysis reveals metabolic alkalosis. ◆ ECG changes include flattened T waves, elevated U waves, and a depressed ST segment.	◆ Monitor cardiac rhythm, vital signs, and pulse oximetry readings. ◆ Administer electrolyte replacement therapy, and monitor laboratory values. ◆ Monitor intake and output, especially when administering I.V. potassium replacement. Urine volume should be greater than 30 ml/hour to prevent rebound hyperkalemia. ◆ Check for signs of hypokalemia-related metabolic alkalosis, including irritability and paresthesia.
Metabolic alkalosis (complication)	◆ Apnea ◆ Atrial tachycardia ◆ Confusion ◆ Cyanosis ◆ Diarrhea ◆ Hypoventilation ◆ Irritability ◆ Nausea ◆ Twitching ◆ Vomiting	◆ ABG analysis reveals pH greater than 7.45 and a bicarbonate level above 29 mEq/L.	◆ Monitor vital signs, respiratory status, and pulse oximetry readings. ◆ Administer oxygen therapy and assist with intubation, if necessary. ◆ Monitor intake and output. ◆ Administer medications, as ordered. ◆ Monitor ABG values.

Hypercalcemia

OVERVIEW

- Excessive levels of serum calcium
- Incidence considerably higher in females than in males and increasing with age
- No gender predominance existing in elevated calcium levels related to cancer

CAUSES

- Certain cancers
- Certain drugs (see *Drugs causing hypercalcemia*)
- Hyperparathyroidism
- Hypervitaminosis D
- Multiple fractures and prolonged immobilization

PATHOPHYSIOLOGY

- Together with phosphorus, calcium is responsible for the formation and structure of bones and teeth and helps to maintain cell structure and function.
- It plays a role in cell membrane permeability and impulse transmission.
- Calcium affects the contraction of cardiac muscle, smooth muscle, and skeletal muscle and participates in the blood-clotting process.
- Patients with squamous cell carcinoma of the lung, myeloma, or breast cancer are especially prone to hypercalcemia.
- Hypophosphatemia and acidosis increase calcium ionization and are associated with hypercalcemia.

CARDIOVASCULAR SYSTEM

- The heart muscle and cardiac conduction system are affected by hypercalcemia, which may lead to arrhythmias such as bradycardia and subsequent cardiac arrest.
- Effects of excess calcium on the heart muscle may lead to hypertension. (See *Disorders affecting management of hypercalcemia*, pages 208 and 209.)

ENDOCRINE SYSTEM

- Hyperparathyroidism, the most common cause of hypercalcemia, occurs when the body excretes more parathyroid hormone than normal, greatly increasing the effects of this hormone on the body.
- Calcium reabsorption from the bones, kidneys, and intestines also increases.

GASTROINTESTINAL SYSTEM

- GI symptoms such as anorexia, nausea, and vomiting may be the first symptoms the patient experiences.
- Excess calcium affects the smooth muscle leading to decreased GI motility, resulting in decreased bowel sounds, constipation, abdominal pain and, possibly, a paralytic ileus.

MUSCULOSKELETAL SYSTEM

- As calcium levels rise, the patient may experience the onset of muscle weakness, hyporeflexia, and decreased muscle tone.
- Pathological fractures and bone pain may result from the excess levels of calcium.

NEUROLOGIC SYSTEM

- Excess calcium levels can affect the nerve cells and the nervous system, leading to drowsiness, lethargy, headaches, depression or apathy, irritability, and confusion. (See *How hypercalcemia develops*.)

RENAL SYSTEM

- The kidneys work overtime to remove excess calcium, which may lead to renal problems such as polyuria, dehydration, and renal failure.
- Renal calculi and other calcifications may develop.

ASSESSMENT

HISTORY

- Underlying cause
- Lethargy
- Weakness
- Anorexia
- Constipation
- Nausea, vomiting
- Polyuria
- Bone pain
- Abdominal upset
- Depression

PHYSICAL FINDINGS

- Confusion (see *Clinical effects of hypercalcemia*)
- Muscle weakness
- Hyporeflexia
- Decreased muscle tone
- Depression

DIAGNOSTIC TEST RESULTS

◆ Serum calcium level is greater than 10.5 mg/dl.
◆ Ionized calcium level is less than 5.3 mg/dl.
◆ Electrocardiography may show shortened QT interval and ventricular arrhythmias.

TREATMENT

GENERAL
◆ Treatment of the underlying cause

ACTIVITY
◆ As tolerated

MEDICATIONS
◆ Normal saline solution
◆ Loop diuretics

SURGERY
◆ Parathyroidectomy

NURSING CONSIDERATIONS

NURSING DIAGNOSES
◆ Anxiety
◆ Decreased cardiac output
◆ Fear
◆ Impaired gas exchange
◆ Ineffective tissue perfusion: Cardiopulmonary
◆ Risk for injury

EXPECTED OUTCOMES
The patient will:
◆ identify strategies to reduce anxiety
◆ maintain adequate cardiac output
◆ discuss fears and concerns
◆ maintain adequate ventilation and oxygenation
◆ exhibit signs of adequate cardiopulmonary perfusion
◆ remain free from injury.

NURSING INTERVENTIONS

◆ Provide safety measures and institute seizure precautions, if appropriate.
◆ Give prescribed I.V. solutions.
◆ Watch for signs of heart failure.
◆ Monitor cardiac rhythm and calcium levels.

After parathyroidectomy
◆ Keep a tracheotomy tray and endotracheal tube setup at the patient's bedside.
◆ Maintain seizure precautions.
◆ Place the patient in semi-Fowler's position.
◆ Support the patient's head and neck with sandbags.
◆ Have the patient ambulate as soon as possible.
◆ Assess for increased neuromuscular activity.
◆ Monitor neck edema.
◆ Assess for Chvostek's and Trousseau's signs.

WARNING *Watch for complaints of tingling in the hands and around the mouth. If these symptoms don't subside quickly, they may be pro-*

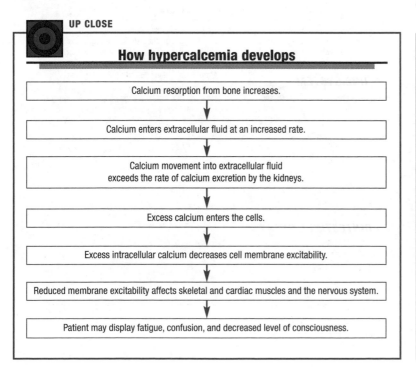

UP CLOSE

How hypercalcemia develops

Calcium resorption from bone increases.

↓

Calcium enters extracellular fluid at an increased rate.

↓

Calcium movement into extracellular fluid exceeds the rate of calcium excretion by the kidneys.

↓

Excess calcium enters the cells.

↓

Excess intracellular calcium decreases cell membrane excitability.

↓

Reduced membrane excitability affects skeletal and cardiac muscles and the nervous system.

↓

Patient may display fatigue, confusion, and decreased level of consciousness.

Clinical effects of hypercalcemia

BODY SYSTEM	EFFECTS
Cardiovascular	◆ Signs of heart block, cardiac arrest, hypertension
Gastrointestinal	◆ Anorexia, nausea, vomiting, constipation, dehydration, polydipsia
Musculoskeletal	◆ Weakness, muscle flaccidity, bone pain, pathologic fractures
Neurologic	◆ Drowsiness, lethargy, headaches, depression or apathy, irritability, confusion
Other	◆ Renal polyuria, flank pain and, eventually, azotemia

(continued)

dromal signs of tetany; so, keep I.V. calcium gluconate or calcium chloride available for emergency administration.

PATIENT TEACHING

Be sure to cover:
◆ disorder, diagnostic testing, and treatment
◆ medication administration, dosage, and possible adverse effects
◆ avoiding over-the-counter drugs that are high in calcium
◆ increasing fluid intake
◆ following a low-calcium diet.

RESOURCES
Organizations
Mayo Clinic: *www.mayoclinic.com*
National Cancer Institute: *www.cancer.gov*
National Library of Medicine: *www.nlm.nih.gov*

Selected references
Delaney, M.F., and Carey, J.J. "Hypercalcemia," *Cleveland Clinic Journal of Medicine* 72(12):1075, December 2005.
Ng, R.W., and Cheng, Y.L. "Calcium Alginate Dressing-Related Hypercalcemia," *Journal of Burn Care & Research* 28(1):203-204, January-February 2007.
Strategies for Managing Multisystem Disorders. Philadelphia: Lippincott Williams & Wilkins, 2006.

Disorders affecting management of hypercalcemia

This chart highlights disorders that affect the management of hypercalcemia.

DISORDER	SIGNS AND SYMPTOMS	DIAGNOSTIC TEST RESULTS	TREATMENT AND CARE
Acute renal failure (complication)	◆ Urine output less than 400 ml/day followed by diuresis of up to 5 L/day ◆ Lethargy ◆ Altered mental status ◆ Headache ◆ Costovertebral pain ◆ Numbness around the mouth ◆ Tingling extremities ◆ Anorexia ◆ Restlessness ◆ Weight gain ◆ Nausea and vomiting ◆ Pallor ◆ Diarrhea	◆ Blood urea nitrogen (BUN) and serum creatinine are increased. ◆ Potassium levels are increased. ◆ Hematocrit, blood pH, bicarbonate, and hemoglobin levels are decreased. ◆ Urine casts and cellular debris are present; specific gravity is decreased.	◆ Treat the underlying cause. ◆ Monitor fluid balance status, including skin turgor, peripheral edema, and intake and output. Monitor urine output hourly, and assess daily weight. ◆ Monitor central venous and pulmonary artery pressures. ◆ Insertion of a temporary dialysis catheter may be necessary for hemodialysis or continuous renal replacement therapy.

DISORDER	SIGNS AND SYMPTOMS	DIAGNOSTIC TEST RESULTS	TREATMENT AND CARE
Hypertension (complication)	◆ Headache ◆ Dizziness ◆ Fatigue ◆ Bounding pulse ◆ Pulsating abdominal mass ◆ Elevated blood pressure ◆ Bruits over the abdominal aorta	◆ Urinalysis may show proteinuria, red blood cells or white blood cells or, possibly, glucose. ◆ Serum potassium levels are less than 3.5 mEq/L. ◆ BUN level is normal or elevated to more than 20 mg/dl. ◆ Serum creatinine levels are normal or elevated to more than 1.5 mg/dl.	◆ Monitor vital signs and laboratory values, especially blood urea nitrogen, creatinine, and electrolytes. ◆ Monitor blood pressure for stability. ◆ Help the patient identify risk factors and modify his lifestyle. Encourage dietary changes. ◆ Advise patient to follow medication regimen in order to control blood pressure. ◆ Help the patient identify stress factors and establish effective coping mechanisms. ◆ Administer thiazide diuretics, angiotensin-converting enzyme inhibitors, angiotensin receptor blockers, and calcium channel blockers.
Renal calculi (complication)	◆ Severe pain that travels from the costovertebral angle to the flank and then to the suprapubic region and external genitalia ◆ Nausea and vomiting ◆ Fever ◆ Chills ◆ Hematuria ◆ Abdominal distention	◆ Kidney-ureter-bladder (KUB) radiography reveals most renal calculi. ◆ Excretory urography helps confirm the diagnosis and determine the size and location of calculi. ◆ Kidney ultrasonography is used to detect obstructive changes, such as unilateral or bilateral hydronephrosis and radiolucent calculi not seen on the KUB radiography. ◆ Urine culture of a midstream specimen may indicate pyuria, a sign of urinary tract infection. ◆ A 24-hour urine collection reveals the presence of calcium oxalate, phosphorus, and uric acid excretion. Three separate collections, along with blood samples, are needed for accurate testing. ◆ Calculus analysis shows mineral content. ◆ Serial blood calcium and phosphorus levels indicate hyperparathyroidism and show an increased calcium level in proportion to normal serum protein levels. ◆ Blood protein levels determine the level of free calcium unbound to protein.	◆ To aid diagnosis, maintain a 24- to 48-hour record of urine pH using nitrazine pH paper. Strain all urine through gauze or a tea strainer, and save all solid material recovered for analysis. ◆ To facilitate spontaneous passage of calculi, encourage the patient to walk, if possible. Also, encourage fluids to maintain a urine output of 3 to 4 qt (3 to 4 L)/day (urine should be very dilute and colorless). ◆ If the patient can't drink the required amount of fluid, give supplemental I.V. fluids. ◆ Record intake and output and daily weight to assess fluid status and renal function. ◆ Medicate the patient for pain when he's passing a calculus. ◆ To help acidify urine, offer fruit juices, especially cranberry juice. *If the patient had calculi surgically removed* ◆ Anticipate that the patient will have an indwelling catheter or a nephrostomy tube. ◆ Unless one of his kidneys was removed, expect bloody drainage from the catheter. ◆ Check dressings regularly for bloody drainage, and know how much drainage to expect. ◆ Immediately report excessive drainage or a rising pulse rate (symptoms of hemorrhage). ◆ Use sterile technique when changing dressings or providing catheter care. ◆ Administer antibiotics for infection. ◆ If lithotripsy is planned, expect to discontinue anticoagulants, aspirin, vitamin E, and platelet inhibitors for 3 days before the procedure.

Hyperchloremia

- Excessive serum levels of the chloride anion
- Usually accompanied by sodium and water retention

CAUSES

- Certain drugs (see *Drugs causing hyperchloremia*)
- Hypernatremia
- Hyperparathyroidism
- Loss of pancreatic secretion
- Metabolic acidosis
- Prolonged diarrhea
- Renal tubular acidosis

PATHOPHYSIOLOGY

- Chloride accounts for two-thirds of all serum anions and is secreted by stomach mucosa as hydrochloric acid; it provides an acid medium that aids digestion and activation of enzymes.
- Chloride helps to maintain acid-base and body water balances, influences the osmolality or tonicity of extracellular fluid, plays a role in the exchange of oxygen and carbon dioxide in red blood cells, and helps activate salivary amylase (which, in turn, activates the digestive process).
- An inverse relationship exists between chloride and bicarbonate. When the level of one goes up, the level of the other goes down. (See *Anion gap and metabolic acidosis*.)

CARDIOVASCULAR SYSTEM

- As the pH drops, central nervous system (CNS) depression affects myocardial function and leads to decreased cardiac output and hypotension.
- Arrhythmias may result from hyperchloremia as a result of untreated acidosis.
- Hypertension may also occur as a result of fluid overload. (See *Disorders*

affecting management of hyperchloremia, page 213.)

ENDOCRINE AND METABOLIC SYSTEMS

- A decrease in the serum bicarbonate level leads to an increase in the chloride level. (See *How hyperchloremia develops*.)
- The patient with diabetes experiencing metabolic acidosis may experience catabolism of fats and excretion of acetone through the lungs, leading to a fruity breath odor.

GASTROINTESTINAL SYSTEM

- Urinary diversion into the sigmoid colon or ileal segment leads to hyperchloremic acidosis and is associated with bicarbonate secretion into the colon in exchange for the reabsorption of urinary chloride.
- In patients with hyperchloremia caused by medications, ion exchange resins that contain sodium can cause chloride to be exchanged for potassium in the bowel. When chloride follows the sodium into the bloodstream, serum chloride levels rise.

INTEGUMENTARY SYSTEM

- Initially, the skin is warm and dry due to peripheral vasodilation but, as shock develops, the skin becomes cool and clammy.

MUSCULOSKELETAL SYSTEM

- Metabolic acidosis may lead to diminished muscle tone and deep tendon reflexes.

NEUROLOGIC SYSTEM

- Metabolic acidosis can produce lethargy, weakness, and diminished thought processes related to CNS depression from the decreased pH level.
- Headache may result from cerebral vessel dilation.

Drugs causing hyperchloremia

These drugs can cause or contribute to hyperchloremia:

- acetazolamide (Diamox)
- ammonium chloride
- sodium polystyrene sulfonate (Kayexalate)
- salicylates (overdose)
- triamterene (Dyrenium).

Anion gap and metabolic acidosis

Hyperchloremia increases the likelihood that a patient will develop hyperchloremic metabolic acidosis.

HOW IT HAPPENS

If a patient with metabolic acidosis has a normal anion gap, the acidosis is probably caused by a loss of bicarbonate ions by the kidneys or the GI tract. In such cases, a corresponding increase in chloride ions also occurs.

Acidosis can also result from an accumulation of chloride ions in the form of acidifying salts. A corresponding decrease in bicarbonate ions occurs at the same time.

RENAL SYSTEM

◆ Renal tubular acidosis is characterized by either bicarbonate loss in the urine or the inability to generate new bicarbonate.
◆ Renal bicarbonate wasting can result from the use of carbonic anhydrase inhibitors.

RESPIRATORY SYSTEM

◆ As acids build in the bloodstream, the lungs compensate by increasing the depth and rate of respirations (Kussmaul's respirations).

ASSESSMENT

HISTORY

◆ Risk factors for high chloride level
◆ Altered level of consciousness

PHYSICAL FINDINGS

◆ Agitation
◆ Pitting edema
◆ Dyspnea
◆ Rapid deep breathing (Kussmaul's respirations)
◆ Weakness
◆ Tachypnea
◆ Hypertension

DIAGNOSTIC TEST RESULTS

◆ Serum chloride level is greater than 108 mEq/L.
◆ With metabolic acidosis, serum pH is less than 7.35, serum carbon dioxide level is less than 22 mEq/L, and the anion gap is normal.
◆ Serum sodium level is greater than 145 mEq/L.

TREATMENT

GENERAL

◆ Treatment of underlying cause
◆ Restoring fluid, electrolyte, and acid-base balance

DIET

◆ Restricted sodium and chloride intake

ACTIVITY

◆ As tolerated

MEDICATIONS

◆ Sodium bicarbonate I.V.
◆ Lactated Ringer's solution
◆ Diuretics

UP CLOSE

How hyperchloremia develops

Chloride intake, absorption, or retention increases.

↓

Water loss may worsen chloride accumulation in extracellular fluid.

↓

Sodium bicarbonate level falls, and sodium level increases.

↓

Patient develops signs and symptoms of metabolic acidosis.

(continued)

NURSING CONSIDERATIONS

NURSING DIAGNOSES

◆ Anxiety
◆ Excess fluid volume
◆ Ineffective breathing pattern
◆ Ineffective tissue perfusion: Cardiopulmonary
◆ Risk for injury

EXPECTED OUTCOMES

The patient will:
◆ express feelings of decreased anxiety
◆ attain and maintain normal fluid and electrolyte balance
◆ maintain effective breathing pattern
◆ maintain adequate cardiac output
◆ remain free from injury.

NURSING INTERVENTIONS

◆ Provide a safe environment.
◆ Give prescribed I.V. fluids.
◆ Evaluate muscle strength and adjust activity level.
◆ Reorient the confused patient when necessary.
◆ Monitor serum electrolyte levels.
◆ Assess respiratory status and neurologic status.
◆ Monitor intake and output, cardiac rhythm, and arterial blood gas levels.
◆ Observe for signs of metabolic alkalosis.

PATIENT TEACHING

Be sure to cover:
◆ disorder, diagnostic testing, and treatment
◆ medication administration, dosage, and possible adverse effects
◆ dietary or fluid restrictions, as indicated.

RESOURCES

Organizations

National Digestive Diseases Information Clearinghouse: *www.niddk.nih.gov/health/digest/nddic.htm*
National Library of Medicine: *www.nlm.nih.gov*

Selected references

Diseases, 4th ed. Philadelphia: Lippincott Williams & Wilkins, 2006.
Story, D.A., et al. "Hyperchloremic Acidosis in the Critically Ill: One of the Strong-Ion Acidosis?" *Anesthesia and Analgesia* 103(1):144-48, July 2006.
Strategies for Managing Multisystem Disorders. Philadelphia: Lippincott Williams & Wilkins, 2006

Disorders affecting management of hyperchloremia

This chart highlights disorders that affect the management of hyperchloremia.

DISORDER	SIGNS AND SYMPTOMS	DIAGNOSTIC TEST RESULTS	TREATMENT AND CARE
Hyperkalemia (complication)	*Mild hyperkalemia* ◆ Diarrhea ◆ Intestinal cramping ◆ Neuromuscular irritability ◆ Restlessness ◆ Tingling lips and fingers *Severe hyperkalemia* ◆ Loss of muscle tone ◆ Muscle weakness ◆ Paralysis	◆ Electrocardiography reveals regular rhythm; rate within normal limits; P wave that has a low amplitude (mild hyperkalemia), that's wide and flattened (moderate hyperkalemia), or indiscernible (severe hyperkalemia); PR interval that's normal or prolonged or not measurable if P wave can't be detected; a widened QRS complex; tall, peaked T wave; shortened QT interval; intraventricular conduction disturbances; and ST-segment elevation (in severe hyperkalemia).	◆ Identify the underlying cause. ◆ Administer I.V. calcium gluconate to decrease neuromuscular irritability, I.V. insulin to facilitate entry of potassium into cells, and I.V. sodium bicarbonate to correct metabolic acidosis. ◆ Administer oral or rectal cation exchange resins (sodium polystyrene sulfonate) that exchange sodium for potassium in the intestine. ◆ Dialysis may be needed with renal failure or severe hyperkalemia. ◆ Monitor serum potassium levels closely. ◆ Identify and manage arrhythmias.
Hypertension (complication)	◆ Headache ◆ Dizziness ◆ Fatigue ◆ Bounding pulse ◆ Pulsating abdominal mass ◆ Elevated blood pressure ◆ Bruits over the abdominal aorta	◆ Urinalysis may show proteinuria, red blood cells or white blood cells or, possibly, glucose. ◆ Serum potassium levels are less than 3.5 mEq/L. ◆ Blood urea nitrogen is normal or elevated to more than 20 mg/dl. ◆ Serum creatinine levels are normal or elevated to more than 1.5 mg/dl.	◆ Monitor blood pressure for stability. ◆ Help the patient identify risk factors and modify his lifestyle. Encourage dietary changes. ◆ Advise the patient to follow medication regimen in order to control blood pressure. ◆ Help the patient identify stress factors and establish effective coping mechanisms. ◆ Administer thiazide diuretics, angiotensin-converting enzyme inhibitors, angiotensin receptor blockers, and calcium channel blockers
Metabolic acidosis (complication)	◆ Headache, lethargy progressing to drowsiness, central nervous system depression, Kussmaul's respirations, hypotension, stupor, and coma ◆ Anorexia, nausea, vomiting, diarrhea and, possibly, dehydration ◆ Warm, flushed skin ◆ Fruity breath odor	◆ Arterial pH is below 7.35. ◆ Partial pressure of arterial carbon dioxide may be normal or less than 34 mm Hg; bicarbonate level may be less than 22 mEq/L. ◆ Serum potassium level is greater than 5.5 mEq/L. ◆ Anion gap is greater than 14 mEq/L.	◆ For severe cases, administer sodium bicarbonate I.V. ◆ Monitor vital signs, laboratory results, pulse oximetry readings, and level of consciousness. ◆ Administer electrolyte supplements and evaluate effects. ◆ Initiate aspiration precautions. ◆ Record intake and output to monitor renal function.

Hyperkalemia

OVERVIEW

- Excessive serum levels of the potassium anion
- Commonly induced by treatments for other disorders
- Affects males and females equally
- Diagnosed in up to 8% of hospitalized patients in the United States

CAUSES

- Adrenal gland insufficiency
- Burns
- Certain drugs (see *Drugs causing hyperkalemia*)
- Crushing injuries
- Decreased urinary excretion of potassium
- Dehydration
- Diabetic acidosis
- Increased intake of potassium
- Large quantities of blood transfusions
- Renal dysfunction or failure
- Severe infection
- Use of potassium-sparing diuretics, such as triamterene, by patients with renal disease

PATHOPHYSIOLOGY

- Slight deviation in serum levels can produce profound clinical consequences.

CARDIOVASCULAR SYSTEM

- Potassium facilitates contraction of both skeletal and smooth muscles, including myocardial contraction.
- Elevated levels of potassium can result in cardiac arrhythmias. (See *Disorders affecting management of hyperkalemia,* pages 217.)

NEUROLOGIC SYSTEM

- Potassium figures prominently in nerve impulse conduction, acid-base balance, enzyme action, and cell membrane function.

MUSCULOSKELETAL SYSTEM

- Potassium imbalance can lead to muscle weakness and flaccid paralysis because of an ionic imbalance in neuromuscular tissue excitability.

ASSESSMENT

HISTORY

- Irritability
- Paresthesia
- Muscle weakness
- Nausea
- Abdominal cramps
- Diarrhea

PHYSICAL FINDINGS

- Hypotension
- Irregular heart rate
- Irregular heart rhythm

DIAGNOSTIC TEST RESULTS

- Serum potassium level is greater than 5 mEq/L.
- Arterial pH is decreased.
- Electrocardiography may show a tall, tented T wave. (See *Clinical effects of hyperkalemia.*)

Drugs causing hyperkalemia

These drugs may increase potassium levels:
- angiotensin-converting enzyme inhibitors
- antibiotics
- beta-adrenergic blockers
- chemotherapeutic drugs
- nonsteroidal anti-inflammatory drugs
- potassium (in excessive amounts)
- spironolactone (Aldactone).

Clinical effects of hyperkalemia

BODY SYSTEM	EFFECTS
Cardiovascular	◆ Tachycardia and later bradycardia, ECG changes (tented and elevated T waves, widened QRS complex, prolonged PR interval, flattened or absent P waves, depressed ST segment), cardiac arrest (with levels > 7 mEq/L)
Gastrointestinal	◆ Nausea, diarrhea, abdominal cramps
Genitourinary	◆ Oliguria, anuria
Musculoskeletal	◆ Muscle weakness, flaccid paralysis
Neurologic	◆ Hyperreflexia progressing to weakness, numbness, tingling, flaccid paralysis
Other	◆ Metabolic acidosis

TREATMENT

GENERAL
- Treatment of the underlying cause
- Hemodialysis or peritoneal dialysis

DIET
- Low-potassium

ACTIVITY
- As tolerated

MEDICATIONS
- Rapid infusion of 10% calcium gluconate (decreases myocardial irritability)
- Insulin and 10% to 50% glucose I.V.
- Sodium polystyrene sulfonate with 70% sorbitol

NURSING CONSIDERATIONS

NURSING DIAGNOSES
- Decreased cardiac output
- Diarrhea
- Risk for injury

EXPECTED OUTCOMES
The patient will:
- maintain adequate cardiac output and hemodynamic stability
- regain normal bowel elimination pattern
- remain free from injury.

NURSING INTERVENTIONS
- Check the serum sample. (See *Avoiding false results.*)
- Give prescribed drugs.
- Insert an indwelling urinary catheter.
- Implement safety measures.
- Be alert for signs of hypokalemia after treatment.
- Monitor serum potassium levels, cardiac rhythm, and intake and output.

Avoiding false results

When your patient's laboratory test result indicates a high potassium level, and the result doesn't make sense, make sure it's a true result. If the sample was drawn using poor technique, the results may be falsely high. These are some of the causes of falsely high potassium levels:
- drawing the sample above an I.V. infusion containing potassium
- using a recently exercised arm or leg for the venipuncture site
- causing hemolysis (cell damage) as the sample is obtained.

(continued)

Be sure to cover:
- disorder, diagnostic testing, and treatment
- medication administration, dosage, and possible adverse effects
- monitoring intake and output
- preventing future episodes of hyperkalemia
- need for potassium-restricted diet.

RESOURCES
Organizations
Mayo Clinic: *www.mayoclinic.com*
The Merck Manuals Online Medical Library: *www.merck.com/mmhe*
National Library of Medicine: *www.nlm.nih.gov*

Selected references
Cheng, C.J., et al. "Perplexing Hyperkalemia," *Nephrology, Dialysis, Transplantation* 21(11):3320-323, November, 2006.

Dursun, I., and Sahin, M. "Difficulties in Maintaining Potassium Homeostasis in Patients with Heart Failure," *Clinical Cardiology* 29(9):388-92, September 2006.

Indermitte, J., et al. "Risk Factors Associated with a High Velocity of the Development of Hyperkalemia in Hospitalised Patients," *Drug Safety* 30(1):71-80, 2007.

Disorders affecting management of hyperkalemia

This chart highlights disorders that affect the management of hyperkalemia.

DISORDER	SIGNS AND SYMPTOMS	DIAGNOSTIC TEST RESULTS	TREATMENT AND CARE
Cardiac arrhythmia (complication)	◆ Palpitations ◆ Chest pain ◆ Dizziness ◆ Weakness, fatigue ◆ Irregular heart rhythm ◆ Hypotension ◆ Syncope ◆ Altered level of consciousness (LOC) ◆ Diaphoresis, pallor, cold, clammy skin	◆ Blood urea nitrogen, serum creatinine, sodium, and potassium levels are elevated. ◆ Arterial blood gas values show decreased arterial pH and bicarbonate levels. ◆ Hematocrit and hemoglobin level are low; red blood cell survival time is decreased. ◆ Aldosterone secretion is increased. ◆ Hyperglycemia and hypertriglyceridemia occur. ◆ Urine reveals proteinuria, glycosuria, red blood cells, leukocytes, casts, and crystals.	◆ Assess airway, breathing, and circulation if life-threatening arrhythmia develops; follow advanced cardiac life support protocols for treatment. ◆ Monitor cardiac rhythm continuously, and obtain serial electrocardiograms (ECGs) to evaluate changes and effects of treatment. ◆ Administer antiarrhythmics and monitor for adverse effects. ◆ Assess cardiovascular system for signs of hypoperfusion; monitor vital signs. ◆ Assist with insertion of temporary pacemaker, or apply transcutaneous pacemaker, if appropriate.
Chronic renal failure (coexisting)	◆ Decreased urine output ◆ Hypotension or hypertension ◆ Altered LOC ◆ Peripheral edema ◆ Cardiac arrhythmias ◆ Bibasilar crackles ◆ Uremic fetor ◆ Poor skin turgor ◆ Pale, yellowish-bronze skin color	◆ Arterial pH is below 7.35. ◆ Partial pressure of arterial carbon dioxide may be normal or less than 34 mm Hg; bicarbonate level may be less than 22 mEq/L. ◆ Serum potassium level is greater than 5.5 mEq/L. ◆ Anion gap is greater than 14 mEq/L.	◆ Give prescribed drugs. ◆ Perform meticulous skin care. ◆ Encourage the patient to express feelings; provide emotional support. ◆ Monitor renal function studies, vital signs, intake and output, and daily weight. ◆ Assess for signs and symptoms of fluid overload.
Metabolic acidosis (complication)	◆ Headache, lethargy progressing to drowsiness, central nervous system depression ◆ Kussmaul's respirations, hypotension, stupor, and coma ◆ Anorexia, nausea, vomiting, diarrhea and, possibly, dehydration ◆ Warm, flushed skin ◆ Fruity breath odor	◆ ECG identifies specific waveform changes associated with the arrhythmia. ◆ Laboratory testing reveals electrolyte abnormalities, hypoxemia, or acid-base abnormalities. ◆ Electrophysiologic testing identifies the mechanism of an arrhythmia and the location of accessory pathways.	◆ For severe cases, administer sodium bicarbonate I.V. ◆ Monitor vital signs, laboratory results, pulse oximetry readings, and LOC. ◆ Administer electrolyte supplements and evaluate effects. ◆ Initiate aspiration precautions. ◆ Record intake and output to monitor renal function.

Hypermagnesemia

- Excessive serum levels of the magnesium cation

CAUSES
- Addison's disease
- Adrenocortical insufficiency
- Chronic renal insufficiency
- Overcorrection of hypomagnesemia
- Overuse of magnesium-containing antacids
- Severe dehydration (resulting oliguria can cause magnesium retention)
- Untreated diabetic ketoacidosis
- Use of laxatives (magnesium sulfate, milk of magnesia, and magnesium citrate solutions), especially with renal insufficiency (see *Drugs and supplements causing hypermagnesemia*)

RISK FACTORS
- Advanced age
- Pregnancy
- Neonate whose mother received magnesium sulfate during labor
- Patient receiving magnesium sulfate to control seizures

PATHOPHYSIOLOGY

- Magnesium enhances neuromuscular integration and stimulates parathyroid hormone secretion, thus regulating intracellular fluid calcium levels.
- Magnesium may also regulate skeletal muscles through its influence on calcium utilization by depressing acetylcholine release at synaptic junctions.
- Magnesium activates many enzymes for proper carbohydrate and protein metabolism, aids in cell metabolism and the transport of sodium and potassium across cell membranes, and influences sodium, potassium, calcium, and protein levels.
- About one-third of magnesium taken into the body is absorbed through the small intestine and is eventually excreted in the urine; remaining unabsorbed magnesium is excreted in the stool.

CARDIOVASCULAR SYSTEM
- Cardiovascular effects of hypermagnesemia are related to its calcium channel blocker effect on the cardiac conduction system and the smooth muscle of blood vessels.
- Bradycardia, atrioventricular block, and asystole may occur. (See *Disorders affecting management of hypermagnesemia*, page 221.)
- Arrhythmias may lead to decreased cardiac output. (See *How hypermagnesemia develops*.)
- A high serum magnesium level may cause vasodilation, which lowers the blood pressure and leads to the patient feeling flushed or warm all over his body.
- Hypotension related to vasodilation occurs early.

RESPIRATORY SYSTEM
- Weakening of the respiratory muscles may lead to slow, shallow, and depressed respirations and may progress to respiratory arrest and the need for mechanical ventilation.

Drugs and supplements causing hypermagnesemia

Monitor your patient's magnesium level closely if he's receiving any of these drugs that can cause hypermagnesemia:
- antacid (Di-Gel, Gaviscon, Maalox)
- laxative (Milk of Magnesia, Haley's M-O, magnesium citrate)
- magnesium supplement (magnesium oxide, magnesium sulfate).

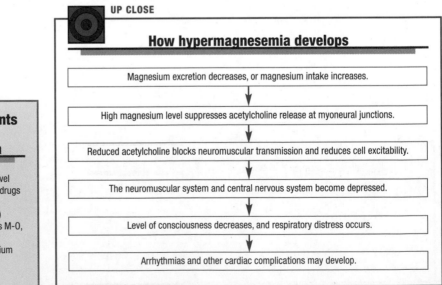

UP CLOSE

How hypermagnesemia develops

Magnesium excretion decreases, or magnesium intake increases.

↓

High magnesium level suppresses acetylcholine release at myoneural junctions.

↓

Reduced acetylcholine blocks neuromuscular transmission and reduces cell excitability.

↓

The neuromuscular system and central nervous system become depressed.

↓

Level of consciousness decreases, and respiratory distress occurs.

↓

Arrhythmias and other cardiac complications may develop.

NEUROMUSCULAR SYSTEM

- Excessive magnesium depresses the central nervous system (CNS). The patient may appear lethargic or drowsy and experience a change in level of consciousness or advance to a coma.
- CNS depression depresses muscle and nerve activities, leading to hypoactive deep tendon reflexes that, without treatment, progress to a loss of the patellar reflex.

HISTORY

- Nausea
- Vomiting
- Drowsiness
- Confusion

PHYSICAL FINDINGS

- Flushed appearance
- Hypotension (see *Clinical effects of hypermagnesemia*)
- Weak pulse
- Muscle weakness
- Hyporeflexia

DIAGNOSTIC TEST RESULTS

- Serum magnesium level is greater than 2.5 mEq/L.
- Electrocardiography may show a prolonged PR interval, widened QRS complex, and tall T waves.

GENERAL

- Identification and correction of the underlying cause
- Peritoneal dialysis or hemodialysis

DIET

- Increased fluid intake

ACTIVITY

- As tolerated

MEDICATIONS

- Loop diuretics, such as furosemide, with impaired renal function
- Calcium gluconate (10%)

Clinical effects of hypermagnesemia

BODY SYSTEM	EFFECTS
Cardiovascular	◆ Bradycardia, weak pulse, hypotension, heart block, cardiac arrest
Neurologic	◆ Drowsiness, flushing, lethargy, confusion, diminished sensorium
Neuromuscular	◆ Diminished reflexes, muscle weakness, flaccid paralysis, respiratory muscle paralysis that may cause respiratory embarrassment

(continued)

NURSING CONSIDERATIONS

NURSING DIAGNOSES
- Anxiety
- Decreased cardiac output
- Impaired gas exchange
- Ineffective tissue perfusion: Renal
- Risk for injury

EXPECTED OUTCOMES
The patient will:
- identify strategies to reduce anxiety
- maintain adequate cardiac output and hemodynamic stability
- maintain adequate ventilation and oxygenation
- exhibit signs of adequate renal perfusion
- remain free from injury.

NURSING INTERVENTIONS
- Provide sufficient fluids for adequate hydration and maintenance of renal function.
- Give prescribed drugs.
- Report abnormal serum electrolyte levels immediately.
- Watch patients receiving a cardiac glycoside and calcium gluconate simultaneously because calcium excess enhances the cardiac glycoside.
- Monitor vital signs, magnesium levels, electrolyte levels, intake and output, and cardiac rhythm.
- Assess neurologic and respiratory status.

PATIENT TEACHING

Be sure to cover:
- disorder, diagnostic testing, and treatment
- avoidance of abusing laxatives and antacids containing magnesium, particularly in elderly patients or those patients with compromised renal function
- hydration requirements
- medication administration, dosage, and possible adverse effects.

RESOURCES
Organizations
The Merck Manuals Online Medical Library: *www.merck.com/mmhe*
National Institute of Diabetes & Digestive & Kidney Diseases: *www.niddk.nih.gov*
National Library of Medicine: *www.nlm.nih.gov*

Selected references
Deshpande, G.G., et al. "Acute Hypermagnesemia in a Child," *American Journal of Health-System Pharmacy* 63(3):262-65, February 2006.
Oneshi, S., and Yoshino, S. "Cathartic-Induced Hypermagnesemia in the Elderly," *Internal Medicine* 45(4):207-10, March 2006.
Strategies for Managing Multisystem Disorders. Philadelphia: Lippincott Williams & Wilkins, 2006.

Disorders affecting management of hypermagnesemia

This chart highlights disorders that affect the management of hypermagnesemia.

DISORDER	SIGNS AND SYMPTOMS	DIAGNOSTIC TEST	TREATMENT AND CARE
Acute respiratory failure (complication)	◆ Tachypnea ◆ Cyanosis ◆ Crackles, rhonchi, wheezing ◆ Diminished breath sounds ◆ Restlessness ◆ Altered mental status ◆ Tachycardia ◆ Increased cardiac output ◆ Increased blood pressure ◆ Cardiac arrhythmias	◆ Arterial blood gas (ABG) values show deteriorating values and a pH below 7.35. ◆ Chest X-ray shows pulmonary disease or condition. ◆ Electrocardiogram (ECG) may show cardiac arrhythmia or right ventricular hypertrophy. ◆ Pulse oximetry shows decreasing arterial oxygen saturation.	◆ Administer oxygen therapy and monitor respiratory status; assist with endotracheal intubation and mechanical ventilation, if necessary. ◆ Assess breath sounds and note changes. ◆ Monitor ABG values and pulse oximetry. ◆ Monitor vital signs and intake and output. ◆ Monitor cardiac rhythm for arrhythmias. ◆ Administer antibiotics, bronchodilators, corticosteroids, positive inotropic agents, diuretics, vasopressors, or antiarrhythmics.
Complete heart block (complication)	◆ Changes in level of consciousness ◆ Changes in mental status ◆ Chest pain ◆ Diaphoresis ◆ Dyspnea ◆ Hypotension ◆ Light-headedness ◆ Pallor ◆ Severe fatigue ◆ Slow peripheral pulse rate	◆ Serum magnesium is 10 mEq/L. ◆ ECG shows ventricular depolarization typically initiated by junctional escape pacemaker (at a rate of 40 to 60 beats/minute); a normal-looking QRS complex, if the block is at the atrioventricular node level; or an intrinsic rate less than 40 beats/minute because of unstable ventricular escape pacemaker located distal to site of block and a wide, bizarre QRS complex.	◆ If the patient has serious signs and symptoms, immediate treatment includes maintaining transcutaneous pacing (most effective) and administering I.V. atropine, dopamine, epinephrine, or a combination of these drugs (for short-term use in emergencies). ◆ If the patient has no symptoms, maintain temporary transvenous pacing until the need for a permanent pacemaker is determined. Make sure patient has a patent I.V. line, administer oxygen, assess for correctable causes of arrhythmia (such as drugs and myocardial ischemia), minimize the patient's activity level, and maintain bed rest.
Hypocalcemia (coexisting)	◆ Anxiety, confusion, irritability ◆ Seizures ◆ Paresthesia of the toes, fingers, or face, especially around the mouth ◆ Twitching ◆ Muscle cramps ◆ Tremors ◆ Laryngospasm ◆ Bronchospasm ◆ Positive Trousseau's or Chvostek's signs ◆ Brittle nails ◆ Dry skin and hair ◆ Diarrhea ◆ Hyperactive deep tendon reflexes ◆ Decreased cardiac output ◆ Cardiac arrhythmias (prolonged ST segment, lengthened QT interval, or decreased myocardial contractility, leading to angina, bradycardia, hypotension, and heart failure)	◆ Total serum calcium level is less than 8.5 mg/dl. ◆ Ionized calcium level is below 4.5 mg/dl. ◆ Albumin level is decreased. ◆ ECG reveals a prolonged ST segment and lengthened QT interval.	◆ Monitor vital signs and respiratory, cardiovascular, and neurologic status. ◆ Watch for stridor, dyspnea, and crowing. ◆ Keep a tracheotomy tray and handheld bag-mask valve at the bedside in case of severe laryngospasm and airway occlusion. ◆ Monitor cardiac rhythm for arrhythmias, especially if the patient is receiving I.V. calcium and digoxin. ◆ Administer calcium replacements, as ordered. ◆ Monitor laboratory results. ◆ Initiate seizure precautions. ◆ Reorient the confused patient, and maintain safety measures.

Hypernatremia

OVERVIEW

- Excessive serum levels of the sodium cation relative to body water
- Occurs in about 1% of hospitalized patients (usually elderly patients)
- Affects males and females equally

CAUSES

- Antidiuretic hormone (ADH) deficiency (diabetes insipidus)
- Certain drugs (see *Drugs causing hypernatremia*)
- Decreased water intake
- Excess adrenocortical hormones, as in Cushing's syndrome
- Excessive I.V. administration of sodium solutions
- Salt intoxication (less common), which may be produced by excessive table salt ingestion

RISK FACTORS

- People who can't drink voluntarily

PATHOPHYSIOLOGY

- Sodium is the major cation (90%) in extracellular fluid, and potassium is the major cation in intracellular fluid.
- During repolarization, the sodium-potassium pump continually shifts sodium into the cells and potassium out of the cells; during depolarization, it does the reverse.
- Sodium cation functions include maintaining tonicity and concentration of extracellular fluid, acid-base balance (reabsorption of sodium ion and excretion of hydrogen ion), nerve conduction and neuromuscular function, glandular secretion, and water balance.
- Increased sodium causes high serum osmolality (increased solute concentrations in the body), which stimulates the hypothalamus to release ADH and initiate the sensation of thirst.

CARDIOVASCULAR SYSTEM

- Fluid shifts out of the cells into the extracellular fluid and results in hypertension and peripheral edema. (See *Disorders affecting management of hypernatremia*, page 225.)

GASTROINTESTINAL SYSTEM

- High serum osmolality due to increased solute concentrations in the blood stimulates the hypothalamus and initiates the thirst mechanism. (See *How hypernatremia develops*.)
- Diarrhea leads to water loss (major cause of hypernatremia in children).

METABOLIC AND ENDOCRINE SYSTEMS

- ADH is secreted by the posterior pituitary gland as the body strives to maintain a normal serum sodium level. ADH causes water to be retained and results in lowering the sodium levels.
- Excessive water loss can occur when the patient experiences fever or heatstroke.

NEUROMUSCULAR SYSTEM

- Fluid shifting from the cells leads to cellular dehydration and significantly affects the central nervous system, leading to agitation, confusion, restlessness, lethargy, stupor, seizures, and—without treatment—coma.

RENAL SYSTEM

- Urine specific gravity increases with hypernatremia as the kidneys attempt to conserve water that's lost through the GI tract, skin, or lungs. If

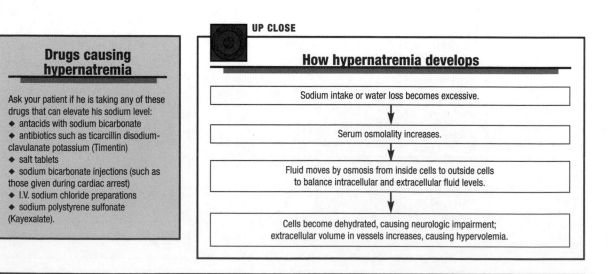

Drugs causing hypernatremia

Ask your patient if he is taking any of these drugs that can elevate his sodium level:
- antacids with sodium bicarbonate
- antibiotics such as ticarcillin disodium-clavulanate potassium (Timentin)
- salt tablets
- sodium bicarbonate injections (such as those given during cardiac arrest)
- I.V. sodium chloride preparations
- sodium polystyrene sulfonate (Kayexalate).

UP CLOSE

How hypernatremia develops

Sodium intake or water loss becomes excessive.

↓

Serum osmolality increases.

↓

Fluid moves by osmosis from inside cells to outside cells to balance intracellular and extracellular fluid levels.

↓

Cells become dehydrated, causing neurologic impairment; extracellular volume in vessels increases, causing hypervolemia.

the physiological defect involves water loss from the kidneys, the urine specific gravity is very low.
◆ Renal impairment may lead to oliguria.

RESPIRATORY SYSTEM
◆ Dyspnea, respiratory arrest, and death may result from a dramatic rise in osmotic pressure.

HISTORY
◆ Fatigue
◆ Restlessness, agitation
◆ Weakness
◆ Disorientation
◆ Lethargy

PHYSICAL FINDINGS
◆ Flushed skin (see *Clinical effects of hypernatremia*)
◆ Dry, swollen tongue
◆ Sticky mucous membranes
◆ Low-grade fever
◆ Twitching
◆ Hypertension, dyspnea (with hypervolemia)
◆ Orthostatic hypotension and oliguria (with hypovolemia)

DIAGNOSTIC TEST RESULTS
◆ Serum sodium level is greater than 145 mEq/L.
◆ Urine sodium level is less than 40 mEq/24 hours, with high serum osmolality.

GENERAL
◆ Treatment of underlying cause
◆ Administration of salt-free solutions (such as dextrose in water) followed by infusion of half-normal saline solution to prevent hyponatremia
◆ Discontinuation of drugs that promote sodium retention

DIET
◆ Sodium restriction
◆ Oral hypotonic fluids

ACTIVITY
◆ As tolerated

MEDICATIONS
◆ Isotonic serum chloride solution
◆ Diuretics
◆ ADH replacement therapy

Clinical effects of hypernatremia

BODY SYSTEM	EFFECTS
Cardiovascular	◆ Hypertension, tachycardia, pitting edema, excessive weight gain
Gastrointestinal	◆ Rough, dry tongue; intense thirst
Genitourinary	◆ Oliguria
Integumentary	◆ Flushed skin; dry, sticky membranes
Neurologic	◆ Fever, agitation, restlessness, seizures
Respiratory	◆ Dyspnea, respiratory arrest, death (from dramatic rise in osmotic pressure)

(continued)

NURSING CONSIDERATIONS

NURSING DIAGNOSES
- Anxiety
- Deficient fluid volume
- Fear
- Ineffective tissue perfusion: Cardiopulmonary
- Risk for injury

EXPECTED OUTCOMES
The patient will:
- identify strategies to reduce anxiety
- maintain adequate fluid volume
- discuss fears and concerns
- exhibit signs of adequate cardiopulmonary perfusion
- remain free from injury.

NURSING INTERVENTIONS
- Obtain a drug history to check for drugs that promote sodium retention.
- Assist with oral hygiene.
- Observe for signs of cerebral edema during fluid replacement therapy.
- Monitor serum sodium levels, intake and output, and neurologic status.

PATIENT TEACHING

Be sure to cover:
- disorder, diagnostic testing, and treatment
- importance of sodium restriction and low-sodium diet
- medication administration, dosage, and possible adverse effects
- signs and symptoms of hypernatremia
- avoiding over-the-counter medications that contain sodium.

RESOURCES
Organizations
The Merck Manuals Online Medical Library: *www.merck.com/mmhe*
National Institute of Diabetes & Digestive & Kidney Diseases: *www.niddk.nih.gov*

Selected references

Machino, T., and Yoshizawa, T. "Brain Shrinkage Due to Acute Hypernatremia," *Neurology* 67(5): 880, September 2006.

Sedlacek, M., et al. "Electrolyte Disturbance in the Intensive Care Unit," *Seminars in Dialysis* 19(6):496-501, November-December 2006.

Strategies for Managing Multisystem Disorders. Philadelphia: Lippincott Williams & Wilkins, 2006.

Sze, L., et al. "Severe Hypernatremia Due to Nephrogenic Diabetes Insipidus—A Life-Threatening Side Effect of Chronic Lithium Therapy," *Experimental and Clinical Endocrinology and Diabetes* 114(10):596-98, November, 2006.

Disorders affecting management of hypernatremia

This chart highlights disorders that affect the management of hypernatremia.

DISORDER	SIGNS AND SYMPTOMS	DIAGNOSTIC TEST RESULTS	TREATMENT AND CARE
Acute respiratory failure (complication)	◆ Tachypnea ◆ Cyanosis ◆ Crackles, rhonchi, wheezing ◆ Diminished breath sounds ◆ Restlessness ◆ Altered mental status ◆ Tachycardia ◆ Increased cardiac output ◆ Increased blood pressure ◆ Cardiac arrhythmias	◆ Arterial blood gas (ABG) values show deteriorating values and a pH below 7.35. ◆ Chest X-ray shows pulmonary disease or condition. ◆ Electrocardiogram may show cardiac arrhythmia or right ventricular hypertrophy. ◆ Pulse oximetry shows decreasing arterial oxygen saturation.	◆ Administer oxygen therapy and monitor respiratory status; assist with endotracheal intubation and mechanical ventilation, if necessary. ◆ Assess breath sounds and note changes. ◆ Monitor ABG values and pulse oximetry. ◆ Monitor vital signs and intake and output. ◆ Monitor cardiac rhythm for arrhythmias. ◆ Administer antibiotics, bronchodilators, corticosteroids, positive inotropic agents, diuretics, vasopressors, or antiarrhythmics.
Dehydration (complication)	◆ Tachycardia ◆ Dry mucous membranes ◆ Poor skin turgor ◆ Decreased blood pressure ◆ Decreased urine output ◆ Lethargy ◆ Delayed capillary refill	◆ Urine specific gravity is elevated. ◆ Blood urea nitrogen (BUN) and creatinine are elevated. ◆ Complete blood count reveals elevated hematocrit.	◆ Encourage small amounts of oral fluids. ◆ Administer I.V. fluids. ◆ Administer electrolyte solutions, oral or I.V., to correct imbalances. ◆ Monitor vital signs, including central and peripheral pulses and capillary refill, approximately every 15 minutes. ◆ Monitor neurologic status for increasing lethargy or seizures.
Hypertension (complication)	◆ Headache ◆ Dizziness ◆ Fatigue ◆ Bounding pulse ◆ Pulsating abdominal mass ◆ Elevated blood pressure ◆ Bruits over the abdominal aorta	◆ Urinalysis may show proteinuria, red blood cells or white blood cells or, possibly, glucose. ◆ Serum potassium levels are less than 3.5 mEq/L. ◆ BUN is normal or elevated to more than 20 mg/dl. ◆ Serum creatinine levels are normal or elevated to more than 1.5 mg/dl.	◆ Monitor blood pressure for stability. ◆ Help the patient identify risk factors and modify his lifestyle ◆ Encourage dietary changes. ◆ Advise the patient to follow his medication regimen to control blood pressure. ◆ Help the patient identify stress factors and establish effective coping mechanisms.

Hyperparathyroidism

OVERVIEW

- Characterized by a greater than normal secretion of parathyroid hormone (PTH)
- Classified as either primary or secondary
- More common in females than in males
- Incidence higher in postmenopausal females
- Onset usually between ages 35 and 65

CAUSES

- Adenoma
- Chronic renal failure
- Decreased intestinal absorption of vitamin D or calcium
- Dietary vitamin D or calcium deficiency
- Genetic disorders
- Idiopathic
- Ingestion of drugs such as phenytoin
- Laxative ingestion
- Multiple endocrine neoplasia
- Osteomalacia

PATHOPHYSIOLOGY

- Overproduction of PTH by a tumor or hyperplastic tissue increases intestinal calcium absorption, reduces renal calcium clearance, and increases bone calcium release. Response to this excess varies with each patient for unknown reasons.
- Hypophosphatemia results when excessive PTH inhibits renal tubular phosphate reabsorption. The hypophosphatemia aggravates hypercalcemia by increasing the sensitivity of the bone to PTH.

CARDIOVASCULAR SYSTEM

- Cardiac arrhythmias, vascular damage, hypertension, and heart failure can occur because of increased levels of calcium.

ENDOCRINE SYSTEM

- Calcium microthrombi can travel to the pancreas causing pancreatitis.

MUSCULOSKELETAL SYSTEM

- Untreated hyperparathyroidism damages the skeleton and kidneys from hypercalcemia.
- Bone and articular problems, such as chondrocalcinosis, osteoporosis, subperiosteal resorption, occasional severe osteopenia, erosions of the juxta-articular surface, subchondral fractures, traumatic synovitis, and pseudogout, may occur. (See *Disorders affecting management of hyperparathyroidism*, pages 228 and 229.)

NEUROLOGIC SYSTEM

- Central nervous system changes can result from parathyroid poisoning and may progress to coma.

RENAL SYSTEM

- Renal complications that result from hypercalcemia include nephrolithiasis; hypercalciuria; and renal calculi, colic, and insufficiency.
- Renal failure can occur as a result of parathyroid poisoning and elevated calcium levels.

RESPIRATORY SYSTEM

- Calcium microthrombi can travel to the lungs causing pulmonary emboli and respiratory distress.

ASSESSMENT

HISTORY

- Recurring nephrolithiasis
- Polyuria
- Hematuria
- Chronic lower back pain
- Fractures
- Osteoporosis
- Constant, severe epigastric pain that radiates to the back
- Abdominal pain
- Anorexia, nausea, and vomiting
- Constipation
- Polydipsia
- Muscle weakness, particularly in the legs
- Lethargy
- Personality disturbances
- Depression
- Overt psychosis
- Cataracts
- Anemia

PHYSICAL FINDINGS

- Muscle weakness and atrophy
- Psychomotor disturbances
- Stupor and, possibly, coma
- Skin necrosis
- Subcutaneous calcification

DIAGNOSTIC TEST RESULTS

In primary disease

- Alkaline phosphatase level is increased.
- Osteocalcin level is increased.
- Tartrate-resistant acid phosphatase levels are increased.
- Serum PTH level is increased.
- Serum calcium level is increased.
- Serum phosphorus level is decreased.
- Urine and serum calcium and serum chloride levels are increased.
- Creatinine level may be increased.
- Basal acid secretion may be increased.
- Serum amylase level may be increased.
- X-rays show diffuse bone demineralization, bone cysts, outer cortical bone absorption, and subperiosteal erosion of the phalanges and distal clavicles.
- X-ray spectrophotometry shows increased bone turnover.
- Esophagography, thyroid scan, parathyroid thermography, ultrasonography, thyroid angiography, computed tomography scan, and magnetic resonance imaging may show location of parathyroid lesions.

In secondary disease

- Serum calcium level is normal or slightly decreased.
- Serum phosphorus level is variable.
- Serum PTH level is increased.

TREATMENT

GENERAL
- With primary disease, treatment to decrease calcium levels
- With renal failure, dialysis
- With secondary disease, treatment to correct underlying cause of parathyroid hypertrophy

DIET
- Increased oral fluid intake

ACTIVITY
- As tolerated

MEDICATIONS
Primary disease
- Bisphosphonates
- Oral sodium or potassium phosphate
- Calcitonin (Miacalcin)
- Plicamycin (Mithracin), if primary disease is metastatic

Secondary disease
- Vitamin D therapy
- Aluminum hydroxide
- Glucocorticoids

Postoperatively
- I.V. magnesium and phosphate
- Sodium phosphate
- Supplemental calcium
- Vitamin D or calcitriol (Calcijex)

SURGERY
- With primary hyperparathyroidism, removal of adenoma or all but one-half of one gland

NURSING CONSIDERATIONS

NURSING DIAGNOSES
- Activity intolerance
- Acute pain
- Anxiety
- Decreased cardiac output
- Disturbed body image
- Excess fluid volume
- Fear
- Imbalanced nutrition: Less than body requirements
- Ineffective coping

EXPECTED OUTCOMES
The patient will:
- perform activities of daily living without excessive fatigue
- express feelings of increased comfort and decreased pain
- verbalize strategies to reduce anxiety
- maintain adequate cardiac output
- express positive feelings about self
- maintain normal fluid volume
- express fears and concerns
- maintain adequate nutrition and hydration
- demonstrate adaptive coping behaviors.

NURSING INTERVENTIONS
- Obtain baseline serum potassium, calcium, phosphate, and magnesium levels before treatment.
- Monitor vital signs, intake and output, and serum calcium levels.
- Monitor respiratory and cardiovascular status.
- Provide at least 3 qt (3 L) of fluid per day.
- Institute safety precautions.
- Schedule frequent rest periods.
- Provide comfort measures.
- Give prescribed drugs.
- Help the patient turn and reposition every 2 hours.
- Support affected extremities with pillows.
- Offer emotional support.
- Help the patient develop effective coping strategies.

After parathyroidectomy
- Keep a tracheotomy tray at the bedside.
- Maintain seizure precautions.
- Place the patient in semi-Fowler's position.
- Support the patient's head and neck with sandbags.
- Have the patient ambulate as soon as possible.
- Monitor for increased neuromuscular irritability.
- **WARNING** *Watch for complaints of tingling in the hands and around the mouth. If these symptoms occur but don't subside quickly, they may be prodromal signs of tetany and may require emergency administra-tion of I.V. calcium gluconate or calcium chloride.*
- Monitor for neck edema and Chvostek's and Trousseau's signs.
- Observe for complications.

PATIENT TEACHING

Be sure to cover:
- disorder, diagnostic testing, and treatment
- medication administration, dosage, and possible adverse effects
- when to notify the practitioner
- signs and symptoms of tetany, respiratory distress, and renal dysfunction
- need for periodic blood tests
- avoidance of calcium-containing antacids and thiazide diuretics
- need to wear medical identification jewelry.

RESOURCES
Organizations
American Association of Clinical Endocrinologists: *www.aace.com*
Endocrine Society: *www.endo-society.org*

Selected references
Donovan, P.I. "Outpatient Parathyroidectomy: A New Paradigm from a Nursing Perspective," *Current Opinion in Oncology* 17(1):28-32, January 2005.
Peregrin, T. "Early Assessment of Secondary Hyperparathyroidism," *Journal of the American Dietetic Association* 106(1):22-23, January 2006.
Strategies for Managing Multisystem Disorders. Philadelphia: Lippincott Williams & Wilkins, 2006.
Zanocco, K., et al. "Cost-Effectiveness Analysis of Parathyroidectomy for Asymptomatic Primary Hyperparathyroidism," *Surgery* 140(6):874-81, December 2006.

(continued)

Disorders affecting management of hyperparathyroidism

This chart highlights disorders that affect the management of hyperparathyroidism.

DISORDER	SIGNS AND SYMPTOMS	DIAGNOSTIC TEST RESULTS	TREATMENT AND CARE
Pancreatitis (complication)	◆ Midepigastric abdominal pain, which can radiate to the back ◆ Mottled skin ◆ Tachycardia ◆ Low-grade fever ◆ Cold, sweaty extremities ◆ Restlessness ◆ Extreme malaise (in chronic pancreatitis)	◆ Serum amylase levels are dramatically elevated—in many cases over 500 units/L. ◆ Urine and pleural fluid analysis amylase are dramatically elevated in ascites. ◆ Serum lipase levels are increased. ◆ Serum calcium levels are decreased (hypocalcemia). ◆ White blood cell counts range from 8,000 to 20,000/µl, with increased polymorphonuclear leukocytes. ◆ Glucose levels are elevated—as high as 500 to 900 mg/dl. ◆ Abdominal X-rays or computed tomography (CT) scans show dilation of the small or large bowel or calcification of the pancreas. ◆ An ultrasound or CT scan reveals an increased pancreatic diameter and helps distinguish acute cholecystitis from acute pancreatitis.	◆ Monitor the patient's vital signs and pulmonary artery pressure or central venous pressure closely. Give plasma or albumin to maintain blood pressure. Record fluid intake and output, check urine output hourly, and monitor electrolyte levels. Assess for crackles, rhonchi, or decreased breath sounds. ◆ For bowel decompression, maintain constant nasogastric suctioning, and give nothing by mouth. ◆ Watch for signs and symptoms of calcium deficiency (tetany, cramps, carpopedal spasm, and seizures). If you suspect hypocalcemia, keep airway and suction apparatus handy, and pad side rails. ◆ Administer analgesics to relieve the patient's pain and anxiety. Remember that anticholinergics reduce salivary and sweat gland secretions. Warn the patient that he may experience dry mouth and facial flushing. *Caution:* Narrow-angle glaucoma contraindicates the use of atropine or its derivatives. ◆ Monitor glucose levels. ◆ Watch for complications of total parenteral nutrition, such as sepsis, hypokalemia, overhydration, and metabolic acidosis. Watch for fever, cardiac irregularities, changes in arterial blood gas measurements, and deep respirations. Use strict aseptic technique when caring for the catheter insertion site.
Pseudogout (complication)	◆ Pain in the great toe ◆ Swollen, red or purple joint with limited movement ◆ Tophi, especially in the outer ears, hands, and feet ◆ Warmth over the joint and extreme tenderness ◆ Fever ◆ Hypertension	◆ Joint aspiration and synovial biopsy detect calcium pyrophosphate crystals. ◆ X-rays show calcium deposits in the fibrocartilage and linear markings along the bone ends. ◆ Blood tests may detect an underlying endocrine or metabolic disorder.	◆ Urge the patient to perform as much self-care as his immobility and pain allow. ◆ Encourage bed rest, but use a bed cradle to keep bed linens off sensitive, inflamed joints. ◆ Carefully evaluate the patient's condition after joint aspiration. ◆ Give pain medication (especially during acute attacks), and monitor the patient's response. ◆ Apply cold packs to inflamed joints to ease discomfort and reduce swelling. ◆ To promote sleep, administer pain medication. ◆ Help the patient identify techniques and activities that promote rest and relaxation. ◆ Administer anti-inflammatory medication and other drugs, and watch for adverse reactions. Be alert for GI disturbances in the patient taking colchicine. ◆ When encouraging fluids, record intake and output accurately. Be sure to monitor serum uric acid levels regularly. Administer sodium bicarbonate or other agents to alkalinize the patient's urine. ◆ Provide a nutritious, but low-purine diet. ◆ Watch for acute gout attacks 24 to 96 hours after surgery. Administering colchicine before and after surgery may help prevent gout attacks.

DISORDER	SIGNS AND SYMPTOMS	DIAGNOSTIC TEST RESULTS	TREATMENT AND CARE
Renal calculi (complication)	◆ Severe pain that travels from the costovertebral angle to the flank and then to the suprapubic region and external genitalia ◆ Nausea ◆ Vomiting ◆ Fever ◆ Chills ◆ Hematuria ◆ Abdominal distention	◆ Kidney-ureter-bladder (KUB) radiography reveals renal calculi. ◆ Excretory urography determines the size and location of calculi. ◆ Kidney ultrasonography detects obstructive changes, such as unilateral or bilateral hydronephrosis and radiolucent calculi not seen on the KUB radiography. ◆ Urine culture of a midstream specimen may indicate pyuria. ◆ A 24-hour urine collection may detect the presence of calcium oxalate, phosphorus, and uric acid excretion. Three separate collections, along with blood samples, are needed for accurate testing. ◆ Calculus analysis shows mineral content. ◆ Serum blood calcium and phosphorus levels show an increased calcium level in proportion to normal serum protein levels. ◆ Blood protein levels determine the level of free calcium unbound to protein.	◆ Maintain a 24- to 48-hour record of urine pH using nitrazine pH paper. Strain urine and save solid material for analysis. ◆ To facilitate spontaneous passage of calculi, encourage patient mobility and fluids. ◆ If the patient can't drink the required amount of fluid, give supplemental I.V. fluids. ◆ Record intake and output and daily weight to assess fluid status and renal function. ◆ Medicate the patient for pain when he's passing a calculus. ◆ To help acidify urine, offer fruit juices, especially cranberry juice, anticipate that the patient will have an indwelling catheter or a nephrostomy tube. ◆ Watch for signs of infection, such as a rising fever or chills, and give antibiotics, as needed. ◆ If lithotripsy is planned, expect to discontinue anticoagulants, aspirin, vitamin E, and platelet inhibitors for 3 days before the procedure.

Hyperphosphatemia

- Excessive serum levels of phosphate
- Reflects the kidney's inability to excrete excess phosphorus
- Occurs most commonly in children, who tend to consume more phosphorus-rich foods and beverages than adults
- Incidence higher in children and adults with renal insufficiency

CAUSES

- Acid-base imbalance
- Certain drugs (see *Drugs and supplements causing hyperphosphatemia*)
- Hypervitaminosis D
- Hypocalcemia
- Hypoparathyroidism
- Overuse of laxatives with phosphates or phosphate enemas
- Renal failure

RISK FACTORS

- Muscle necrosis
- Infection
- Heat stroke
- Trauma
- Chemotherapy

Drugs and supplements causing hyperphosphatemia

These drugs may cause hyperphosphatemia:
- enemas such as Fleet enemas
- laxatives containing phosphorus or phosphate
- oral phosphorus supplements
- parenteral phosphorus supplements (sodium phosphate, potassium phosphate)
- vitamin D supplements.

- Phosphorus exists in combination with calcium in teeth and bones.
- In extracellular fluid, the phosphate ion supports many metabolic functions: B vitamin use, acid-base homeostasis, bone formation, nerve and muscle activity, cell division, transmission of hereditary traits, and metabolism of carbohydrates, proteins, and fats.
- Renal tubular reabsorption of phosphate is inversely regulated by calcium levels—an increase in phosphorus causes a decrease in calcium. An imbalance causes hypophosphatemia or hyperphosphatemia.
- The pathophysiologic processes involved in hyperphosphatemia can vary depending on the cause of the condition. (See *Disorders affecting management of hyperphosphatemia*, pages 232 and 233.)

CARDIOVASCULAR SYSTEM

- Arrhythmias, palpitations, and an irregular heart rate may be related to hypocalcemia of calcium-phosphate calcification.

ENDOCRINE AND METABOLIC SYSTEMS

- Hyperphosphatemia in renal failure results in acidosis; because acidosis favors increased calcium ionization, patients are less prone to develop hypocalcemia.

INTEGUMENTARY SYSTEM

- Calcium-phosphate calcification can lead to soft-tissue calcification causing dry, itchy skin with papular eruptions.
- Calcification of ocular vessels can lead to conjunctivitis and corneal haziness that progresses to impaired vision.

NEUROMUSCULAR SYSTEM

- Associated hypocalcemia can lead to signs of tetany such as tingling of the tips of the fingers and around the mouth. These sensations may increase in severity and spread along the limbs and to the face, resulting in numbness, muscle spasms, and pain.
- Hyperreflexia, mental status changes, muscle weakness, or seizures may develop because of hypocalcemia.

RENAL SYSTEM

- Oliguria related to acute or chronic renal failure may develop.
- Precipitation of calcium phosphate can lead to progressive renal impairment.

RESPIRATORY SYSTEM

- The patient may experience respiratory compromise related to lung tissue calcification.
- Hyperphosphatemia commonly leads to respiratory acidosis.

ASSESSMENT

HISTORY
- Anorexia
- Decreased mental status
- Nausea and vomiting
- Excessive use of antacids or oral phosphate binders
- Use of laxatives or enemas

PHYSICAL FINDINGS
- Hyperreflexia
- Hypocalcemic electrocardiogram changes
- Muscle weakness and cramps
- Papular eruptions
- Paresthesia
- Presence of Chvostek's or Trousseau's sign
- Abdominal spasm
- Tetany
- Visual impairment
- Conjunctivitis

DIAGNOSTIC TEST RESULTS
- Serum phosphorus level is greater than 4.5 mg/dl.
- Serum calcium level is less than 8.9 mg/dl.
- Blood urea nitrogen and creatinine levels are increased.
- X-ray studies reveal skeletal changes caused by osteodystrophy in chronic hyperphosphatemia.
- Electrocardiography may show changes characteristic of hypercalcemia.

TREATMENT

GENERAL
- Treatment of the underlying cause
- Peritoneal dialysis or hemodialysis (if severe)
- Discontinuation of drugs associated with hyperphosphatemia
- I.V. saline solution

DIET
- Low in phosphorus

ACTIVITY
- As tolerated

MEDICATIONS
- Diuretic carbonic anhydrase inhibitor
- Calcium salts
- Phosphate-binding antacids

NURSING CONSIDERATIONS

NURSING DIAGNOSES
- Acute pain
- Anxiety
- Risk for injury

EXPECTED OUTCOMES
The patient will:
- express feelings of increased comfort and decreased pain
- express feelings of decreased anxiety
- remain free from injury.

NURSING INTERVENTIONS
- Provide safety measures.
- Be alert for signs of hypocalcemia.
- Give prescribed drugs.
- Give antacids with meals to increase their effectiveness.
- Prepare the patient for dialysis, if appropriate.
- Assist with selecting a low-phosphorus diet.
- Monitor vital signs, phosphorus and calcium levels, intake and output, and renal studies.

Foods high in phosphorus

These foods are high in phosphorus:
- beans
- bran
- chocolate
- dark-colored sodas
- fish and seafood
- ice cream
- lentils
- meat
- milk, cheese, yogurt
- nuts
- peanut butter
- poultry
- seeds
- whole grains.

PATIENT TEACHING

Be sure to cover:
- disorder, diagnostic testing, and treatment
- medication administration, dosage, and possible adverse effects
- need to avoid preparations that contain phosphorus
- need to avoid high-phosphorus foods. (See *Foods high in phosphorus*.)

RESOURCES
Organizations
American Association of Kidney Patients: *www.aakp.org*
National Institute of Diabetes & Digestive & Kidney Diseases: *www.niddk.nih.gov*

Selected references
Achinger, S., and Avus, J. "Left Ventricular Hypertrophy: Is Hyperphosphatemia Among Dialysis Patients a Risk Factor?" *Journal of the American Society of Nephrology* 17(12suppl3):S255-61, December 2006.
Kuhlmann, M.K. "Practical Approaches to Management of Hyperphosphatemia; Can We Improve the Current Situation?," *Blood Purification* 25(1):120-24, January 2007.
Schucker, J.J., and Ward, K.E. "Hyperphosphatemia and Phosphate Binders," *American Journal of Health-System Pharmacy* 62(22):2355-361, November 2005.
Strategies for Managing Multisystem Disorders. Philadelphia: Lippincott Williams & Wilkins, 2006.

(continued)

Disorders affecting management of hyperphosphatemia

This chart highlights disorders that affect the management of hyperphosphatemia.

DISORDER	SIGNS AND SYMPTOMS	DIAGNOSTIC TEST RESULTS	TREATMENT AND CARE
Heart failure (complication)	◆ Cough that produces pink, frothy sputum ◆ Cyanosis of the lips and nail beds ◆ Pale, cool, clammy skin ◆ Diaphoresis ◆ Jugular vein distention ◆ Ascites ◆ Pulsus alternans ◆ Tachycardia ◆ Hepatomegaly ◆ Decreased pulse pressure ◆ Third and fourth heart sounds (S_3 and S_4) ◆ Moist, basilar crackles ◆ Rhonchi ◆ Expiratory wheezing ◆ Decreased pulse oximetry ◆ Peripheral edema ◆ Decreased urinary output	◆ B-type natriuretic peptide immunoassay is elevated. ◆ Chest X-ray shows increased pulmonary vascular markings, interstitial edema, or pleural effusions and cardiomegaly. ◆ Electrocardiography (ECG) reveals heart enlargement or ischemia, tachycardia, extrasystole, or atrial fibrillation. ◆ Pulmonary artery pressure, pulmonary artery wedge pressure, and left ventricular end-diastolic pressure are elevated in the presence of left-sided heart failure; right atrial or central venous pressure is elevated in right-sided heart failure.	◆ Administer supplemental oxygen and mechanical ventilation, if needed. ◆ Place the patient in Fowler's position. ◆ Administer diuretics, inotropic drugs, vasodilators, angiotensin-converting enzyme inhibitors, angiotensin receptor blockers, cardiac glycosides, beta-adrenergic blockers, and electrolyte supplements. ◆ Initiate cardiac monitoring. ◆ Recurrent heart failure from valvular dysfunction may require surgery. ◆ A ventricular assist device may be needed. ◆ Maintain adequate cardiac output, and monitor hemodynamic stability. ◆ Assess for deep vein thrombosis, and apply antiembolism stockings.
Hypocalcemia (complication)	◆ Anxiety, confusion, irritability ◆ Seizures ◆ Paresthesia of the toes, fingers, or face, especially around the mouth ◆ Twitching ◆ Muscle cramps ◆ Tremors ◆ Laryngospasm ◆ Bronchospasm ◆ Positive Trousseau's or Chvostek's signs ◆ Brittle nails ◆ Dry skin and hair ◆ Diarrhea ◆ Hyperactive deep tendon reflexes ◆ Decreased cardiac output ◆ Arrhythmias (prolonged ST segment, lengthened QT interval [risk of torsades de pointes] or decreased myocardial contractility, leading to angina, bradycardia, hypotension, and heart failure)	◆ Total serum calcium level is less than 8.5 mg/dl. ◆ Ionized calcium level is below 4.5 mg/dl. ◆ Albumin level is low. ◆ ECG reveals a prolonged ST segment and lengthened QT interval.	◆ Monitor vital signs and assess the patient frequently. ◆ Monitor respiratory status, including rate, depth, and rhythm. ◆ Watch for stridor, dyspnea, and crowing. ◆ If the patient shows overt signs of hypocalcemia, keep a tracheotomy tray and a handheld resuscitation bag at the bedside in case laryngospasm occurs. ◆ Place your patient on a cardiac monitor, and evaluate him for changes in heart rate and rhythm, such as ventricular tachycardia or heart block. ◆ Check the patient for Chvostek's sign or Trousseau's sign. ◆ Monitor the patient receiving I.V. calcium for arrhythmias, especially if he's also taking digoxin. Calcium and digoxin have similar effects on the heart. ◆ Administer I.V. calcium replacement therapy carefully. Ensure the patency of the I.V. line because infiltration can cause tissue necrosis and sloughing. ◆ Administer oral replacements. Give calcium supplements 1 to 1½ hours after meals. If GI upset occurs, give the supplement with milk. ◆ Monitor pertinent laboratory test results, including calcium levels, albumin levels, and other electrolyte levels. Check the ionized calcium level after every 4 units of blood transfused. ◆ Encourage the older patient to take a calcium supplement and to exercise as much as he can tolerate to prevent calcium loss from bones. ◆ Initiate seizure precautions such as padding bedside rails. ◆ Reorient the confused patient. Provide a calm, quiet environment.

Disorders affecting management of hyperphosphatemia *(continued)*

DISORDER	SIGNS AND SYMPTOMS	DIAGNOSTIC TEST RESULTS	TREATMENT AND CARE
Respiratory acidosis (complication)	◆ Apprehension ◆ Confusion ◆ Decreased deep tendon reflexes ◆ Diaphoresis ◆ Dyspnea with rapid, shallow respirations ◆ Headache ◆ Nausea or vomiting ◆ Restlessness ◆ Tachycardia ◆ Tremors ◆ Warm, flushed skin	◆ Arterial blood gas (ABG) analysis reveals pH below 7.35 and partial pressure of arterial carbon dioxide above 45 mm Hg. ◆ HCO_3^- level varies depending on how long the acidosis has been present. In the patient with acute respiratory acidosis, HCO_3^- level may be normal; in the patient with chronic respiratory acidosis, it may be above 26 mEq/L. ◆ Serum electrolyte levels reveal a potassium level greater than 5 mEq/L.	◆ Maintain a patent airway. Provide adequate humidification to ensure moist secretions. ◆ Monitor vital signs and assess cardiac rhythm as respiratory acidosis can cause tachycardia, alterations in respiratory rate and rhythm, hypotension, and arrhythmias. ◆ Continue to assess respiratory patterns. Immediately report changes. Prepare for mechanical ventilation, if indicated. ◆ Monitor the patient's neurologic status, and report significant changes. ◆ Monitor the patient's cardiac function because respiratory acidosis may progress to shock and cardiac arrest. ◆ Report variations in ABG values, pulse oximetry, or serum electrolyte levels. ◆ Administer antibiotics or bronchodilators. ◆ Administer oxygen. Generally, lower concentrations of oxygen are given to patients with chronic obstructive pulmonary disease because the medulla of these patients is accustomed to high carbon dioxide levels. ◆ Perform tracheal suctioning, incentive spirometry, postural drainage, and coughing and deep breathing, as indicated. ◆ Make sure the patient takes in enough oral and I.V fluids, and maintain accurate intake and output records. ◆ Provide reassurance to the patient and family. ◆ Keep in mind that sedatives can decrease his respiratory rate. ◆ Institute safety measures, as needed, to protect a confused patient.

Hyperpituitarism

- Chronic, progressive disease marked by hormonal dysfunction and startling skeletal overgrowth
- Prognosis dependent on cause
- Life expectancy usually reduced
- Appears in two forms:
- Acromegaly: occurs equally in males and females and usually occurs between ages 30 and 50
- Gigantism: affects infants and children
- Also referred to as *growth hormone (GH) excess*

CAUSES

- Excessive GH-releasing hormone
- Excessive GH secretion
- GH-producing adenoma of the anterior pituitary gland
- Possible genetic cause

PATHOPHYSIOLOGY

- Progressive excessive secretion of pituitary GH occurs.
- Acromegaly occurs after epiphyseal closure, causing bone thickening and transverse growth and visceromegaly.
- Gigantism occurs before epiphyseal closure with excess GH, causing proportional overgrowth of all body tissues.
- A large tumor may cause loss of other trophic hormones, such as thyroid-stimulating hormone, luteinizing hormone, follicle-stimulating hormone, and corticotropin, which may cause dysfunction of target organs. (See *Disorders affecting management of hyperpituitarism,* pages 236 and 237.)

CARDIOVASCULAR SYSTEM

- Excess GH causes enlargement of internal organs, which can result in cardiovascular disease, arteriosclerosis, hypertension, left-sided heart failure, and acromegalic cardiomyopathy with arrhythmias.

ENDOCRINE SYSTEM

- Gigantism and acromegaly can cause signs of glucose intolerance and clinically apparent diabetes mellitus because of the insulin-antagonistic character of GH.

MUSCULOSKELETAL SYSTEM

- Excessive GH secretion may lead to arthritis, carpal tunnel syndrome, osteoporosis, and kyphosis.
- In acromegaly, the excess GH increases bone density and width and the proliferation of connective and soft tissues.
- In pituitary gigantism—because the epiphyseal plates aren't closed—the excess GH stimulates linear growth.

NEUROLOGIC SYSTEM

- Acromegaly may result in blindness and severe neurologic disturbances due to compression of surrounding tissues by the tumor.
- Bilateral temporal hemianopsia is common because of optic chiasm compression.

HISTORY

- Gradual onset of acromegaly
- Relatively abrupt onset of gigantism
- Soft-tissue swelling
- Hypertrophy of the face and extremities
- Diaphoresis, oily skin
- Fatigue, sleep disturbances
- Weight gain
- Headaches, decreased vision
- Decreased libido, impotence
- Oligomenorrhea, infertility
- Joint pain
- Hypertrichosis
- Irritability, hostility, and other psychological disturbances

PHYSICAL FINDINGS

- Enlarged jaw, thickened tongue
- Enlarged and weakened hands and feet
- Coarsened facial features
- Oily or leathery skin
- Prominent supraorbital ridge
- Deep, hollow-sounding voice
- Cartilaginous and connective tissue overgrowth
- Skeletal abnormalities

DIAGNOSTIC TEST RESULTS

- GH radioimmunoassay shows increased plasma GH levels and levels of insulin-like growth factor I.
- Glucose suppression test fails to suppress the hormone level to below the accepted norm of 2 ng/ml.
- Skull X-rays, computed tomography scan, or magnetic resonance imaging show location of pituitary tumor, cortical thickening, and enlargement of frontal sinuses.
- Bone X-rays show a thickening of the cranium and long bones and osteoarthritis in the spine.

TREATMENT

GENERAL
◆ Treatment to curb overproduction of GH
◆ Pituitary radiation therapy

DIET
◆ Well-balanced

ACTIVITY
◆ As tolerated

MEDICATIONS
◆ Thyroid, cortisone, and gonadal hormone therapy (postoperatively) if entire pituitary removed
◆ GH synthesis inhibitor
◆ Long-acting analogue of somatostatin

SURGERY
◆ Transsphenoidal hypophysectomy

NURSING CONSIDERATIONS

NURSING DIAGNOSES
◆ Activity intolerance
◆ Acute pain
◆ Chronic low self-esteem
◆ Disturbed body image
◆ Disturbed sensory perception: Visual
◆ Impaired oral mucous membrane
◆ Impaired physical mobility
◆ Ineffective coping
◆ Sexual dysfunction

EXPECTED OUTCOMES
The patient will:
◆ perform activities of daily living within the confines of the disorder
◆ express feelings of increased comfort and decreased pain
◆ voice positive feelings related to self-esteem
◆ express positive feelings related to body image
◆ maintain optimal functioning within the limits of his visual disturbance
◆ maintain intact oral mucous membranes

◆ maintain joint mobility and range of motion (ROM)
◆ demonstrate effective coping skills
◆ verbalize feelings regarding actual or perceived sexual impairment.

NURSING INTERVENTIONS
◆ Provide emotional support.
◆ Provide reassurance that mood changes result from hormonal imbalances and can be reduced with treatment.
◆ Give prescribed drugs.
◆ Provide comfort measures.
◆ Perform or assist with ROM exercises.
◆ Evaluate muscle weakness.
◆ Institute safety precautions.
◆ Provide meticulous skin care.
◆ Assist with early postoperative ambulation.
◆ Monitor vital signs, intake and output, and serum glucose levels.

⚠ **WARNING** *Report large increases in urine output after surgery, which may indicate diabetes insipidus.*

◆ Observe for signs and symptoms of hyperglycemia.

After surgery
◆ Assess for signs and symptoms of increased intracranial pressure (ICP) and intracranial bleeding.
◆ Monitor respiratory status.
◆ Assess surgical incisions and dressings.
◆ Observe for signs and symptoms of complications.

PATIENT TEACHING

Be sure to cover:
◆ disorder, diagnostic testing, and treatment
◆ medication administration, dosage, and possible adverse effects
◆ when to notify the practitioner
◆ avoidance of activities that increase ICP
◆ deep breathing through the mouth if nasal packing is in place postoperatively
◆ hormone replacement therapy, if ordered
◆ importance of wearing a medical identification bracelet
◆ follow-up examinations
◆ possibility of tumor recurrence
◆ available psychological counseling to help deal with body image changes and sexual dysfunction, as needed
◆ information on how to contact an acromegaly center for further information and support.

RESOURCES
Organizations
Endocrine Society: *www.endo-society.org*
Pituitary Network Association: *www.pituitary.com*

Selected references
Ezzat, S. "Pharmacological Options in the Treatment of Acromegaly," *Current Opinion in Investigational Drugs* 6(10):1023-1027, October 2005.

Lombardi, G., et al. "Acromegaly and the Cardiovascular System," *Neuroendocrinology* 83(3-4): 211-17, 2006.

Strategies for Managing Multisystem Disorders. Philadelphia: Lippincott Williams & Wilkins, 2006.

Waxler, R. "Acromegaly," *American Journal of Orthodontics and Dentofacial Orthopedics* 131(1):6, January 2007.

(continued)

Disorders affecting management of hyperpituitarism

This chart highlights disorders that affect the management of hyperpituitarism.

DISORDER	SIGNS AND SYMPTOMS	DIAGNOSTIC TEST RESULTS	TREATMENT AND CARE
Diabetes mellitus (complication)	◆ Weight loss despite voracious hunger ◆ Weakness ◆ Vision changes ◆ Frequent skin and urinary tract infections ◆ Dry, itchy skin ◆ Poor skin turgor ◆ Dry mucous membranes ◆ Dehydration ◆ Decreased peripheral pulses ◆ Cool skin temperature ◆ Decreased reflexes ◆ Orthostatic hypotension ◆ Muscle wasting ◆ Loss of subcutaneous fat ◆ Fruity breath odor from ketoacidosis	◆ Fasting plasma glucose level is 126 mg/dl or greater, or a random blood glucose level is 200 mg/dl or greater on at least two occasions. ◆ Blood glucose level is 200 mg/dl or greater 2 hours after ingestion of 75 grams of oral dextrose. ◆ An ophthalmologic examination may show diabetic retinopathy.	◆ Keep a snack available in case the patient becomes hypoglycemic. ◆ Keep accurate records of vital signs, weight, fluid intake, urine output, and calorie intake. ◆ Monitor serum glucose and urine acetone levels. ◆ Monitor the patient for acute complications of diabetic therapy, especially hypoglycemia (vagueness, slow cerebration, dizziness, weakness, pallor, tachycardia, diaphoresis, seizures, and coma); immediately give carbohydrates in the form of fruit juice, hard candy, or honey; if the patient is unconscious, give glucagon or I.V. dextrose. ◆ Be alert for signs of hyperosmolar coma (polyuria, thirst, neurologic abnormalities, and stupor). This hyperglycemic crisis requires I.V. fluids and insulin replacement. ◆ Monitor the effects of diabetes on the cardiovascular system—such as cerebrovascular, coronary artery, and peripheral vascular impairment—and on the peripheral and autonomic nervous systems. ◆ Provide meticulous skin care, and watch for manifestations of urinary tract and vaginal infections.
Heart failure (complication)	◆ Cough that produces pink, frothy sputum ◆ Cyanosis of the lips and nail beds ◆ Pale, cool, clammy skin ◆ Diaphoresis ◆ Jugular vein distention ◆ Ascites ◆ Pulsus alternans ◆ Tachycardia ◆ Hepatomegaly ◆ Decreased pulse pressure ◆ Third and fourth heart sounds (S_3 and S_4) ◆ Moist, basilar crackles ◆ Rhonchi ◆ Expiratory wheezing ◆ Decreased pulse oximetry ◆ Peripheral edema ◆ Decreased urinary output	◆ B-type natriuretic peptide immunoassay is elevated. ◆ Chest X-ray shows increased pulmonary vascular markings, interstitial edema, or pleural effusions and cardiomegaly. ◆ Electrocardiography reveals heart enlargement or ischemia, tachycardia, extrasystole, or atrial fibrillation. ◆ Pulmonary artery pressure, pulmonary artery wedge pressure, and left ventricular end-diastolic pressure are elevated in the presence of left-sided heart failure; right atrial or central venous pressure is elevated in right-sided heart failure.	◆ Administer supplemental oxygen and mechanical ventilation, if needed. ◆ Place the patient in Fowler's position. ◆ Administer diuretics, inotropic drugs, vasodilators, angiotensin-converting enzyme inhibitors, angiotensin receptor blockers, cardiac glycosides, beta-adrenergic blockers, and electrolyte supplements. ◆ Initiate cardiac monitoring. ◆ Recurrent heart failure from valvular dysfunction may require surgery. ◆ A ventricular assist device may be needed. ◆ Maintain adequate cardiac output, and monitor hemodynamic stability. ◆ Assess for deep vein thrombosis, and apply antiembolism stockings.

Disorders affecting management of hyperpituitarism *(continued)*

DISORDER	SIGNS AND SYMPTOMS	DIAGNOSTIC TEST RESULTS	TREATMENT AND CARE
Osteoporosis (complication)	◆ Dowager's hump ◆ Back pain (thoracic and lumbar) ◆ Loss of height ◆ Unsteady gait ◆ Joint pain ◆ Weakness	◆ Dual photon or dual energy X-ray absorptiometry can detect bone loss. ◆ X-ray reveals characteristic degeneration in the lower vertebrae. ◆ Parathyroid levels may be elevated. ◆ Bone biopsy allows direct examination of changes in bone cells and the rate of bone turnover.	◆ Provide supportive devices such as a back brace. ◆ Encourage lifestyle modifications, such as weight loss, exercise program, and dietary modifications. ◆ Offer analgesics and heat for pain relief. ◆ Administer calcium and vitamin D supplements to stimulate bone formation. ◆ Give sodium fluoride to stimulate bone formation; give calcitonin to reduce bone resorption and slow the decline in bone mass.

Hypertension

- Intermittent or sustained elevation of diastolic or systolic blood pressure
- Usually beginning as benign disease, slowly progressing to accelerated or malignant state
- Two major types: essential (also called *primary* or *idiopathic*) and secondary
- Essential hypertension: accounts for 90% to 95% of cases
- Secondary hypertension: results from renal disease or another identifiable cause
- Malignant hypertension (medical emergency): severe, fulminant form commonly arising from both types
- Affects 15% to 20% of adults in the United States

CAUSES
- Exact cause unknown

RISK FACTORS
- Family history
- History of coronary artery disease
- History of diabetes mellitus or renal disease
- Blacks in the United States
- Stress
- Obesity
- High-sodium, high–saturated fat diet
- Use of tobacco
- Use of hormonal contraceptives
- Excessive alcohol intake
- Sedentary lifestyle
- Aging

- Arterial blood pressure is a product of total peripheral resistance and cardiac output.
- Cardiac output is increased by conditions that increase heart rate, stroke volume, or both. Peripheral resistance is increased by factors that increase blood viscosity or reduce the lumen size of vessels, especially the arterioles.

SEVERAL THEORIES
- Changes in arteriolar bed cause increased peripheral vascular resistance.
- Abnormally increased tone in the sympathetic nervous system originates in the vasomotor system centers, causing increased peripheral vascular resistance.
- Increased blood volume results from renal or hormonal dysfunction.
- Increased arteriolar thickening is caused by genetic factors, leading to increased peripheral vascular resistance.
- Abnormal renin release results in the formation of angiotensin II, which constricts the arterioles and increases blood volume. (See *How hypertension develops.)*
- In secondary hypertension, damage to the kidney from chronic glomerulonephritis or renal artery stenosis interferes with sodium excretion, the renin-angiotensin-aldosterone system, or renal perfusion, causing blood pressure to increase.

CARDIOVASCULAR SYSTEM
- Prolonged hypertension increases the heart's workload as resistance to left ventricular ejection increases.
- To increase contractile force, the left ventricle hypertrophies, raising the heart's oxygen demands and workload.
- Cardiac dilation and failure may occur when hypertrophy can no longer maintain sufficient cardiac output.
- Because hypertension promotes coronary atherosclerosis, the heart may be further compromised by reduced blood flow to the myocardium, resulting in angina or myocardial infarction (MI).
- Hypertension causes vascular damage, leading to accelerated atherosclerosis and target organ damage, such as retinal injury, renal failure, stroke, and aortic aneurysm and dissection. (See *Disorders affecting management of hypertension,* pages 242 and 243.)

NEUROLOGIC SYSTEM
- As organ damage occurs, cerebral perfusion decreases and stress on vessel walls increases.
- Arterial spasm and ischemia lead to transient ischemic attacks.
- Weakening of the vessel intima leads to possible aneurysm formation and intracranial hemorrhage.

HISTORY

◆ In many cases, no symptoms; disorder revealed incidentally during evaluation for another disorder or during a routine blood pressure screening program
◆ Symptoms that reflect the effect of hypertension on the organ systems
◆ Awakening with a headache in the occipital region, which subsides spontaneously after a few hours
◆ Dizziness, fatigue, confusion
◆ Palpitations, chest pain, dyspnea
◆ Epistaxis
◆ Hematuria
◆ Blurred vision

PHYSICAL FINDINGS

◆ Bounding pulse
◆ S_4
◆ Peripheral edema in late stages
◆ Hemorrhages, exudates, and papilledema of the eye in late stages if hypertensive retinopathy present
◆ Pulsating abdominal mass, suggesting an abdominal aneurysm
◆ Elevated blood pressure on at least two consecutive occasions after initial screenings
◆ Bruits over the abdominal aorta and femoral arteries or the carotids

UP CLOSE

How hypertension develops

Increased blood volume, cardiac rate, and stroke volume or arteriolar vasoconstriction that increases peripheral resistance causes blood pressure to rise. Hypertension may also result from the breakdown or inappropriate response of the following intrinsic regulatory mechanisms.

RENIN-ANGIOTENSIN SYSTEM

Renal hypoperfusion causes the release of renin. Angiotensinogen, a liver enzyme, converts the renin to angiotensin I, which increases preload and afterload. Angiotensin I then converts to angiotensin II in the lungs. A powerful vasoconstrictor, angiotensin II also helps increase preload and afterload by stimulating the adrenal cortex to secrete aldosterone. This serves to increase sodium reabsorption. Next comes hypertonic-stimulated release of antidiuretic hormone from the pituitary gland. This, in turn, increases water absorption, plasma volume, cardiac output, and blood pressure.

AUTOREGULATION

Several intrinsic mechanisms work to change an artery's diameter to maintain tissue and organ perfusion, despite fluctuations in systemic blood pressure. Mechanisms include stress relaxation and capillary fluid shift.

During stress relaxation, blood vessels gradually dilate when blood pressure rises to reduce peripheral resistance. During capillary fluid shift, plasma moves between vessels and extravascular spaces to maintain intravascular volume.

When blood pressure decreases, baroreceptors in the aortic arch and carotid sinuses decrease their inhibition of the medulla's vasomotor center. This action increases sympathetic stimulation of the heart by norepinephrine. This, in turn, increases cardiac output by strengthening the contractile force, increasing the heart rate, and augmenting peripheral resistance by vasoconstriction. Stress can also stimulate the sympathetic nervous system to increase cardiac output and peripheral vascular resistance.

BLOOD VESSEL DAMAGE

Sustained hypertension damages blood vessels (as pictured below). Vascular injury begins with alternating areas of dilation and constriction in the arterioles. Increased intra-arterial pressure damages the endothelium (see illustration, below left). Independently, angiotensin induces endothelial wall contraction (see middle illustration below), allowing plasma to leak through interendothelial spaces. Eventually, plasma constituents deposited in the vessel wall cause medial necrosis (see illustration, below right).

VASCULAR DAMAGE

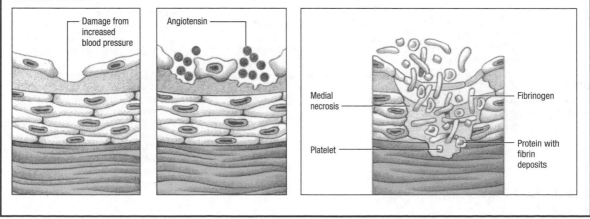

Damage from increased blood pressure

Angiotensin

Medial necrosis

Platelet

Fibrinogen

Protein with fibrin deposits

(continued)

DIAGNOSTIC TEST RESULTS

◆ Urinalysis may show protein, red blood cells, or white blood cells, suggesting renal disease; or may reflect glucose, suggesting diabetes mellitus.
◆ Serum potassium levels less than 3.5 mEq/L may indicate adrenal dysfunction (primary hyperaldosteronism).
◆ Blood urea nitrogen levels normal or elevated to more than 20 mg/dl and serum creatinine levels normal or elevated to more than 1.5 mg/dl suggest renal disease.
◆ Excretory urography reveals renal atrophy, indicating chronic renal disease; one kidney more than 5⅛" (1.6 cm) shorter than the other suggests unilateral renal disease.
◆ Chest X-rays demonstrate cardiomegaly.
◆ Renal arteriography shows renal artery stenosis.
◆ Electrocardiography may show left ventricular hypertrophy or ischemia.
◆ Oral captopril challenge test may reveal renovascular hypertension.
◆ Ophthalmoscopy reveals arteriovenous nicking and, in hypertensive encephalopathy, edema.

TREATMENT

GENERAL

◆ Lifestyle modification, such as weight control, limiting alcohol intake, regular exercise, and smoking cessation
◆ For a patient with secondary hypertension, correction of the underlying cause and control of hypertensive effects (see *Antihypertension therapy*)

DIET

◆ Low in saturated fat and sodium
◆ Adequate intake of calcium, magnesium, and potassium

ACTIVITY

◆ Regular exercise

MEDICATIONS

◆ Diuretics
◆ Beta-adrenergic blockers
◆ Calcium channel blockers
◆ Angiotensin-converting enzyme inhibitors
◆ Alpha-receptor antagonists
◆ Vasodilators
◆ Angiotensin-receptor blockers
◆ Aldosterone antagonist

NURSING CONSIDERATIONS

NURSING DIAGNOSES

◆ Fatigue
◆ Ineffective coping
◆ Ineffective tissue perfusion: Cardiopulmonary
◆ Noncompliance (therapeutic regimen)
◆ Risk for injury

EXPECTED OUTCOMES

The patient will:
◆ express feelings of increased energy
◆ demonstrate adaptive coping behaviors
◆ maintain adequate cardiac output and hemodynamic stability
◆ comply with the therapy regimen
◆ remain free from injury.

NURSING INTERVENTIONS

◆ Give prescribed drugs.
◆ Encourage dietary changes, as appropriate.
◆ Help the patient identify risk factors and modify his lifestyle, as appropriate.
◆ Monitor vital signs.
◆ Assess for signs and symptoms of target end-organ damage.
◆ Observe for complications.
◆ Evaluate response to treatment, and observe for adverse effects of antihypertensives.

PATIENT TEACHING

Be sure to cover:
◆ disorder, diagnostic testing, and treatment
◆ how to use a self-monitoring blood pressure cuff and to record the reading in a journal for review by the practitioner
◆ importance of compliance with antihypertensive therapy and establishing a daily routine for taking prescribed drugs
◆ need to report adverse effects of drugs
◆ need to avoid high-sodium antacids and over-the-counter cold and sinus medications containing harmful vasoconstrictors
◆ examining and modifying lifestyle, as indicated to reduce risks
◆ need for a routine exercise program, particularly aerobic walking
◆ dietary restrictions
◆ importance of follow-up care
◆ contact information for stress-reduction therapies or support groups, as needed
◆ available weight-reduction or smoking-cessation groups, as needed.

RESOURCES

Organizations

American Heart Association: *www.americanheart.org*
American Medical Association: *www.ama-assn.org*

Selected references

Frost, K., and Topp, R. "A Physical Activity RX for the Hypertensive Patient," *The Nurse Practitioner* 31(4):29-37, April 2006.
Kennedy, S. "Essential Hypertension: Treatment and Monitoring Update," *Community Practitioner* 79(2):64-66, February 2006.
Nettina, S.M. *Lippincott Manual of Nursing Practice*, 8th ed. Philadelphia: Lippincott Williams & Wilkins, 2006.
Woods, A. "Advances in Hypertensive Management," *Nursing* 36(10 Suppl): 1-3, Fall 2006.

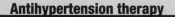

Antihypertension therapy

The algorithm below illustrates the approach to the treatment of hypertension recommended by the National Institutes of Health. The progression of therapy is based on the patient's achievement toward target blood pressure goal.

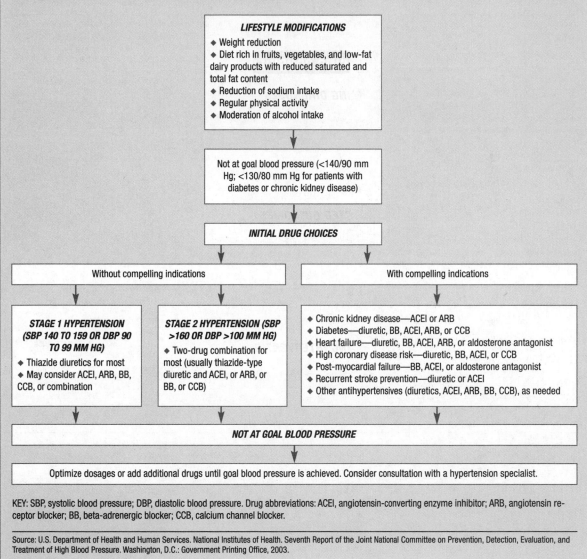

LIFESTYLE MODIFICATIONS

- ◆ Weight reduction
- ◆ Diet rich in fruits, vegetables, and low-fat dairy products with reduced saturated and total fat content
- ◆ Reduction of sodium intake
- ◆ Regular physical activity
- ◆ Moderation of alcohol intake

Not at goal blood pressure (<140/90 mm Hg; <130/80 mm Hg for patients with diabetes or chronic kidney disease)

INITIAL DRUG CHOICES

Without compelling indications

With compelling indications

STAGE 1 HYPERTENSION (SBP 140 TO 159 OR DBP 90 TO 99 MM HG)

- ◆ Thiazide diuretics for most
- ◆ May consider ACEI, ARB, BB, CCB, or combination

STAGE 2 HYPERTENSION (SBP >160 OR DBP >100 MM HG)

- ◆ Two-drug combination for most (usually thiazide-type diuretic and ACEI, or ARB, or BB, or CCB)

- ◆ Chronic kidney disease—ACEI or ARB
- ◆ Diabetes—diuretic, BB, ACEI, ARB, or CCB
- ◆ Heart failure—diuretic, BB, ACEI, ARB, or aldosterone antagonist
- ◆ High coronary disease risk—diuretic, BB, ACEI, or CCB
- ◆ Post-myocardial failure—BB, ACEI, or aldosterone antagonist
- ◆ Recurrent stroke prevention—diuretic or ACEI
- ◆ Other antihypertensives (diuretics, ACEI, ARB, BB, CCB), as needed

NOT AT GOAL BLOOD PRESSURE

Optimize dosages or add additional drugs until goal blood pressure is achieved. Consider consultation with a hypertension specialist.

KEY: SBP, systolic blood pressure; DBP, diastolic blood pressure. Drug abbreviations: ACEI, angiotensin-converting enzyme inhibitor; ARB, angiotensin receptor blocker; BB, beta-adrenergic blocker; CCB, calcium channel blocker.

Source: U.S. Department of Health and Human Services. National Institutes of Health. Seventh Report of the Joint National Committee on Prevention, Detection, Evaluation, and Treatment of High Blood Pressure. Washington, D.C.: Government Printing Office, 2003.

(continued)

Disorders affecting management of hypertension

This chart highlights disorders that affect the management of hypertension.

DISORDER	SIGNS AND SYMPTOMS	DIAGNOSTIC TEST RESULTS	TREATMENT AND CARE
Aortic aneurysm (complication)	◆ Pallor ◆ Diaphoresis ◆ Dyspnea ◆ Cyanosis ◆ Leg weakness or transient paralysis ◆ Abrupt onset of intermittent neurologic deficits ◆ Hoarseness ◆ Dyspnea ◆ Throat pain ◆ Dysphagia ◆ Dry cough *Dissecting ascending aneurysm* ◆ Pain most intense at its onset that may extend to neck, shoulders, lower back, and abdomen ◆ Boring, tearing, or ripping sensation in the thorax or the right anterior chest *Dissecting descending aneurysm* ◆ Sharp, tearing pain located between the shoulder blades that commonly radiates to the chest *Dissecting transverse aneurysm* ◆ Sharp, boring, and tearing pain that radiates to the shoulders	◆ Abdominal ultrasonography or echocardiography determines the size, shape, and location of the aneurysm. ◆ Aortography shows condition of vessels proximal and distal to aneurysm.	◆ Manage blood pressure with beta-adrenergic blockers, angiotensin-converting enzyme (ACE) inhibitors, and diuretics. For severe hypertensive episode, give nitroprusside. ◆ Monitor aneurysm growth with serial ultrasounds. ◆ Encourage lifestyle modifications, such as smoking cessation, weight loss, and diet modification, as appropriate. ◆ Advise the patient to seek medical attention for abdominal or back pain.
Cardiac arrhythmia (complication)	◆ Palpitations ◆ Chest pain ◆ Dizziness ◆ Weakness, fatigue ◆ Irregular heart rhythm ◆ Hypotension ◆ Syncope ◆ Altered level of consciousness (LOC) ◆ Diaphoresis, pallor, cold, clammy skin	◆ Electrocardiography identifies specific waveform changes associated with the arrhythmia. ◆ Laboratory testing reveals electrolyte abnormalities, hypoxemia, or acid-base abnormalities. ◆ Electrophysiologic testing identifies the mechanism of an arrhythmia and the location of accessory pathways.	◆ Assess airway, breathing, and circulation if life-threatening arrhythmia develops; follow advanced cardiac life support protocols for treatment. ◆ Monitor cardiac rhythm continuously and obtain serial electrocardiograms to evaluate changes and effects of treatment. ◆ Administer antiarrhythmics and monitor for adverse effects. ◆ Assess cardiovascular status for signs of hypoperfusion; monitor vital signs. ◆ Assist with insertion of temporary pacemaker or apply transcutaneous pacemaker, if appropriate.

DISORDER	SIGNS AND SYMPTOMS	DIAGNOSTIC TEST RESULTS	TREATMENT AND CARE
Chronic renal failure (complication)	◆ Muscle twitching ◆ Paresthesia ◆ Bone pain ◆ Pruritus ◆ Decreased urine output ◆ Stomatitis ◆ Lethargy ◆ Seizures ◆ Brittle nails and hair ◆ Kussmaul's respirations ◆ Uremic frost ◆ Ecchymosis ◆ Weight gain	◆ Glomerular filtration rate (GFR) is decreased or urinalysis shows albuminuria, proteinuria, glycosuria, erythrocytes, and leukocytes. ◆ Serum creatinine may increase by 2 mg/dl or more over a 2-week period. ◆ Creatinine clearance is decreased. ◆ Blood urea nitrogen (BUN) suddenly increases. ◆ Uric acid is elevated. ◆ Potassium level is elevated. ◆ Arterial blood gas (ABG) analysis may show metabolic acidosis.	◆ ACE inhibitors and angiotensin receptor blockers to achieve target blood pressure of less than 130/80 mm Hg. ◆ Therapeutic goals to reduce the deterioration of renal function and prevent stroke. ◆ Loop diuretics may be used in patients with advanced renal disease. ◆ Monitor creatinine clearance, BUN, uric acid, and GFR. ◆ Monitor potassium levels to detect hyperkalemia. ◆ Monitor ABG studies for metabolic acidosis. ◆ Be alert for drug toxicity and adverse reactions. ◆ Advise the patient taking loop diuretics about maintaining a sodium-restricted diet.
Diabetes mellitus (coexisting)	◆ Weight loss ◆ Anorexia ◆ Polyphagia ◆ Acetone breath ◆ Weakness ◆ Fatigue ◆ Dehydration ◆ Pain ◆ Paresthesia ◆ Polyuria ◆ Polydipsia ◆ Kussmaul's respirations ◆ Mottled extremities ◆ Blurred vision	◆ Fasting blood glucose is 126 mg/dl or higher, or a random blood glucose level is 200 mg/dl or higher on at least two occasions. ◆ Blood glucose level is 200 mg/dl or higher 2 hours after ingestion of 75 grams of dextrose.	◆ Thiazide diuretics, ACE inhibitors, beta-adrenergic blockers, angiotensin receptor blockers, and calcium channel blockers help reduce the risk of cardiovascular disease and stroke. ◆ Encourage lifestyle modifications, such as smoking cessation, weight loss, and dietary modifications, as appropriate. ◆ Monitor blood glucose levels. ◆ Advise the patient to watch for changes in vision and signs of infection, diabetic neuropathy, and cardiac distress. ◆ Advise the patient to perform good foot care and to watch for altered skin integrity or delayed wound healing. ◆ Monitor potassium levels and assess for signs of dehydration, if a diuretic is prescribed.
Metabolic acidosis (complication)	◆ Headache, lethargy progressing to drowsiness, central nervous system depression ◆ Kussmaul's respirations, hypotension, stupor, and coma ◆ Anorexia, nausea, vomiting, diarrhea and, possibly, dehydration ◆ Warm, flushed skin ◆ Fruity breath odor	◆ Arterial pH is below 7.35. ◆ Partial pressure of arterial carbon dioxide may be normal or less than 34 mm Hg; bicarbonate level may be less than 22 mEq/L. ◆ Serum potassium level is greater than 5.5 mEq/L. ◆ Anion gap is greater than 14 mEq/L.	◆ For severe cases, administer sodium bicarbonate I.V. ◆ Monitor vital signs, laboratory results, pulse oximetry readings, and LOC. ◆ Administer electrolyte supplements and evaluate effects. ◆ Initiate aspiration precautions. ◆ Record intake and output to monitor renal function.

Hyperthermia LIFE-THREATENING DISORDER

OVERVIEW

- Elevation of body temperature over 99° F (37.2° C)
- Heat exhaustion: acute heat injury with hyperthermia caused by dehydration
- Heat stroke: extreme hyperthermia with thermoregulatory failure
- Affects males and females equally
- Incidence increasing among older patients and neonates during excessively hot summer days
- Also known as *heat syndrome*

CAUSES

- Behavior
- Dehydration
- Drugs, such as phenothiazines, anticholinergics, and amphetamines (see *Malignant hyperthermia*)
- Endocrine disorders
- Excessive clothing
- Excessive physical activity
- Heart disease
- Hot environment without ventilation
- Illness
- Inadequate fluid intake
- Infection (fever)
- Lack of acclimatization
- Neurologic disorder
- Sudden discontinuation of Parkinson's disease medications

RISK FACTORS

- Obesity
- Salt and water depletion
- Alcohol use
- Poor physical condition
- Age
- Socioeconomic status

PATHOPHYSIOLOGY

- Body temperature is normally coordinated by the hypothalamus.
- Regulation of temperature is through evaporation (30% of body's heat loss) or vasodilation. When heat is generated or gained by the body faster than it can dissipate, the thermoregulatory mechanism is stressed and eventually fails, which causes hyperthermia to accelerate.
- Cerebral edema and cerebrovascular congestion occurs.
- Cerebral perfusion pressure increases and decreases cerebral blood flow.
- Tissue damage occurs when temperature exceeds 107.6° F (42° C), resulting in tissue necrosis, organ dysfunction, and failure. (See *Disorders affecting management of hyperthermia*, pages 246 and 247.)

CARDIOVASCULAR SYSTEM

- If body temperature remains elevated, blood flow is redistributed to the periphery, fluid and electrolyte losses occur through sweat, and cardiac output is decreased.
- If left untreated, excessive body temperature can lead to hypovolemic shock, cardiogenic shock, and cardiac arrhythmias.

GASTROINTESTINAL SYSTEM

- Fulminant hepatic failure may result from massive destruction of liver tissue following prolonged hyperthermia.

HEMATOLOGIC SYSTEM

- Disseminated intravascular coagulation may result from the extensive destruction of endothelial surfaces caused by hyperthermia, causing the direct release of tissue plasminogen activator and generation of plasmin.

NEUROLOGIC SYSTEM

- Level of consciousness (LOC) changes as cerebral perfusion diminishes.

RENAL SYSTEM

- Prolonged hyperthermia may result in rhabdomyolysis related to the hypermetabolic state of muscles, resulting in myoglobinuria and, possibly, renal failure.

RESPIRATORY SYSTEM

- Prolonged hyperthermia results in acidosis, central nervous system (CNS) stimulation, and hypoxia, causing respiratory failure.

ASSESSMENT

HISTORY
Heat exhaustion

- Prolonged activity in a very warm or hot environment
- Muscle cramps
- Nausea and vomiting
- Thirst
- Weakness
- Headache
- Fatigue
- Sweating
- Tachycardia

Heatstroke

- Exposure to high temperature and humidity without air circulation
- Same signs as heat exhaustion

Malignant hyperthermia

Malignant hyperthermia is an inherited condition of hypermetabolism that occurs after exposure to certain drugs, including anesthetic agents such as succinylcholine or halothane. Drugs such as cocaine, diuretics, barbiturates, hallucinogens, and tricyclic antidepressants may depress hypothalamus activity, produce skin vasoconstriction (thus decreasing the ability to dissipate heat, causing a systemwide blockage of sweat production), and block the body's cardiovascular responses to heat, which increases cardiac output.

The number of malignant hyperthermia cases has increased in part because of "designer drug" use. For example, people attending raves (dance parties that last from one to several days) use various illicit drugs to avoid sleeping. Many patients suffer water intoxication and malignant hyperthermia. Frequent monitoring of electrolyte levels in addition to controlling core temperature is crucial. Also, obtaining a sample of the drug taken allows for chemical analysis of the substance, which may help guide treatment.

- Blurred vision
- Confusion
- Hallucinations
- Decreased muscle coordination
- Syncope

PHYSICAL FINDINGS
Heat exhaustion
- Rectal temperature greater than 100° F (37.8° C)
- Pale skin
- Thready, rapid pulse
- Cool, moist skin
- Decreased blood pressure
- Irritability
- Syncope
- Impaired judgment
- Hyperventilation

Heatstroke
- Rectal temperature of at least 104° F (40° C)
- Red, diaphoretic, hot skin in early stages
- Gray, dry, hot skin in later stages
- Tachycardia
- Slightly elevated blood pressure in early stages
- Decreased blood pressure in later stages
- Tachypnea
- Decreased LOC
- Signs of CNS dysfunction
- Altered mental status
- Hyperpnea
- Cheyne-Stokes respirations
- Anhidrosis (late sign)

DIAGNOSTIC TEST RESULTS
- Hypernatremia or hyponatremia and hyperkalemia or hypokalemia, depending on cause and severity of hypertension.
- Arterial blood gas levels may indicate respiratory alkalosis.
- Lactic acid level is increased.
- Complete blood count may reveal leukocytosis and thrombocytopenia.
- Coagulation studies may show increased bleeding and clotting times.
- Urinalysis may show concentrated urine and proteinuria with tubular casts and myoglobinuria.
- Blood urea nitrogen may be elevated.

- Creatine kinase, lactate dehydrogenase, and aldolase levels may be elevated.
- Serum calcium level may be decreased.
- Serum phosphorus level may be decreased.
- Myoglobinuria may indicate rhabdomyolosis.

TREATMENT

GENERAL
Heat exhaustion
- Cool environment
- Oral or I.V. fluid administration

Heatstroke
- Lowering of body temperature as rapidly as possible
- Evaporation, hypothermia blankets, and ice packs to the groin, axillae, and neck
- Supportive respiratory and cardiovascular measures

DIET
- Increased hydration; cool liquids only
- Avoidance of caffeine and alcohol

ACTIVITY
- Minimal activity until body temperature decreases

NURSING CONSIDERATIONS

NURSING DIAGNOSES
- Decreased cardiac output
- Deficient fluid volume
- Hyperthermia
- Impaired gas exchange
- Impaired home maintenance

EXPECTED OUTCOMES
The patient will:
- exhibit signs of adequate cardiac output
- express understanding of the need to maintain adequate fluid intake
- maintain a normal body temperature
- maintain adequate ventilation and oxygenation

- express understanding of how to prevent recurrent episodes of hyperthermia.

NURSING INTERVENTIONS
- Perform rapid cooling procedures.
- Provide supportive measures.
- Administer adequate fluid replacement.
- Give prescribed drugs.
- Monitor vital signs, pulse oximetry readings, intake and output, and cardiac rhythm.
- Observe for complications.
- Assess LOC.
- Monitor myoglobin test results.

PATIENT TEACHING

Be sure to cover:
- disorder, diagnostic testing, and treatment
- how to avoid reexposure to high temperatures
- need to maintain adequate fluid intake
- need to wear loose clothing
- activity limitation in hot weather
- referral to social services, if appropriate.

RESOURCES
Organizations
National Center for Injury Prevention and Control: *www.cdc.gov/ncipc*
National Institutes of Health: *www.nih.gov*

Selected references
Dinman, S. "Pharmacy Department: Malignant Hyperthermia," *Plastic Surgical Nursing* 26(4):206-207, October-December 2006.
Glazer, J.L. "Management of Heatstroke and Heat Exhaustion," *American Family Physician* 71(11):2133-140, June 2005.
Sucholeiki, R. "Heatstroke," *Seminars in Neurology: Tropical Neurology* 25(3):307-14, September 2005.
Thompson, H., et al. "Intensive Care Unit Management of Fever Following Traumatic Brain Injury," *Intensive Critical Care Nurse* 23(2):91-96, April 2007.

(continued)

Disorders affecting management of hyperthermia

This chart highlights disorders that affect the management of hyperthermia.

DISORDER	SIGNS AND SYMPTOMS	DIAGNOSTIC TEST RESULTS	TREATMENT AND CARE
Acute renal failure (complication)	◆ Urine output less than 400 ml/day for 1 to 2 weeks followed by diuresis (excretion of 3 to 5 L/day) for 2 to 3 weeks ◆ Lethargy ◆ Drowsiness ◆ Stupor ◆ Coma ◆ Irritability ◆ Headache ◆ Costovertebral pain ◆ Numbness around the mouth ◆ Tingling extremities ◆ Anorexia ◆ Restlessness ◆ Weight gain ◆ Nausea and vomiting ◆ Pallor ◆ Epistaxis ◆ Ecchymosis ◆ Diarrhea or constipation ◆ Stomatitis ◆ Thick, tenacious sputum	◆ Blood urea nitrogen (BUN) and serum creatinine levels are increased. With rhabdomyolysis, a creatinine increase greater than 5 mg/dl/day may occur because muscle is a major source of creatine, which is the precursor of creatinine. ◆ Potassium levels are increased. ◆ Hematocrit, blood pH, bicarbonate, and hemoglobin levels are decreased. ◆ Urine casts and cellular debris are present; specific gravity is decreased.	◆ Monitor fluid balance status, including skin turgor; evidence of peripheral, sacral, or periorbital edema; and intake and output. Monitor urine output every hour, and assess daily weights. ◆ Anticipate insertion of a central venous catheter or pulmonary artery catheter to assess hemodynamic status. ◆ Insertion of a temporary dialysis catheter may be necessary for hemodialysis or continuous renal replacement therapy, depending on the patient's condition. ◆ Monitor results of laboratory and diagnostic tests, especially BUN and creatinine levels, arterial blood gas studies, and serum electrolyte levels.
Cardiac arrhythmia (complication)	◆ Palpitations ◆ Chest pain ◆ Dizziness ◆ Weakness, fatigue ◆ Irregular heart rhythm ◆ Hypotension ◆ Syncope ◆ Altered level of consciousness (LOC) ◆ Diaphoresis, pallor, cold, clammy skin	◆ Electrocardiography identifies specific waveform changes associated with the arrhythmia. ◆ Laboratory testing reveals electrolyte abnormalities, hypoxemia, or acid-base abnormalities. ◆ Electrophysiologic testing identifies the mechanism of an arrhythmia and the location of accessory pathways.	◆ Assess airway, breathing, and circulation if life-threatening arrhythmia develops; follow advanced cardiac life support protocols for treatment. ◆ Monitor cardiac rhythm continuously, and obtain serial electrocardiograms to evaluate changes and effects of treatment. ◆ Administer antiarrhythmics and monitor for adverse effects. ◆ Assess cardiovascular status for signs of hypoperfusion; monitor vital signs. ◆ Assist with insertion of temporary pacemaker or apply transcutaneous pacemaker, if appropriate.
Disseminated intravascular coagulation (complication)	◆ Petechiae ◆ Ecchymosis ◆ Prolonged bleeding after venipuncture ◆ Hemorrhage ◆ Oliguria ◆ Anxiety ◆ Restlessness ◆ Purpura ◆ Acrocyanosis ◆ Joint pain ◆ Dyspnea ◆ Hemoptysis ◆ Crackles	◆ Platelet count is decreased, usually less than 100,000/µl. ◆ Fibrinogen levels are less than 150 mg/dl. ◆ Prothrombin time (PT) is greater than 15 seconds. ◆ Partial thromboplastin time (PTT) is greater than 60 seconds. ◆ Fibrin degradation products are increased, commonly greater than 45 mcg/ml. ◆ D-dimer test is positive at less than 1:8 dilution. ◆ Fibrin monomers are positive. ◆ Levels of factors V and VIII are diminished. ◆ Red blood cell smear shows fragmentation. ◆ Hemoglobin is less than 10 g/dl.	◆ Assess the patient for bleeding and blood loss. Administer fluid replacement and blood products, as indicated. ◆ Be alert for signs of pulmonary emboli. Watch hemodynamic parameters closely; decreased values suggest hemorrhage, whereas increased values suggest emboli. ◆ Fresh frozen plasma administration allows for replacement of clotting factors and inhibitors. Cryoprecipitate is the drug of choice if the patient's fibrinogen levels are significantly decreased. ◆ Obtain serial hemoglobin and hematocrit levels; monitor results of coagulation studies, including PTT, PT, fibrinogen levels, fibrin split products, and platelet counts. ◆ Monitor intake and output hourly. Monitor renal status for signs of acute renal failure.

Disorders affecting management of hyperthermia *(continued)*

DISORDER	SIGNS AND SYMPTOMS	DIAGNOSTIC TEST RESULTS	TREATMENT AND CARE
Hypovolemic shock (complication)	◆ Pale skin color ◆ Decreased LOC ◆ Hypotension ◆ Tachycardia ◆ Cool, clammy skin ◆ Urine output less than 25 ml/hour	◆ Central venous pressure, pulmonary wedge pressure, and cardiac output are decreased. ◆ Hematocrit, hemoglobin, and red blood cell and platelet counts are low. ◆ Serum potassium, sodium, lactic dehydrogenase, blood urea nitrogen, and creatinine are elevated. ◆ Urine specific gravity is increased. ◆ Arterial blood gas analysis shows respiratory acidosis.	◆ Assess extent of fluid loss; administer fluid and blood replacement, as indicated. ◆ Administer supplemental oxygen. ◆ Monitor vital signs and intake and output. ◆ Monitor respiratory status and pulse oximetry. ◆ Assist with endotracheal intubation, if necessary.

Hyperthyroidism

- Alteration in thyroid function, in which thyroid hormones (TH) exert greater than normal responses
- Form of thyrotoxicosis, in which excess THs are secreted by thyroid gland
- Graves' disease (also known as *toxic diffuse goiter*):
- Autoimmune disease; most common form of hyperthyroidism
- Most common between ages 30 and 60; more common in females than in males
- Increased incidence among monozygotic twins
- Only 5% of hyperthyroid patients younger than age 15 affected
- More common in those with a family history of thyroid abnormalities
- Thyrotoxicoses not associated with hyperthyroidism: subacute thyroiditis, ectopic thyroid tissue, and ingestion of excessive TH
- Also known as *thyrotoxicosis*

CAUSES
- Genetic and immunologic factors
- Graves' disease
- Increased thyroid-stimulating hormone (TSH) secretion
- Thyroid cancer
- Toxic multinodular goiter

RISK FACTORS
- Diabetic ketoacidosis
- Excessive iodine intake
- Infection
- Stress
- Surgery
- Toxemia of pregnancy

PATHOPHYSIOLOGY

- In Graves' disease, thyroid-stimulating antibodies bind to and stimulate the TSH receptors of the thyroid gland.
- It's associated with the production of autoantibodies possibly caused by a defect in suppressor T-lymphocyte function that allows the formation of these autoantibodies.
- Hyperthyroidism affects every body system. (See *Disorders affecting management of hyperthyroidism*, page 251.)

CARDIOVASCULAR SYSTEM
- Hyperthyroidism causes tachycardia; full, bounding pulse; wide pulse pressure; cardiomegaly; increased cardiac output and blood volume; visible point of maximal impulse; paroxysmal supraventricular tachycardia and atrial fibrillation (especially in elderly people); and occasionally, systolic murmur at the left sternal border.

EYES
- The combined effects of accumulation of mucopolysaccharides and fluids in the retro-orbital tissues may force the eyeball outward (exophthalmos) and the lid to retract, producing the characteristic staring gaze of hyperthyroidism.
- Inflammation of conjunctivae, corneas, or eye muscles may occur.
- Diplopia and increased tearing may occur.
- The eyes may not be able to close, causing the exposed corneal surfaces to become dry and irritated.

GASTROINTESTINAL SYSTEM
- Increased GI mobility and peristalsis may cause anorexia, nausea and vomiting, increased defecation, soft stools or, with severe disease, diarrhea and liver and spleen enlargement.

INTEGUMENTARY SYSTEM
- Skin becomes smooth, warm, and flushed; the patient sleeps with minimal covering and little clothing.
- Fine, soft hair; premature graying; and increased hair loss occurs in both sexes.
- Nails become friable and onycholysis (distal nail becomes separated from the bed) develops.
- Pretibial myxedema (dermopathy) produces thickened skin, accentuated hair follicles, and raised red patches of skin that are itchy and sometimes painful with occasional nodule formation. Microscopic examination shows increased mucin deposits.

NEUROLOGIC SYSTEM
- Increased T4 secretion accelerates cerebral function, causing difficulty in concentrating.
- Excitability or nervousness occurs because of an increased basal metabolic rate.
- Increased activity in the spinal cord area that controls muscle tone leads to fine tremor, shaky handwriting, and clumsiness.
- Emotional instability and mood swings range from occasional outbursts to overt psychosis.

MUSCULOSKELETAL SYSTEM
- Weakness, fatigue, and muscle atrophy may develop.
- Generalized or localized paralysis is associated with hypokalemia.
- Occasionally, acropachy—soft-tissue swelling, accompanied by underlying bone changes where new bone formation occurs—develops.

REPRODUCTIVE SYSTEM
- In females, oligomenorrhea or amenorrhea, decreased fertility, and higher incidence of spontaneous abortions may occur.
- In males, gynecomastia (due to increased estrogen levels) may occur.
- In both sexes, libido is diminished.

RESPIRATORY SYSTEM
◆ Cardiac decompensation and increased cellular oxygen use cause an increased respiratory rate and dyspnea on exertion and at rest.

ASSESSMENT

HISTORY
◆ Nervousness, tremor
◆ Heat intolerance
◆ Weight loss despite increased appetite
◆ Sweating
◆ Frequent bowel movements
◆ Palpitations
◆ Poor concentration
◆ Shaky handwriting
◆ Clumsiness
◆ Emotional instability and mood swings
◆ Thin, brittle nails
◆ Hair loss
◆ Nausea and vomiting
◆ Weakness and fatigue
◆ Oligomenorrhea or amenorrhea
◆ Fertility problems
◆ Diminished libido
◆ Diplopia

PHYSICAL FINDINGS
◆ Enlarged thyroid (goiter)
◆ Exophthalmos (Graves' disease)
◆ Tremor
◆ Smooth, warm, flushed skin
◆ Fine, soft hair
◆ Premature graying and increased hair loss
◆ Friable nails and onycholysis
◆ Pretibial myxedema
◆ Thickened skin
◆ Accentuated hair follicles
◆ Tachycardia at rest
◆ Full, bounding pulses
◆ Arrhythmias, especially atrial fibrillation
◆ Wide pulse pressure
◆ Possible systolic murmur
◆ Dyspnea
◆ Hepatomegaly
◆ Hyperactive bowel sounds
◆ Weakness, especially in proximal muscles, and atrophy
◆ Possible generalized or localized paralysis
◆ Gynecomastia in males
◆ Increased tearing

DIAGNOSTIC TEST RESULTS
◆ Radioimmunoassay shows increased serum triiodothyronine and thyroxine concentrations.
◆ Serum protein-bound iodine level increases.
◆ Serum cholesterol and total lipid levels decrease.
◆ TSH level decreases.
◆ Thyroid scan shows increased uptake of radioactive iodine (^{131}I).
◆ Ultrasonography shows subclinical ophthalmopathy.

TREATMENT

GENERAL
◆ Eye care, such as sunglasses, cool compresses, and lubricating drops (for Graves' disease)

DIET
◆ Adequate caloric and fluid intake

ACTIVITY
◆ As tolerated

MEDICATIONS
◆ Treatment with ^{131}I: a single oral dose; treatment of choice for women past reproductive age or men and women not planning to have children
◆ TH antagonists
◆ Beta-adrenergic antagonists
◆ Corticosteroids
◆ Sedatives

SURGERY
◆ Subtotal (partial) thyroidectomy
◆ Orbital decompression

(continued)

NURSING DIAGNOSES
- Decreased cardiac output
- Diarrhea
- Disturbed body image
- Imbalanced nutrition: Less than body requirements
- Ineffective coping
- Risk for deficient fluid volume
- Risk for imbalanced body temperature

EXPECTED OUTCOMES
The patient will:
- maintain normal cardiac output
- have normal bowel movements
- express positive feelings about body image
- maintain adequate nutrition and hydration with no further weight loss
- demonstrate adaptive coping behaviors
- maintain an adequate fluid balance
- remain normothermic.

NURSING INTERVENTIONS
- Monitor vital signs, daily weight, intake and output, neck circumference, and serum electrolyte results.
- Check for hyperglycemia and glycosuria while on corticosteroids.
- Observe cardiac rhythm for arrhythmias and ST-segment changes and signs and symptoms of heart failure.
- Minimize physical and emotional stress.
- Balance rest periods with activity.
- Keep the patient's room cool and quiet and the lights dim.
- Encourage the patient to dress in loose-fitting, cotton clothing.
- Consult a dietitian to ensure a nutritious diet with adequate calories and fluids.
- Offer small, frequent meals.
- Provide meticulous skin care.
- Reassure the patient and his family that mood swings and nervousness usually subside with treatment.
- Encourage verbalization of feelings.
- Help the patient identify and develop coping strategies.
- Offer emotional support.
- Give prescribed drugs.
- Avoid excessive palpation of the thyroid.
- Note frequency and characteristics of stools.

After thyroidectomy
- Change dressings and perform wound care, as ordered.
- Keep the patient in semi-Fowler's position.
- Support the patient's head and neck with sandbags.
- Observe for signs and symptoms of hemorrhage into the neck.
- Note dysphagia or hoarseness.
- Monitor for signs and symptoms of hypocalcemia.

Be sure to cover:
- disorder, diagnostic testing, and treatment
- medication administration, dosage, and possible adverse effects
- when to notify the practitioner
- need for regular medical follow-up visits
- need for lifelong TH replacement
- importance of wearing medical identification jewelry
- precautions with ^{131}I therapy
- signs and symptoms of hypothyroidism and hyperthyroidism
- eye care for ophthalmopathy.

RESOURCES
Organizations
American Association of Clinical Endocrinologists: *www.aace.com*
Endocrine and Metabolic Diseases Information Service: *www.endocrine.niddk.nih.gov*
Endocrine Society: *www.endo-society.org*

Selected references
Franklyn, J.A., et al. "Thyroid Function and Mortality in Patients Treated for Hyperthyroidism," *JAMA* 294(1):71-80, July 2005.
Liles, A., and Harrell, K. "Common Thyroid Disorders: A Review of Therapies," *Advance for Nurse Practitioners* 14(1):29-32, January 2006.
Noble, N.A. "Thyroid Storm," *Journal of Perianesthesia Nursing* 21(2):119-22, April 2006.
Strategies for Managing Multisystem Disorders. Philadelphia: Lippincott Williams & Wilkins, 2006.

Disorders affecting management of hyperthyroidism

This chart highlights disorders that affect the management of hyperthyroidism.

DISORDER	SIGNS AND SYMPTOMS	DIAGNOSTIC TEST RESULTS	TREATMENT AND CARE
Cardiac arrhythmias (complication)	*Supraventricular tachycardia* ◆ Rapid apical pulse rate ◆ Rapid peripheral pulse rate ◆ Regular or irregular rhythm, depending on the type of atrial tachycardia ◆ Sudden feeling of palpitations, especially with paroxysmal atrial tachycardia ◆ Decreased cardiac output and possible hypotension and syncope from persistent tachycardia and rapid ventricular rate *Atrial fibrillation* ◆ Irregularly irregular pulse rhythm with normal or abnormal heart rate ◆ Radial pulse rate slower than apical pulse rate ◆ Palpable peripheral pulse with the stronger contractions of atrial fibrillation ◆ Hypotension ◆ Light-headedness	◆ Electrocardiography reveals cardiac arrhythmias—usually paroxysmal supraventricular tachycardia or atrial fibrillation. ◆ Chest X-ray may show heart failure.	◆ Monitor heart rhythm continuously. ◆ Monitor vital signs. ◆ Chemical conversion may include administration of adenosine (Adenocard), diltiazem (Cardizem), procainamide (Procanbid), or amiodarone (Cordarone) I.V. ◆ Synchronized electrical conversion may be needed; premedicate the patient with sedatives and heparin, as appropriate. ◆ Continue treatment with beta-adrenergic blockers, calcium channel blockers, digoxin, or antiarrhythmics. ◆ Administer anticoagulants, as appropriate. ◆ Encourage follow-up care with a cardiologist.
Osteoporosis (complication)	◆ Dowager's hump (kyphosis) ◆ Back pain (thoracic and lumbar) ◆ Loss of height ◆ Unsteady gait ◆ Joint pain ◆ Weakness	◆ X-ray reveals characteristic degeneration in the lower vertebrae. ◆ Parathyroid levels may be elevated. ◆ Bone biopsy allows direct examination of changes in bone cells and the rate of bone turnover. ◆ Dual photon or dual energy X-ray absorptiometry can detect bone loss; bone mineral density is 2.5 or more below the young adult reference mean.	◆ Provide supportive devices such as a back brace. ◆ Encourage lifestyle modifications, such as weight loss, exercise program, and dietary modifications, as appropriate. ◆ Offer analgesics and heat for pain relief. ◆ Give calcium and vitamin D supplements to help support normal bone metabolism. ◆ Give sodium fluoride to stimulate bone formation. ◆ Calcitonin may reduce bone resorption and slow the decline in bone mass.
Thyroid storm (complication)	◆ Marked tachycardia ◆ Vomiting ◆ Stupor ◆ Vascular collapse ◆ Hypotension ◆ Irritability ◆ Restlessness ◆ Visual disturbances (diplopia) ◆ Tremor ◆ Weakness ◆ Angina ◆ Shortness of breath ◆ Cough ◆ Swollen extremities ◆ Warm, moist, flushed skin ◆ Hyperthermia ◆ Coma ◆ Death	◆ Diagnosis is based on clinical findings for immediate treatment. ◆ Triiodothyronine (T_3) and thyroxine (T_4) are elevated; free T_4 is elevated; T_3 resin uptake is increased. ◆ Thyroid-stimulating hormone is suppressed. ◆ 24-hour iodine uptake is elevated.	◆ Monitor patients with a history of hyperthyroidism for thyroid storm. ◆ Monitor vital signs. ◆ Provide supplemental oxygen and ventilation support, as needed. ◆ Administer antiadrenergic and antithyroid drugs. ◆ Provide supportive, symptomatic care.

Hypocalcemia

OVERVIEW

- Deficient serum levels of calcium
- Occurs equally in males and females and affects people of all ages

CAUSES

- Hypomagnesemia
- Hypoparathyroidism
- Inadequate dietary intake of calcium and vitamin D
- Malabsorption or loss of calcium from the GI tract
- Overcorrection of acidosis
- Pancreatic insufficiency
- Renal failure
- Severe infections or burns

PATHOPHYSIOLOGY

- Together with phosphorous, calcium is responsible for the formation and structure of bones and teeth.
- Calcium helps maintain cell structure and function and plays a role in cell membrane permeability and impulse transmission.
- It affects the contraction of cardiac muscle, smooth muscle, and skeletal muscle and also participates in the blood-clotting process.
- Pathophysiologic processes involved in hypocalcemia vary depending on the cause. (See *Disorders affecting management of hypocalcemia*, pages 254 and 255.)

CARDIOVASCULAR SYSTEM

- Arrhythmias, palpitations, decreased cardiac output, and an irregular heart rate may occur because of the lack of calcium and the direct effect on the contractility of the cardiac muscle.
- The presence of hypomagnesemia and hypokalemia can potentiate the cardiac and neurologic effects of hypocalcemia.

GASTROINTESTINAL SYSTEM

- Increased nervous system excitability can lead to diarrhea.

INTEGUMENTARY SYSTEM

- Calcium-phosphate calcification can lead to soft-tissue calcification, causing dry, itchy skin with papular eruptions.
- Calcification of the ocular vessels can lead to conjunctivitis and corneal haziness, which may progress to impaired vision.

NEUROMUSCULAR SYSTEM

- Hypocalcemia can lead to symptoms of tetany, which includes parasthesia in the fingertips and around the mouth. Parasthesia may increase in severity and spread up the arms and to the face, leading to numbness, muscle spasms, and pain.
- Hypocalcemia may lead to hyperreflexia, mental status changes, irritability, confusion, muscle weakness, or seizures.
- Carpopedal spasms, laryngeal spasms, and abdominal muscle cramps or spasms may occur.
- Fractures may occur because of the loss of calcium from the bones.

RENAL SYSTEM

- Precipitation of calcium phosphate can lead to progressive renal impairment.
- Oliguria related to acute or chronic renal failure may occur.

RESPIRATORY SYSTEM

- Hypocalcemia may cause respiratory compromise related to lung tissue calcification.

ASSESSMENT

HISTORY

- Underlying cause
- Anxiety
- Irritability
- Seizures
- Muscle cramps
- Diarrhea

PHYSICAL FINDINGS

- Twitching (see *Clinical effects of hypocalcemia*)
- Carpopedal spasm
- Tetany
- Hypotension
- Confusion
- Positive Chvostek's and Trousseau's signs (see *Eliciting signs of hypocalcemia*)

DIAGNOSTIC TEST RESULTS

- Serum calcium level is less than 8.5 mg/dl.
- Ionized calcium level is less than 4.5 mg/dl.
- Electrocardiography shows lengthened QT interval, prolonged ST segment, and arrhythmias.

TREATMENT

GENERAL

- Treatment of the underlying cause
- Seizure precautions
- Cardiac monitoring

Clinical effects of hypocalcemia

BODY SYSTEM	EFFECTS
Cardiovascular	- Arrhythmias, hypotension
Gastrointestinal	- Increased GI motility, diarrhea
Musculoskeletal	- Paresthesia, tetany or painful tonic muscle spasms, facial spasms, abdominal cramps, muscle cramps, spasmodic contractions
Neurologic	- Anxiety, irritability, twitching around mouth, laryngospasm, seizures, Chvostek's sign, Trousseau's sign
Other	- Blood-clotting abnormalities

DIET

◆ High in calcium and vitamin D

ACTIVITY

◆ As tolerated

MEDICATIONS

◆ Oral calcium and vitamin D supplements
◆ Calcium gluconate I.V.

NURSING CONSIDERATIONS

NURSING DIAGNOSES

◆ Anxiety
◆ Decreased cardiac output
◆ Fear
◆ Impaired gas exchange
◆ Ineffective tissue perfusion: Cardiopulmonary
◆ Risk for injury

EXPECTED OUTCOMES

The patient will:
◆ identify strategies to reduce anxiety
◆ maintain adequate cardiac output
◆ discuss fears and concerns
◆ maintain adequate ventilation and oxygenation
◆ exhibit signs of adequate cardiopulmonary perfusion
◆ remain free from injury.

NURSING INTERVENTIONS

◆ Monitor cardiac rhythm and calcium levels.
◆ Observe for seizures.
◆ Provide safety measures; institute seizure precautions, if appropriate.
◆ Give prescribed calcium replacement.
◆ Monitor I.V. sites if administering calcium I.V. (infiltration causes sloughing).

PATIENT TEACHING

Be sure to cover:
◆ disorder, diagnostic testing, and treatment
◆ medication administration, dosage, and adverse effects
◆ importance of following a high-calcium diet
◆ referral to a dietitian and social services, if indicated.

RESOURCES
Organizations

Endocrine and Metabolic Diseases Information Service: *www.endocrine.niddk.nih.gov*
Mayo Clinic: *www.mayoclinic.com*
National Library of Medicine: *www.nlm.nih.gov*

Selected references

Bellazzini, M.A., and Howes, D.S. "Pediatric Hypocalcemia Seizures: A Case of Rickets," *Journal of Emergency Medicine* 28(2):161-64, February 2005.

McCusker, L., et al. "Hypocalcemia in a Patient with Congenital Heart Disease," *Journal of the Royal Society of Medicine* 100(1):51-53, January 2007.

Sedlacek, M., et al. "Electrolyte Disturbances in the Intensive Care Unit," *Seminars in Dialysis* 19(6):496-501, November-December 2006.

Strategies for Managing Multisystem Disorders. Philadelphia: Lippincott Williams & Wilkins, 2006.

Vivien, B., et al. "Early Hypocalcemia in Severe Trauma," *Critical Care Medicine* 33(9):1946-952, September 2005.

Eliciting signs of hypocalcemia

When the patient complains of muscle spasms and paresthesia in his limbs, try eliciting Chvostek's and Trousseau's signs—indications of tetany associated with calcium deficiency.

Follow the procedures described here, keeping in mind the discomfort they typically cause. If you detect these signs, notify the practitioner immediately. During these tests, watch the patient for laryngospasm, monitor his cardiac status, and have resuscitation equipment nearby.

CHVOSTEK'S SIGN

To elicit this sign, tap the patient's facial nerve just in front of the earlobe and below the zygomatic arch or between the zygomatic arch and the corner of the mouth, as shown at right.

A positive response (indicating latent tetany) ranges from simple mouth-corner twitching to twitching of all facial muscles on the side tested. Simple twitching may be normal in some patients. However, a more pronounced response usually confirms Chvostek's sign.

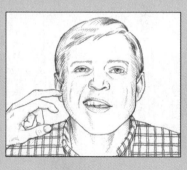

TROUSSEAU'S SIGN

In this test, occlude the brachial artery by inflating a blood pressure cuff on the patient's upper arm to a level between diastolic and systolic blood pressure. Maintain this inflation for 3 minutes while observing the patient for carpal spasm (shown at right), which is Trousseau's sign.

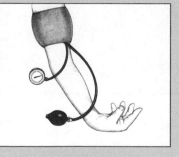

(continued)

Disorders affecting management of hypocalcemia

This chart highlights disorders that affect the management of hypocalcemia.

DISORDER	SIGNS AND SYMPTOMS	DIAGNOSTIC TEST RESULTS	TREATMENT AND CARE
Cardiac arrhythmia (complication)	◆ Palpitations ◆ Chest pain ◆ Dizziness ◆ Weakness, fatigue ◆ Irregular heart rhythm ◆ Hypotension ◆ Syncope ◆ Altered level of consciousness ◆ Diaphoresis, pallor, cold, clammy skin	◆ Electrocardiogram identifies specific waveform changes associated with the arrhythmia. ◆ Laboratory testing reveals electrolyte abnormalities, hypoxemia, or acid-base abnormalities. ◆ Electrophysiologic testing identifies the mechanism of an arrhythmia and the location of accessory pathways.	◆ Assess airway, breathing, and circulation if life-threatening arrhythmia develops; follow advanced cardiac life support protocols for treatment. ◆ Monitor cardiac rhythm continuously, and obtain serial electrocardiograms to evaluate changes and effects of treatment. ◆ Administer antiarrhythmics and monitor for adverse effects. ◆ Assess cardiovascular status for signs of hypoperfusion; monitor vital signs. ◆ Assist with insertion of temporary pacemaker or apply transcutaneous pacemaker, if appropriate.
Heart failure (complication)	◆ Cough that produces pink, frothy sputum ◆ Cyanosis of the lips and nail beds ◆ Pale, cool, clammy skin ◆ Diaphoresis ◆ Jugular vein distention ◆ Ascites ◆ Pulsus alternans ◆ Tachycardia ◆ Hepatomegaly ◆ Decreased pulse pressure ◆ Third and fourth heart sounds (S_3 and S_4) ◆ Moist, basilar crackles ◆ Rhonchi ◆ Expiratory wheezing ◆ Decreased pulse oximetry ◆ Peripheral edema ◆ Decreased urinary output	◆ B-type natriuretic peptide immunoassay is elevated. ◆ Chest X-ray shows increased pulmonary vascular markings, interstitial edema, or pleural effusions and cardiomegaly. ◆ Electrocardiography reveals heart enlargement or ischemia, tachycardia, extrasystole, or atrial fibrillation. ◆ Pulmonary artery pressure, pulmonary artery wedge pressure, and left ventricular end-diastolic pressure are elevated in the presence of left-sided heart failure; right atrial or central venous pressure is elevated in right-sided heart failure.	◆ Administer supplemental oxygen and mechanical ventilation, if needed. ◆ Place the patient in Fowler's position. ◆ Administer diuretics, inotropic drugs, vasodilators, angiotensin-converting enzyme inhibitors, angiotensin receptor blockers, cardiac glycosides, beta-adrenergic blockers, and electrolyte supplements. ◆ Initiate cardiac monitoring. ◆ Recurrent heart failure from valvular dysfunction may require surgery. ◆ A ventricular assist device may be needed. ◆ Maintain adequate cardiac output, and monitor hemodynamic stability. ◆ Assess for deep vein thrombosis, and apply antiembolism stockings.
Seizure (complication)	◆ Aura ◆ Loss of consciousness ◆ Dyspnea ◆ Fixed and dilated pupils ◆ Incontinence	◆ EEG shows abnormal wave patterns and the focus of the seizure activity. ◆ Magnetic resonance imaging may show pathologic changes. ◆ Brain mapping identifies seizure areas.	◆ Ensure patient safety; initiate seizure precautions. ◆ Monitor neurologic and respiratory status. ◆ Observe and document the seizure activity (body movement, respiratory pattern, duration of seizure, loss of consciousness, incontinence, and pupillary response changes). ◆ Administer medications. ◆ Monitor vital signs, intake and output, and laboratory values.

DISORDER	SIGNS AND SYMPTOMS	DIAGNOSTIC TEST RESULTS	TREATMENT AND CARE
Torsades de pointes (complication)	◆ Tachycardia ◆ Hypotension ◆ Poor peripheral pulse ◆ Possibly unconscious with no pulse or respirations	◆ Electrocardiography reveals irregular or regular ventricular rhythm, a ventricular rate of 150 to 250 beats/minute, an unidentifiable P wave, and a wide QRS complex that's usually a phasic variation in electrical polarity (shown by complexes that point downward for several beats).	◆ Monitor cardiac status. ◆ The condition may progress quickly to ventricular fibrillation. Monitor the patient's hemodynamic status, although the patient may be hemodynamically stable with a normal pulse and blood pressure. ◆ Anticipate that the physician will initiate mechanical overdrive pacing. ◆ Be prepared to administer magnesium. ◆ Electrical cardioversion may be used if the patient doesn't respond to other treatments.

Hypochloremia

OVERVIEW

- Deficient serum levels of the chloride anion
- May affect levels of sodium, potassium, calcium, and other electrolytes
- Causes bicarbonate levels to rise (in compensation)

CAUSES

- Addison's disease
- Administration of dextrose I.V. without electrolytes
- Certain drugs (see *Drugs causing hypochloremia*)
- Chloride-deficient formula (for infants)
- Loss of hydrochloric acid in gastric secretions due to vomiting, gastric suctioning, or gastric surgery
- Prolonged diarrhea or diaphoresis
- Prolonged use of mercurial diuretics
- Salt-restricted diets
- Untreated diabetic ketoacidosis

RISK FACTORS

- Cystic fibrosis
- Pyloric obstruction
- Draining fistula
- Ileostomy
- Heart failure

Drugs causing hypochloremia

These kinds of diuretics may cause hypochloremia:
- loop (such as furosemide [Lasix])
- osmotic (such as mannitol [Osmitrol])
- thiazide (such as hydrochlorothiazide [Esidrix]).

PATHOPHYSIOLOGY

- Chloride accounts for two-thirds of all serum anions.
- Chloride is secreted by the stomach's mucosa as hydrochloric acid; it provides an acid medium that aids digestion and activation of enzymes.
- Chloride balance affects many body systems. It participates in maintaining acid-base and body water balances, influences the osmolality or tonicity of extracellular fluid, plays a role in the exchange of oxygen and carbon dioxide in red blood cells, and helps activate salivary amylase (which, in turn, activates the digestive process). (See *Disorders affecting management of hypochloremia*, page 259.)

CARDIOVASCULAR SYSTEM

- As the pH increases, myocardial function may be affected, leading to arrhythmias.

ENDOCRINE AND METABOLIC SYSTEMS

- Accumulation of bicarbonate ions in the extracellular fluid raises the pH level, leading to hypochloremic metabolic alkalosis.

GASTROINTESTINAL SYSTEM

- Excessive loss of fluid through the GI tract can lead to hypochloremic metabolic alkalosis.

INTEGUMENTARY SYSTEM

- Excessive diaphoresis can cause hypochloremia.

NEUROLOGIC SYSTEM

- Hypochloremia can affect the neurologic system by increasing excitability, irritability, or agitation, leading to hyperactive deep tendon reflexes; muscle hypertonicity; tetany; muscle cramps; twitching; and weakness.
- Late-developing neurologic signs of hypochloremia include seizures and coma.

RESPIRATORY SYSTEM

- Hyperchloremic metabolic alkalosis results in a high pH. To compensate, respirations become slow and shallow as the body attempts to retain carbon dioxide and restore the pH level to a normal range.
- Untreated hypochloremia may lead to respiratory arrest.

ASSESSMENT

HISTORY
- Risk factors for low chloride levels
- Agitation
- Irritability

PHYSICAL FINDINGS
- Muscle weakness
- Twitching
- Tetany
- Shallow, depressed breathing
- Hyperactive deep tendon reflexes
- Muscle cramps
- Cardiac arrhythmias

DIAGNOSTIC TEST RESULTS
- Serum chloride level is less than 98 mEq/L.
- Serum sodium level is less than 135 mEq/L.
- Supportive values in metabolic alkalosis:
- Serum pH is greater than 7.45.
- Serum carbon dioxide level is greater than 32 mEq/L.

TREATMENT

GENERAL
- Treatment of underlying condition
- Treatment of associated metabolic acidosis or electrolyte imbalances

DIET
- High-sodium with foods high in chloride

ACTIVITY
- As tolerated

MEDICATIONS
- Normal saline I.V. solution
- Ammonium chloride
- Potassium chloride (for metabolic acidosis)

NURSING CONSIDERATIONS

NURSING DIAGNOSES
- Anxiety
- Ineffective breathing pattern
- Ineffective tissue perfusion: Cardiopulmonary
- Risk for injury

EXPECTED OUTCOMES
The patient will:
- express feelings of decreased anxiety
- maintain effective breathing pattern
- maintain adequate cardiac output
- remain free from injury.

NURSING INTERVENTIONS
- Observe level of consciousness.
- Assess muscle strength, movement, and respiratory status.
- Monitor cardiac rhythm, arterial blood gas levels, and serum electrolyte levels.
- Report signs of metabolic alkalosis.
- Offer foods high in chloride. (See *Dietary sources of chloride.*)
- Provide environmental safety.
- Give prescribed I.V. fluids and drugs.

Dietary sources of chloride

These foods provide chloride:
- fruits
- vegetables
- table salt
- salty foods
- processed meats
- canned vegetables.

(continued)

Be sure to cover:
- disorder, diagnostic testing, and treatment
- medication administration, dosage, and possible adverse effects
- signs and symptoms of electrolyte imbalance
- dietary supplements.

RESOURCES
Organizations
Endocrine and Metabolic Diseases Information Service: *www.endocrine.niddk.nih.gov*

National Institute of Diabetes & Digestive & Kidney Diseases: *www.niddk.nih.gov*

Selected references
Khanna, A., and Kurtzman, N. "Metabolic Alkalosis," *Journal of Nephrology* 19(Suppl 9):S86-96, March-April 2006.

Sedlacek, M., et al. "Electrolyte Disturbances in the Intensive Care Unit," *Seminars in Dialysis* 19(6):496-501, November-December 2006.

Strategies for Managing Multisystem Disorders. Philadelphia: Lippincott Williams & Wilkins, 2006.

Disorders affecting management of hypochloremia

This chart highlights disorders that affect the management of hypochloremia.

DISORDER	SIGNS AND SYMPTOMS	DIAGNOSTIC TEST RESULTS	TREATMENT AND CARE
Acute respiratory failure (complication)	◆ Tachypnea ◆ Cyanosis ◆ Crackles, rhonchi, wheezing ◆ Diminished breath sounds ◆ Restlessness ◆ Altered mental status ◆ Tachycardia ◆ Increased cardiac output ◆ Increased blood pressure ◆ Cardiac arrhythmias	◆ Arterial blood gas (ABG) values show deteriorating values. ◆ Chest X-ray shows pulmonary disease or condition. ◆ Pulse oximetry shows decreasing arterial oxygen consumption.	◆ Administer oxygen therapy and monitor respiratory status; assist with endotracheal intubation and mechanical ventilation, if necessary. ◆ Assess breath sounds and note changes. ◆ Monitor ABG values and pulse oximetry. ◆ Monitor vital signs and intake and output. ◆ Monitor cardiac rhythm for arrhythmias. ◆ Administer antibiotics, bronchodilators, corticosteroids, positive inotropic agents, diuretics, vasopressors, or antiarrhythmics.
Metabolic alkalosis (complication)	◆ Anorexia ◆ Apathy ◆ Confusion ◆ Cyanosis ◆ Hypotension ◆ Loss of reflexes ◆ Muscle twitching ◆ Nausea and vomiting ◆ Paresthesia ◆ Polyuria ◆ Weakness ◆ Cardiac arrhythmias ◆ Decreased rate and depth of respirations	◆ ABG values show pH greater than 7.45, HCO_3^- greater than 26 mEq/L, and partial pressure of carbon dioxide greater than 45 mm Hg (indicates attempts at respiratory compensation). ◆ Potassium level is less than 3.5 mEq/L. ◆ Calcium level is less than 8.9 mg/dl. ◆ Chloride level is less than 98 mEq/L. ◆ Electrocardiography may show a low T wave merging with a P wave and atrial or sinus tachycardia.	◆ Administer potassium chloride and normal saline solution I.V. ◆ Monitor electrolytes and ABG results. ◆ Monitor respiratory status and cardiac rhythm; administer oxygen, as needed. ◆ Discontinue diuretics. ◆ Administer oral or I.V. acetazolamide (Diamox). ◆ Monitor vital signs, pulse oximetry readings, and intake and output. ◆ Initiate seizure precautions.
Seizure (complication)	◆ Aura ◆ Loss of consciousness ◆ Dyspnea ◆ Fixed and dilated pupils ◆ Incontinence	◆ EEG shows abnormal wave patterns and the focus of the seizure activity. ◆ Magnetic resonance imaging may show pathologic changes. ◆ Brain mapping identifies seizure areas.	◆ Observe and record the seizure activity (initial movement, respiratory pattern, duration of seizure, loss of consciousness, aura, incontinence, and pupillary changes). ◆ Assess postictal state. ◆ Protect the patient from falls. ◆ Assess neurologic and respiratory status. ◆ Administer medications. ◆ Maintain seizure precautions. ◆ Monitor and record vital signs, intake and output, neurovital signs, and laboratory studies.

Hypokalemia LIFE-THREATENING DISORDER

OVERVIEW

- Deficient serum levels of the potassium anion
- Normal range: 3.5 to 5 mEq/L; slight decrease can have profound consequences
- Affects up to 20% of hospitalized patients, but is significant in only 4% to 5% of these patients
- Up to 14% of all outpatients mildly affected
- Affects about 80% of patients who receive diuretics
- Affects males and females equally

CAUSES

- Acid-base imbalances
- Certain drugs, especially potassium-wasting diuretics, steroids, and certain sodium-containing antibiotics (carbenicillin) (see *Drugs causing hypokalemia*)
- Chronic renal disease, with tubular potassium wasting
- Cushing's syndrome
- Excessive GI or urinary losses, such as vomiting, gastric suction, diarrhea, dehydration, anorexia, or chronic laxative abuse
- Excessive ingestion of licorice
- Hyperglycemia
- Low-potassium diet
- Primary hyperaldosteronism
- Prolonged potassium-free I.V. therapy
- Severe serum magnesium deficiency
- Trauma (injury, burns, or surgery)

PATHOPHYSIOLOGY

- Potassium is a major cation in the intracellular fluid; therefore, a deficit in this electrolyte can have a significant impact on the body. (See *Disorders affecting management of hypokalemia*, page 263.)
- Potassium facilitates contraction of both skeletal and smooth muscles, including myocardial contraction.
- Potassium figures prominently in nerve impulse conduction, acid-base balance, enzyme action, and cell membrane function.
- Potassium imbalance can lead to muscle weakness and flaccid paralysis because of an ionic imbalance in neuromuscular tissue excitability.

CARDIOVASCULAR SYSTEM

- Abnormalities of the electrophysiology and contractility of the heart muscle lead to orthostatic hypotension and a weak and irregular pulse, possibly resulting in cardiac arrest.

ENDOCRINE AND METABOLIC SYSTEMS

- Hypokalemia impairs insulin release and organ sensitivity to insulin, which contributes to worsening hyperglycemia in patients with diabetes.
- Vomiting can lead to metabolic alkalosis related to gastric acid loss and the movement of potassium ions into the cell as hydrogen ions move out of the cell.

GASTROINTESTINAL SYSTEM

- Anorexia, nausea, vomiting, prolonged gastric emptying, and paralytic ileus may result from a weakness of the GI tract's smooth muscle.

NEUROMUSCULAR SYSTEM

- Neurologic involvement includes muscle weakness, especially in the legs, which eventually leads to paresthesia and leg cramps.
- Deep tendon reflexes may be decreased or absent.

RENAL SYSTEM

- The patient may experience polyuria, nocturia, dilute urine, and polydipsia related to the inability to concentrate urine.
- Cell function is affected, which can produce rhabdomyolysis—a breakdown of muscle fibers leading to myoglobin in the urine.

RESPIRATORY SYSTEM

- The effects on the neurologic system can subsequently lead to paralysis of the respiratory muscles and to respiratory failure.

Drugs causing hypokalemia

These drugs can deplete potassium and cause hypokalemia:
- adrenergics, such as albuterol (Proventil) and epinephrine
- antibiotics, such as amphotericin B, carbenicillin (Geocillin), and gentamicin
- cisplatin
- corticosteroids
- diuretics, such as furosemide and thiazide
- insulin
- laxatives (when used excessively).

HISTORY

◆ Muscle weakness
◆ Paresthesia
◆ Abdominal cramps
◆ Anorexia
◆ Nausea, vomiting
◆ Constipation
◆ Polyuria

PHYSICAL FINDINGS

◆ Hyporeflexia (see *Clinical effects of hypokalemia*)
◆ Weak, irregular pulse
◆ Orthostatic hypotension
◆ Decreased bowel sounds

DIAGNOSTIC TEST RESULTS

◆ Serum potassium level is less than 3.5 mEq/L.
◆ Bicarbonate and pH levels are elevated.
◆ Serum glucose level is slightly elevated.
◆ Electrocardiogram may show a flattened T wave and a depressed ST segment and U wave.

GENERAL

◆ Treatment of the underlying cause

DIET

◆ High potassium

ACTIVITY

◆ As tolerated

MEDICATIONS

◆ Potassium chloride supplements (I.V. or orally)

WARNING *A patient taking a diuretic may be switched to a potassium-sparing diuretic to prevent excessive urinary loss of potassium.*

Clinical effects of hypokalemia

BODY SYSTEM	EFFECTS
Cardiovascular	◆ Dizziness, hypotension, arrhythmias, electrocardiogram changes (flattened T waves, elevated U waves, decreased ST segments), cardiac arrest (with levels < 2.5 mEq/L)
Gastrointestinal	◆ Nausea, vomiting, anorexia, diarrhea, abdominal distention, paralytic ileus or decreased peristalsis
Genitourinary	◆ Polyuria
Musculoskeletal	◆ Muscle weakness and fatigue, leg cramps
Neurologic	◆ Malaise, irritability, confusion, mental depression, speech changes, decreased reflexes, respiratory paralysis
Other	◆ Metabolic alkalosis

(continued)

NURSING DIAGNOSES
- Decreased cardiac output
- Diarrhea
- Fatigue
- Risk for injury

EXPECTED OUTCOMES
The patient will:
- maintain adequate cardiac output and hemodynamic stability
- regain normal bowel elimination pattern
- express feelings of increased energy
- remain free from injury.

NURSING INTERVENTIONS
- Monitor serum potassium levels, cardiac rhythm, intake and output, and vital signs.
- Assess respiratory status.
- Give prescribed drugs.
- Implement safety measures.
- Be alert for signs of hyperkalemia after treatment.
- Administer I.V. fluids.
- Encourage foods high in potassium. (See *Dietary sources of potassium.*)

    WARNING *A patient taking a cardiac glycoside, especially if he's also taking a diuretic, should be monitored closely for hypokalemia, which can potentiate the action of the cardiac glycoside, thus causing toxicity.*

Be sure to cover:
- disorder, diagnostic testing, and treatment
- medication administration, dosage, and possible adverse effects
- how to monitor intake and output
- preventing future episodes of hypokalemia
- need for a high-potassium diet
- warning signs and symptoms to report to the practitioner.

RESOURCES
Organizations
American Heart Association: *www.americanheart.org*
The Merck Manuals Online Medical Library: *www.merck.com/mmhe*
National Institute of Diabetes & Digestive & Kidney Diseases: *www.niddk.nih.gov*
National Library of Medicine: *www.nlm.nih.gov*

Selected references
Miller, J. "Potassium in the Balance: Understanding Hyperkalemia and Hypokalemia," *LPN* 2(5):42-49, October 2006.
Sedlacek, M., et al. "Electrolyte Disturbances in the Intensive Care Unit," *Seminars in Dialysis* 19(6):496-501, November-December 2006.
Stern, E. "Hypokalemia," *AJN* 105(4):15, April 2005.
Strategies for Managing Multisystem Disorders. Philadelphia: Lippincott Williams & Wilkins, 2006.

Dietary sources of potassium

These foods are high in potassium:
- fruits, especially apricots, figs, and bananas and prune juice
- beans and legumes
- green, leafy vegetables, especially spinach
- milk and ice cream
- nuts and seeds
- potatoes
- tomatoes
- bran products.

Disorders affecting management of hypokalemia

This chart highlights disorders that affect the management of hypokalemia.

DISORDER	SIGNS AND SYMPTOMS	DIAGNOSTIC TEST RESULTS	TREATMENT AND CARE
Cardiac arrhythmia (complication)	◆ Palpitations ◆ Chest pain ◆ Dizziness ◆ Weakness, fatigue ◆ Irregular heart rhythm ◆ Hypotension ◆ Syncope ◆ Altered level of consciousness ◆ Diaphoresis, pallor, cold, clammy skin	◆ Electrocardiogram (ECG) identifies specific waveform changes associated with the arrhythmia. ◆ Laboratory testing reveals electrolyte abnormalities, hypoxemia, or acid-base abnormalities. ◆ Electrophysiologic testing identifies the mechanism of an arrhythmia and the location of accessory pathways.	◆ Assess airway, breathing, and circulation if life-threatening arrhythmia develops; follow advanced cardiac life support protocols for treatment. ◆ Monitor cardiac rhythm continuously and obtain serial ECGs to evaluate changes and effects of treatment. ◆ Administer antiarrhythmics and monitor for adverse effects. ◆ Assess cardiovascular status for signs of hypoperfusion; monitor vital signs. ◆ Assist with insertion of temporary pacemaker, or apply transcutaneous pacemaker, if appropriate.
Respiratory arrest (complication)	◆ Absence of spontaneous breathing ◆ No rise or fall of the chest ◆ Inability to feel the movement of air from the mouth or nose ◆ Cyanosis	◆ Arterial blood gas analysis identifies hypoxemia or hypercapnia.	◆ Assess for respirations, circulation, and airway patency. Initiate basic life support in the absence of circulation and respirations and in the presence of a patent airway. ◆ Assess breath sounds; observe for "seesaw" respirations. ◆ Administer oxygen; monitor oxygen saturation using pulse oximetry. ◆ Continually assess for stridor, cyanosis, and changes in level of consciousness. ◆ Prepare for endotracheal intubation or a tracheostomy if the airway can't be established. ◆ Anticipate cardiac arrest; initiate or continue cardiac monitoring. ◆ Place an I.V. line for fluid and medication administration if one isn't already in place. ◆ Administer medications.
Rhabdomyolysis (complication)	◆ Abnormal urine color (dark, red, or cola colored) ◆ Muscle tenderness ◆ Weakness of the affected muscle ◆ Muscle stiffness or aching (myalgia) ◆ Unintentional weight gain ◆ Seizures ◆ Joint pain ◆ Fatigue	◆ Urine myoglobin level exceeds 0.5 mg/dl. ◆ Creatinine kinase level is elevated (0.5 to 0.95 mg/dl) from muscle damage. ◆ Blood urea nitrogen, creatinine, creatine, and phosphate levels are elevated. ◆ Intracompartmental venous pressure measurements are elevated. ◆ Computed tomography, magnetic resonance imaging, and bone scintigraphy are used to detect muscle necrosis. ◆ Urinalysis may reveal casts. ◆ Serum potassium is elevated.	◆ Treat the underlying disorder. ◆ Assess for and prevent renal failure. ◆ Place the patient on bed rest to prevent further muscle breakdown. ◆ Administer I.V. fluids. ◆ Monitor intake and output. ◆ Monitor renal studies, urine myoglobin levels, electrolytes, and acid-base balance. ◆ If renal failure occurs, prepare the patient for dialysis or slow, continuous renal replacement therapy. ◆ Administer anti-inflammatory agents, diuretics, corticosteroids, and analgesics, as appropriate. ◆ Prepare the patient for an immediate fasciotomy and debridement if compartment venous pressures exceed 25 mm Hg.

Hypomagnesemia LIFE-THREATENING DISORDER

OVERVIEW

- Deficient serum levels of the magnesium cation
- Relatively common imbalance
- Occurs in 10% to 20% of hospitalized patients and in 50% to 60% of patients in the intensive care unit
- Occurs in 25% of outpatients with diabetes
- Occurs in 30% to 80% of alcoholics
- Affects males and females equally

CAUSES

- Administration of parenteral fluids without magnesium salts
- Certain drugs (see *Drugs causing hypomagnesemia*)
- Chronic alcoholism
- Chronic diarrhea
- Diabetic acidosis
- Excessive release of adrenocortical hormones
- Hyperaldosteronism
- Hypercalcemia
- Hyperparathyroidism
- Hypoparathyroidism
- Malabsorption syndrome
- Nasogastric suctioning
- Postoperative complications after bowel resection
- Prolonged diuretic therapy
- Severe dehydration
- Starvation or malnutrition

RISK FACTORS

- Sepsis
- Serious burns
- Wounds requiring debridement

PATHOPHYSIOLOGY

- Magnesium is the second most abundant intracellular cation.
- It's active in cellular metabolism and is important for neuromuscular transmission.
- Magnesium is also closely related to calcium, phosphorus, and potassium; thus, changes in magnesium levels can affect multiple body systems.

CARDIOVASCULAR SYSTEM

- Myocardial irritability can lead to cardiac arrhythmias, which can cause a decrease in cardiac output. (See *Disorders affecting management of hypomagnesemia*, page 267.)
- Arrhythmias triggered by a low serum magnesium level include atrial fibrillation, heart block, paroxysmal atrial tachycardia, premature ventricular contractions, supraventricular tachycardia, torsades de pointes, ventricular fibrillation, and ventricular tachycardia.

GASTROINTESTINAL SYSTEM

- Insufficient magnesium can cause anorexia, dysphagia, and nausea and vomiting.

NEUROLOGIC SYSTEM

- Decreased serum magnesium increases the irritability of nerve tissue, possibly leading to altered level of consciousness (LOC), ataxia, confusion, delusions, depression, emotional lability, hallucinations, insomnia, psychosis, seizures, or vertigo.

NEUROMUSCULAR SYSTEM

- As the body compensates for low serum magnesium levels, magnesium moves out of the cells, causing skeletal muscles to become weak and nerves to become hyperirritable.
- Increased nerve irritability can lead to leg and foot cramps, hyperactive deep tendon reflexes, twitching, tremors, tetany, and Chvostek's and Trousseau's signs.

RENAL SYSTEM

- Hypokalemia is a common finding with hypomagnesemia because the kidneys can't conserve potassium in the presence of a magnesium deficiency.

RESPIRATORY SYSTEM

- Respiratory muscles may be affected, possibly leading to respiratory difficulties, respiratory failure, or laryngeal stridor.

Drugs causing hypomagnesemia

Monitor your patient's magnesium level if he's taking any of these drugs that can cause or contribute to hypomagnesemia:

- aminoglycoside antibiotic, such as amikacin, gentamicin, streptomycin, or tobramycin
- amphotericin B
- cisplatin
- cyclosporine
- insulin
- laxative
- loop or thiazide diuretics, such as bumetanide, furosemide, or torsemide
- pentamidine isethionate.

ASSESSMENT

HISTORY
◆ Dysphagia
◆ Nausea
◆ Vomiting
◆ Drowsiness
◆ Confusion
◆ Leg and foot cramps

PHYSICAL FINDINGS
◆ Tachycardia
◆ Hypertension (see *Clinical effects of hypomagnesemia*)
◆ Muscle weakness, tremors, twitching
◆ Hyperactive deep tendon reflexes
◆ Chvostek's and Trousseau's signs
◆ Cardiac arrhythmia

DIAGNOSTIC TEST RESULTS
◆ Serum magnesium level is less than 1.5 mEq/L.
◆ Serum potassium or calcium level is below normal.
◆ Electrocardiography may show abnormalities, such as prolonged QT interval and atrioventricular block.

TREATMENT

GENERAL
◆ Treatment of the underlying cause
◆ Cardiac monitoring
◆ Seizure precautions

DIET
◆ Foods high in magnesium (see *Dietary sources of magnesium*)

ACTIVITY
◆ As tolerated

MEDICATIONS
◆ Magnesium oxide
◆ Magnesium sulfate (I.M. or I.V.)

NURSING CONSIDERATIONS

NURSING DIAGNOSES
◆ Anxiety
◆ Decreased cardiac output
◆ Imbalanced nutrition: Less than body requirements
◆ Risk for injury

EXPECTED OUTCOMES
The patient will:
◆ identify strategies to reduce anxiety
◆ maintain adequate cardiac output and hemodynamic stability
◆ maintain daily calorie requirements
◆ remain free from injury.

NURSING INTERVENTIONS
◆ Monitor vital signs, magnesium levels, electrolyte levels, and intake and output.
◆ Assess cardiac rhythm, LOC, and respiratory status.
◆ Institute seizure precautions.
◆ Give prescribed drugs.
◆ Report abnormal serum electrolyte levels immediately.

WARNING *A low magnesium level may increase a patient's retention of digoxin (Lanoxin). Be alert for signs of digoxin toxicity.*

◆ Ensure patient safety.
◆ Reorient the patient, as needed.
◆ Encourage foods high in magnesium.

Clinical effects of hypomagnesemia

BODY SYSTEM	EFFECTS
Cardiovascular	Arrhythmias, vasomotor changes (vasodilation and hypotension) and, occasionally, hypertension
Neurologic	Confusion, delusions, hallucinations, seizures
Neuromuscular	Hyperirritability, tetany, leg and foot cramps, Chvostek's sign (facial muscle spasms induced by tapping the branches of the facial nerve)

Dietary sources of magnesium

These foods are high in magnesium:
◆ fish, especially tuna and halibut
◆ fruits, especially bananas, figs, and prunes
◆ grains
◆ milk and yogurt
◆ nuts
◆ beans
◆ vegetables, especially artichokes, spinach, and tomatoes.

(continued)

Be sure to cover:
◆ disorder, diagnostic testing, and treatment
◆ medication administration, dosage, and possible adverse effects
◆ avoidance of drugs that deplete magnesium, such as diuretics and laxatives
◆ need to adhere to a high-magnesium diet
◆ danger signs and when to report them
◆ referral to Alcoholics Anonymous, if appropriate.

RESOURCES
Organizations
Endocrine and Metabolic Diseases Information Service: *www.endocrine.niddk.nih.gov*
The Merck Manuals Online Medical Library: *www.merck.com/mmhe*
National Institute of Diabetes & Digestive & Kidney Diseases: *www.niddk.nih.gov*
National Library of Medicine: *www.nlm.nih.gov*

Selected references
Richette, P., et al. "Hypomagnesemia and Chondrocalcinosis in Short Bowel Syndrome," *Journal of Rheumatology* 32(12):2434-436, December 2005.
Shechter, M., and Shechter, A. "Magnesium and Myocardial Infarction," *Clinical Calcium* 15(11):111-15, November 2005.
Strategies for Managing Multisystem Disorders. Philadelphia: Lippincott Williams & Wilkins, 2006.
Tong, G.M., and Rude, R.K. "Magnesium Deficiency in Critical Illness," *Journal of Intensive Care Medicine* 20(1):3-17, January-February 2005.

Disorders affecting management of hypomagnesemia

This chart highlights disorders that affect the management of hypomagnesemia.

DISORDER	SIGNS AND SYMPTOMS	DIAGNOSTIC TEST RESULTS	TREATMENT AND CARE
Acute respiratory failure (complication)	◆ Tachypnea ◆ Cyanosis ◆ Crackles, rhonchi, wheezing ◆ Diminished breath sounds ◆ Restlessness ◆ Altered mental status ◆ Tachycardia ◆ Increased cardiac output ◆ Increased blood pressure ◆ Cardiac arrhythmias	◆ Arterial blood gas (ABG) values show deteriorating values. ◆ Chest X-ray shows pulmonary disease or condition. ◆ Electrocardiogram may show cardiac arrhythmia or right ventricular hypertrophy. ◆ Pulse oximetry shows decreasing arterial oxygen saturation.	◆ Administer oxygen therapy and monitor respiratory status; assist with endotracheal intubation and mechanical ventilation, if necessary. ◆ Assess breath sounds and note changes. ◆ Monitor ABG values and pulse oximetry. ◆ Monitor vital signs and intake and output. ◆ Monitor cardiac rhythm for arrhythmias. ◆ Administer antibiotics, bronchodilators, corticosteroids, positive inotropic agents, diuretics, vasopressors, or antiarrhythmics.
Cardiac arrhythmia (complication)	◆ May be asymptomatic ◆ Dizziness ◆ Hypotension ◆ Syncope ◆ Weakness ◆ Cool, clammy skin ◆ Altered level of consciousness (LOC) ◆ Reduced urine output ◆ Shortness of breath ◆ Chest pain	◆ Electrocardiography detects arrhythmias as well as ischemia and infarction that may result in arrhythmias. ◆ Laboratory testing may reveal electrolyte abnormalities, acid-base abnormalities, or drug toxicities that may cause arrhythmias. ◆ Holter monitoring, event monitoring, and loop recording can detect arrhythmias and effectiveness of drug therapy during a patient's daily activities. ◆ Exercise testing may detect exercise-induced arrhythmias. ◆ Electrophysiologic testing identifies the mechanism of an arrhythmia and the location of accessory pathways; it also assesses the effectiveness of antiarrhythmics, radiofrequency ablation, and implanted cardioverter-defibrillators.	◆ When life-threatening arrhythmias develop, rapidly assess LOC, respirations, and pulse rate. ◆ Initiate cardiopulmonary resuscitation, if indicated. ◆ Evaluate cardiac output resulting from arrhythmias. ◆ If the patient develops heart block, prepare for cardiac pacing. ◆ Administer antiarrhythmics; prepare to assist with medical procedures, if indicated. ◆ Assess intake and output every hour; insert an indwelling urinary catheter, as indicated, to ensure accurate urine measurement. ◆ Document arrhythmias in a monitored patient, and assess for possible causes and effects. ◆ If the patient's pulse is abnormally rapid, slow, or irregular, watch for signs of hypoperfusion, such as hypotension and diminished urine output. ◆ Monitor for predisposing factors, such as fluid and electrolyte imbalance, or possible drug toxicity.
Seizures (complication)	◆ Aura ◆ Loss of consciousness ◆ Dyspnea ◆ Fixed and dilated pupils ◆ Incontinence	◆ EEG shows abnormal wave patterns and the focus of the seizure activity. ◆ Magnetic resonance imaging may show pathologic changes. ◆ Brain mapping identifies seizure areas.	◆ Observe and record the seizure activity (initial movement, respiratory pattern, duration of seizure, loss of consciousness, aura, incontinence, and pupillary changes). ◆ Assess postictal state. ◆ Protect the patient from falls. ◆ Assess neurologic and respiratory status. ◆ Administer anticonvulsants. ◆ Maintain seizure precautions. ◆ Monitor and record vital signs, intake and output, neurovital signs, and laboratory studies.

Hyponatremia

- Deficient serum levels of the sodium cation in relation to body water
- Occurs in about 1% of hospitalized patients
- More common in the very young and very old
- Affects males and females equally

CAUSES

- Adrenal gland insufficiency (Addison's disease) or hypoaldosteronism
- Certain drugs, such as chlorpropamide and clofibrate (see *Drugs causing hyponatremia*)
- Cirrhosis of the liver with ascites
- Diarrhea
- Excessive perspiration or fever
- Excessive water intake
- Infusion of I.V. dextrose in water without other solutes
- Low-sodium diet, usually in combination with one of the other causes
- Malnutrition or starvation
- Suctioning
- Syndrome of inappropriate antidiuretic hormone (SIADH), resulting from brain tumor, stroke, pulmonary disease, or neoplasm with ectopic antidiuretic hormone (ADH) production
- Tap water enemas
- Trauma, surgery (wound drainage), or burns
- Use of potent diuretics
- Vomiting

PATHOPHYSIOLOGY

- Sodium is the major cation (90%) in extracellular fluid; potassium, the major cation in intracellular fluid.
- During repolarization, the sodium-potassium pump continually shifts sodium into the cells and potassium out of the cells; during depolarization, it does the reverse.
- Sodium cation functions include maintaining tonicity and concentration of extracellular fluid, acid-base balance (reabsorption of sodium ion and excretion of hydrogen ion), nerve conduction and neuromuscular function, glandular secretion, and water balance. Thus, hyponatremia has extensive effects on several body systems.

CARDIOVASCULAR SYSTEM

- Associated hypovolemia results in hypotension, tachycardia, vasomotor collapse, and a thready pulse. Central venous pressure and pulmonary artery pressure may be decreased.
- Patients with associated hypervolemia may exhibit edema, jugular vein distention, hypertension, and a rapid, bounding pulse. Central venous pressure and pulmonary artery pressure may be elevated.

INTEGUMENTARY SYSTEM

- Hypovolemia with depletional hyponatremia can cause dry mucous membranes and poor skin turgor related to fluid volume deficits.

METABOLIC AND ENDOCRINE SYSTEMS

- Loss or gain of body fluids may result in weight gain from fluid retention or weight loss from a fluid volume deficit.
- Excessive release of ADH from a disorder of the posterior pituitary leads to SIADH.

NEUROMUSCULAR SYSTEM

- Hyponatremia leads to nerve conduction problems, such as headache, twitching, tremors, and muscle weakness.
- Changes in level of consciousness (LOC) may start as a shortened attention span and progress to lethargy and confusion; as the condition worsens, stupor, seizures, and coma may develop. (See *Disorders affecting management of hyponatremia,* page 271.)

RENAL SYSTEM

- Oliguria or anuria may occur related to renal failure or decreased renal function.

RESPIRATORY SYSTEM

- Severe hyponatremia may lead to cyanosis from inadequate oxygenation.

Drugs causing hyponatremia

Drugs can contribute to the development of hyponatremia by potentiating the action of antidiuretic hormone, by causing syndrome of inappropriate antidiuretic hormone secretion, or by inhibiting sodium reabsorption in the kidney (diuretics).

ANTICONVULSANTS

- carbamazepine (Tegretol)

ANTIDIABETICS

- chlorpropamide (Diabinese)
- utolbutamide (rarely)

ANTINEOPLASTICS

- cyclophosphamide (Cytoxan)
- vincristine

ANTIPSYCHOTICS

- fluphenazine (Prolixin)
- thioridazine
- thiothixene (Navane)

DIURETICS

- bumetanide (Bumex)
- ethacrynic acid (Edecrin)
- furosemide (Lasix)
- thiazides

SEDATIVES

- barbiturates
- morphine

HISTORY
◆ Altered LOC
◆ Nausea
◆ Headache
◆ Muscle weakness
◆ Abdominal cramps

PHYSICAL FINDINGS
◆ Orthostatic hypotension (see *Clinical effects of hyponatremia*)
◆ Dry mucous membranes
◆ Poor skin turgor
◆ Rapid, bounding pulse
◆ Muscle twitching

DIAGNOSTIC TEST RESULTS
◆ Serum sodium level is less than 135 mEq/L.
◆ Urine specific gravity is less than 1.010.
◆ Serum osmolality is less than 280 mOsm/kg (dilute blood).
◆ Urine specific gravity is increased and urine sodium is elevated (0.2 mEq/L).

GENERAL
◆ Treatment of the underlying cause
◆ Cardiac monitoring

DIET
◆ Restricted fluid intake
◆ Adequate sodium

ACTIVITY
◆ As tolerated

MEDICATIONS
◆ Oral sodium supplements
◆ Demeclocycline or lithium (Eskalith)
◆ Administration of normal saline solution
◆ Hypertonic (3% or 5%) saline solutions (with serum sodium levels below 110 mEq/L)

NURSING DIAGNOSES
◆ Anxiety
◆ Fear
◆ Ineffective tissue perfusion: Cardiopulmonary
◆ Risk for imbalanced fluid volume
◆ Risk for injury

EXPECTED OUTCOMES
The patient will:
◆ identify strategies to reduce anxiety
◆ discuss fears and concerns
◆ exhibit signs of adequate cardiopulmonary perfusion
◆ attain and maintain normal fluid volume and electrolyte balance
◆ remain free from injury.

NURSING INTERVENTIONS
◆ Monitor vital signs, serum sodium levels, urine specific gravity, and intake and output.
◆ Assess neurologic status.
◆ Restrict fluid intake.
◆ Give prescribed I.V. fluids.
◆ Provide a safe environment.

Clinical effects of hyponatremia

BODY SYSTEM	EFFECTS
Cardiovascular	◆ Hypotension; tachycardia; with severe deficit, vasomotor collapse, thready pulse
Gastrointestinal	◆ Nausea, vomiting, abdominal cramps
Genitourinary	◆ Oliguria or anuria
Integumentary	◆ Cold, clammy skin; decreasing skin turgor
Neurologic	◆ Anxiety, headaches, muscle twitching and weakness, seizures
Respiratory	◆ Cyanosis with severe deficiency

(continued)

PATIENT TEACHING

Be sure to cover:
- disorder, diagnostic testing, and treatment
- medication administration, dosage, and possible adverse effects
- dietary changes and fluid restrictions
- monitoring daily weight
- signs and symptoms to report to the practitioner.

RESOURCES
Organizations
Endocrine and Metabolic Diseases Information Service: *www.endocrine.niddk.nih.gov*

Mayo Clinic: *www.mayoclinic.com*

National Institute of Diabetes & Digestive & Kidney Diseases: *www.niddk.nih.gov*

National Library of Medicine: *www.nlm.nih.gov*

Selected references
Chen, S., et al. "Evaluation and Treatment of Hyponatremia; An Emerging Role for Vasopression Receptor Antagonists," *Nature Clinical Practice: Nephrology* 3(2): 82-95, February 2007.

Rottmann, C.N. "SSRIs and the Syndrome of Inappropriate Antidiuretic Hormone Secretion," *AJN* 107(1):51-58, January 2007.

Strategies for Managing Multisystem Disorders. Philadelphia: Lippincott Williams & Wilkins, 2006.

Disorders affecting management of hyponatremia

This chart highlights disorders that affect the management of hyponatremia.

DISORDER	SIGNS AND SYMPTOMS	DIAGNOSTIC TEST RESULTS	TREATMENT AND CARE
Adrenal hypofunction (coexisting)	◆ Poor coordination ◆ Bronze discoloration of skin and darkening of scars ◆ Areas of vitiligo ◆ Increased pigmentation of mucous membrane ◆ Weak, irregular pulse ◆ Hypotension ◆ Craving for salty foods ◆ Muscle weakness ◆ Fatigue ◆ Weight loss	◆ Rapid corticotropin stimulation test may show low levels, which indicates a secondary disorder; elevated levels indicate a primary disorder. ◆ Plasma cortisol level is less than 10 mcg/dl in the morning and even lower in the evening. ◆ Serum sodium and fasting blood glucose levels are decreased. ◆ Computed tomography scan of the abdomen shows adrenal calcification.	◆ Encourage increased fluid intake, and administer I.V. fluids, as ordered. ◆ Monitor vital signs, intake and output, and electrolyte levels. ◆ Provide small, frequent, high-protein meals. ◆ Administer corticosteroids. ◆ Monitor blood glucose levels.
Cerebral edema (complication)	◆ Headache (especially new onset) ◆ Irritability ◆ Altered behavior ◆ Drowsiness ◆ Decreasing level of consciousness ◆ Bradycardia ◆ Hypertension	◆ Computed tomography scan and magnetic resonance imaging (MRI) rule out herniation or neoplasms that would cause altered mental status and may show evidence of brain edema.	◆ Administer osmotic diuretics and monitor serum osmolarity. ◆ Elevate the head of the patient's bed to 30 degrees. ◆ Maintain head alignment. ◆ Monitor vital signs and neurologic status.
Seizures (complication)	◆ Aura ◆ Loss of consciousness ◆ Dyspnea ◆ Fixed and dilated pupils ◆ Incontinence	◆ EEG shows abnormal wave patterns and the focus of the seizure activity. ◆ MRI may show pathologic changes. ◆ Brain mapping identifies seizure areas.	◆ Observe and record the seizure activity (initial movement, respiratory pattern, duration of seizure, loss of consciousness, aura, incontinence, and pupillary changes). ◆ Assess postictal state. ◆ Protect the patient from falls. ◆ Assess neurologic and respiratory status. ◆ Administer anticonvulsants. ◆ Maintain seizure precautions. ◆ Monitor and record vital signs, intake and output, neurologic vital signs, and laboratory studies.

Hypoparathyroidism

OVERVIEW

- Deficiency in parathyroid hormone (PTH) secretion by the parathyroid glands or the decreased action of PTH in the periphery
- May be acute or chronic
- Classified as idiopathic, acquired, or reversible
- Idiopathic and reversible forms most common in children
- Acquired form most common in older patients who have undergone thyroid gland surgery

CAUSES

- Abnormalities of the calcium-sensor receptor
- Accidental removal of or injury to one or more parathyroid glands during surgery
- Amyloidosis
- Autoimmune genetic disorder
- Congenital absence or malformation of the parathyroid glands
- Delayed maturation of parathyroid function
- Hemochromatosis
- Hypomagnesemia-induced impairment of hormone secretion
- Ischemia or infarction of the parathyroid glands during surgery
- Massive thyroid irradiation
- Neoplasms
- Sarcoidosis
- Suppression of normal gland function due to hypercalcemia
- Trauma
- Tuberculosis

PATHOPHYSIOLOGY

- PTH normally maintains serum calcium levels by increasing bone resorption and by stimulating renal conversion of vitamin D to its active form, which enhances GI absorption of calcium and bone resorption.
- PTH also maintains the inverse relationship between serum calcium and phosphate levels by inhibiting phosphate reabsorption in the renal tubules and enhancing calcium reabsorption.
- Abnormal PTH production in hypoparathyroidism disrupts this delicate balance. (See *Disorders affecting management of hypoparathyroidism,* page 275.)

NEUROLOGIC SYSTEM

- Decreased calcium levels result in neuromuscular irritability, which may cause paresthesia, muscle twitching, tetany, and seizures.

CARDIOVASCULAR SYSTEM

- Prolonged QTc intervals cause cardiac arrhythmias due to decreased calcium levels and interference with myocardial contraction.

RESPIRATORY SYSTEM

- Potentially life-threatening laryngospasm and stridor may result from decreased calcium levels that result from increased phosphorus levels.

ASSESSMENT

HISTORY

- Neck surgery or irradiation
- Malabsorption disorders
- Alcoholism
- Tingling in the fingertips, around the mouth and, occasionally, in the feet
- Muscle tension and spasms
- Feeling like throat is constricted
- Dysphagia
- Difficulty walking, frequent falls
- Nausea, vomiting, abdominal pain
- Constipation or diarrhea
- Personality changes
- Fatigue

PHYSICAL FINDINGS

- Brittle nails
- Dry skin
- Coarse hair, alopecia
- Transverse and longitudinal ridges in the fingernails
- Loss of eyelashes and fingernails
- Stained, cracked, and decayed teeth
- Tetany
- Positive Chvostek's and Trousseau's signs
- Increased deep tendon reflexes
- Irregular, slow, or rapid pulse

DIAGNOSTIC TEST RESULTS

- Radioimmunoassay for PTH is decreased.
- Serum and urine calcium levels are decreased.
- Serum phosphate level is increased.
- Urine creatinine level is decreased.
- Computed tomography scan shows frontal lobe and basal ganglia calcifications.
- X-rays show increased bone density and bone malformation.
- Electrocardiography shows a prolonged QTc interval.

TREATMENT

GENERAL
- Treatment of underlying cause
- Supportive care for an acute, life-threatening attack or hypoparathyroid tetany

DIET
- High-calcium, low-phosphorus

ACTIVITY
- As tolerated

MEDICATIONS
- Vitamin D
- Supplemental calcium
- Calcitriol (Rocaltrol)

Acute, life-threatening tetany
- I.V. administration of 10% calcium gluconate, 10% calcium gluceptate, or 10% calcium chloride
- Sedatives
- Anticonvulsants

SURGERY
- To treat underlying cause such as a tumor

NURSING CONSIDERATIONS

NURSING DIAGNOSES
- Anxiety
- Decreased cardiac output
- Disturbed body image
- Impaired skin integrity
- Ineffective breathing pattern
- Ineffective coping
- Risk for injury
- Risk for peripheral neurovascular dysfunction

EXPECTED OUTCOMES
The patient will:
- identify strategies to reduce anxiety
- maintain normal cardiac output
- express positive feelings about body image
- maintain skin integrity
- maintain adequate ventilation
- demonstrate adaptive coping behaviors
- remain free from injury
- recognize signs and symptoms of neurovascular impairment.

NURSING INTERVENTIONS
- Monitor vital signs, intake and output, and serum calcium and phosphorus levels.
- Assess electrocardiogram for QT-interval changes and arrhythmias.
- Observe for signs and symptoms of decreased cardiac output.
- Give prescribed drugs.
- Maintain a patent I.V. line.
- Keep emergency equipment readily available.
- Maintain seizure precautions.
- Provide meticulous skin care.
- Institute safety precautions.
- Encourage the patient to express his feelings.
- Offer emotional support.
- Help the patient develop effective coping strategies.
- Assess for Chvostek's and Trousseau's signs.

WARNING *Closely monitor the patient receiving digoxin and calcium because calcium potentiates the effect of digoxin. Stay alert for signs of digoxin toxicity.*

(continued)

Be sure to cover:
♦ disorder, diagnostic testing, and treatment
♦ medication administration, dosage, and possible adverse effects
♦ when to notify the practitioner
♦ follow-up care
♦ signs and symptoms of complications
♦ periodic checks of serum calcium levels
♦ referral to a mental health professional for additional counseling, if necessary.

RESOURCES
Organizations
American Association of Clinical Endocrinologists: *www.aace.com*
Endocrine Society: *www.endo-society.org*

Selected references
Adorni, A., et al. "Extensive Brain Calcification and Dementia in Postsurgical Hypoparathyroidism," *Neurology* 65(9):1501, November 2005.

Diseases, 4th ed. Philadelphia: Lippincott Williams & Wilkins, 2006.

Epstein, M., et al. "Proton-Pump Inhibitors and Hypomagnasemic Hypoparathyroidism," *New England Journal of Medicine* 355(17):1834-836, October 2006.

Even, L., et al. "Nocturnal Calcium, Phosphorus, and Parathyroid Hormone in the Diagnosis of Concealed and Subclinical Hypoparathyroidism," *European Journal of Endocrinology* 156(1):113-16, January 2007.

Heymann, R.S., et al. "Anaplastic Thyroid Carcinoma with Thyrotoxicosis and Hypoparathyroidism," *Endocrine Practice* 11(4):281-84, July-August 2005.

Disorders affecting management of hypoparathyroidism

This chart highlights disorders that affect the management of hypoparathyroidism.

DISORDER	SIGNS AND SYMPTOMS	DIAGNOSTIC TEST RESULTS	TREATMENT AND CARE
Cardiac arrhythmia (complication)	◆ Palpitations ◆ Chest pain ◆ Dizziness ◆ Weakness, fatigue ◆ Irregular heart rhythm ◆ Hypotension ◆ Syncope ◆ Altered level of consciousness ◆ Diaphoresis, pallor, cold, clammy skin	◆ Electrocardiogram (ECG) identifies specific waveform changes associated with the arrhythmia. ◆ Laboratory testing reveals electrolyte abnormalities, hypoxemia, or acid-base abnormalities. ◆ Electrophysiologic testing identifies the mechanism of an arrhythmia and the location of accessory pathways.	◆ Assess airway, breathing, and circulation if life-threatening arrhythmia develops; follow advanced cardiac life support protocols for treatment. ◆ Monitor cardiac rhythm continuously, and obtain serial ECGs to evaluate changes and effects of treatment. ◆ Administer antiarrhythmics and monitor for adverse effects. ◆ Assess cardiovascular status for signs of hypoperfusion; monitor vital signs. ◆ Assist with insertion of temporary pacemaker, or apply transcutaneous pacemaker, if appropriate
Hyperphosphatemia (coexisting)	◆ Anorexia ◆ Nausea and vomiting ◆ Altered mental status ◆ Hyperreflexia ◆ Muscle weakness and cramps ◆ Paresthesia ◆ Chvostek's or Trousseau's sign ◆ Tetany	◆ Serum phosphorus level is greater than 4.5 mg/dl. ◆ Serum calcium level is less than 8.9 mg/dl. ◆ Blood urea nitrogen and creatinine levels are increased. ◆ ECG may show changes characteristic of hypocalcemia.	◆ Provide safety measures. ◆ Monitor vital signs, phosphorus, and calcium levels. ◆ Administer calcium replacements. ◆ Assess for signs and symptoms of hypocalcemia.
Hypocalcemia (coexisting)	◆ Irritability ◆ Seizures ◆ Muscle cramps ◆ Chvostek's or Trousseau's sign ◆ Hypotension ◆ Confusion ◆ Carpopedal spasm ◆ Tetany	◆ Serum calcium level is less than 8.5 mg/dl. ◆ Ionized calcium level is less than 4.5 mg/dl. ◆ ECG shows lengthened QT interval, prolonged ST segment, and arrhythmias.	◆ Provide safety measures; initiate seizure precautions, if appropriate. ◆ Administer calcium replacements. ◆ Monitor cardiac rhythm and vital signs. ◆ Monitor calcium levels.
Seizures (complication)	◆ Aura ◆ Loss of consciousness ◆ Dyspnea ◆ Fixed and dilated pupils ◆ Incontinence	◆ EEG slows abnormal wave patterns and the focus of the seizure activity. ◆ Magnetic resonance imaging may show pathologic changes. ◆ Brain mapping identifies seizure areas.	◆ Ensure patient safety; initiate seizure precautions. ◆ Monitor neurologic and respiratory status. ◆ Observe and document the seizure activity (body movement, respiratory pattern, duration of seizure, loss of consciousness, incontinence, and pupillary changes). ◆ Administer medications. ◆ Monitor vital signs, intake and output, and laboratory values.

Hypophosphatemia

- Deficient serum phosphate levels
- Incidence varies according to underlying cause

CAUSES

- Chronic diarrhea
- Certain drugs (see *Drugs causing hypophosphatemia*)
- Diabetic acidosis
- Hyperparathyroidism with resultant hypercalcemia
- Hypomagnesemia
- Inadequate dietary intake
- Intestinal malabsorption
- Malnutrition, resulting from a prolonged catabolic state or chronic alcoholism
- Renal tubular defects
- Tissue damage in which phosphorus is released by injured cells
- Use of parenteral nutrition solution with inadequate phosphate content
- Vitamin D deficiency

Drugs causing hypophosphatemia

These drugs may cause hypophosphatemia:
- acetazolamide (Diamox), thiazide diuretics (chlorothiazide [Diuril] and hydrochlorothiazide [Esidrix]), loop diuretics (bumetanide [Bumex] and furosemide [Lasix]), and other diuretics
- antacids, such as aluminum carbonate, aluminum hydroxide, calcium carbonate, and magnesium oxide
- insulin
- laxatives.

PATHOPHYSIOLOGY

- Phosphorus exists primarily in inorganic combinations with calcium in teeth and bones.
- In extracellular fluid, the phosphate ion supports several metabolic functions: utilization of B vitamins, acid-base homeostasis, bone formation, nerve and muscle activity, cell division, transmission of hereditary traits, and metabolism of carbohydrates, proteins, and fats.
- Renal tubular reabsorption of phosphate is inversely regulated by calcium levels—an increase in phosphorus causes a decrease in calcium. An imbalance causes hypophosphatemia or hyperphosphatemia.

CARDIOVASCULAR SYSTEM

- The heart's contractility is decreased because of low energy stores of adenosine triphosphate (ATP) and hypotension, possibly resulting in low cardiac output.
- Severe hypophosphatemia may lead to cardiomyopathy, which can be reversed with treatment.
- The patient may experience chest pain due to mechanisms that lead to decreased oxygen delivery to the myocardium.

IMMUNE AND HEMATOLOGIC SYSTEMS

- Because of structural and functional changes to the red blood cells, hypophosphatemia may lead to hemolytic anemia.
- Lack of ATP results in decreased leukocyte production, making the patient susceptible to infection.
- Chronic hypophosphatemia affects platelet function, resulting in bruising and bleeding.

MUSCULOSKELETAL SYSTEM

- Osteomalacia, loss of bone density, and bone pain may occur with prolonged hypophosphatemia and can result in pathological fractures.

NEUROMUSCULAR SYSTEM

- Lack of ATP may lead to muscle weakness, malaise, slurred speech, dysphagia, and a weakened hand grasp. The patient may also experience myalgia.
- Lack of ATP may affect the central nervous system, causing paresthesia, irritability, apprehension, and confusion that may progress to seizures and coma.
- Severe cases of hypophosphatemia may alter muscle cell activity by inhibiting the release of muscle enzymes from the cells into the extracellular fluid, resulting in rhabdomyolysis. (See *Disorders affecting management of hypophosphatemia*, pages 278 and 279.)

RESPIRATORY SYSTEM

- Respiratory failure may result from weakened respiratory muscles and poor contractility of the diaphragm.
- Respirations may be shallow and ineffective, leading to poor oxygenation and cyanosis.

ASSESSMENT

HISTORY
- Anorexia
- Memory loss
- Muscle and bone pain
- Fractures
- Chest pain

PHYSICAL FINDINGS
- Tremor and weakness in speaking voice
- Confusion
- Bruising and bleeding

DIAGNOSTIC TEST RESULTS
- Serum phosphorus level is less than 2.5 mg/dl.

TREATMENT

GENERAL
- Treatment of the underlying cause
- Discontinuation of drugs that may cause hypophosphatemia

DIET
- High-phosphorus

ACTIVITY
- As tolerated

MEDICATIONS
- Phosphate salt tablets or capsules
- Potassium phosphate I.V.

NURSING CONSIDERATIONS

NURSING DIAGNOSES
- Acute pain
- Anxiety
- Impaired gas exchange
- Risk for injury

EXPECTED OUTCOMES
The patient will:
- express feelings of increased comfort and decreased pain
- identify strategies to reduce anxiety
- maintain adequate ventilation and oxygenation
- remain free from injury.

NURSING INTERVENTIONS
- Provide safety measures.
- Give prescribed phosphorus replacement.
- Assist with ambulation and activities of daily living.
- Encourage intake of foods high in phosphorus. (See *Dietary sources of phosphorus.*)
- Assess respiratory and neurologic status.
- Monitor phosphorus and calcium levels and intake and output.

PATIENT TEACHING

Be sure to cover:
- disorder, diagnostic testing, and treatment
- medication administration, dosage, and adverse effects
- importance of adhering to a high-phosphorus diet
- referral to a dietitian and social services, if indicated.

RESOURCES
Organizations
Alcoholics Anonymous: *www.alcoholicsanonymous.org*
Endocrine and Metabolic Diseases Information Service: *www.endocrine.niddk.nih.gov*
National Institute of Diabetes & Digestive & Kidney Diseases: *www.niddk.nih.gov*
National Library of Medicine: *www.nlm.nih.gov*

Selected references
Gaasbeek, A., and Meinders, A.E. "Hypophosphatemia: An Update on Its Etiology and Treatment," *American Journal of Medicine* 118(10):1094-1101, October 2005.

Heames, R., and Cope, R. "Hypophosphatemia Causing Profound Cardiac Failure after Cardiac Surgery," *Anaesthesia* 61(12):1211-213, December 2006.

Marinella, M.A. "Refeeding Syndrome and Hypophosphatemia," *Journal of Intensive Care Medicine* 20(3):155-59, May-June 2005.

Strategies for Managing Multisystem Disorders. Philadelphia: Lippincott Williams & Wilkins, 2006.

Dietary sources of phosphorus

These foods are high in phosphorus:
- instant breakfast products
- bran muffins and cereal
- homemade waffles
- milk and yogurt
- fruits, especially raisins and bananas
- fish
- beans
- nuts
- lentils

(continued)

Disorders affecting management of hypophosphatemia

This chart highlights disorders that affect the management of hypophosphatemia.

DISORDER	SIGNS AND SYMPTOMS	DIAGNOSTIC TEST RESULTS	TREATMENT AND CARE
Cardiac arrhythmia (complication)	◆ Possibly asymptomatic ◆ Dizziness ◆ Hypotension ◆ Syncope ◆ Weakness ◆ Cool, clammy skin ◆ Altered level of consciousness (LOC) ◆ Reduced urine output ◆ Shortness of breath ◆ Chest pain	◆ ECG detects arrhythmias as well as ischemia and infarction that may result in arrhythmias. ◆ Laboratory testing may reveal electrolyte abnormalities, acid-base abnormalities, or drug toxicities that may cause arrhythmias. ◆ Holter monitoring, event monitoring, and loop recording can detect arrhythmias and effectiveness of drug therapy during a patient's daily activities. ◆ Exercise testing may detect exercise-induced arrhythmias. ◆ Electrophysiologic testing identifies the mechanism of the arrhythmia.	◆ When life-threatening arrhythmias develop, rapidly assess LOC, respirations, and pulse rate. ◆ Initiate cardiopulmonary resuscitation, if indicated. ◆ Evaluate cardiac output resulting from arrhythmias. ◆ If the patient develops heart block, prepare for cardiac pacing. ◆ Administer antiarrhythmics; prepare to assist with medical procedures, if indicated. ◆ Assess intake and output every hour; insert an indwelling urinary catheter, as indicated, to ensure accurate urine measurement. ◆ Document arrhythmias in a monitored patient and assess for possible causes and effects. ◆ If the patient's pulse is abnormally rapid, slow, or irregular, watch for signs of hypoperfusion, such as hypotension and diminished urine output. ◆ Monitor for predisposing factors, such as fluid and electrolyte imbalance, or possible drug toxicity.
Metabolic acidosis (complication)	◆ Confusion ◆ Decreased deep tendon reflexes ◆ Dull headache ◆ Hyperkalemic signs and symptoms (including abdominal cramping, diarrhea, muscle weakness, and electrocardiogram [ECG] changes) ◆ Hypotension ◆ Kussmaul's respirations ◆ Lethargy ◆ Warm, dry skin	◆ Arterial blood gas (ABG) analysis reveals a pH below 7.35. Partial pressure of arterial carbon dioxide may be less than 35 mm Hg. ◆ Serum potassium levels are usually elevated. ◆ Blood glucose and serum ketone levels rise in patients with diabetic ketoacidosis (DKA). ◆ Plasma lactate levels rise in patients with lactic acidosis. ◆ The anion gap is increased. (Normal anion gap is 8 to 14 mEq/L.) ◆ ECG reveals changes associated with hyperkalemia, such as tall T waves, prolonged PR intervals, and widened QRS complexes.	◆ Monitor vital signs and assess cardiac rhythm. ◆ Prepare for mechanical ventilation or dialysis, as required. ◆ Monitor the patient's neurologic status closely because changes can occur rapidly. Notify the physician of changes in the patient's condition. ◆ Insert an I.V. line and maintain patent I.V. access. Have a large-bore catheter in place for emergency situations. ◆ Administer I.V. fluids, vasopressors, antibiotics, and other medications (such as sodium bicarbonate). ◆ Position the patient to promote chest expansion and facilitate breathing. If the patient is stuporous, turn him frequently. ◆ Take steps to help eliminate the underlying cause. For example, administer insulin and I.V. fluids to reverse DKA. ◆ Watch for secondary changes that hypovolemia may cause, such as declining blood pressure. ◆ Monitor the patient's renal function by recording intake and output. ◆ Watch for changes in the serum electrolyte levels, and monitor ABG results throughout treatment to check for overcorrection. ◆ Orient the patient, as needed. If he's confused, take steps to ensure his safety, such as keeping his bed in the lowest position.

Disorders affecting management of hypophosphatemia *(continued)*

DISORDER	SIGNS AND SYMPTOMS	DIAGNOSTIC TEST RESULTS	TREATMENT AND CARE
Rhabdomyolysis (complication)	◆ Abnormal urine color (dark, red, or cola colored) ◆ Muscle tenderness ◆ Weakness of the affected muscle ◆ Muscle stiffness or aching (myalgia) ◆ Unintentional weight gain ◆ Seizures ◆ Joint pain ◆ Fatigue	◆ Urine myoglobin level exceeds 0.5 mg/dl. ◆ Creatinine kinase level is elevated (0.5 to 0.95 mg/dl) from muscle damage. ◆ Blood urea nitrogen, creatinine, creatine, and phosphate levels are elevated. ◆ Intracompartmental venous pressure measurements are elevated. ◆ Computed tomography, magnetic resonance imaging, and bone scintigraphy detect muscle necrosis. ◆ Urinalysis may reveal casts. ◆ Serum potassium is elevated.	◆ Treat the underlying disorder. ◆ Assess for and prevent renal failure. ◆ Place the patient on bed rest to prevent further muscle breakdown. ◆ Administer I.V. fluids. ◆ Monitor intake and output. ◆ Monitor renal studies, urine myoglobin levels, electrolytes, and acid-base balance. ◆ In the presence of renal failure, prepare the patient for dialysis or slow, continuous renal replacement therapy. ◆ Administer anti-inflammatory agents, diuretics, corticosteroids, and analgesics. ◆ Prepare patient for an immediate fasciotomy and debridement, if compartment venous pressures exceed 25 mm Hg.

Hypopituitarism

- Partial or complete failure of the anterior pituitary gland to produce its vital hormones: luteinizing hormone (LH), follicle-stimulating hormone (FSH), thyroid-stimulating hormone (TSH), corticotropin, growth hormone (GH), and prolactin
- May be primary or secondary, resulting from dysfunction of the hypothalamus
- Development of clinical features typically slow in onset and not apparent until 75% of the pituitary gland is destroyed
- Prognosis good with adequate replacement therapy and correction of the underlying cause
- Relatively rare
- Affects adults and children
- Affects males and females equally
- Panhypopituitarism: absence of all hormone production; fatal without treatment

CAUSES
- Congenital defects
- Deficiency of hypothalamus-releasing hormones
- Granulomatous disease
- Idiopathic
- Infection
- Partial or total hypophysectomy by surgery, irradiation, or chemical agents
- Pituitary gland hypoplasia or aplasia
- Pituitary infarction
- Trauma
- Tumor

PATHOPHYSIOLOGY

- The pituitary gland is extremely vulnerable to ischemia and infarction because it's highly vascular.
- Any event that leads to circulatory collapse and compensatory vasospasm may result in gland ischemia, tissue necrosis, or edema.
- Expansion of the pituitary within the fixed compartment of the sella turcica further impedes blood supply to the pituitary. (See *Disorders affecting management of hypopituitarism,* page 283.)

ENDOCRINE SYSTEM
- Lack of pituitary function can result in diminished hormone production, which can affect various body functions and growth, based on which hormone production is affected
- Space-occupying lesions that affect the hypothalamus may result in syndrome of inappropriate antidiuretic hormone secretion, causing fluid and electrolyte imbalances.

REPRODUCTIVE SYSTEM
- Lack of gonadotropin can result in stunted sexual organ growth, impotence, and infertility.

MUSCULOSKELETAL SYSTEM
- Diminished or absent GH results in stunted growth of long bones, beginning in infancy.
- Failure to thrive may occur.

NEUROLOGIC SYSTEM
- Hypopituitarism caused by space-occupying tumors may cause headaches and vision disturbances.

ASSESSMENT

HISTORY
- Signs and symptoms dependent on which pituitary hormones are deficient, patient's age, and severity of disorder

Gonadotropin (FSH and LH) deficiency in females
- Amenorrhea
- Dyspareunia
- Infertility
- Reduced libido

Gonadotropin (FSH and LH) deficiency in males
- Impotence
- Reduced libido

TSH deficiency
- Cold intolerance
- Constipation
- Menstrual irregularity
- Lethargy
- Severe growth retardation in children despite treatment

Corticotropin deficiency
- Fatigue
- Nausea, vomiting, anorexia
- Weight loss

Prolactin deficiency
- Absent postpartum lactation
- Amenorrhea

PHYSICAL FINDINGS
GH deficiency
- Physical signs possibly not apparent in neonate
- Growth retardation usually apparent at age 6 months

In children
- Chubbiness from fat deposits in the lower trunk
- Short stature
- Delayed secondary tooth eruption
- Delayed puberty
- Average height of 48″ (1.2 m), with normal proportions

Gonadotropin (FSH and LH) deficiency in females
◆ Breast atrophy
◆ Sparse or absent axillary and pubic hair
◆ Dry skin

Gonadotropin (FSH and LH) deficiency in males
◆ Decreased muscle strength
◆ Testicular softening and shrinkage
◆ Retarded secondary sexual hair growth

TSH deficiency
◆ Dry, pale, puffy skin
◆ Slow thought processes
◆ Bradycardia

Corticotropin deficiency
◆ Depigmentation of skin and nipples
◆ Hypothermia and hypotension during periods of stress

Prolactin deficiency
◆ Sparse or absent growth of pubic and axillary hair

Panhypopituitarism
◆ Mental abnormalities, including lethargy and psychosis
◆ Physical abnormalities, including orthostatic hypotension and bradycardia

DIAGNOSTIC TEST RESULTS
◆ Serum thyroxine level is decreased in diminished thyroid gland function due to lack of TSH.
◆ Radioimmunoassay shows decreased plasma levels of some or all of the pituitary hormones.
◆ Increased prolactin levels may indicate a lesion in the hypothalamus or pituitary stalk.
◆ Computed tomography scans, magnetic resonance imaging, or cerebral angiography show intrasellar or extrasellar tumors.
◆ Oral administration of metyrapone shows the source of low hydroxycorticosteroid levels.

◆ Insulin administration shows low levels of corticotropin, indicating pituitary or hypothalamic failure.
◆ Dopamine antagonist administration evaluates prolactin secretory reserve.
◆ I.V. administration of gonadotropin-releasing hormone distinguishes pituitary and hypothalamic causes of gonadotropin deficiency.
◆ Provocative testing shows persistently low GH and insulin-like growth factor-1 levels, confirming GH deficiency.

TREATMENT

GENERAL
◆ If caused by a lesion or tumor, removal, radiation, or both, followed by possible lifelong hormone replacement therapy
◆ Endocrine substitution therapy for affected organs

DIET
◆ High-calorie, high-protein

ACTIVITY
◆ Regular exercise
◆ Rest periods for fatigue

MEDICATIONS
◆ Hormone replacement therapy

AGE FACTOR *Children with hypopituitarism may also need adrenal and thyroid hormone replacement and, as they approach puberty, sex hormones.*

SURGERY
◆ Pituitary tumor removal

(continued)

NURSING CONSIDERATIONS

NURSING DIAGNOSES
- Chronic low self-esteem
- Delayed growth and development
- Disturbed body image
- Disturbed sensory perception: Visual
- Hypothermia
- Imbalanced nutrition: Less than body requirements
- Ineffective coping
- Risk for infection
- Sexual dysfunction

EXPECTED OUTCOMES
The patient will:
- verbalize feelings of positive self-esteem
- demonstrate age-appropriate skills and behavior to the extent possible
- express positive feelings about self
- maintain optimal functioning within the limits of the visual impairment
- maintain normal body temperature
- maintain appropriate body weight
- seek help from peer support groups or professional counselors to increase adaptive coping behaviors
- remain free from signs and symptoms of infection
- verbalize feelings regarding impaired sexual function.

NURSING INTERVENTIONS
- Monitor vital signs.
- Assess neurologic status.
- Observe for signs and symptoms of pituitary apoplexy, a medical emergency.
- Give prescribed drugs.
- Encourage maintenance of adequate calorie intake.
- Offer small, frequent meals.
- Keep the patient warm.
- Institute safety precautions.
- Provide emotional support.
- Encourage the patient to express his feelings.
- Monitor laboratory tests for hormonal deficiencies.
- Obtain calorie intake and monitor daily weight.

PATIENT TEACHING

Be sure to cover (with the patient and family):
- disorder, diagnostic testing, and treatment
- long-term hormone replacement therapy and adverse reactions
- when to notify the practitioner
- regular follow-up appointments
- energy-conservation techniques
- need for adequate rest
- need for a balanced diet
- referral to psychological counseling or to community resources, if indicated.

RESOURCES
Organizations
American Association of Clinical Endocrinologists: *www.aace.com*
National Organization for Rare Diseases: *www.rarediseases.org*

Selected references
Agha, A., et al. "The Natural History of Post-Traumatic Hypopituitarism: Implications for Assessment and Treatment," *American Journal of Medicine* 118(12):1416, December 2005.

Hanberg, A. "Common Disorders of the Pituitary Gland: Hyposecretion versus Hypersecretion," *Journal of Infusion Nursing* 28(1):36-44, January-February 2005.

Mondok, A., et al. "Treatment of Pituitary Tumors: Radiation," *Endocrine* 28(1):77-85, October 2005.

Morton, A., and Kannan, S. "Peripartum Cardiomyopathy in a Woman with Hypopituitarism," *BJOG* 113(1):123-24, January 2006.

Disorders affecting management of hypopituitarism

This chart highlights disorders that affect the management of hypopituitarism.

DISORDER	SIGNS AND SYMPTOMS	DIAGNOSTIC TEST RESULTS	TREATMENT AND CARE
Adrenal hypofunction (complication)	◆ Bronze discoloration of skin and darkening of scars ◆ Areas of vitiligo ◆ Increased pigmentation of mucous membrane ◆ Weak, irregular pulse ◆ Hypotension ◆ Craving for salty foods ◆ Muscle weakness ◆ Fatigue ◆ Weight loss	◆ Rapid corticotropin stimulation test may show low levels, which indicates a secondary disorder; elevated levels indicate a primary disorder. ◆ Plasma cortisol level is less than 10 mcg/dl in the morning and even lower in the evening. ◆ Serum sodium and fasting blood glucose levels are decreased. ◆ Computed tomography (CT) scan of the abdomen shows adrenal calcification.	◆ Encourage increased fluid intake, and administer I.V. fluids, as ordered. ◆ Monitor vital signs, intake and output, and electrolyte levels. ◆ Provide small, frequent, high-protein meals. ◆ Administer corticosteroids. ◆ Monitor blood glucose levels.
Diabetes insipidus (complication)	◆ Extreme polyuria—usually 4 to 6 L/day of dilute urine but sometimes as much as 30 L/day, with a low specific gravity (less than 1.005) ◆ Polydipsia, particularly for cold, iced drinks ◆ Nocturia ◆ Fatigue (in severe cases) ◆ Dehydration, characterized by weight loss, poor tissue turgor, dry mucous membranes, constipation, muscle weakness, dizziness, tachycardia, and hypotension	◆ Urinalysis reveals almost colorless urine of low osmolality (less than 200 mOsm/kg) and low specific gravity (less than 1.005). ◆ A water deprivation test confirms the diagnosis by demonstrating renal inability to concentrate urine (evidence of antidiuretic hormone deficiency). ◆ If the patient has central diabetes insipidus, subcutaneous injection of 5 units of vasopressin produces decreased urine output with increased specific gravity.	◆ Monitor intake and output. ◆ Administer I.V. fluid replacement. ◆ Monitor vital signs and assess for signs and symptoms of dehydration. ◆ Administer medications, as ordered, and evaluate effect on urine output. ◆ Measure urine specific gravity. ◆ Provide skin and mouth care.
Hypothyroidism (complication)	◆ Fatigue ◆ Unexplained weight gain ◆ Anorexia ◆ Hoarseness ◆ Periorbital edema; puffy face, hands, and feet ◆ Dry, sparse hair with patchy hair loss ◆ Dry, flaky skin ◆ Thick, brittle nails ◆ Possible goiter ◆ Hypotension ◆ Muscle weakness ◆ Poor coordination	◆ Radioimmunoassay shows decreased serum levels of triiodothyronine and thyroxine. ◆ Serum thyroid-stimulating hormone level decreases with hypothalamic or pituitary insufficiency. ◆ Serum cholesterol, alkaline phosphatase, and triglyceride levels are elevated. ◆ Skull X-rays, CT scan, and magnetic resonance imaging show pituitary or hypothalamic lesions.	◆ Provide a high-fiber, low-fat, low-cholesterol diet. ◆ Administer thyroid replacement therapy. ◆ Provide postoperative care, as indicated. ◆ Maintain fluid balance; monitor intake and output. ◆ Monitor vital signs and laboratory results.

Hypothermia

- Core body temperature below 95° F (35° C)
- Affects chemical changes in the body
- May be classified as mild, 89.6° to 95° F (32° to 35° C); moderate, 86° to 89.6° F (30° to 32° C); or severe, 77° to 86° F (25° to 30° C), which may be fatal

CAUSES

- Near drowning
- Prolonged exposure to cold temperatures
- Disease or disability that alters the patient's homeostasis
- Administration of large amounts of cold blood or blood products

RISK FACTORS

- Lack of insulating body fat
- Wet or inadequate clothing
- Drug or alcohol abuse
- Cardiac disease
- Smoking
- Fatigue
- Malnutrition and depletion of caloric reserves
- Age (incidence highest in children and elderly people)

PATHOPHYSIOLOGY

- Cold temperatures cause metabolic changes that slow the functions of most major organ systems. (See *Disorders affecting management of hypothermia,* pages 287 to 289.)
- Severe hypothermia results in depression of cerebral blood flow, diminished oxygen requirements, reduced cardiac output, and decreased arterial pressure.

CARDIOVASCULAR SYSTEM

- Peripheral vasoconstriction, an increase in cardiac afterload, and elevated myocardial oxygen consumption result in initial tachycardia then bradycardia and myocardial depression, which lead to decreased cardiac output and hypotension.
- Hypothermia causes metabolic changes that induce cardiac arrhythmias such as ventricular fibrillation.

ENDOCRINE SYSTEM

- Cold stimulates the release of catecholamines, which produce thermogenesis.
- Corticosteroid levels become elevated.
- Hyperglycemia may result from an increase in catecholamines, a decrease in insulin activity, and a decrease in renal excretion of glucose.

GASTROINTESTINAL SYSTEM

- GI smooth-muscle motility decreases, resulting in acute gastric dilation, paralytic ileus, and distention of the colon.
- GI secretions and free acid production are decreased.
- Cold-associated hemorrhages—called *Wischnevsky's lesions*—develop in the pancreatic and gastric mucosa.
- Liver function decreases, eventually leading to an impaired ability to metabolize drugs, metabolites, or conjugate steroids.

IMMUNE SYSTEM

- Cold temperatures inhibit immune function, resulting in cold-induced immunosuppression.

RENAL SYSTEM

- Renal function is depressed because of a fall in systemic blood pressure.
- Renal vascular resistance rises, leading to a further decrease in renal flow and glomerular filtration.

RESPIRATORY SYSTEM

- The brain stem is impaired by hypothermia, which results in respiratory compromise and diminished oxygen requirements and a decreased respiratory minute volume.
- Tissues retain carbon dioxide, resulting in respiratory acidosis.
- Respiratory ciliary motility decreases.
- Lung compliance decreases.
- The potential for noncardiogenic pulmonary edema increases.
- Elasticity of the thorax decreases.
- Physiologic and anatomic dead spaces are increased.

HISTORY
- History revealing cause, temperature to which the patient was exposed, and length of exposure

Mild hypothermia
- Amnesia

Moderate hypothermia
- Unresponsive

Severe hypothermia
- Appears lifeless
- Cardiac arrhythmias or cardiac arrest

WARNING *If a patient has hypothermia, use an esophageal or rectal probe that reads as low as 77° F (25° C) to determine an accurate core body temperature. Core body temperature can also be determined using a pulmonary artery catheter.*

PHYSICAL FINDINGS
- Vary with the patient's body temperature

Mild hypothermia
- Severe shivering
- Slurred speech

Moderate hypothermia
- Unresponsive
- Peripheral cyanosis
- Muscle rigidity
- Signs of shock

Severe hypothermia
- No palpable pulse
- No audible heart sounds
- Possible dilated pupils
- State of rigor mortis
- Ventricular fibrillation
- Loss of deep tendon reflexes

DIAGNOSTIC TEST RESULTS
- Technetium pertechnetate scanning shows perfusion defects and deep-tissue damage and can be used to identify nonviable bone.
- Doppler and plethysmographic studies help determine pulses and the extent of frostbite after thawing.
- Laboratory testing during treatment of moderate or severe hypothermia includes a complete blood count, coagulation profile, urinalysis, and serum amylase, electrolyte, hemoglobin, glucose, liver enzyme, blood urea nitrogen, creatinine, and arterial blood gas levels.

TREATMENT

GENERAL
- Passive rewarming (patient rewarms on his own)
- Active external rewarming (using heating blankets, warm-water immersion, heated objects such as water bottles, and radiant heat)
- Active core rewarming (using heated I.V. fluids, genitourinary tract irrigation, extracorporeal rewarming, hemodialysis, and peritoneal, gastric, and mediastinal lavage)
- Cardiopulmonary resuscitation, as needed, until rewarming raises the core temperature to at least 89.6° F (32° C)
- Depending on test results, administration of oxygen, endotracheal intubation, controlled ventilation, I.V. fluids, and treatment of metabolic acidosis

DIET
- Nothing by mouth until condition is stable

ACTIVITY
- As tolerated once stable

MEDICATIONS
- Emergency medications for cardiac arrhythmias per advanced cardiac life support protocol

(continued)

NURSING DIAGNOSES

◆ Acute pain
◆ Decreased cardiac output
◆ Disturbed thought processes
◆ Impaired gas exchange
◆ Ineffective tissue perfusion: Peripheral
◆ Risk for aspiration
◆ Risk for injury

EXPECTED OUTCOMES

The patient will:

◆ express feelings of increased comfort and decreased pain
◆ maintain adequate cardiac and organ perfusion
◆ maintain appropriate thought processes
◆ maintain adequate ventilation and oxygenation
◆ exhibit signs of adequate peripheral circulation
◆ not aspirate
◆ remain free from injury.

NURSING INTERVENTIONS

◆ Remove wet clothing.
◆ Provide rewarming techniques.
◆ Administer I.V.fluids, as ordered.
◆ Monitor vital signs, pulse oximetry readings, and cardiac rhythm.
◆ Treat underlying disorders, as indicated.

Be sure to cover:

◆ disorder, diagnostic testing, and treatment
◆ how to avoid hypothermic situations
◆ need for alcohol and drug rehabilitation, as appropriate
◆ referral for social services, if needed.

RESOURCES

Organizations

National Center for Injury Prevention and Control: *www.cdc.gov/ncipc*
National Institutes of Health: *www.nih.gov*

Selected references

Day, M.P. "Hypothermia: A Hazard for All Seasons," *Nursing* 36(12):44-47, December 2006.
Holden, M., and Flynn Makic, M. "Clinically Induced Hypothermia: Why Chill Your Patient?" *AACN Advanced Critical Care* 17(2):125-32, April-June 2006.
Wehmer, M. "Warm Up to Your Patients," *OR Nurse* 1(1):21-30, January 2007.

Disorders affecting management of hypothermia

This chart highlights disorders that affect the management of hypothermia.

DISORDER	SIGNS AND SYMPTOMS	DIAGNOSTIC TEST RESULTS	TREATMENT AND CARE
Aspiration pneumonia (complication)	◆ Fever ◆ Chills ◆ Sweats ◆ Pleuritic chest pain ◆ Cough ◆ Sputum production ◆ Hemoptysis ◆ Dyspnea ◆ Headache ◆ Fatigue ◆ Bronchial breath sounds over areas of consolidation ◆ Crackles ◆ Increased tactile fremitus ◆ Unequal chest wall expansion	◆ Chest X-rays show infiltrates, confirming the diagnosis. ◆ Sputum specimen for Gram stain and culture and sensitivity tests show acute inflammatory cells. ◆ White blood cell count indicates leukocytosis in bacterial pneumonia and a normal or low count in viral or mycoplasmal pneumonia. ◆ Blood cultures reflect bacteremia and help determine the causative organism. ◆ Arterial blood gas (ABG) levels vary depending on the severity of pneumonia and the underlying lung state. ◆ Bronchoscopy or transtracheal aspiration allows the collection of material for culture. Pleural fluid culture may also be obtained. ◆ Pulse oximetry may show a reduced level of arterial oxygen saturation.	◆ Maintain a patent airway and adequate oxygenation. Measure the patient's ABG levels, especially if he's hypoxic. Administer supplemental oxygen if his partial pressure of arterial oxygen falls below 55 to 60 mm Hg. If he has an underlying chronic lung disease, give oxygen cautiously. ◆ With severe pneumonia that requires endotracheal intubation or a tracheostomy with or without mechanical ventilation, provide thorough respiratory care and suction as needed, using sterile technique, to remove secretions. ◆ Obtain sputum specimens as needed. Use suction if the patient can't produce a specimen. ◆ Administer antibiotics and pain medication. Administer I.V. fluids and electrolyte replacement for fever and dehydration. ◆ Provide a high-calorie, high-protein diet of soft foods to offset the calories the patient uses to fight the infection. If necessary, supplement oral feedings with nasogastric (NG) tube feedings or parenteral nutrition. ◆ To prevent aspiration during NG tube feedings, elevate the patient's head, check the tube position, and administer the feeding slowly. Don't give large volumes at one time because this can cause vomiting. ◆ Monitor the patient's fluid intake and output. ◆ Institute infection control precautions. ◆ Provide a quiet, calm environment, with frequent rest periods.

(continued)

DISORDER	SIGNS AND SYMPTOMS	DIAGNOSTIC TEST RESULTS	TREATMENT AND CARE
Cardiac arrhythmia (complication)	◆ Palpitations ◆ Chest pain ◆ Dizziness ◆ Weakness, fatigue ◆ Irregular heart rhythm ◆ Hypotension ◆ Syncope ◆ Altered level of consciousness ◆ Diaphoresis, pallor, cold, clammy skin	◆ Electrocardiogram (ECG) identifies specific waveform changes associated with the arrhythmia. ◆ Laboratory testing reveals electrolyte abnormalities, hypoxemia, or acid-base abnormalities. ◆ Electrophysiologic testing identifies the mechanism of an arrhythmia and the location of accessory pathways.	◆ Assess airway, breathing, and circulation if life-threatening arrhythmia develops; follow advanced cardiac life support protocols for treatment. ◆ Monitor cardiac rhythm continuously, and obtain serial ECGs to evaluate changes and effects of treatment. ◆ Administer antiarrhythmics and monitor for adverse effects. ◆ Assess cardiovascular system for signs of hypoperfusion; monitor vital signs. ◆ Assist with insertion of temporary pacemaker, or apply transcutaneous pacemaker, if appropriate.
Metabolic acidosis (complication)	◆ Headache, lethargy progressing to drowsiness, central nervous system depression ◆ Kussmaul's respirations, hypotension, stupor, and coma ◆ Anorexia, nausea, vomiting, diarrhea and, possibly, dehydration ◆ Warm, flushed skin ◆ Fruity breath odor	◆ Arterial pH is below 7.35. ◆ Partial pressure of arterial carbon dioxide may be normal or less than 34 mm Hg; bicarbonate level may be less than 22 mEq/L. ◆ Serum potassium level is greater than 5.5 mEq/L. ◆ Anion gap is greater than 14 mEq/L.	◆ For severe cases, administer sodium bicarbonate I.V. ◆ Monitor vital signs, laboratory results, pulse oximetry readings, and level of consciousness. ◆ Administer electrolyte supplements and evaluate effects. ◆ Initiate aspiration precautions. ◆ Record intake and output to monitor renal function.
Pancreatitis (complication)	◆ Steady epigastric pain centered close to the umbilicus, radiating between the 10th thoracic and 6th lumbar vertebrae ◆ Pain unrelieved by vomiting *With severe attack* ◆ Extreme pain ◆ Persistent vomiting ◆ Abdominal rigidity ◆ Diminished bowel activity ◆ Crackles at lung bases ◆ Left pleural effusion ◆ Extreme malaise ◆ Restlessness ◆ Mottled skin ◆ Tachycardia ◆ Low-grade fever (100° to 102° F [37.8° to 38.9° C]) ◆ Possible ileus ◆ Cold, sweaty extremities	◆ Serum amylase level is dramatically elevated (in many cases over 500 U/L), which confirms pancreatitis and rules out perforated peptic ulcer, acute cholecystitis, appendicitis, and bowel infarction or obstruction. ◆ Urine and pleural fluid analysis amylase is dramatically elevated in ascites. Characteristically, amylase levels return to normal 48 hours after onset of pancreatitis, despite continuing symptoms. ◆ Serum lipase levels are increased, which rise more slowly than serum amylase. ◆ Serum calcium levels are decreased (hypocalcemia) from fat necrosis and formation of calcium soaps. ◆ White blood cell counts range from 8,000 to 20,000/µl, with increased polymorphonuclear leukocytes. ◆ Glucose levels will be elevated—as high as 500 to 900 mg/dl, indicating hyperglycemia. ◆ Abdominal X-rays or computed tomography (CT) scans show dilation of the small or large bowel or calcification of the pancreas. ◆ An ultrasound or CT scan reveals an increased pancreatic diameter and helps distinguish acute cholecystitis from acute pancreatitis.	◆ After the emergency phase, continue I.V. therapy for 5 to 7 days to provide adequate electrolytes and protein solutions that don't stimulate the pancreas. ◆ If the patient can't tolerate oral feedings, total parenteral nutrition (TPN) or nonstimulating elemental lavage feedings may be needed. ◆ With extreme cases, laparotomy to drain the pancreatic bed, 95% pancreatectomy, or a combination of cholecystectomy-gastrostomy, feeding jejunostomy, and drainage may be needed. ◆ Give plasma or albumin, if ordered, to maintain blood pressure. ◆ Record intake and output, check urine output hourly, and monitor electrolyte levels. ◆ Watch for signs of calcium deficiency, such as tetany, cramps, carpopedal spasm, and seizures. ◆ If you suspect hypocalcemia, keep airway and suction apparatus readily available and pad the side rails. ◆ Administer analgesics as needed to relieve the patient's pain and anxiety. ◆ Watch for complications of TPN, such as sepsis, hypokalemia, overhydration, and metabolic acidosis.

DISORDER	SIGNS AND SYMPTOMS	DIAGNOSTIC TEST RESULTS	TREATMENT AND CARE
Renal failure (complication)	◆ Oliguria (initially) ◆ Azotemia ◆ Anuria (rare) ◆ Electrolyte imbalance ◆ Metabolic acidosis ◆ Anorexia ◆ Nausea and vomiting ◆ Diarrhea or constipation ◆ Dry mucous membranes ◆ Headache ◆ Confusion ◆ Seizures ◆ Drowsiness ◆ Irritability ◆ Coma ◆ Dry skin ◆ Pruritus ◆ Pallor ◆ Purpura ◆ Uremic frost ◆ Hypotension (early) ◆ Hypertension with arrhythmias (later) ◆ Fluid overload ◆ Heart failure ◆ Systemic edema ◆ Anemia ◆ Altered clotting mechanisms ◆ Pulmonary edema ◆ Kussmaul's	◆ Blood urea nitrogen, serum creatinine, and potassium levels are elevated. ◆ Bicarbonate level, hematocrit, hemoglobin, and pH are decreased. ◆ Urine studies show casts, cellular debris, and decreased specific gravity; in glomerular diseases, proteinuria and urine osmolality that's close to serum osmolality; urine sodium level is less than 20 mEq/L if oliguria results from decreased perfusion, or more than 40 mEq/L if the cause is intrarenal. ◆ Creatinine clearance tests measuring glomerular filtration rate reflect the number of remaining functioning nephrons. ◆ ECG reveals tall, peaked T waves; widening QRS; and disappearing P waves if hyperkalemia is present. ◆ Ultrasonography, abdominal and kidney-ureter-bladder X-rays, excretory urography, renal scan, retrograde pyelography, CT scan, and nephrotomography reveal abnormalities of the urinary tract.	◆ Measure intake and output, including body fluids, NG output, and diarrhea; weigh the patient daily. ◆ Measure hemoglobin level and hematocrit, and replace blood components. ◆ Monitor vital signs; check and report for signs of pericarditis (pleuritic chest pain, tachycardia, pericardial friction rub), inadequate renal perfusion (hypotension), and acidosis. ◆ Maintain proper electrolyte balance. Monitor potassium levels, and monitor for hyperkalemia (malaise, anorexia, paresthesia or muscle weakness) and ECG changes. ◆ If the patient receives hypertonic glucose and insulin infusions, monitor potassium and glucose levels. If giving sodium polystyrene sulfonate rectally, make sure the patient doesn't retain it and become constipated; doing so prevents bowel perforation. ◆ Maintain nutritional status with a high-calorie, low-protein, low-sodium, and low-potassium diet and vitamin supplements. ◆ Monitor the patient carefully during peritoneal dialysis. ◆ If the patient requires hemodialysis, monitor the venous access site, and assess the patient and laboratory work carefully.

Hypothyroidism

OVERVIEW

- Characterized by decreased circulating levels of or resistance to free thyroid hormone (TH)
- Classified as primary or secondary
- Severe hypothyroidism known as *myxedema*
- More prevalent in females
- In United States, incidence increasing in people older than age 40

CAUSES

- Amyloidosis
- Antithyroid drugs
- Autoimmune thyroiditis (Hashimoto's) (most common cause)
- Congenital defects
- Drugs, such as iodides and lithium
- Endemic iodine deficiency
- External radiation to the neck
- Hypothalamic failure to produce thyrotropin-releasing hormone
- Idiopathic
- Inflammatory conditions
- Pituitary failure to produce thyroid-stimulating hormone (TSH)
- Pituitary tumor
- Postpartum pituitary necrosis
- Radioactive iodine therapy
- Sarcoidosis
- Thyroid gland surgery

PATHOPHYSIOLOGY

- The thyroid gland synthesizes and secretes the iodinated hormones, thyroxine (T_4) and triiodothyronine (T_3). THs are necessary for normal growth and development and act on many tissues to increase metabolic activity and protein synthesis.
- In primary hypothyroidism, a decrease in TH production is a result of the loss of thyroid tissue, which results in an increased secretion of TSH that leads to a goiter.
- In secondary hypothyroidism, the pituitary typically fails to synthesize or secrete adequate amounts of TSH, or target tissues fail to respond to normal blood levels of TH.
- Either type may progress to myxedema, which is clinically more severe and considered a medical emergency. (See *Managing myxedema coma.*)
- Chronic autoimmune thyroiditis, also called *chronic lymphocytic thyroiditis,* occurs when autoantibodies destroy thyroid gland tissue.
- Subacute thyroiditis, painless thyroiditis, and postpartum thyroiditis are self-limited conditions that usually follow an episode of hyperthyroidism.

CARDIOVASCULAR SYSTEM

- Cardiovascular involvement includes decreased cardiac output resulting in slow pulse rate, signs of poor peripheral circulation and, occasionally, an enlarged heart, eventually leading to heart failure.
- Fluid retention may lead to periorbital edema.

GASTROINTESTINAL SYSTEM

- Unexplained weight gain may be attributed to fluid retention in the myxedematous tissues.
- Constipation, anorexia, and abdominal distention occur; these conditions may eventually lead to megacolon.

Managing myxedema coma

Myxedema coma is a medical emergency that's commonly fatal. Progression is usually gradual, but when stress aggravates severe or prolonged hypothyroidism, coma may develop abruptly. Examples of severe stress are infection, exposure to cold, and trauma. Other precipitating factors include thyroid medication withdrawal and the use of a sedative, an opioid, or an anesthetic.

Patients in myxedema coma have significantly depressed respirations, so their partial pressure of carbon dioxide in arterial blood may increase. Decreased cardiac output and worsening cerebral hypoxia may also occur. The patient is stuporous and hypothermic, and vital signs reflect bradycardia and hypotension.

LIFESAVING INTERVENTIONS

If your patient becomes comatose, begin these interventions as soon as possible:
- Maintain airway patency with ventilatory support, if necessary.
- Maintain circulation through I.V. fluid replacement.
- Provide continuous electrocardiogram monitoring.
- Monitor arterial blood gas levels to detect hypoxia and metabolic acidosis.
- Warm the patient by wrapping him in blankets. Don't use a warming blanket because it might increase peripheral vasodilation, causing shock.
- Monitor body temperature, until stable, with a low-reading thermometer.
- Replace thyroid hormone by administering large doses of I.V. levothyroxine, as ordered. Monitor vital signs because rapid correction of hypothyroidism can cause adverse cardiac reactions.
- Monitor intake and output and daily weight. With treatment, urine output should increase and body weight should decrease; if not, report this to the practitioner.
- Replace fluids and other substances such as glucose. Monitor serum electrolyte levels.
- Administer a corticosteroid, as ordered.
- Check for possible sources of infection, such as blood, sputum, or urine, which may have precipitated coma. Treat infections or any other underlying illness.

GENITOURINARY SYSTEM

◆ Menorrhagia and decreased libido occur because of altered prolactin levels; these conditions may lead to infertility.

INTEGUMENTARY SYSTEM

◆ Decreased sweating occurs.
◆ The epidermis thins and hyperkeratosis occurs.
◆ Increased dermal glycoaminoglycan content traps water and gives rise to skin thickening without pitting (myxedema).
◆ Dry, flaky, inelastic skin develops.
◆ Hair patterns and eyebrows change.
◆ Nails become dry and brittle.

MUSCULOSKELETAL SYSTEM

◆ Ataxia, nystagmus, and reflexes with delayed relaxation time (especially in the Achilles tendon) occur because of endocrine effects.

NEUROLOGIC SYSTEM

◆ Metabolic effects disrupt the central nervous system (CNS), leading to weakness, fatigue, forgetfulness, sensitivity to cold, and decreased mental stability.
◆ CNS effects can progress to myxedema coma. Progression is usually gradual but may develop abruptly. Such stresses as hypoventilation, hypoglycemia, hyponatremia, hypotension, and hypothermia in those with severe or prolonged hypothyroidism increase the risk. (See *Disorders affecting management of hypothyroidism*, page 293.)

ASSESSMENT

HISTORY

◆ Vague and varied symptoms that have developed slowly over time
◆ Energy loss, fatigue
◆ Forgetfulness
◆ Sensitivity to cold
◆ Unexplained weight gain
◆ Constipation
◆ Anorexia
◆ Decreased libido
◆ Menorrhagia
◆ Paresthesia
◆ Joint stiffness
◆ Muscle cramping

PHYSICAL FINDINGS

◆ Slight mental slowing to severe obtundation
◆ Thick, dry tongue
◆ Hoarseness; slow, slurred speech
◆ Dry, flaky, inelastic skin
◆ Puffy face, hands, and feet
◆ Periorbital edema; drooping upper eyelids
◆ Dry, sparse hair with patchy hair loss
◆ Loss of outer third of eyebrow
◆ Thick, brittle nails with transverse and longitudinal grooves
◆ Ataxia, intention tremor; nystagmus
◆ Doughy skin that feels cool
◆ Weak pulse and bradycardia
◆ Muscle weakness
◆ Sacral or peripheral edema
◆ Delayed reflex relaxation time
◆ Possible goiter
◆ Absent or decreased bowel sounds
◆ Hypotension
◆ A gallop or distant heart sounds
◆ Adventitious breath sounds
◆ Abdominal distention or ascites

DIAGNOSTIC TEST RESULTS

◆ Radioimmunoassay show decreased serum levels of T_3 and T_4.
◆ Serum TSH level increases with thyroid insufficiency and decreases with hypothalamic or pituitary insufficiency.
◆ Serum cholesterol, alkaline phosphatase, and triglycerides levels are elevated.
◆ Serum electrolyte levels show low serum sodium levels in myxedema coma.
◆ Arterial blood gas results show decreased pH and increased partial pressure of carbon dioxide in myxedema coma.
◆ Skull X-rays, computed tomography scan, and magnetic resonance imaging show pituitary or hypothalamic lesions.

TREATMENT

GENERAL

◆ Treatment of underlying cause
◆ Need for long-term thyroid replacement

DIET

◆ Low-fat, low-cholesterol, high-fiber, low-sodium
◆ Possibly, fluid restriction

ACTIVITY

◆ As tolerated

MEDICATIONS

◆ Synthetic hormone levothyroxine
◆ Synthetic liothyronine

SURGERY

◆ For underlying cause such as pituitary tumor

(continued)

NURSING CONSIDERATIONS

NURSING DIAGNOSES
◆ Chronic low self-esteem
◆ Constipation
◆ Decreased cardiac output
◆ Disturbed body image
◆ Excess fluid volume
◆ Ineffective coping
◆ Ineffective tissue perfusion: Cardiopulmonary
◆ Risk for impaired skin integrity

EXPECTED OUTCOMES
The patient will:
◆ express feelings about self-esteem
◆ resume a normal bowel elimination pattern
◆ maintain adequate cardiac output
◆ express positive feelings about self
◆ maintain balanced fluid volume
◆ demonstrate adaptive coping behaviors
◆ remain hemodynamically stable
◆ maintain skin integrity.

NURSING INTERVENTIONS
◆ Monitor vital signs, intake and output, and daily weight.
◆ Assess cardiovascular and respiratory status.
◆ Give prescribed drugs.
◆ Provide adequate rest periods.
◆ Apply antiembolism stockings.
◆ Encourage coughing and deep-breathing exercises.
◆ Maintain fluid restrictions and a low-salt diet.
◆ Provide a high-bulk, low-calorie diet.
◆ Reorient the patient, as needed.
◆ Offer support and encouragement.
◆ Provide meticulous skin care.
◆ Keep the patient warm, as needed.
◆ Encourage the patient to express his feelings.
◆ Help the patient develop effective coping strategies.
◆ Note any edema.
◆ Assess bowel sounds, abdominal distention, and frequency of bowel movements.
◆ Observe for signs and symptoms of hyperthyroidism.

PATIENT TEACHING

Be sure to cover:
◆ disorder, diagnostic testing, and treatment
◆ medication administration, dosage, and possible adverse effects
◆ when to notify the practitioner
◆ physical and mental changes
◆ signs and symptoms of myxedema
◆ need for lifelong hormone replacement therapy
◆ need to wear a medical identification bracelet
◆ importance of keeping accurate records of daily weight
◆ need for a well-balanced, high-fiber, low-sodium diet
◆ energy-conservation techniques
◆ referral to a mental health professional for additional counseling, if needed.

RESOURCES
Organizations
American Foundation of Thyroid Patients: *www.thyroidfoundation.org*
American Thyroid Association: *www.thyroid.org*
Thyroid Foundation of America, Inc.: *www.tsh.org*

Selected references
Holcomb, S.S. "Detecting Thyroid Disease," *Nursing* 35(10 Suppl):4-8, October 2005.
Liles, A., and Harrell, K. "Common Thyroid Disorders; A Review of Therapies," *Advance for Nurse Practitioners* 14(1):29-32, January 2006.
Porsche, R., and Brenner, Z. "Amiodarone-Induced Thyroid Dysfunction," *Critical Care Nurse* 26(3):34-41, June 2006.
Strategies for Managing Multisystem Disorders. Philadelphia: Lippincott Williams & Wilkins, 2006.

Disorders affecting management of hypothyroidism

This chart highlights disorders that affect the management of hypothyroidism.

DISORDER	SIGNS AND SYMPTOMS	DIAGNOSTIC TEST RESULTS	TREATMENT AND CARE
Heart failure (complication)	◆ Cough that produces pink, frothy sputum ◆ Cyanosis of the lips and nail beds ◆ Pale, cool, clammy skin ◆ Diaphoresis ◆ Jugular vein distention ◆ Ascites ◆ Pulsus alternans ◆ Tachycardia ◆ Hepatomegaly ◆ Decreased pulse pressure ◆ Third and fourth heart sounds (S_3 and S_4) ◆ Moist, basilar crackles ◆ Rhonchi ◆ Expiratory wheezing ◆ Decreased pulse oximetry ◆ Peripheral edema ◆ Decreased urinary output	◆ B-type natriuretic peptide immunoassay is elevated. ◆ Chest X-ray shows increased pulmonary vascular markings, interstitial edema, or pleural effusions and cardiomegaly. ◆ Electrocardiography reveals heart enlargement or ischemia, tachycardia, extrasystole, or atrial fibrillation. ◆ Pulmonary artery pressure, pulmonary artery wedge pressure, and left ventricular end-diastolic pressure are elevated in the presence of left-sided heart failure; right atrial or central venous pressure is elevated in right-sided heart failure.	◆ Administer supplemental oxygen and mechanical ventilation, if needed. ◆ Place the patient in Fowler's position. ◆ Administer diuretics, inotropic drugs, vasodilators, angiotensin-converting enzyme inhibitors, angiotensin receptor blockers, cardiac glycosides, beta-adrenergic blockers, and electrolyte supplements. ◆ Initiate cardiac monitoring. ◆ Recurrent heart failure from valvular dysfunction may require surgery. ◆ A ventricular assist device may be needed. ◆ Maintain adequate cardiac output, and monitor hemodynamic stability. ◆ Assess for deep vein thrombosis, and apply antiembolism stockings.
Myxedema coma (complication)	◆ Progressive stupor ◆ Hypoventilation ◆ Hypoglycemia ◆ Hyponatremia ◆ Hypotension ◆ Hypothermia	◆ Serum sodium levels are low, pH is decreased, and partial pressure of arterial carbon dioxide is increased.	◆ Check frequently for signs of decreased cardiac output (such as decreased urine output). ◆ Monitor the patient's temperature until he's stable. Provide extra blankets and clothing and a warm room to compensate for hypothermia. Rapid rewarming may cause vasodilatation and vascular collapse. ◆ Record intake and output and daily weight. As treatment begins, urine output should increase and body weight decrease; if not, report this immediately. ◆ Turn the edematous, bedridden patient every 2 hours, and provide skin care, particularly around bony prominences, at lease once per shift. ◆ Avoid sedation when possible or reduce dosage of sedatives because hypothyroidism delays metabolism of many drugs. ◆ Monitor serum electrolyte levels carefully when administering I.V. fluids. ◆ Monitor vital signs carefully when administering levothyroxine because rapid correction of hypothyroidism can cause adverse cardiac effects. Report chest pain or tachycardia immediately. Watch for hypertension and heart failure in the older patient. ◆ Check arterial blood gas values for hypercapnia, metabolic acidosis, and hypoxia to determine whether the patient requires ventilatory assistance. ◆ Administer corticosteroids. ◆ Because myxedema coma may have been precipitated by an infection, check possible sources of the infection, such as blood and urine, and obtain sputum cultures.

Hypovolemic shock

- Reduced intravascular blood volume that causes circulatory dysfunction and inadequate tissue perfusion resulting from loss of blood, plasma, or fluids
- Potentially life-threatening
- Incidence dependent on cause
- Affects all ages and males and females equally
- Occurs more frequently and is less likely to be tolerated in elderly patients

CAUSES
- Acute blood loss (about one-fifth of total volume)
- Acute pancreatitis
- Ascites
- Burns
- Dehydration, as from excessive perspiration, severe diarrhea, protracted vomiting, diabetes insipidus, diuresis, or inadequate fluid intake
- Diuretic abuse
- Intestinal obstruction
- Peritonitis

Checking for early hypovolemic shock

Orthostatic vital signs and tilt test results can help in assessing for the possibility of impending hypovolemic shock.

ORTHOSTATIC VITAL SIGNS
Measure the patient's blood pressure and pulse rate while he's lying in a supine position, sitting, and standing. Wait at least 1 minute between each position change. A systolic blood pressure decrease of 10 mm Hg or more between positions or a pulse rate increase of 10 beats/minute or more is a sign of volume depletion and impending hypovolemic shock.

TILT TEST
With the patient lying in a supine position, raise his legs above heart level. If his blood pressure increases significantly, the test is positive, indicating volume depletion and impending hypovolemic shock.

PATHOPHYSIOLOGY

- When fluid is lost from the intravascular space, venous return to the heart is reduced.
- This decreases ventricular filling, which leads to a drop in stroke volume.
- Cardiac output falls, causing reduced perfusion to tissues and organs.
- Tissue anoxia prompts a shift in cellular metabolism from aerobic to anaerobic pathways.
- This produces an accumulation of lactic acid, resulting in metabolic acidosis.

CARDIOVASCULAR SYSTEM
- Tachycardia and bounding pulse occur related to sympathetic stimulation.
- Hypotension occurs as compensatory mechanisms begin to fail.
- Narrowed pulse pressure is associated with reduced stroke volume.
- Weak, thready pulse is caused by decreased cardiac output.
- Rapidly falling blood pressure occurs as a result of decompensation.

HEMATOLOGIC SYSTEM
- Disseminated intravascular coagulation (DIC) may develop due to an imbalance of homeostasis mechanisms as coagulation factors are activated. (See *Disorders affecting management of hypovolemic shock,* pages 296 and 297.)

INTEGUMENTARY SYSTEM
- Cool, pale skin is associated with vasoconstriction; continued shock results in cold, clammy skin.
- Cyanosis occurs as a result of hypoxia.

NEUROLOGIC SYSTEM
- Restlessness and irritability occur related to cerebral hypoxia.
- Unconsciousness and absent reflexes are caused by reduced cerebral perfusion, acid-base imbalance, or electrolyte abnormalities.

RENAL SYSTEM
- Reduced urinary output occurs secondary to vasoconstriction. Reduced urinary output continues to occur as a result of poor renal perfusion.
- Anuria is related to renal failure.

RESPIRATORY SYSTEM
- Tachypnea occurs to compensate for hypoxia.
- Shallow respirations occur as the patient weakens.
- Slow, shallow, or Cheyne-Stokes respirations occur secondary to respiratory center depression.
- Metabolic acidosis with an accumulation of lactic acid develops as a result of tissue anoxia as cellular metabolism shifts from aerobic to anaerobic pathways.

ASSESSMENT

HISTORY
- Disorders or conditions that reduce blood volume, such as GI hemorrhage, trauma, and severe diarrhea and vomiting
- With existing cardiac disease, possible anginal pain because of decreased myocardial perfusion and oxygenation

PHYSICAL FINDINGS
- Pale, cool, clammy skin
- Decreased sensorium
- Rapid, shallow respirations
- Urine output usually less than 20 ml/hour
- Rapid, thready pulse
- Mean arterial pressure less than 60 mm Hg in adults (in chronic hypotension, mean pressure may fall below 50 mm Hg before signs of shock)
- Orthostatic vital signs and tilt test results consistent with hypovolemic shock (see *Checking for early hypovolemic shock*)

DIAGNOSTIC TEST RESULTS
- Hematocrit is low, and hemoglobin levels and red blood cell and platelet counts are decreased.

- Serum potassium, sodium, lactate dehydrogenase, creatinine, and blood urea nitrogen levels are elevated.
- Urine specific gravity (greater than 1.020) and urine osmolality are increased.
- pH and partial pressure of arterial oxygen are decreased, and partial pressure of arterial carbon dioxide is increased.
- Aspiration of gastric contents through a nasogastric tube identifies internal bleeding.
- Occult blood tests are positive.
- Coagulation studies show coagulopathy from DIC.
- Chest or abdominal X-rays help to identify internal bleeding sites.
- Gastroscopy helps to identify internal bleeding sites.
- Invasive hemodynamic monitoring shows reduced central venous pressure, right atrial pressure, pulmonary artery pressure, pulmonary artery wedge pressure, and cardiac output.

TREATMENT

GENERAL
- In severe cases, an intra-aortic balloon pump, ventricular assist device, or pneumatic antishock garment
- Bleeding control by direct application of pressure and related measures
- Supplemental oxygen therapy, intubation, or mechanical ventilation, if indicated

DIET
- Possible parenteral nutrition or tube feedings

ACTIVITY
- Bed rest

MEDICATIONS
- Prompt and vigorous blood and fluid replacement
- Positive inotropics
- Oxygen therapy

SURGERY
- Possibly, to correct underlying problem

NURSING CONSIDERATIONS

NURSING DIAGNOSES
- Anxiety
- Decreased cardiac output
- Deficient fluid volume
- Disabled family coping
- Impaired gas exchange
- Ineffective tissue perfusion: Cardiopulmonary, cerebral, renal
- Risk for infection
- Risk for injury

EXPECTED OUTCOMES
The patient (or family) will:
- verbalize strategies to reduce anxiety
- maintain adequate cardiac output and hemodynamic stability
- maintain adequate fluid volume
- express feelings and develop adequate coping mechanisms
- maintain adequate ventilation and oxygenation
- maintain adequate cardiopulmonary, cerebral, and renal perfusion as evidenced by palpable pulses, no signs of respiratory distress, normal mentation, and normal urine output
- remain free from signs and symptoms of infection
- remain free from injury.

NURSING INTERVENTIONS
- Check for a patent airway and adequate circulation. Start cardiopulmonary resuscitation, as indicated.
- Monitor vital signs, peripheral pulses, and intake and output.
- Assess cardiac rhythm and hemodynamic readings.
- Give prescribed I.V. solutions or blood products, as indicated.
- Insert an indwelling urinary catheter.
- Give prescribed oxygen.
- Provide emotional support to the patient and family.

- Monitor coagulation studies, complete blood count, electrolyte measurements, and arterial blood gas levels.

PATIENT TEACHING

Be sure to cover:
- disorder, diagnostic testing, and treatment
- medication administration, dosage, and possible adverse effects.
- risks associated with blood transfusions
- purpose of all equipment such as mechanical ventilation
- dietary restrictions

RESOURCES
Organizations
American Heart Association: *www.americanheart.org*
National Heart, Lung, and Blood Institute: *www.nhlbi.nih.gov*

Selected references
Cottingham, C., and Bridges, E. "Resuscitation of Traumatic Shock: A Hemodynamic Review," *AACN Advanced Critical Care* 17(3):317-26, July-September 2006.
Kelley, D.M. "Hypovolemic Shock: An Overview," *Critical Care Nursing Quarterly* 28(1):2-19, January-March 2005.
Nettina, S.M. *Lippincott Manual of Nursing Practice*, 8th ed. Philadelphia: Lippincott Williams & Wilkins, 2006.
Yanagawa, Y., et al. "Early Diagnosis of Hypovolemic Shock by Sonographic Measurement of Inferior Vena Cava in Trauma Patients," *Journal of Trauma-Injury Infection & Critical Care* 58(4):825-29, April 2005.

(continued)

Disorders affecting management of hypovolemic shock

This chart highlights disorders that affect the management of hypovolemic shock.

DISORDER	SIGNS AND SYMPTOMS	DIAGNOSTIC TEST RESULTS	TREATMENT AND CARE
Acute respiratory failure (complication)	◆ Tachypnea ◆ Cyanosis ◆ Crackles, rhonchi, wheezing ◆ Diminished breath sounds ◆ Restlessness ◆ Altered mental status ◆ Tachycardia ◆ Increased cardiac output ◆ Increased blood pressure ◆ Cardiac arrhythmias	◆ Arterial blood gas (ABG) values show deteriorating values and a pH below 7.35. ◆ Chest X-ray shows pulmonary disease or condition. ◆ Electrocardiogram (ECG) may show cardiac arrhythmia or right ventricular hypertrophy. ◆ Pulse oximetry shows decreasing arterial oxygen saturation.	◆ Administer oxygen therapy and monitor respiratory status; assist with endotracheal intubation and mechanical ventilation, if necessary. ◆ Assess breath sounds and note changes. ◆ Monitor ABG values and pulse oximetry. ◆ Monitor vital signs and intake and output. ◆ Monitor cardiac rhythm for arrhythmias. ◆ Administer antibiotics, bronchodilators, corticosteroids, positive inotropic agents, diuretics, vasopressors, or antiarrhythmics.
Disseminated intravascular coagulation (complication)	◆ Bleeding from puncture sites ◆ Petechiae ◆ Ecchymoses ◆ Hematoma ◆ Nausea and vomiting ◆ Severe muscle, back, and abdominal pain ◆ Chest pain ◆ Hemoptysis	◆ Platelet count is less than 100,000/µl. ◆ Fibrinogen level is less than 150 mg/dl. ◆ Prothrombin time (PT) is greater than 15 seconds. ◆ Fibrin degradation products level is greater than 45 mcg/ml. ◆ D-dimer is elevated. ◆ Blood urea nitrogen and creatinine levels are elevated.	◆ Treat the underlying cause. ◆ Administer fresh frozen plasma, platelets, cryoprecipitate, and packed red blood cells to combat bleeding and blood loss. ◆ Monitor vital signs at least every 30 minutes. ◆ Administer supplemental oxygen, as indicated. ◆ Assess level of consciousness hourly and when the patient's condition changes. ◆ Monitor serial hemoglobin, hematocrit, partial thromboplastin time, PT, fibrinogen levels, fibrinogen degradation products, and platelet counts. ◆ Administer low-dose heparin infusions, vitamin K, and folate. ◆ Institute safety precautions to minimize bleeding.
Myocardial infarction (MI) (complication)	◆ Persistent, crushing, substernal chest pain that may radiate ◆ Cool extremities, perspiration, anxiety, and restlessness ◆ Initially, elevated blood pressure and pulse; if cardiac output is reduced, decreased blood pressure ◆ Bradycardia ◆ Fatigue and weakness ◆ Nausea and vomiting ◆ Shortness of breath and crackles ◆ Low-grade temperature ◆ Jugular vein distention	◆ Serial 12-lead ECG may reveal characteristic changes such as serial ST-segment depression in non–Q-wave MI and ST-segment elevation in Q-wave MI. ECG can also identify the location of MI, arrhythmias, hypertrophy, and pericarditis. ◆ Serial cardiac enzymes and proteins (CK-MB, troponin T and I, and myoglobin) may show a characteristic rise and fall. ◆ Laboratory testing may reveal elevated white blood cell count, C-reactive protein level, and erythrocyte sedimentation rate. ◆ Echocardiography may show ventricular wall motion abnormalities and may detect septal or papillary muscle rupture.	◆ Monitor and record the patient's ECG, blood pressure, temperature, and heart and breath sounds. ◆ Assess and record the severity and duration of pain, and administer analgesics. Avoid I.M. injections. ◆ Check blood pressure after giving nitroglycerin, especially the first dose. ◆ Frequently monitor ECG to detect rate changes or arrhythmias. Place rhythm strips in the patient's chart periodically for evaluation. ◆ During episodes of chest pain, obtain 12-lead ECG, blood pressure, and pulmonary artery measurements. Monitor for changes. ◆ Watch for signs and symptoms of fluid retention. Carefully monitor daily weight, intake and output, respirations, serum enzyme levels, and blood pressure. ◆ Auscultate for adventitious breath sounds periodically, for S_3 or S_4 gallops, and for new-onset heart murmurs. ◆ Organize care and activities to maximize periods of uninterrupted rest. ◆ Ask the dietary department to provide a clear liquid diet until nausea subsides. A low-cholesterol, low-sodium, low-fat, high-fiber diet may be prescribed.

DISORDER	SIGNS AND SYMPTOMS	DIAGNOSTIC TEST RESULTS	TREATMENT AND CARE
Myocardial infarction (MI) (complication) *(continued)*	◆ Third (S_3) and fourth (S_4) heart sounds ◆ Loud, holosystolic murmur ◆ Reduced urine output	◆ Chest X-rays may show left-sided heart failure or cardiomegaly caused by ventricular dilation. ◆ Nuclear imaging scanning can identify areas of infarction. ◆ Cardiac catheterization may be used to identify the involved coronary artery and provide information on ventricular function and pressures and volumes within the heart.	◆ Provide a stool softener to prevent straining during defecation, which causes vagal stimulation and may slow the heart rate. Allow the patient to use a bedside commode, and provide as much privacy as possible. ◆ Assist the patient with range-of-motion exercises. If completely immobilized by a severe MI, turn him often. ◆ Antiembolism stockings help prevent venostasis and thrombophlebitis. ◆ Provide emotional support and help reduce stress and anxiety; administer sedatives, as needed.

Lupus erythematosus

- Chronic inflammatory disorder of the connective tissues that appears in two forms: discoid lupus erythematosus, which affects only the skin; and systemic lupus erythematosus (SLE), which affects multiple organ systems as well as the skin and can be fatal (see *Discoid lupus erythematosus*)
- Recurring remissions and exacerbations with SLE, especially common during the spring and summer
- Prognosis improved with early detection and treatment; remains poor for patients who develop cardiovascular, renal, or neurologic complications or severe bacterial infections
- With SLE, 14 to 50 people affected per 100,000 population in the United States
- Affects more females than males
- Affects all ages, but peak incidence occurs in young adulthood

CAUSES

- Exact cause unknown, but involves several risk factors

RISK FACTORS

- Family history
- Physical or mental stress
- Streptococcal or viral infections
- Altered T and B lymphocyte function
- Exposure to sunlight or ultraviolet light
- Human leukocyte antigens complement deficiency
- Immunization
- Hormonal contraceptive use
- Pregnancy
- Abnormal estrogen metabolism
- Drug therapies, such as procainamide (Pronestyl), hydralazine (Apresoline), and anticonvulsants

PATHOPHYSIOLOGY

- Autoimmunity is believed to be the prime mechanism involved in SLE.
- The body produces antibodies against components of its own cells, such as the antinuclear antibody (ANA), and immune complex disease follows.
- Patients with SLE may produce antibodies against many different tissue components, such as red blood cells (RBCs), neutrophils, platelets, lymphocytes, or almost any organ or tissue in the body. (See *Disorders affecting management of lupus erythematosus,* pages 302 and 303.)

CARDIOPULMONARY SYSTEM

- Immune complexes may be deposited in the vascular tissue (of the heart and lungs), leading to pericarditis, myocarditis, valvular disease, pleural effusions, pleuritis, pneumonitis, chronic interstitial lung disease, and pulmonary embolism.
- Raynaud's phenomenon may occur because of vasculitis.

GENITOURINARY SYSTEM

- Immune complexes may be deposited in the renal tissue, leading to glomerulonephritis, interstitial nephritis, nephritic syndrome and, possibly, renal failure.

HEMATOLOGIC SYSTEM

- The development of autoantibodies against blood cell components—such as RBCs, white blood cells (WBCs), platelets, and lymphocytes—and subsequent deposition of immune complexes can affect overall blood cell function, causing anemia, leukopenia, thrombocytopenia, and lymphopenia.
- Immune complexes may be deposited in the lymph nodes, causing lymphadenopathy.

Discoid lupus erythematosus

Discoid lupus erythematosus (DLE) is a form of lupus erythematosus that's marked by chronic skin eruptions. DLE can cause scarring and permanent disfigurement if left untreated. About 5% of patients with DLE later develop systemic lupus erythematosus (SLE). An estimated 60% of patients with DLE are females in their late 20s or older. The disease seldom occurs in children. Its exact cause isn't known, but evidence suggests an autoimmune process.

CLINICAL FINDINGS

The patient with DLE has lesions that appear as raised, red, scaling plaques with follicular plugging and central atrophy. The raised edges and sunken centers give the lesions a coinlike appearance. Although these lesions can appear anywhere on the body, they usually erupt on the face, scalp, ears, neck, and arms or on any part of the body that is exposed to sunlight. Such lesions can resolve completely or may cause hypopigmentation or hyperpigmentation, atrophy, and scarring. Facial plaques sometimes assume the butterfly pattern characteristic of SLE. Hair becomes brittle and may fall out in patches.

DIAGNOSTIC TEST RESULTS

As a rule, the patient's history and the rash are enough to form the diagnosis. Positive findings in the LE cell test (in which polymorphonuclear leukocytes engulf cell nuclei to form so-called LE cells) occur in less than 10% of patients. Positive skin biopsy results of lesions typically disclose immunoglobulins or complement components. SLE must be ruled out.

TREATMENT AND CARE

As in SLE, drug treatment consists of topical, intralesional, and systemic medications. In addition, patients require education about the following: avoiding prolonged exposure to the sun, fluorescent lighting, and reflected sunlight; use of protective clothing and sunscreens; avoidance of outdoor activity during peak sunlight periods (between 10 a.m. and 2 p.m.); and the need to report changes in the lesions.

INTEGUMENTARY SYSTEM

◆ As autoantibodies are produced and immune complexes are formed, they're deposited in the layers of the skin, causing an inflammatory response and tissue injury, resulting in the classic butterfly rash and lesions, such as hives and cyanotic discolorations.

◆ Deposition of the immune complexes may cause erythema of the nailbeds, splinter hemorrhages, and hair loss.

MUSCULOSKELETAL SYSTEM

◆ Deposition of immune complexes into joint tissue may cause arthritis and arthralgias. As the disease progresses, tendons, ligaments, and joint capsules may become affected, leading to deformity and loss of function.

NEUROLOGIC SYSTEM

◆ SLE may cause acute vasculitis in the cerebral blood vessels, leading to impaired cerebral blood flow and, ultimately, hemorrhage or stroke.

◆ Antibodies may be developed to specifically attack neuronal cells and phospholipids, damaging blood vessels and causing cerebral blood clots.

◆ Seizure disorders, mental dysfunction (confusion, decreased cognition, and altered levels of consciousness), and psychosis (emotional lability involving extremes of euphoria and depression) may occur.

ASSESSMENT

HISTORY

◆ History of a contributing factor
◆ Fever
◆ Weight loss
◆ Malaise
◆ Fatigue
◆ Polyarthralgia
◆ Rash
◆ Abdominal pain
◆ Headaches, irritability, and depression (common)
◆ Nausea, vomiting, diarrhea, or constipation
◆ Irregular menstrual periods or amenorrhea during the active phase of SLE

PHYSICAL FINDINGS

◆ Rashes (see *Signs of systemic lupus erythematosus*)
◆ Joint involvement, similar to rheumatoid arthritis (although the arthritis of lupus is usually nonerosive)
◆ Skin lesions, most commonly an erythematous rash in areas exposed to light (classic butterfly rash over the nose and cheeks in less than 50% of patients) or a scaly, papular rash (mimics psoriasis), especially in sun-exposed areas (see *Recognizing butterfly rash,* page 300)
◆ Vasculitis (especially in the digits), possibly leading to infarctive lesions, necrotic leg ulcers, or digital gangrene
◆ Patchy alopecia and painless ulcers of the mucous membranes
◆ Lymph node enlargement (diffuse or local and nontender)

DIAGNOSTIC TEST RESULTS

◆ Results of anti–double-stranded deoxyribonucleic acid antibody (anti-dsDNA) test (most specific test for SLE) correlate with disease activity, especially renal involvement, and help monitor response to therapy (anti-dsDNA may be low or absent in remission).
◆ Complete blood count (CBC) with differential possibly shows anemia and a decreased WBC count.
◆ CBC shows a decreased platelet count.
◆ Erythrocyte sedimentation rate is elevated.
◆ CBC reveals hypergammaglobulinemia.
◆ ANA and lupus erythematosus cell test results are positive in active SLE.

Signs of systemic lupus erythematosus

Diagnosing systemic lupus erythematosus (SLE) is difficult because it often mimics other diseases; symptoms may be vague and vary greatly among patients.

For these reasons, the American Rheumatism Association issued a list of criteria for classifying SLE, to be used primarily for consistency in epidemiologic surveys. Usually, four or more of these signs are present at some time during the course of the disease:

◆ malar (over the cheeks of the face) or discoid (patch red) rash
◆ photosensitivity
◆ oral or nasopharyngeal ulcerations
◆ nonerosive arthritis (of two or more peripheral joints)
◆ pleuritis or pericarditis
◆ profuse proteinuria (more than 0.5 g/day) or excessive cellular casts in the urine
◆ seizures or psychoses
◆ hemolytic anemia, leukopenia, lymphopenia, or thrombocytopenia
◆ abnormal antinuclear antibody titer
◆ elevated anti–double-stranded deoxyribonucleic acid antibodies and anti–Smith antibodies
◆ positive anticardiolipin (or antiphospholipid) antibody test
◆ positive LE prep test
◆ positive lupus anticoagulant test
◆ false positive serologic test for syphilis.

(continued)

- Urine study results may show RBCs and WBCs, urine casts and sediment, and significant protein loss (greater than 0.5 g/24 hours).
- Blood study results show decreased serum complement (C3 and C4) levels, indicating active disease.
- Lupus anticoagulant and anticardiolipin test results are positive in some patients (usually in patients prone to antiphospholipid syndrome of thrombosis, abortion, and thrombocytopenia).
- Chest X-ray may show pleurisy or lupus pneumonitis.
- Electrocardiography may show a conduction defect with cardiac involvement or pericarditis.
- Biopsy of the kidney determines disease stage and extent of renal involvement.

TREATMENT

GENERAL
- Symptomatic
- Dialysis or kidney transplantation for renal failure

DIET
- Restrictions based on extent of disorder

ACTIVITY
- As tolerated
- Frequent rest periods

MEDICATIONS
- Nonsteroidal anti-inflammatory drugs, including aspirin
- Topical corticosteroid creams, such as hydrocortisone buteprate (Pandel) or triamcinolone (Aristocort)
- Intralesional corticosteroids or antimalarials such as hydroxychloroquine sulfate (Plaquenil)
- Systemic corticosteroids
- Methotrexate (Trexall)

Recognizing butterfly rash

In the classic butterfly rash of systemic lupus erythematosus, lesions appear on the cheeks and the bridge of the nose, creating a characteristic butterfly pattern. The rash may vary in severity from malar erythema (redness of the cheeks) to discoid lesions (plaques).

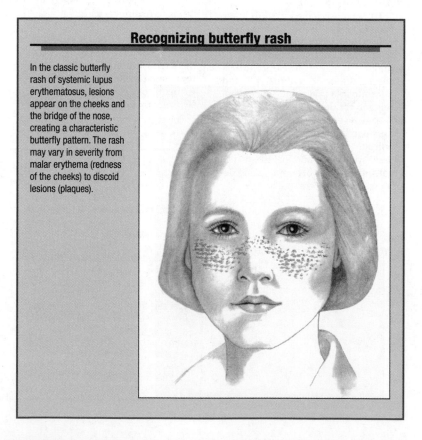

NURSING DIAGNOSES

- Acute pain
- Constipation
- Decreased cardiac output
- Diarrhea
- Disturbed body image
- Fatigue
- Imbalanced nutrition: Less than body requirements
- Impaired oral mucous membrane
- Impaired physical mobility
- Impaired skin integrity
- Impaired tissue integrity
- Impaired urinary elimination
- Ineffective breathing pattern
- Risk for infection

EXPECTED OUTCOMES

The patient will:

- express feelings of increased comfort and decreased pain
- pass soft, regular stool without straining
- maintain adequate cardiac output
- resume a normal bowel elimination pattern
- verbalize feelings about a changed body image
- express feelings of increased energy
- show no signs of malnutrition
- maintain intact oral mucous membranes
- maintain joint mobility and range of motion (ROM)
- maintain skin integrity
- have reduced pain, redness, and swelling at the site of impaired tissue
- maintain fluid balance; intake will equal output
- maintain an effective breathing pattern
- remain free from infection
- report alterations in sensation or pain in the extremities.

NURSING INTERVENTIONS

- Provide a balanced diet. For renal involvement, provide a low-sodium, low-protein diet.
- Provide frequent rest periods.
- Explain all tests and procedures.
- Apply heat packs to relieve joint pain and stiffness.
- Encourage regular exercise to maintain full ROM and prevent contractures.
- Observe for signs and symptoms of complications.
- Monitor vital signs, intake and output, and laboratory reports.

Be sure to cover:

- disorder, diagnostic testing, and treatment
- medication administration, dosage, and possible adverse effects
- ROM exercises as well as body alignment and postural techniques
- referral for physical therapy and occupational counseling, if needed
- information about the Lupus Foundation of America and the Arthritis Foundation.

RESOURCES

Organizations

Arthritis Foundation: *www.arthritis.org*
Lupus Foundation of America: *www.lupus.org*

Selected references

Botwinik, J., and Kessenich, C. "Systemic Erythematosus: An Overview," *Advance for Nurse Practitioners* 14(7):51-53, July 2006.

Childs, S. "The Pathogenesis of Systemic Lupus Erythematosus," *Orthopaedic Nursing* 25(2):140-45, March-April 2006.

Chu, Y.T., and Chiou, S.S. "Painless Massive Ascites and Hypoalbuminemia as the Major Manifestations of Systemic Lupus Erythematosus," *Journal of Microbiology, Immunology, and Infection* 39(1):78-81, February 2006.

Shirato, S. "How CAM Helps Systemic Lupus Erythematosus," *Holistic Nursing Practice* 19(1):36-39, January-February 2005.

(continued)

Disorders affecting management of lupus erythematosus

This chart highlights disorders that affect the management of lupus erythematosus.

DISORDER	SIGNS AND SYMPTOMS	DIAGNOSTIC TEST RESULTS	TREATMENT AND CARE
Acute renal failure (complication)	◆ Oliguria, azotemia and, rarely, anuria ◆ Electrolyte imbalance and metabolic acidosis ◆ Anorexia, nausea, vomiting, diarrhea or constipation, stomatitis, bleeding, hematemesis, dry mucous membranes, and uremic breath ◆ Headache, drowsiness, irritability, confusion, peripheral neuropathy, seizures, and coma ◆ Dry skin, pruritus, pallor, purpura and, rarely, uremic frost ◆ Hypotension (early); hypertension, arrhythmias, fluid overload, heart failure, systemic edema, anemia, and altered clotting mechanisms (later) ◆ Pulmonary edema ◆ Kussmaul's respirations	◆ Blood studies show elevated blood urea nitrogen (BUN), serum creatinine, and potassium levels; decreased bicarbonate level, hematocrit, and hemoglobin levels; and low blood pH. ◆ Urine studies show casts, cellular debris, and decreased specific gravity; urine sodium level is more than 40 mEq/L. ◆ Creatinine clearance test measures glomerular filtration rate and reflects the number of remaining functioning nephrons. ◆ Electrocardiography (ECG) shows tall, peaked T waves; widening QRS complex; and disappearing P waves if hyperkalemia is present.	◆ Measure and record intake and output, including body fluids; weigh the patient daily. ◆ Anticipate fluid restriction to minimize edema. ◆ Assess hemoglobin levels and hematocrit, and replace blood components. ◆ Monitor vital signs. Watch for and report signs of pericarditis, inadequate renal perfusion (hypotension), and acidosis. ◆ Maintain proper electrolyte balance. Strictly monitor potassium levels. ◆ Administer medications, such as diuretic therapy to treat oliguric phase; sodium polystyrene sulfonate (Kayexalate) to reverse hyperkalemia; and hypertonic glucose, insulin, and I.V. sodium bicarbonate for severe hyperkalemic symptoms. ◆ Prepare for hemodialysis or peritoneal dialysis to correct electrolyte and fluid imbalances. ◆ Assess the patient frequently, especially during emergency treatment to lower potassium levels. ◆ If the patient receives hypertonic glucose and insulin infusions, monitor potassium and glucose levels. ◆ If sodium polystyrene sulfonate is used rectally, make sure the patient doesn't retain it and become constipated to prevent bowel perforation. ◆ Maintain nutritional status. Provide a high-calorie, low-protein, low-sodium, and low-potassium diet and vitamin supplements. Give the anorexic patient small, frequent meals. ◆ Encourage frequent coughing and deep breathing, and perform passive range-of-motion exercises. ◆ Provide good mouth care frequently.
Pericarditis (complication)	◆ Pericardial friction rub (best heard when the patient leans forward and exhales) ◆ Sharp and typically sudden pain, usually starting over the sternum and radiating to the neck (especially the left trapezius ridge), shoulders, back, and arms ◆ Shallow, rapid respirations ◆ Mild fever ◆ Dyspnea, orthopnea, and tachycardia as fluid builds up in the pericardial space ◆ Muffled and distant heart sounds ◆ Pallor, clammy skin, hypotension, pulsus paradoxus, neck vein distention and, eventually, cardiovascular collapse ◆ Fluid retention, ascites, hepatomegaly, jugular vein distention, and other signs of chronic right-sided heart failure ◆ Pericardial knock in early diastole along the left sternal border	◆ ECG may reveal diffuse ST-segment elevation in the limb leads and most precordial leads, downsloping PR segments and upright T waves present in most leads, QRS segments possibly diminished when pericardial effusion exists, and arrhythmias, such as atrial fibrillation and sinus arrhythmias. ◆ Laboratory testing may reveal an elevated erythrocyte sedimentation rate or a normal or elevated white blood cell count. ◆ BUN may detect uremia as a cause. ◆ Echocardiography may show an echo-free space between the ventricular wall and the pericardium and reduced pumping action of the heart. ◆ Chest X-rays may be normal with acute pericarditis. The cardiac silhouette may be enlarged with a water bottle shape caused by fluid accumulation if pleural effusion is present.	◆ Maintain bed rest as long as fever and pain persist to reduce metabolic needs. ◆ Administer medications, such as nonsteroidal anti-inflammatory drugs (NSAIDs), to relieve pain and reduce inflammation; give corticosteroids if NSAIDs are ineffective and no infection exists. ◆ Prepare for pericardiocentesis to remove excess fluid from the pericardial space, or for partial or total pericardectomy, if indicated. ◆ Place the patient in an upright position to relieve dyspnea and chest pain. ◆ Administer supplemental oxygen as indicated. ◆ Monitor for signs of cardiac compression or cardiac tamponade and possible complications of pericardial effusion, which include decreased blood pressure, increased central venous pressure, and pulsus paradoxus.

DISORDER	SIGNS AND SYMPTOMS	DIAGNOSTIC TEST RESULTS	TREATMENT AND CARE
Pleural effusion (complication)	◆ Dyspnea ◆ Dry cough ◆ Pleural friction rub ◆ Possible pleuritic pain that worsens with coughing or deep breathing ◆ Dullness on percussion ◆ Tachycardia ◆ Tachypnea ◆ Decreased chest motion and breath sounds	◆ Thoracentesis reveals pleural fluid with specific gravity greater than 1.02 and ratio of protein in pleural fluid to serum equal to or greater than 0.5. Pleural fluid lactate dehydrogenase (LD) is equal to or greater than 200 IU; ratio of LD in pleural fluid to LD in serum is equal to or greater than 0.6. ◆ Fluid aspiration is positive for LE cells. ◆ Chest X-ray shows radiopaque fluid in dependent regions.	◆ Prepare for thoracentesis and chest tube insertion, if indicated. ◆ Monitor vital signs closely during thoracentesis. If fluid is removed too quickly, the patient may experience bradycardia, hypotension, pain, pulmonary edema, or even cardiac arrest. ◆ Watch for respiratory distress or pneumothorax after thoracentesis. ◆ Administer oxygen. ◆ Encourage deep-breathing exercises to promote lung expansion and the use of incentive spirometry to promote deep breathing. ◆ Provide meticulous chest tube care (if inserted), and use sterile technique for changing dressings around the tube insertion site. Monitor chest tube patency. ◆ Record the amount, color, and consistency of tube drainage.
Stroke (complication)	◆ Headache with no known cause ◆ Numbness or weakness of the face, arm, or leg, especially on one side of the body ◆ Confusion, trouble speaking or understanding ◆ Trouble seeing or walking, dizziness, and loss of coordination	◆ Magnetic resonance imaging or computed tomography scan shows evidence of thrombosis or hemorrhage. ◆ Brain scan reveals ischemia (may not be positive for up to 2 weeks after the stroke). ◆ Lumbar puncture may reveal blood in the cerebrospinal fluid (if hemorrhagic). ◆ Carotid ultrasound may detect a blockage, stenosis, or reduced blood flow. ◆ Angiography can help pinpoint the site of occlusion or rupture. ◆ EEG may help localize the area of damage.	◆ Administer medications, such as antiplatelet agents to prevent recurrent stroke (but not in hemorrhagic stroke) and benzodiazepines or anticonvulants to treat or prevent seizures. ◆ Maintain a patent airway and provide oxygen. ◆ If unconscious, the patient may aspirate saliva; place the patient in a lateral position to promote drainage, or suction as needed. ◆ Insert an artificial airway, and start mechanical ventilation or supplemental oxygen, if needed. ◆ Check the patient's vital signs and neurologic status. Monitor blood pressure, level of consciousness, motor function (voluntary and involuntary movements), senses, speech, skin color, and temperature. ◆ Assess gag reflex before offering oral fluids. Maintain fluid intake orally or with I.V. therapy as appropriate.

Lyme disease

- Disorder caused by a spirochete
- Affects all ages and both sexes
- More common during the summer months

CAUSES

- The spirochete *Borrelia burgdorferi*, carried by the minute tick *Ixodes dammini* (also called *I. scapularis*) or another tick in the Ixodidae family

PATHOPHYSIOLOGY

- A tick injects spirochete-laden saliva into the bloodstream or deposits fecal matter on the skin.
- After incubating for 3 to 32 days, the spirochetes migrate outward on the skin, causing a rash, and disseminate to other skin sites or organs through the bloodstream or lymphatic system.
- Spirochetes may survive for years in the joints or die after triggering an inflammatory response in the host.
- Typically, Lyme disease has three stages. (See *Stages of Lyme disease.*)

CARDIOVASCULAR SYSTEM

- Usually, weeks to months after the tick bite, the spirochete can disseminate through the bloodstream and travel to the heart, causing myocarditis.
- The conduction system becomes damaged secondary to the myocarditis, resulting in atrioventricular block, possibly progressing to complete heart block.

INTEGUMENTARY SYSTEM

- Spirochetes migrate to the skin, where they set off an inflammatory response, producing the characteristic rash.

MUSCULOSKELETAL SYSTEM

- Commonly, the spirochete invades the soft tissue and joint spaces of the musculoskeletal system, causing an inflammatory response that ultimately leads to the development of a chronic inflammatory infiltrate in the lining below the synovial fluid.
- Typically, only one joint or a few joints are affected, primarily the large weight-bearing joints such as the knees.
- Recurrent attacks may lead to chronic arthritis with severe cartilage and bone erosion. (See *Disorders affecting management of Lyme disease*, page 307.)

NEUROLOGIC SYSTEM

- The spirochete can travel through the bloodstream to the nervous system, where an inflammatory response occurs in the meningeal lining of the peripheral and cranial nerves, resulting in lymphocytic meningitis; cranial neuropathy, which causes facial nerve palsy; and radiculoneuritis, which causes numbness, tingling, and aching pain.
- The spirochete can invade the eye structures causing follicular conjunctivitis, keratitis, periorbital edema, photophobia, and subconjunctival hemorrhage.

Stages of Lyme disease

Lyme disease typically occurs in three stages. The signs and symptoms, however, may take years to develop. It may be impossible to delineate exactly when one stage ends and another stage starts. Additionally, not all patients pass through each stage.

STAGE 1: EARLY, LOCALIZED STAGE

Erythema migrans, or the "bull's-eye" rash, heralds stage 1 Lyme disease. It begins as a red macule or papule that typically develops at the site of a tick bite. This lesion tends to feel hot and itchy and may grow to more than 20″ (51 cm) in diameter. Within a few days, more lesions may erupt along with a malar rash, conjunctivitis, or diffuse urticaria. In 3 to 4 weeks, lesions are replaced by small, red blotches, which persist for several more weeks.

Malaise and fatigue are constant, but other findings (headache, fever, chills, myalgias, and regional lymphadenopathy) are intermittent. Less common effects are meningeal irritation, mild encephalopathy, migrating musculoskeletal pain, and hepatitis. A persistent sore throat and dry cough may appear several days before erythema migrans.

STAGE 2: EARLY, DISSEMINATED STAGE

Weeks to months later, the second stage begins with neurologic abnormalities—fluctuating meningoencephalitis with peripheral and cranial neuropathy—that usually resolve after days or months. Facial palsy is especially noticeable.

Cardiac abnormalities, such as a brief, fluctuating atrioventricular heart block, may also develop.

STAGE 3: LATE STAGE

Characterized by arthritis, stage 3 begins weeks or years later. Migrating musculoskeletal pain leads to frank arthritis with marked swelling, especially in the large joints. Recurrent attacks may precede chronic arthritis with severe cartilage and bone erosion.

ASSESSMENT

HISTORY
- Recent exposure to ticks
- Onset of symptoms in warmer months
- Severe headache and stiff neck with rash eruption
- Fever (up to 104° F [40° C]) and chills

PHYSICAL FINDINGS
- Regional lymphadenopathy
- Tenderness in the skin lesion site or the posterior cervical area

Early stage
- Tachycardia or irregular heartbeat
- Mild dyspnea
- Erythema migrans
- Headache
- Myalgia
- Arthralgia

Later stage
- Neurologic signs such as memory impairment
- Bell's palsy
- Intermittent arthritis (see *Differentiating Lyme disease*)
- Cardiac symptoms, such as heart failure, pericarditis, and dyspnea
- Neurologic symptoms, such as memory impairment and myelitis
- Fibromyalgia
- Ocular signs such as conjunctivitis

Differentiating Lyme disease

Lyme disease, or chronic neuroborreliosis, needs to be differentiated from chronic fatigue syndrome and fibromyalgia, which is difficult late in the disease because of chronic pain and fatigue. The other diseases produce more generalized and disabling symptoms; also, patients lack evidence of joint inflammation, have normal neurologic test results, and have a greater degree of anxiety and depression than do patients with Lyme disease.

DIAGNOSTIC TEST RESULTS
- Results of assays for anti–*B. burgdorferi* (anti–B) show evidence of previous or current infection.
- Enzyme-linked immunosorbent assay technology or indirect fluorescence assay show immunoglobulin (Ig) M levels that peak 3 to 6 weeks after infection; IgG antibodies detected several weeks after infection may continue to develop for several months and generally persist for years. (See *Lyme disease serology*.)
- Results of Western blot assay show serologic evidence of past or current infection with *B. burgdorferi*.
- Polymerase chain reaction test is used when joint and cerebrospinal fluid involvement are present and detects the genetic material found in the Lyme disease bacteria.

WARNING *Serologic testing isn't useful early in the course of Lyme disease because of its low sensitivity. It may be more useful in later disease stages, when sensitivity and specificity of the test are improved.*

- Analysis of cerebrospinal fluid obtained by lumbar puncture may show antibodies to *B. burgdorferi*.
- Biopsy of skin specimen may be performed to detect *B. burgdorferi*.

TREATMENT

GENERAL
- Prompt tick removal using proper technique

DIET
- No restrictions

ACTIVITY
- Rest periods, as needed

MEDICATIONS
- I.V. or oral antibiotics (initiated as soon as possible after infection)

Lyme disease serology

Serologic tests for Lyme disease, both indirect immunofluorescent and enzyme-linked immunosorbent assays, measure antibody response to the *Borrelia burgdorferi* spirochete and indicate current infection or past exposure. Serologic tests can identify 50% of patients with early-stage Lyme disease, all patients with later complications of carditis, neuritis, and arthritis, as well as patients in remission.

Positive serologic tests for Lyme disease can help confirm diagnosis, but their results aren't definitive because the tests can't detect infection until a sufficient amount of antibodies are produced, which may take as long as 2 to 4 months after the tick bite. In fact, more than 15% of patients with Lyme disease fail to develop any antibodies. Additionally, other treponemal diseases and high rheumatoid factor titers can cause false-positive results.

(continued)

NURSING CONSIDERATIONS

NURSING DIAGNOSES

- Acute pain
- Fatigue
- Hyperthermia
- Impaired physical mobility
- Impaired skin integrity
- Risk for infection

EXPECTED OUTCOMES

The patient will:

- express increased comfort and decreased pain
- return to a normal energy level during recovery
- remain afebrile
- attain the highest degree of mobility possible
- experience a decrease in the size of the rash
- remain free from further signs or symptoms of infection.

NURSING INTERVENTIONS

- Plan care to provide adequate rest.
- Give prescribed drugs.
- Assist with range-of-motion and strengthening exercises (with arthritis).
- Encourage verbalization and provide support.
- Monitor skin lesions and response to treatment.
- Observe for adverse drug reactions and signs and symptoms of complications.

PATIENT TEACHING

Be sure to cover:

- disorder, diagnostic testing, and treatment
- medication administration, dosage, and possible adverse effects
- importance of follow-up care and reporting recurrent or new symptoms to the practitioner
- methods for preventing Lyme disease, such as avoiding tick-infested areas, covering the skin with clothing, using insect repellants, inspecting exposed skin for attached ticks at least every 4 hours, and removing ticks promptly
- information about the vaccine for persons at risk for contracting Lyme disease
- if the patient is in the late stages of the disease, referral to a dermatologist, neurologist, cardiologist, or infectious disease specialist, as indicated.

RESOURCES
Organizations

Centers for Disease Control and Prevention: *www.cdc.gov*

Harvard University Consumer Health Information: *www.intelihealth.com*

National Health Information Center: *www.health.gov/nhic*

National Institute of Allergy and Infectious Diseases: *www.niaid.nih.gov*

National Library of Medicine: *www.nlm.nih.gov*

SELECTED REFERENCES

Bratton, R.L., and Corey, R. "Tick-Borne Disease," *American Family Physician* 71(12):2323-330, June 2005.

Corapi, K., et al. "Strategies for Primary and Secondary Prevention of Lyme Disease," *Nature Clinical Practice: Rheumatology* 3(1):20-25, January 2007.

Kasper, D.L., et al., eds. *Harrison's Principles of Internal Medicine,* 16th ed. New York: McGraw-Hill Book Co., 2005.

Phillips, S.E., et al. "Rash Decisions about Southern Tick-Associated Rash Illness and Lyme Disease," *Clinical Infectious Diseases* 42(2):306-307, January 2006.

Disorders affecting management of Lyme disease

This chart highlights disorders that affect the management of Lyme disease.

DISORDER	SIGNS AND SYMPTOMS	DIAGNOSTIC TEST RESULTS	TREATMENT AND CARE
Arthritis (complication)	◆ Fatigue ◆ Malaise ◆ Anorexia and weight loss ◆ Low-grade fever ◆ Lymphadenopathy ◆ Vague articular symptoms that become specific, localized, bilateral, and symmetric ◆ Stiffening of affected joints ◆ Joint pain and tenderness ◆ Feeling of warmth at joint ◆ Diminished joint function and deformities ◆ Stiff, weak, or painful muscles	◆ X-rays show bone changes, such as demineralization and soft-tissue swelling. ◆ Synovial fluid analysis shows increased volume and turbidity but decreased viscosity and elevated white blood cell counts. ◆ Serum protein electrophoresis possibly shows elevated serum globulin levels. ◆ Erythrocyte sedimentation rate (ESR) and C-reactive protein levels may be elevated. ◆ Complete blood count usually reveals moderate anemia, slight leukocytosis, and slight thrombocytosis.	◆ Administer salicylates or nonsteroidal anti-inflammatory drugs. ◆ Assess all joints carefully. Look for deformities, contractures, immobility, and an inability to perform everyday activities. ◆ Monitor vital signs. Note weight changes, sensory disturbances, and patient's level of pain. ◆ Administer analgesics and watch for adverse effects. ◆ Provide meticulous skin care. Check for pressure ulcers and skin breakdown.
Facial nerve palsy (complication)	◆ Unilateral facial weakness or paralysis, with aching at the jaw angle ◆ Drooping mouth, causing drooling on the affected side ◆ Distorted taste perception over the affected anterior portion of the tongue ◆ Markedly impaired ability to close the eye on the weak side ◆ Incomplete eye closure and Bell's phenomenon (eye rolling upward as eye is closed) ◆ Inability to raise the eyebrow, smile, show the teeth, or puff out the cheek on the affected side	◆ No specific diagnostic test findings are noted; diagnosis is based on clinical findings. ◆ After 10 days, electromyography helps predict the level of expected recovery by distinguishing temporary conduction defects from a pathologic interruption of nerve fibers.	◆ Administer prescribed prednisone therapy. ◆ Apply moist heat to the affected side of the face to reduce pain. ◆ Massage the patient's face with a gentle upward motion two to three times daily for 5 to 10 minutes, and teach him how to perform this massage. ◆ Apply a facial sling to improve lip alignment. Tape eye shut at night to prevent corneal abrasions. ◆ Give the patient frequent and complete mouth care. Remove residual food that collects between the cheeks and gums.
Myocarditis (complication)	◆ Nonspecific symptoms, such as fatigue, dyspnea, palpitations, and fever ◆ Mild, continuous pressure or soreness in the chest (occasionally) ◆ Tachycardia ◆ Third and fourth heart sound gallops (S_3 and S_4) ◆ Possible murmur of mitral insufficiency ◆ Pericardial friction rub	◆ Laboratory testing may reveal elevated levels of creatine kinase (CK), CK-MB, troponin I, troponin T, aspartate aminotransferase, and lactate dehydrogenase. ◆ White blood cell count is increased. ◆ ESR is elevated. ◆ Electrocardiography may reveal diffuse ST-segment and T-wave abnormalities, conduction defects (prolonged PR interval, bundle-branch block, or complete heart block), supraventricular arrhythmias, and ventricular extrasystoles. ◆ Chest X-rays may show an enlarged heart and pulmonary vascular congestion. ◆ Echocardiography may demonstrate some degree of left ventricular dysfunction. ◆ Radionuclide scanning may identify inflammatory and necrotic changes characteristic of myocarditis.	◆ Administer antipyretics to reduce fever and decrease stress on the heart, diuretics to decrease fluid retention, antiarrhythmics, and anticoagulants to prevent thromboembolism. ◆ Institute bed rest to reduce oxygen demands and the heart's workload, and restrict activity to minimize myocardial oxygen consumption. ◆ Administer supplemental oxygen therapy. ◆ Assess cardiovascular status frequently, watching for signs of heart failure, such as dyspnea, hypotension, and tachycardia. Check for changes in cardiac rhythm or conduction. ◆ Monitor sodium intake; anticipate sodium restriction to decrease fluid retention. ◆ Prepare for insertion of cardiac assist devices or transplantation as a last resort in severe cases that resist treatment.

Marfan syndrome

OVERVIEW

- Rare multisystem disorder of the connective tissue
- Results from microfibril defects and causes ocular, skeletal, and cardiovascular anomalies
- May result in death at any point between early infancy and adulthood related to cardiovascular complications
- Occurs in 1 out of every 5,000 to 10,000 people and affects males and females of all racial and ethnic groups equally

CAUSES

- Autosomal dominant trait of chromosome 15 that's caused by mutations in fibrillin-1 gene located on this chromosome
- In 75% of patients, syndrome inherited from a biological parent; in remaining 25%, mutation in the fibrillin-1 gene occurring spontaneously in the egg or sperm from which the patient was conceived

PATHOPHYSIOLOGY

- The gene on chromosome 15 is responsible for the genetic code for fibrillin—a glycoprotein component of connective tissue that comprises the extracellular matrix of many tissues.
- Many copies of fibrillin protein combine to make microfibrils, which are abundant in large blood vessels, the suspensory ligaments of the ocular lenses, and the bones.
- Fibrillin-1 mutations can lead to abnormal microfibrils and ultimately affect the elasticity or structure of connective tissues.
- Tissues subject to stress, such as in the aorta, eye, and skin, are especially vulnerable. Mutations of fibrillin-1 also cause overgrowth of long bones. (See *Disorders affecting management of Marfan Syndrome,* pages 310 and 311.)

CARDIOVASCULAR SYSTEM

- The medial layer of the arteries, specifically the aorta, are weakened. The arterial wall shows a loss of elastic fibers and enlargement of smooth-muscle cells.
- The aorta can't withstand the high-pressure blood flow. Subsequently, dilation of the aorta can occur, leading to an aneurysm that can rupture into the pericardial or retroperitoneal cavity.
- The mitral valve leaflets may be affected, leading to mitral insufficiency and mitral valve prolapse.

EYES

- Suspensory fibers that hold the lens in place are weakened as a result of the disorder.
- Other ocular structures may be affected because of the increased globe length, resulting from weakened connective tissue support. Subsequently, myopia and retinal detachment can occur.

MUSCULOSKELETAL SYSTEM

- Typically, the body is long and thin (especially the extremities) due to the overgrowth of bones.
- The lower body from the pubis to the soles of the feet is usually longer than the upper body.
- The skull bones are long, with a protruding frontal bone.
- The ribs form pectus excavatum (funnel chest) or pectus carinatum (pigeon chest).
- Arms span exceeds height.
- The laxity of the connective tissue leads to weakness in the tendons, ligaments, and joint capsules, resulting in hyperextensibility of the joints, dislocations, hernia, and kyphoscoliosis.

ASSESSMENT

HISTORY

- Positive family history in one parent
- Joint dislocations or "double-jointedness"
- Visual problems
- Palpitations
- Shortness of breath

PHYSICAL FINDINGS

- Taller than average for his family (in the 95th percentile for his age), with the upper half of his body shorter than average and the lower half longer
- Long, slender fingers (arachnodactyly) with positive wrist (Walker) and thumb (Steinberg) sign
- Defects of sternum (funnel chest or pigeon breast), chest asymmetry, scoliosis, and kyphosis
- Loose, hyperextensible joints with possible dislocation
- Abnormal heart sounds
- Cardiac arrhythmia (primary feature)
- Abdominal bruit
- Nearsightedness
- Possible lens displacement (ocular hallmark of the syndrome)
- Stretch marks in the absence of marked weight change or pregnancy

DIAGNOSTIC TEST RESULTS

◆ In the absence of family history, diagnosis requires documentation of at least one major finding in two body systems and one minor finding in a third body system.
◆ Skin culture detects fibrillin.
◆ X-rays confirm skeletal abnormalities.
◆ Echocardiogram shows dilation of the aortic root.
◆ Magnetic resonance imaging identifies aortic dissection.
◆ Deoxyribonucleic acid linkage analysis shows evidence of mutation. This test is performed if multiple family members are affected.

TREATMENT

GENERAL
◆ Symptomatic care
◆ For patients with scoliosis whose curvature is greater than 20 degrees, mechanical bracing and physical therapy
◆ Genetic counseling

DIET
◆ No restrictions

ACTIVITY
◆ Avoidance of competitive and contact sports

WARNING *High school and college athletes (particularly basketball players) who fit the criteria for Marfan syndrome should undergo a careful clinical and cardiac examination before being allowed to play sports to avoid sudden death from dissecting aortic aneurysm or other cardiac complications.*

◆ Avoid isometric exercises.

MEDICATIONS
◆ Beta-adrenergic blockers
◆ Calcium channel blockers

SURGERY
◆ Aneurysm repair to prevent rupture
◆ Surgical correction of ocular deformities to improve vision
◆ Aortic valve and mitral valve replacement
◆ Rod insertion if scoliosis curvature is greater than 45 degrees

NURSING CONSIDERATIONS

NURSING DIAGNOSES
◆ Decreased cardiac output
◆ Disturbed body image
◆ Risk for activity intolerance
◆ Risk for injury

EXPECTED OUTCOMES
The patient will:
◆ maintain adequate cardiac output
◆ verbalize feelings concerning body image and voice acceptance
◆ participate in activities without negative outcomes
◆ remain free from injury.

NURSING INTERVENTIONS
◆ Monitor vital signs, pulse oximetry readings, and cardiac rhythm.
◆ Assess cardiovascular status.
◆ Assist with activities of daily living, if indicated.
◆ Administer medications and evaluate effects.
◆ Provide preoperative and postoperative care, as appropriate.

PATIENT TEACHING

Be sure to cover:
◆ disorder, diagnostic testing, and treatment
◆ medication administration, dosage, and possible adverse effects
◆ activity restrictions
◆ need for eye care
◆ increased risks during pregnancy
◆ importance of follow-up care
◆ importance of wearing medical identification bracelet
◆ referral for genetic counseling
◆ referral to the National Marfan Foundation for additional information.

RESOURCES
Organization
The National Marfan Foundation: *www.marfan.org*

Selected references
Chaffins, D. "Marfan Syndrome," *Radiologic Technology* 78(3):222-36, January-February 2007.
Nicholson, C. "Cardiovascular Care of Patients with Marfan Syndrome," *Nursing Standard* 19(27):38-44, March 2005.
Rybczynski, M., et al. "Tissue Doppler Imaging Identifies Myocardial Dysfunction in Adults with Marfan Syndrome," *Clinical Cardiology* 30(1):19-24, January 2007.

(continued)

Disorders affecting management of Marfan syndrome

This chart highlights disorders that affect the management of Marfan syndrome.

DISORDER	SIGNS AND SYMPTOMS	DIAGNOSTIC TEST RESULTS	TREATMENT AND CARE
Cardiac arrhythmia (complication)	◆ Palpitations ◆ Chest pain ◆ Dizziness ◆ Weakness, fatigue ◆ Irregular heart rhythm ◆ Hypotension ◆ Syncope ◆ Altered level of consciousness ◆ Diaphoresis, pallor, cold, clammy skin	◆ Electrocardiogram (ECG) identifies specific waveform changes associated with the arrhythmia. ◆ Laboratory testing reveals electrolyte abnormalities, hypoxemia, or acid-base abnormalities. ◆ Electrophysiologic testing identifies the mechanism of an arrhythmia and the location of accessory pathways.	◆ Assess airway, breathing, and circulation if life-threatening arrhythmia develops; follow advanced cardiac life support protocols for treatment. ◆ Monitor cardiac rhythm continuously and obtain serial ECGs to evaluate changes and effects of treatment. ◆ Administer antiarrhythmics and monitor for adverse effects. ◆ Assess cardiovascular status for signs of hypoperfusion; monitor vital signs. ◆ Assist with insertion of temporary pacemaker, or apply transcutaneous pacemaker, if appropriate.
Dissecting aortic aneurysm (complication)	◆ Sudden, severe abdominal or lumbar pain that radiates to the flank and groin ◆ Severe and persistent abdominal pain mimicking renal or ureteral colic pain ◆ Massive hematemesis ◆ Melena ◆ Systolic bruit over the aorta ◆ Hypotension ◆ Tachycardia ◆ Cool, clammy skin	◆ Complete blood count (CBC) may reveal leukocytosis and decreased hemoglobin and hematocrit. ◆ Transesophageal echocardiogram provides visualization of the thoracic aorta and is usually combined with Doppler flow studies to provide information about blood flow. ◆ Abdominal ultrasonography or echocardiography can determine the aneurysm size, shape, length, and location. ◆ Anteroposterior and lateral X-rays of the chest or abdomen can detect aortic calcification and widened areas of the aorta. ◆ Computed tomography scan and magnetic resonance imaging can identify the aneurysm size and its effect on nearby organs. ◆ Aortography helps determine the aneurysm's approximate size and patency of the visceral vessels.	◆ Insert or assist with insertion of an arterial line to allow for continuous blood pressure monitoring; assist with insertion of a pulmonary artery catheter to assess hemodynamic balance. ◆ Insert a large-bore I.V. catheter, and begin fluid resuscitation. ◆ Administer nitroprusside (Nitropress) I.V., usually to maintain a mean arterial pressure of 70 to 80 mm Hg; also administer propranolol (Inderal) I.V. at a rate of 1 mg every 5 minutes (to a maximum initial dose not exceeding 0.15 mg/kg of body weight) to reduce left ventricular ejection velocity until the heart rate ranges from 60 to 80 beats/minute. ◆ If the patient is experiencing acute pain, administer morphine 2 to 10 mg I.V. ◆ Assess the patient's vital signs frequently, especially blood pressure; monitor blood pressure and pulse in extremities and compare findings bilaterally. ◆ Assess cardiovascular status frequently, including arterial blood gas (ABG) values, heart rate, rhythm, ECG, and cardiac enzyme levels. A myocardial infarction can occur if an aneurysm ruptures along the coronary arteries. ◆ Monitor urine output hourly. ◆ Evaluate CBC for evidence of blood loss, reflected in decreased hemoglobin level, hematocrit, and red blood cell count. ◆ Prepare the patient for emergency surgery.

Disorders affecting management of Marfan syndrome *(continued)*

DISORDER	SIGNS AND SYMPTOMS	DIAGNOSTIC TEST RESULTS	TREATMENT AND CARE
Mitral insufficiency (complication)	◆ Orthopnea and dyspnea ◆ Fatigue ◆ Angina, palpitations, and tachycardia ◆ Peripheral edema ◆ Jugular vein distention and hepatomegaly (right-sided heart failure) ◆ Crackles ◆ Pulmonary edema ◆ Holosystolic murmur at apex; a possible split second heart sound and third heart sound (S_3 and S_4)	◆ Cardiac catheterization reveals mitral insufficiency with increased left ventricular end-diastolic volume and pressure, increased atrial pressure and pulmonary artery wedge pressure, and decreased cardiac output. ◆ Chest X-rays show left atrial and ventricular enlargement and pulmonary venous congestion. ◆ Echocardiography reveals abnormal valve leaflet motion and left atrial enlargement. ◆ ECG may show left atrial and ventricular hypertrophy, sinus tachycardia, and atrial fibrillation.	◆ Assess the patient's vital signs, ABG values, pulse oximetry, intake and output, daily weights, blood chemistry studies, chest X-rays, and ECG. ◆ Promote measures to reduce activity level and decrease myocardial oxygen demands. ◆ Place the patient in an upright position to relieve dyspnea, if needed. ◆ Administer oxygen to prevent tissue hypoxia. ◆ Administer drug therapy, including digoxin, diuretics, and vasodilators to combat heart failure; anticoagulants to prevent thrombus formation; and nitroglycerin to relieve angina. ◆ Institute continuous cardiac monitoring to evaluate for arrhythmias if they occur; administer appropriate therapy per facility policy and physician's order. ◆ Observe for signs and symptoms of left-sided heart failure, pulmonary edema, and adverse reactions to drug therapy. ◆ Prepare for valvular surgery, if indicated.
Retinal detachment (complication)	◆ Floaters ◆ Light flashes ◆ Sudden, painless vision loss that may be described as a curtain that eliminates a portion of the visual field	◆ Ophthalmoscopic examination through a well-dilated pupil confirms the diagnosis. In severe detachment, examination reveals folds in the retina and a ballooning out of the area. ◆ Indirect ophthalmoscopy is used to search the retina for tears and holes. ◆ Ocular ultrasonography may be needed if the lens is opaque or if the vitreous humor is cloudy.	◆ Restrict eye movements through bed rest and sedation. ◆ If the patient's macula is threatened, position his head so the tear or hole is below the rest of the eye before surgical intervention. ◆ Prepare patient for surgical repair (cryotherapy, laser therapy, scleral buckling, pneumatic retinopexy, or vitrectomy). ◆ Provide emotional support. ◆ Position the patient facedown if gas has been injected to maintain pressure on the retina.

Metabolic acidosis LIFE-THREATENING DISORDER

OVERVIEW

- Acid-base disorder that's characterized by excess acid and deficient bicarbonate (HCO_3^-) caused by an underlying nonrespiratory disorder
- Children more vulnerable because their metabolic rates are rapid and ratios of water to total-body weight are low
- Fatal, if severe or left untreated

CAUSES

- Excessive production of metabolic acids, such as fat metabolism, in the absence of usable carbohydrates
- Anaerobic carbohydrate metabolism that forces a shift from aerobic to anaerobic metabolism, causing a corresponding increase in lactic acid level (see *Understanding lactic acidosis*)
- Underexcretion of metabolized acids or inability to conserve base caused by renal insufficiency and failure
- Diarrhea, intestinal malabsorption, or loss of sodium bicarbonate from the intestines, causing the bicarbonate buffer system to shift to the acidic side
- Salicylate intoxication; exogenous poisoning; or, less frequently, addisonism
- Inhibited secretion of acid caused by hypoaldosteronism or the use of potassium-sparing diuretics (see *Conditions that may cause metabolic acidosis*)

PATHOPHYSIOLOGY

- The underlying mechanisms in metabolic acidosis are a loss of HCO_3^- from extracellular fluid, an accumulation of metabolic acids, or a combination of the two; the condition may also be related to an overproduction of ketone bodies.
- Fatty acids are converted to ketone bodies when glucose supplies have been used and the body draws on fat stores for energy. Lactic acidosis can cause or worsen metabolic acidosis.
- If the patient's anion gap (measurement of the difference between the amount of sodium and the amount of bicarbonate in the blood) is greater than 14 mEq/L, then the aci-

---

UP CLOSE

Understanding lactic acidosis

Lactate, produced as a result of carbohydrate metabolism, is metabolized by the liver. The normal lactate level is 0.93 to 1.65 mEq/L. With tissue hypoxia, however, cells are forced to switch to anaerobic metabolism and more lactate is produced. When lactate accumulates in the body faster than it can be metabolized, lactic acidosis occurs. It can happen at any time the demand for oxygen in the body is greater than its availability.

The causes of lactic acidosis include septic shock, cardiac arrest, pulmonary disease, seizures, and strenuous exercise.

The latter two cause transient lactic acidosis. Hepatic disorders can also cause lactic acidosis because the liver can't metabolize lactate.

TREATMENT

Treatment focuses on eliminating the underlying cause. If pH is below 7.1, sodium bicarbonate may be given. Use caution when administering sodium bicarbonate, however, because it may cause alkalosis.

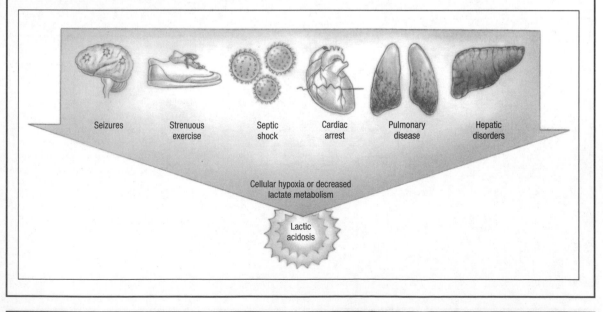

Seizures Strenuous exercise Septic shock Cardiac arrest Pulmonary disease Hepatic disorders

Cellular hypoxia or decreased lactate metabolism

Lactic acidosis

---

dosis is due to an accumulation of metabolic acids (unmeasured anions).

◆ If the metabolic acidosis is associated with a normal anion gap (8 to 14 mEq/L), loss of HCO_3^- may be the cause. (See *What happens in metabolic acidosis,* page 314.)

CARDIOVASCULAR SYSTEM

◆ As the pH drops and the balance of electrolytes is altered, membrane excitability in the cells of the heart muscle and blood vessels is altered, resulting in depressed myocardial function and decreased cardiac output and blood pressure.

◆ Arrhythmias may occur because of the shifts in electrolytes (especially potassium and calcium).

◆ Initially, vasodilation occurs as the blood vessels of the skin are less receptive to sympathetic stimuli. Skin is warm, flushed, and dry.

◆ As metabolic acidosis progresses, shock ensues, leading to cold and clammy skin.

GASTROINTESTINAL SYSTEM

◆ Excessive hydrogen ions diffuse into the cells of the GI system, and potassium is released into the blood.

Conditions that may cause metabolic acidosis

The following conditions may result in metabolic acidosis if left uncontrolled, untreated, or not treated appropriately.
◆ Diabetes mellitus
◆ Renal failure
◆ Myocardial infarction with cardiac pump failure
◆ Pulmonary disease
◆ Hepatic disease
◆ Dieting
◆ Drug usage or overdose
◆ Crohn's disease
◆ Shock
◆ Anemia
◆ Ureteroenterostomy
◆ Hypoaldosteronism

◆ The elevated potassium levels disrupt the normal balance of electrolytes and ultimately affect nerve impulse transmission to the muscles of the GI tract, resulting in colic and diarrhea.

NEUROLOGIC SYSTEM

◆ As the pH drops, central nervous system (CNS) depression occurs.

◆ Excessive hydrogen ions diffuse into the cells of the CNS, and potassium is released into the blood.

◆ Elevated potassium levels disrupt neuromuscular transmission. Subsequently, weakness or flaccid paralysis, numbness, and tingling in the extremities can occur.

◆ The continued decrease in pH depresses the excitability of the cell membranes and disrupts the balance of other electrolytes, including sodium and calcium, leading to reduced excitability of the nerve cells. The patient's level of consciousness (LOC) may deteriorate from confusion to stupor and coma.

◆ A neuromuscular examination may show diminished muscle tone and deep tendon reflexes.

RESPIRATORY SYSTEM

◆ As acid builds up in the bloodstream, the lungs compensate by blowing off carbon dioxide.

◆ Hyperventilation, especially increased depth of respirations (Kussmaul's respirations), is the first clue to metabolic acidosis.

◆ A patient with diabetes who experiences Kussmaul's respirations may have a fruity odor to his breath, which stems from catabolism of fats and excretion of acetone through the lungs.

◆ If the pH remains low, stimulation of the chemoreceptors continues to maintain hyperventilation as a means to blow off carbon dioxide. If hyperventilation continues, respiratory failure may occur. (See *Disorders affecting management of metabolic acidosis,* pages 316 and 317.)

ASSESSMENT

HISTORY

◆ Presence of risk factors, including associated disorders and the use of medications that contain alcohol or aspirin

◆ Change in LOC, ranging from lethargy, drowsiness, and confusion to stupor and coma

◆ Generalized weakness

PHYSICAL FINDINGS

◆ Decreased deep tendon reflexes and muscle tone
◆ Dull headache
◆ Hyperkalemic signs and symptoms, including abdominal cramping, diarrhea, muscle weakness, and electrocardiogram changes
◆ Hypotension
◆ Arrhythmias
◆ Kussmaul's respirations
◆ Lethargy
◆ Warm, dry skin
◆ Fruity breath odor in patients with underlying diabetes mellitus
◆ Signs of dehydration, such as poor skin turgor and dry mucous membranes

DIAGNOSTIC TEST RESULTS

◆ Arterial blood gas studies reveal an arterial pH less than 7.35 (as low as 7.10 in severe acidosis), a partial pressure of carbon dioxide ($Paco_2$) that's normal or less than 34 mm Hg as respiratory compensatory mechanisms take hold, and a HCO_3^- level of 22 mEq/L.

◆ Urine pH is less than 4.5 in the absence of renal disease (as the kidneys excrete acid to raise blood pH).

◆ Potassium level is greater than 5.5 mEq/L from chemical buffering.

◆ Glucose level is greater than 150 mg/dl.

◆ Serum ketone bodies are present in patients with diabetes.

◆ Lactic acid level is elevated in lactic acidosis.

(continued)

What happens in metabolic acidosis

This series of illustrations shows how metabolic acidosis develops at the cellular level.

As hydrogen ions (H+) start to accumulate in the body, chemical buffers (plasma bicarbonate [HCO_3^-] and proteins) in the cells and extracellular fluid bind with them. No signs are detectable at this stage.

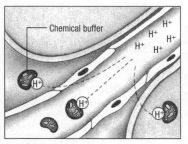

Excess H+ that the buffers can't bind with decrease pH and stimulate chemoreceptors in the medulla to increase respiratory rate. Increased respiratory rate lowers partial pressure of arterial carbon dioxide ($Paco_2$), which allows more H+ to bind with HCO_3^-. Respiratory compensation occurs within minutes but isn't sufficient to correct the imbalance. Look for a pH level below 7.35, a bicarbonate level below 22 mEq/L, a decreasing $Paco_2$ level, and rapid, deeper respirations.

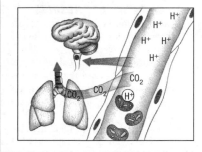

Healthy kidneys try to compensate for acidosis by secreting excess H+ into the renal tubules. Those ions are buffered by phosphate or ammonia and then are excreted into the urine in the form of a weak acid. Look for acidic urine.

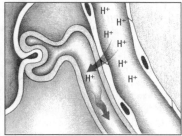

Each time a H+ is secreted into the renal tubules, a sodium (Na) ion and an HCO_3^- are absorbed from the tubules and returned to the blood. Look for pH and HCO_3^- levels that slowly return to normal.

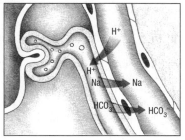

Excess H+ in the extracellular fluid diffuse into cells. To maintain the balance of the charge across the membrane, the cells release potassium ions into the blood. Look for signs and symptoms of hyperkalemia, including colic and diarrhea, weakness or flaccid paralysis, tingling and numbness in the extremities, bradycardia, a tall T wave, a prolonged PR interval, and a widened QRS complex.

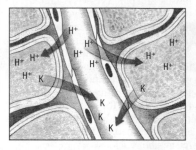

Excess H+ alter the normal balance of potassium (K), sodium (Na), and calcium ions (Ca), leading to reduced excitability of nerve cells. Look for signs and symptoms of progressive central nervous system depression (lethargy, dull headache, confusion, stupor, and coma).

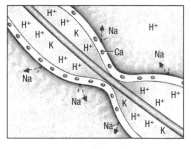

- Anion gap is greater than 14 mEq/L in high anion gap metabolic acidosis, lactic acidosis, ketoacidosis, aspirin overdose, alcohol poisoning, renal failure, or other conditions characterized by accumulation of organic acids, sulfates, or phosphates; 12 mEq/L or less in normal anion gap metabolic acidosis from HCO_3^- loss, GI or renal loss, increased acid load (hyperalimentation fluids), rapid I.V. saline solution administration, or other conditions characterized by loss of HCO_3^-.

TREATMENT

GENERAL
- Treatment of underlying cause
- Endotracheal intubation and mechanical ventilation, if needed
- Dialysis

DIET
- Based on condition and underlying cause

ACTIVITY
- Bed rest until stable

MEDICATIONS
- I.V. sodium bicarbonate (if severe)
- Electrolyte supplements
- I.V. lactated Ringer's solution
- Antidiarrheals
- Vasopressors
- Antianxiety agents

NURSING CONSIDERATIONS

NURSING DIAGNOSES
- Anxiety
- Decreased cardiac output
- Fear
- Impaired gas exchange
- Ineffective breathing pattern
- Risk for injury

EXPECTED OUTCOMES
The patient will:
- demonstrate adequate coping mechanisms and verbalize decreased anxiety
- maintain adequate perfusion of tissues and organs
- express feelings of decreased fear
- maintain adequate ventilation and oxygenation
- maintain effective breathing pattern
- remain free from injury.

NURSING INTERVENTIONS
- Monitor vital signs, pulse oximetry, intake and output, and arterial blood gas results.
- Assess neurologic, cardiovascular, and respiratory status.
- Monitor electrolytes.
- Orient the patient frequently, and reduce unnecessary environmental stimuli.
- Implement safety measures, especially if the patient is confused or comatose.
- Reposition every 2 hours, and provide skin care.

PATIENT TEACHING

Be sure to cover:
- disorder, diagnostic testing, and treatment
- underlying cause of disorder and how to prevent reccurence
- medication administration, dosage, and possible adverse effects
- referral to appropriate agencies for supportive care and further teaching.

RESOURCES
Organizations
Mayo Clinic: *www.mayoclinic.com*
National Institutes of Health: *www.nih.gov*

Selected references
Schoolwerth, A., et al. "Acid-Base Disturbance in the Intensive Care Unit: Metabolic Acidosis," *Seminars in Dialysis* 19(6):492-95, November-December 2006.
Sinert, R., et al. "Effect of Normal Saline Solution on the Diagnostic Utility of Base Deficit in Identifying Major Injury in Trauma Patients," *Academic Emergency Medicine* 13(12):1269-274, December 2006.
Strategies in Managing Multisystem Disorders. Philadelphia: Lippincott Williams & Wilkins, 2006.

(continued)

Disorders affecting management of metabolic acidosis

This chart highlights disorders that affect the management of metabolic acidosis.

DISORDER	SIGNS AND SYMPTOMS	DIAGNOSTIC TEST RESULTS	TREATMENT AND CARE
Cardiac arrhythmia (complication)	◆ Palpitations ◆ Chest pain ◆ Dizziness ◆ Weakness and fatigue ◆ Irregular heart rhythm ◆ Hypotension ◆ Syncope ◆ Altered level of consciousness (LOC) ◆ Diaphoresis ◆ Pallor ◆ Cold, clammy skin	◆ 12-lead electrocardiogram (ECG) identifies specific waveform changes associated with the arrhythmia.	◆ Evaluate the monitored patient's ECG regularly for arrhythmias, and assess hemodynamic parameters, as indicated. Document arrhythmias and notify the physician immediately. ◆ Assess an unmonitored patient for rhythm disturbances. If the patient's pulse rate is abnormally rapid, slow, or irregular, watch for signs of hypoperfusion, such as hypotension and diminished urine output. ◆ As ordered, obtain an EGG tracing in an unmonitored patient to confirm and identify the type of arrhythmia present. ◆ Administer medications and monitor the patient for adverse effects. ◆ If a life-threatening arrhythmia develops, rapidly assess the patient's LOC, pulse and respiratory rates, and hemodynamic parameters. Monitor EGG continuously. Be prepared to initiate cardiopulmonary resuscitation or cardioversion, if indicated.
Hyperkalemia (complication)	◆ Abdominal cramping ◆ Diarrhea ◆ Hypotension ◆ Irregular pulse rate; tachycardia changing to bradycardia ◆ Irritability ◆ Muscle weakness, especially of the lower extremities ◆ Nausea ◆ Paresthesia	◆ Laboratory testing reveals hyperkalemia, electrolyte abnormalities, hypoxemia, or acid-base abnormalities. ◆ Serum potassium level is greater than 5 mEq/L. ◆ ECG changes include a tall, tented T wave; widened QRS complex; prolonged PR interval; flattened or absent P wave; and depressed ST segment. ◆ Arterial blood gas (ABG) analysis reveals decreased pH and metabolic acidosis.	◆ Assess vital signs. Anticipate continuous cardiac monitoring if the patient's serum potassium level exceeds 6 mEq/L. ◆ Monitor the patient's intake and output; report an output of less than 30 ml/hour. ◆ Administer a slow calcium gluconate I.V. infusion to counteract the myocardial depressant effects of hyperkalemia. ◆ For a patient receiving repeated insulin and glucose treatment, check for signs and symptoms of hypoglycemia, including muscle weakness, syncope, hunger, and diaphoresis. ◆ Administer sodium polystyrene sulfonate, and monitor serum sodium levels, which may rise; assess for signs of heart failure. Encourage the patient to retain sodium polystyrene sulfonate enemas for 30 to 60 minutes. Monitor the patient for hypokalemia when administering the drug on 2 or more consecutive days. ◆ Monitor bowel sounds and the number and character of bowel movements. ◆ Monitor serum potassium level and related laboratory test results. ◆ If the patient has acute hyperkalemia that doesn't respond to other treatments, prepare for dialysis. ◆ If the patient has muscle weakness, implement safety measures. ◆ Assess for signs of hypokalemia after treatment.

DISORDER	SIGNS AND SYMPTOMS	DIAGNOSTIC TEST RESULTS	TREATMENT AND CARE
Respiratory failure (complication)	◆ Diminished chest movement ◆ Restlessness, irritability, and confusion ◆ Decreased LOC ◆ Pallor; possible cyanosis of lips, nail beds, or mucous membranes ◆ Tachypnea, tachycardia (strong and rapid initially, but thready and irregular in later stages) ◆ Cold, clammy skin and frank diaphoresis, especially around the forehead and face ◆ Diminished breath sounds; possible adventitious breath sounds ◆ Possible cardiac arrhythmias	◆ ABG analysis indicates early respiratory failure when partial pressure of arterial oxygen is low (usually less than 70 mm Hg) and partial pressure of arterial carbon dioxide is high (greater than 45 mm Hg). ◆ Serial vital capacity reveals readings less than 800 ml. ◆ ECG may demonstrate arrhythmias. ◆ Pulse oximetry reveals a decreased oxygen saturation level. Mixed venous oxygen saturation levels less than 50% indicate impaired tissue oxygenation.	◆ Institute oxygen therapy immediately. ◆ Prepare for endotracheal (ET) intubation and mechanical ventilation, if needed; anticipate the need for high-frequency or pressure ventilation to force airways open. ◆ Administer drug therapy, such as bronchodilators to open airways, corticosteroids to reduce inflammation, continuous I.V. solutions of positive inotropic agents (which increase cardiac output) and vasopressors (which induce vasoconstriction) to maintain blood pressure, and diuretics to reduce fluid overload and edema. ◆ Assess the patient's respiratory status at least every 2 hours, or more often, as indicated. ◆ Monitor the patient for a positive response to oxygen therapy, such as improved breathing, color, and ABG values. Monitor oximetry and capnography values to detect important changes in the patient's condition. ◆ Position the patient for optimal breathing. ◆ Maintain a normothermic environment to reduce the patient's oxygen demand. ◆ Monitor vital signs, heart rhythm, and fluid intake and output. ◆ If intubated, auscultate the lungs to check for accidental intubation of the esophagus or the mainstem bronchus. ◆ Perform suctioning using strict aseptic technique when the patient is intubated. Note the amount and quality of lung secretions, and look for changes in the patient's status. ◆ Check cuff pressure on the ET tube to prevent erosion from an overinflated cuff. Normal cuff pressure is about 20 mm Hg. ◆ Implement measures to prevent nasal tissue necrosis. Position and maintain the nasotracheal tube midline in the nostrils and reposition daily. Tape the tube securely, but use skin protection measures and nonirritating tape to prevent skin breakdown. ◆ Provide a means of communication for patients who are intubated and alert.

Metabolic alkalosis LIFE-THREATENING DISORDER

OVERVIEW

- Acid-base disorder that's characterized by low levels of acid or high bicarbonate (HCO_3^-) levels
- May cause metabolic, respiratory, and renal responses, producing characteristic symptoms (most notably, hypoventilation)
- Always secondary to an underlying cause
- With early diagnosis and prompt treatment, good prognosis; however, if left untreated, may lead to coma and death

CAUSES

- Loss of acid, retention of base, or renal mechanisms linked to low potassium and chloride levels (see *Conditions that may cause metabolic alkalosis*)

Conditions that may cause metabolic alkalosis

The following conditions may result in metabolic alkalosis if left uncontrolled, untreated, or not treated appropriately.
- Chronic vomiting, such as with anorexia nervosa or bulimia
- Nasogastric tube drainage or lavage without adequate electrolyte replacement
- Fistulas
- Use of steroids or certain diuretics (furosemide [Lasix], thiazides, and ethacrynic acid [Edecrin])
- Massive blood transfusions
- Cushing's syndrome, primary hyperaldosteronism, and Bartter's syndrome, which lead to sodium and chloride retention and urinary loss of potassium and hydrogen.
- Excessive intake of bicarbonate of soda or other antacids (usually for treatment of gastritis or peptic ulcer)
- Excessive intake of absorbable alkali (as in milk alkali syndrome, commonly seen in patients with peptic ulcers)
- Excessive amounts of I.V. fluids with high bicarbonate or lactate levels
- Respiratory insufficiency
- Low chloride or potassium level
- Cystic fibrosis

PATHOPHYSIOLOGY

- Underlying mechanisms include a loss of hydrogen ions (acid), a gain in HCO_3^-, or both.
- A partial pressure of arterial carbon dioxide ($Paco_2$) level greater than 45 mm Hg (possibly as high as 60 mm Hg) indicates that the lungs are compensating for the alkalosis.
- The kidneys are more effective at compensating; however, they're far slower than the lungs. As a result, numerous body systems may be affected. (See *What happens in metabolic alkalosis*.)

CARDIOVASCULAR SYSTEM

- As a result of electrolyte imbalances (such as hypokalemia) cardiac muscle contraction and electrical conductivity are altered, which may lead to the development of arrhythmias.
- The risk of arrhythmias is further complicated by the decreased calcium influx in the cardiac muscle secondary to the accompanying hypocalcemia.

GENITOURINARY SYSTEM

- When the blood HCO_3^- rises to 28 mEq/L or more, the amount filtered by the renal glomeruli exceeds the reabsorptive capacity of the renal tubules.
- Excess HCO_3^- is excreted in the urine, and hydrogen ions are retained.
- To maintain electrochemical balance, sodium ions and water are excreted with the bicarbonate ions.

NEUROLOGIC SYSTEM

- When hydrogen ion levels in extracellular fluid are low, hydrogen ions diffuse passively out of the cells and, to maintain the balance of charge across the cell membrane, extracellular potassium ions move into the cells.
- As intracellular hydrogen ion levels fall, calcium ionization decreases and nerve cells become more permeable to sodium ions.

- As sodium ions move into the cells, they trigger neural impulses, first in the peripheral nervous system and then in the central nervous system. Subsequently, hypocalcemia and seizures occur. (See *Disorders affecting management of metabolic alkalosis*, page 321.)

RESPIRATORY SYSTEM

- Chemical buffers in the extracellular fluid and intracellular fluid bind HCO_3^- that accumulates in the body.
- Excess unbound HCO_3^- raises blood pH, which depresses chemoreceptors in the medulla, inhibiting respiration and raising $Paco_2$.
- Carbon dioxide combines with water to form carbonic acid. Low oxygen levels limit respiratory compensation.

ASSESSMENT

HISTORY

- History of underlying condition
- Change in mental status or personality

PHYSICAL FINDINGS

- Anorexia
- Apathy
- Confusion
- Cyanosis
- Hypotension
- Loss of reflexes
- Muscle twitching
- Nausea and vomiting
- Paresthesia
- Polyuria
- Weakness
- Cardiac arrhythmias (occurring with hypokalemia)
- Positive Trousseau's and Chvostek's signs
- Tetany, if serum calcium levels are borderline or low
- Decreased rate and depth of respirations (This mechanism is limited because of the development of hypoxemia, which stimulates ventilation.)

DIAGNOSTIC TEST RESULTS

◆ Arterial blood gas studies reveal a blood pH greater than 7.45, HCO_3^- greater than 26 mEq/L, and $Paco_2$ greater than 45 mm Hg (indicates attempts at respiratory compensation).

◆ Potassium level is less than 3.5 mEq/L, calcium level is less than 8.9 mg/dl, and chloride level is less than 98 mEq/L.

◆ Urine pH is about 7, and urine is alkaline after the renal compensatory mechanism begins to excrete HCO_3^-.

◆ Electrocardiography (ECG) may show a low T wave merging with a P wave and atrial or sinus tachycardia.

UP CLOSE

What happens in metabolic alkalosis

This series of illustrations shows how metabolic alkalosis develops at the cellular level.

As bicarbonate ions (HCO_3^-) start to accumulate in the body, chemical buffers (in extracellular fluid and cells) bind with them. No signs are detectable at this stage.

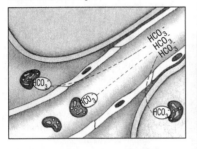

Excess HCO_3^- that doesn't bind with chemical buffers elevates serum pH levels, which in turn depresses chemoreceptors in the medulla. Depression of those chemoreceptors causes a decrease in respiratory rate, which increases partial pressure of arterial carbon dioxide ($Paco_2$). The additional carbon dioxide (CO_2) combines with water (H_2O) to form carbonic acid (H_2CO_3). *Note:* Lowered oxygen levels limit respiratory compensation. Look for a serum pH level above 7.45, a HCO_3^- level above 26 mEq/L, a rising $Paco_2$, and slow, shallow respirations.

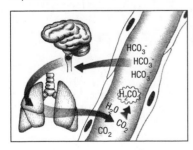

When the HCO_3^- level exceeds 28 mEq/L, the renal glomeruli can no longer reabsorb excess amounts. The excess HCO_3^- is excreted in urine; hydrogen ions (H+) are retained. Look for alkaline urine and pH and bicarbonate levels that slowly return to normal.

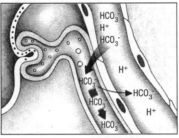

To maintain electrochemical balance, the kidneys excrete excess sodium ions (Na), water, and HCO_3^-. Look for polyuria initially, then signs and symptoms of hypovolemia, including thirst and dry mucous membranes.

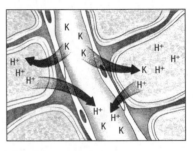

Lowered H+ levels in the extracellular fluid cause the ions to diffuse out of the cells. To maintain the balance of charge across the cell membrane, extracellular potassium ions (K) move into the cells. Look for signs and symptoms of hypokalemia, including anorexia, muscle weakness, loss of reflexes, and others.

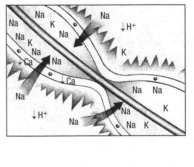

As H+ levels decline, calcium (Ca) ionization decreases. That decrease in ionization makes nerve cells more permeable to sodium ions. Sodium ions moving into nerve cells stimulate neural impulses and produce overexcitability of the peripheral and central nervous systems. Look for tetany, belligerence, irritability, disorientation, and seizures.

(continued)

TREATMENT

GENERAL
- Treatment of underlying cause
- Endotracheal intubation and mechanical ventilation, if needed
- Dialysis

DIET
- Based on condition and underlying cause

ACTIVITY
- Bed rest until stable

MEDICATIONS
- Hydrochloric acid
- Potassium chloride supplement
- Acetazolamide (Diamox)
- Angiotensin-converting enzyme inhibitor (captopril [Capoten])
- I.V. fluids
- Corticosteroids (dexamethasone [Decadron])

NURSING CONSIDERATIONS

NURSING DIAGNOSES
- Anxiety
- Decreased cardiac output
- Fear
- Impaired gas exchange
- Ineffective breathing pattern
- Risk for injury

EXPECTED OUTCOMES
The patient will:
- demonstrate adequate coping mechanisms and verbalize decreased anxiety
- maintain adequate cardiac output
- express feelings of decreased fear
- demonstrate adequate ventilation and oxygenation
- maintain effective breathing pattern
- remain free from injury.

NURSING INTERVENTIONS
- Monitor vital signs, intake and output, electrolyte levels, and ABG values.
- Monitor ECG for arrhythmias; administer supplemental oxygen, if indicated.
- Complete a neurologic assessment with reorientation, as necessary.
- Provide seizure precautions and safety measures for the patient with altered thought processes.

PATIENT TEACHING

Be sure to cover:
- disorder, diagnostic testing, and treatment
- medication administration, dosage, and possible adverse effects
- underlying cause of disorder and how to prevent recurrence
- referral to appropriate agencies for supportive care and further teaching.

RESOURCES
Organizations
Mayo Clinic: *www.mayoclinic.com*
National Institutes of Health: *www.nih.gov*

Selected references
Khanna, A., and Kurtzman, N. "Metabolic Alkalosis," *Journal of Nephrology* 19(Suppl 9):S86-96, March-April 2006.
Kirsch, B., et al. "Metabolic Alkalosis in a Hemodialysis Patient: Successful Treatment with a Proton Pump Inhibitor," *Clinical Nephrology* 66(5):391-94, November 2006.
Strategies for Managing Multisystem Disorders. Philadelphia: Lippincott Williams & Wilkins, 2006.

Disorders affecting management of metabolic alkalosis

This chart highlights disorders that affect the management of metabolic alkalosis.

DISORDER	SIGNS AND SYMPTOMS	DIAGNOSTIC TEST RESULTS	TREATMENT AND CARE
Hypocalcemia (complication)	◆ Anxiety ◆ Irritability ◆ Twitching around the mouth ◆ Laryngospasm ◆ Seizures ◆ Muscle cramps ◆ Paresthesia of the face, fingers, or toes ◆ Tetany ◆ Positive Chvostek's and Trousseau's signs ◆ Hypotension ◆ Arrhythmias ◆ Hyperactive deep tendon reflexes	◆ Serum calcium level is less than 8.5 mg/dl. ◆ Ionized calcium level is usually below 4.5 mg/dl. ◆ Platelet count is decreased. ◆ Electrocardiography shows lengthened QT interval, prolonged ST segment, and arrhythmias. ◆ Serum protein levels may reveal possible changes because half of the serum calcium is bound to albumin.	◆ Assess cardiovascular status and neurologic status for changes; monitor vital signs frequently. ◆ Monitor respiratory status, including rate, depth, and rhythm. ◆ Keep a tracheotomy tray and a handheld resuscitation bag at the bedside in case laryngospasm occurs. ◆ Institute cardiac monitoring and evaluate for changes in heart rate and rhythm. ◆ Assess for Chvostek's sign or Trousseau's sign. ◆ Administer I.V. calcium replacement therapy carefully. Check magnesium and phosphate levels because a low magnesium level must be corrected before I.V. calcium can be effective; if the phosphate level is too high, calcium won't be absorbed. ◆ Ensure the patency of the I.V. line because infiltration can cause tissue necrosis and sloughing. ◆ Give calcium supplements 1 to 1½ hours after meals. If GI upset occurs, give the supplement with milk. ◆ Monitor laboratory test results, including calcium levels, albumin, and magnesium levels. ◆ Institute seizure precautions and safety measures to prevent injury.
Seizures (generalized tonic-clonic) (complication)	◆ Loud cry upon start of seizure ◆ Changes in level of consciousness ◆ Body stiffening, alternating between muscle spasm and relaxation ◆ Tongue biting ◆ Incontinence ◆ Labored breathing, apnea, and cyanosis ◆ Upon wakening, possible confusion and difficulty talking ◆ Drowsiness, fatigue, and headache ◆ Muscle soreness and weakness	◆ EEG reveals paroxysmal abnormalities; high, fast voltage spikes are present in all leads. ◆ Serum chemistry blood studies may reveal hypoglycemia, electrolyte imbalances, elevated liver enzymes, or elevated alcohol levels. ◆ Arterial blood gas (ABG) analysis provides baseline levels for oxygenation and acid-base status.	◆ Establish and maintain the patient's airway; assess respiratory status, including rate, depth, and rhythm of respirations. Observe for accessory muscle use or labored respirations. ◆ Assess neurologic status to establish a baseline and then frequently reassess the patient, at least every 5 to 10 minutes initially, until stabilized. ◆ Assess oxygen saturation with pulse oximetry and ABG analysis; administer supplemental oxygen, as indicated; have endotracheal intubation equipment and ventilatory assistance readily available at the bedside. ◆ Monitor vital signs, and anticipate continuous direct intra-arterial blood pressure monitoring, if appropriate. ◆ Institute continuous cardiac monitoring to evaluate for arrhythmias. ◆ Monitor blood glucose levels for hypoglycemia and administer glucose; prepare to treat the underlying cause. ◆ Administer anticonvulsants I.V. Expect to administer fast-acting agents first, followed by long-acting agents. Monitor the patient's response. ◆ If seizures continue, prepare for general anesthesia with pentobarbital (Nembutal), propofol (Diprivan), or midazolam (Versed). ◆ Institute seizure precautions and safety measures.

Metabolic syndrome

- Cluster of symptoms triggered by insulin resistance, including abdominal fat, obesity, high blood pressure, and high levels of blood glucose, triglycerides, and cholesterol
- Associated with increased risk of diabetes, heart disease, and stroke
- Often goes unrecognized
- Affects an estimated 47 million people in the United States
- Most common in Mexican Americans (highest rate at 32%)
- In Black and Mexican-American individuals, females more susceptible than males; otherwise, males and females equally affected
- Also known as *syndrome X, insulin resistance syndrome, dysmetabolic syndrome,* and *multiple metabolic syndrome*

CAUSES
- Genetic predisposition

RISK FACTORS
- Obesity
- High-fat, high-carbohydrate diet
- Insufficient physical activity
- Aging
- Hyperinsulinemia/impaired glucose tolerance
- Previous heart attack

- The body breaks food down into basic components, one of which is glucose.
- Glucose provides energy for cellular activity.
- Excess glucose is stored in cells for future use and is guided into storage cells by insulin, which is secreted by the pancreas.
- In those with metabolic syndrome, glucose doesn't respond to insulin's attempt to guide it into storage cells. This is called *insulin resistance.*
- To overcome this resistance, the pancreas produces excess insulin, which causes damage to arterial lining.
- Excessive insulin secretion also promotes fat storage deposits and prevents fat breakdown.
- This series of events can lead to diabetes, blood clots, and coronary events. (See *Disorders affecting management of metabolic syndrome,* page 325.)

CARDIOVASCULAR SYSTEM
- Interference with normal fat breakdown can result in plaque buildup in vessels, resulting in hypertension and cardiovascular disease.

ENDOCRINE SYSTEM
- Excess insulin is excreted in an attempt to overcome insulin resistance and is a precursor to type 2 diabetes mellitus.

HISTORY
- Familial history
- Hypertension
- High low-density lipoproteins (LDL) and triglyceride levels
- Low high-density lipoproteins (HDL) levels
- Abdominal obesity
- Sedentary lifestyle
- Poor diet

PHYSICAL FINDINGS
- Abdominal obesity (see *Why abdominal obesity is dangerous*)

DIAGNOSTIC TEST RESULTS
- Glucose level is elevated.
- LDL and triglyceride levels are increased.
- HDL level is decreased.
- Blood tests show hyperinsulinemia.
- Serum uric acid level is elevated.
- Blood pressure is greater than 130/85 mm Hg.

Why abdominal obesity is dangerous

People with excess weight around the waist have a greater risk of developing metabolic syndrome than people with excess weight around the hips. That's because intra-abdominal fat tends to be more resistant to insulin than fat in other areas of the body. Insulin resistance increases the release of free fatty acid into the portal system, leading to increased apolipoprotein B, increased low-density lipoprotein, decreased high-density lipoprotein, and increased triglyceride levels. As a result, the risk of cardiovascular disease increases.

TREATMENT

GENERAL
◆ Weight-reduction program

DIET
◆ Low alcohol intake
◆ Low-cholesterol
◆ High in complex carbohydrates (grains, beans, vegetables, fruit) and low in refined carbohydrates (soda, table sugar, high-fructose corn syrup)

ACTIVITY
◆ Daily physical activity of at least 20 minutes

MEDICATIONS
◆ Oral antidiabetic agents
◆ Antihypertensives
◆ Cholesterol-lowering antihyperlipemics

NURSING CONSIDERATIONS

NURSING DIAGNOSES
◆ Fatigue
◆ Imbalanced nutrition: More than body requirements
◆ Risk for injury

EXPECTED OUTCOMES
The patient will:
◆ express feelings of increased energy
◆ identify appropriate food choices according to a prescribed diet and maintain a healthy weight
◆ remain free from injury.

NURSING INTERVENTIONS
◆ Promote lifestyle changes and give appropriate support.
◆ Monitor vital signs and laboratory values.
◆ Provide emotional support.

PATIENT TEACHING

Be sure to cover:
◆ disorder, diagnostic testing, and treatment
◆ medication administration, dosage, and possible adverse effects
◆ principles of a healthy diet, reference to a weight-reduction program, if indicated
◆ relationship of diet, inactivity, and obesity to metabolic syndrome
◆ benefits of increased physical activity
◆ importance of follow-up care.

(continued)

RESOURCES
Organizations
American Diabetes Association:
www.diabetes.org
American Heart Association:
www.americanheart.org
Cleveland Clinic Health Information Center: *www.clevelandclinic.org/health*

Selected references
Bell-Anderson, K., and Samman, S. "Nutrition and Metabolism: Race, Sex, and the Metabolic Syndrome," *Current Opinion in Lipidology* 17(1):82-84, February 2006.

Bhatheja, R., and Bhatt, D. "Clinical Outcomes in Metabolic Syndromes," *Journal of Cardiovascular Nursing* 21(4): 298-2305, July-August 2006.

Harrell, J., et al. "Obesity and Metabolic Syndrome in Children and Adolescents," *Journal of Cardiovascular Nursing* 21(4):322-30, July-August 2006.

Venkatapuram, S., and Shannon, R.P. "Managing Atherosclerosis in Patients with Type 2 Diabetes and Metabolic Syndrome," *American Journal of Therapeutics* 13(1):64-71, January-February 2006.

Wong, N. "The Metabolic Syndrome and Preventive Cardiology: Working Together to Reduce Cardiometabolic Risks," *Metabolic Syndrome and Related Disorders* 4(4):233-36, December 2006.

Disorders affecting management of metabolic syndrome

This chart highlights disorders that affect the management of metabolic syndrome.

DISORDER	SIGNS AND SYMPTOMS	DIAGNOSTIC TEST RESULTS	TREATMENT AND CARE
Coronary artery disease (complication)	◆ Angina or feeling of burning, squeezing or tightness in the chest that may radiate to the left arm, neck, jaw, or shoulder blade ◆ Nausea and vomiting ◆ Cool extremities and pallor ◆ Diaphoresis ◆ Xanthelasma	◆ Electrocardiogram (ECG) may be normal between anginal episodes. During angina, it may show ischemic changes (T-wave inversion, ST depression, arrhythmia). ◆ Computed tomography may identify calcium deposits in coronary arteries. ◆ Stress testing may detect ST-segment changes. ◆ Coronary angiography reveals location and degree of stenosis, obstruction, and collateral circulation. ◆ Rest perfusion imaging rules out myocardial infarction.	◆ Assess level of pain, vital signs, and pulse oximetry during anginal attack. ◆ Provide oxygen therapy, obtain ECG, and administer medication during an attack. ◆ Explain all testing and answer questions regarding procedures and findings. ◆ Provide teaching regarding diagnosis, medication use, and follow-up care. ◆ Encourage lifestyle changes, as appropriate.
Diabetes mellitus (complication)	◆ Weight loss despite voracious hunger ◆ Weakness ◆ Vision changes ◆ Frequent skin and urinary tract infections ◆ Dry, itchy skin ◆ Poor skin turgor ◆ Dry mucous membranes ◆ Dehydration, despite increased thirst ◆ Polyuria ◆ Decreased peripheral pulses ◆ Cool skin temperature ◆ Decreased reflexes ◆ Orthostatic hypotension ◆ Muscle wasting ◆ Loss of subcutaneous fat ◆ Fruity breath odor from ketoacidosis	◆ Fasting blood glucose level is 126 mg/dl or greater, or a random blood glucose level is 200 mg/dl or greater on at least two occasions. ◆ Blood glucose level is 200 mg/dl or greater 2 hours after ingestion of 75 grams of oral dextrose. ◆ Ophthalmic examination may reveal diabetic retinopathy.	◆ Monitor blood glucose and urine acetone levels. ◆ Monitor intake and output; encourage increased fluid intake or provide I.V. fluids. ◆ Administer insulin or antidiabetic agents, as prescribed. ◆ Provide nutritional counseling and assistance with dietary choices. ◆ Provide teaching on disorder, treatment, and follow-up care. ◆ Assess skin for break in integrity. Provide teaching on skin and foot care. ◆ Assess for signs and symptoms of complications.
Hypertension (complication)	◆ Usually asymptomatic ◆ Elevated blood pressure readings on at least two consecutive occasions ◆ Occipital headache ◆ Epistaxis ◆ Bruits ◆ Dizziness ◆ Confusion ◆ Fatigue ◆ Blurry vision ◆ Nocturia ◆ Edema	◆ Serial blood pressure measurements reveal elevations of 140/90 mm Hg or greater on two or more separate occasions. ◆ Urinalysis may show protein, casts, red blood cells, or white blood cells; blood urea nitrogen and serum creatinine levels may be elevated. ◆ ECG may reveal ventricular hypertrophy or ischemia. ◆ Echocardiography may reveal left ventricular hypertrophy.	◆ Monitor blood pressure readings, response to antihypertensives, and laboratory readings. ◆ Encourage lifestyle modifications or change, especially weight loss, diet, and exercise. ◆ Monitor for complications, such as stroke, myocardial infarction, and renal disease. ◆ Administer medications, as ordered.

Myocardial infarction LIFE-THREATENING DISORDER

OVERVIEW

- Reduced blood flow through one or more coronary arteries causing myocardial ischemia and necrosis
- Infarction site dependent on the vessels involved
- Males more susceptible than premenopausal females
- Incidence increasing among females who smoke and take hormonal contraceptives
- Incidence in postmenopausal females similar to that in males
- Also called *MI* and *heart attack*

CAUSES

- Atherosclerosis
- Coronary artery stenosis or spasm
- Platelet aggregation
- Thrombosis

RISK FACTORS

- Increased age (40 to 70)
- Diabetes mellitus
- Elevated serum triglyceride, low-density lipoprotein, and cholesterol levels and decreased serum high-density lipoprotein levels
- Excessive intake of saturated fats, carbohydrates, or salt
- Hypertension
- Obesity
- Family history of coronary artery disease (CAD)
- Sedentary lifestyle
- Smoking
- Stress or type A personality
- Use of drugs, such as amphetamines or cocaine

PATHOPHYSIOLOGY

- One or more coronary arteries become occluded.
- If coronary occlusion causes ischemia lasting longer than 30 to 45 minutes, irreversible myocardial cell damage and muscle death occur.
- Every MI has a central area of necrosis surrounded by an area of hypoxic injury. This injured tissue is potentially viable and may be salvaged if circulation is restored, or it may progress to necrosis. (See *Understanding MI.*)
- Coronary artery occlusion typically progresses through three stages:
  - *ischemia:* the first indication of an imbalance between blood flow and oxygen demand
  - *injury:* prolonged ischemia damages the heart
  - *infarction:* indicates death of myocardial cells.
- All infarcts—areas of damage due to MI—consist of three zones: a central area of necrosis, a zone of injury surrounding the necrosis and consisting of potentially viable hypoxic injury, and an area of viable ischemic tissue surrounding the zone of injury. (See *Zones of myocardial infarction,* page 328.)
- Although ischemia begins immediately, the size of the infarct may be limited if circulation is restored within 6 hours.
- Although MI principally involves the heart, all body systems can be affected as a result of changes in heart contractility and blood flow. Many patients have coexisting disorders that place them at high risk for additional problems. (See *Disorders affecting management of MI,* pages 332 to 335.)

CARDIOVASCULAR SYSTEM

- After MI, the infarcted myocardial cells release cardiac enzymes and proteins.
- Within 24 hours, the infarcted muscle becomes edematous and cyanotic.
- During the ensuing days, leukocytes infiltrate the necrotic area and begin to remove necrotic cells, thinning the ventricular wall.
- Scar formation begins by the third week after MI. By the sixth week, scar tissue is well established.
- The scar tissue that forms on the necrotic area inhibits contractility. When contractility is inhibited, the compensatory mechanisms (vascular constriction, increased heart rate, and renal retention of sodium and water) try to maintain cardiac output.
- Ventricular dilation may occur in a process called *remodeling.*
- Functionally, an MI may cause reduced contractility with abnormal wall motion, altered left ventricular compliance, reduced stroke volume, reduced ejection fraction, and elevated left ventricular end-diastolic pressure.
- The backup of fluid results in heart failure.

MUSCULOSKELETAL SYSTEM

- Decreased perfusion to skeletal muscles results in fatigue and weakness of muscles.
- Hypoxemia of the skeletal muscle tissue secondary to decreased perfusion leads to lactic acidosis.

NEUROLOGIC SYSTEM

- Anxiety and restlessness as well as cool extremities and perspiration may occur due to the release of catecholamines and stimulation of the sympathetic nervous system.
- Stimulation of vasovagal reflexes or vomiting centers may cause nausea and vomiting.

RENAL SYSTEM

- Reduced urine output occurs secondary to reduced renal perfusion.
- Secretion of aldosterone and antidiuretic hormones increases, leading to fluid conservation.

Understanding MI

With a myocardial infarction (MI), blood supply to the myocardium is interrupted. Here's what happens:

Injury to the endothelial lining of the coronary arteries causes platelets, white blood cells, fibrin, and lipids to gather at the injured site, as shown below. Foam cells, or resident macrophages, gather beneath the damaged lining and absorb oxidized cholesterol, forming a fatty streak that narrows the arterial lumen.

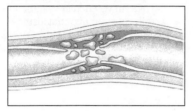

As the arterial lumen narrows, collateral circulation develops, which helps to maintain myocardial perfusion distal to the obstructed vessel lumen. The illustration below shows collateral circulation.

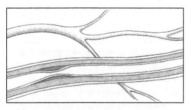

When myocardial demand for oxygen is more than the collateral circulation can supply, myocardial metabolism shifts from aerobic to anaerobic, producing lactic acid (A), which stimulates nerve endings, as shown below.

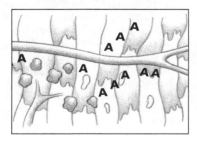

Lacking oxygen, the myocardial cells die, decreasing contractility, stroke volume, and blood pressure.

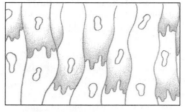

Hypotension stimulates baroreceptors, which in turn stimulate the adrenal glands to release epinephrine and norepinephrine as shown below. These catecholamines (C) increase heart rate and cause peripheral vasoconstriction, further increasing myocardial oxygen demand.

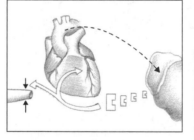

Damaged cell membranes in the infarcted area allow intracellular contents into the vascular circulation, as shown below. Ventricular arrhythmias then develop with elevated serum levels of potassium, creatine kinase (CK), CK-MB, aspartate, aminotransferase, and lactate dehydrogenase.

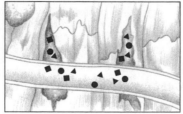

All myocardial cells are capable of spontaneous depolarization and repolarization, so the electrical conduction system may be affected by infarct, injury, or ischemia. The illustration below shows an injury site.

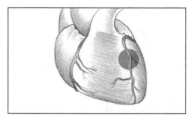

Extensive damage to the left ventricle may impair its ability to pump, allowing blood to back up into the left atrium and, eventually, into the pulmonary veins and capillaries, as shown in the illustration below. Crackles may be heard in the lungs on auscultation. Pulmonary artery wedge pressure is increased.

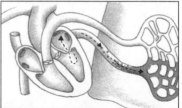

As back pressure rises, fluid crosses the alveolar-capillary membrane, impeding diffusion of oxygen (O_2) and carbon dioxide (CO_2). Arterial blood gas measurements may show decreased partial pressure of arterial oxygen and arterial pH and increased partial pressure of arterial carbon dioxide.

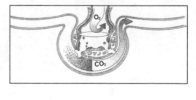

(continued)

RESPIRATORY SYSTEM

◆ Shortness of breath and crackles may occur due to heart failure and decreased oxygenation.
◆ The backup of fluid results in pulmonary edema and, possibly, acute respiratory distress syndrome.

ASSESSMENT

HISTORY

◆ Possible CAD with increasing anginal frequency, severity, or duration
◆ Persistent, crushing substernal pain or pressure possibly radiating to the left arm, jaw, neck, and shoulder blades, and possibly persisting for 12 or more hours (cardinal symptom of MI)
◆ In females, unusual fatigue, shortness of breath, weakness, and dizziness
◆ Pain possibly absent in elderly patients or those with diabetes; pain possibly mild and with confusion and indigestion in others
◆ Feeling of impending doom, fatigue, nausea, vomiting, and shortness of breath
◆ Sudden death (may be the first and only indication of MI)

PHYSICAL FINDINGS

◆ Extreme anxiety and restlessness
◆ Dyspnea
◆ Diaphoresis
◆ Tachycardia
◆ Hypertension
◆ Bradycardia and hypotension in inferior MI
◆ An S_4, an S_3, and paradoxical splitting of S_2 in ventricular dysfunction
◆ Systolic murmur of mitral insufficiency
◆ Pericardial friction rub in transmural MI or pericarditis
◆ Low-grade fever during ensuing days
◆ Dizziness
◆ Weakness

DIAGNOSTIC TEST RESULTS

◆ Serum creatine kinase (CK) level and CK-MB isoenzyme are elevated.
◆ Serum lactate dehydrogenase levels are elevated.
◆ White blood cell count usually appears elevated on the second day and through 1 week.
◆ Myoglobin is detected as soon as 2 hours after MI.
◆ Troponin I level is elevated.
◆ Nuclear medicine scans identify acutely damaged muscle.
◆ Echocardiography shows ventricular wall dyskinesia and helps to evaluate the ejection fraction.
◆ Serial 12-lead electrocardiography (ECG) readings may be normal or inconclusive during the first few hours after an MI. Characteristic abnormalities include serial ST-segment depression in subendocardial MI and ST-segment elevation and Q waves (representing scarring and necrosis) in transmural MI.
◆ Pulmonary artery catheterization may detects left- or right-sided heart failure.

Zones of myocardial infarction

Characteristic electrocardiographic changes are associated with each of the three zones in myocardial infarction.

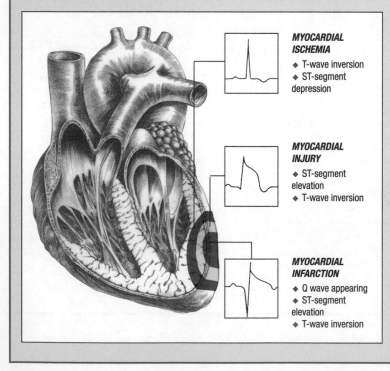

MYOCARDIAL ISCHEMIA

◆ T-wave inversion
◆ ST-segment depression

MYOCARDIAL INJURY

◆ ST-segment elevation
◆ T-wave inversion

MYOCARDIAL INFARCTION

◆ Q wave appearing
◆ ST-segment elevation
◆ T-wave inversion

TREATMENT

GENERAL
◆ Pacemaker implantation or electrical cardioversion for unstable arrhythmias
◆ Intra-aortic balloon pump for cardiogenic shock

DIET
◆ Low-fat, low-cholesterol
◆ Calorie restriction, if indicated

ACTIVITY
◆ Bed rest with bedside commode
◆ Gradual increase in activity, as tolerated

MEDICATIONS
◆ Aspirin (see *Treating myocardial infarction,* pages 330 and 331)
◆ Oxygen
◆ Nitrates
◆ I.V. morphine
◆ I.V. thrombolytic therapy started within 3 hours of onset of symptoms
◆ Antiarrhythmics, antianginals
◆ Calcium channel blockers
◆ I.V. heparin
◆ Inotropic agents
◆ Beta-adrenergic blockers
◆ Angiotensin-converting enzyme inhibitors
◆ Stool softeners
◆ Diuretics

SURGERY
◆ Surgical revascularization (coronary artery bypass graft)
◆ Percutaneous revascularization (percutaneous transluminal coronary angioplasty and stenting)

NURSING CONSIDERATIONS

NURSING DIAGNOSES
◆ Activity intolerance
◆ Acute pain
◆ Anxiety
◆ Decreased cardiac output
◆ Excess fluid volume
◆ Fatigue
◆ Imbalanced nutrition: Less than body requirements
◆ Ineffective coping
◆ Ineffective denial
◆ Ineffective sexuality patterns
◆ Ineffective tissue perfusion: Cardiopulmonary

EXPECTED OUTCOMES
The patient will:
◆ perform activities of daily living without excessive fatigue or exhaustion
◆ express feelings of increased comfort and decreased pain
◆ verbalize strategies to reduce anxiety and stress
◆ maintain adequate cardiac output
◆ develop no complications of fluid volume excess
◆ verbalize the importance of balancing activity, as tolerated, with rest
◆ achieve ideal weight
◆ exhibit adequate coping skills
◆ recognize his acute condition and accept the lifestyle changes he needs to make
◆ voice feelings about changes in sexual patterns
◆ maintain hemodynamic stability and develop no arrhythmias.

NURSING INTERVENTIONS
◆ Assess pain level and give prescribed analgesics. Record the severity, location, type, and duration of pain.
◆ Check the patient's blood pressure before and after giving nitroglycerin.
◆ Obtain ECG during chest pain episodes.
◆ Organize patient care and activities to provide uninterrupted rest.
◆ Provide a low-cholesterol, low-sodium diet with caffeine-free beverages.
◆ Help with range-of-motion exercises.
◆ Provide emotional support and help to reduce stress and anxiety.
◆ Provide sheath care after percutaneous transluminal coronary angioplasty or cardiac catheterization. Watch for bleeding. Keep the leg with the sheath insertion site immobile. Maintain strict bed rest. Check peripheral pulses in affected leg per facility policy.

◆ Monitor cardiac rhythm, serial ECGs, vital signs, pulse oximetry, and laboratory test results.

⚡ **WARNING** *Assess for crackles, cough, tachypnea, and edema, which may indicate impending left-sided heart failure.*
◆ Monitor daily weight and intake and output.

PATIENT TEACHING

Be sure to cover:
◆ disorder, diagnostic testing, and treatment
◆ medication administration, dosage, possible adverse effects, and signs of toxicity to watch for
◆ dietary restrictions
◆ progressive resumption of sexual activity and exercise
◆ appropriate responses to symptoms
◆ types of chest pain to report
◆ referral to a cardiac rehabilitation program
◆ available smoking-cessation or weight-reduction programs.

RESOURCES
Organization
American Heart Association: *www.americanheart.org*

Selected references
Albert, M., et al. "Impact of Traditional and Novel Risk Factors on the Relationship Between Socioeconomic Status and Incidence of Cardiovascular Events," *Circulation* 114(24):2619-626, December 2006.
Day, W., and Batten, L. "Cardiac Rehabilitation for Women: One Size Does Not Fit All," *The Australian Journal of Advanced Nursing* 24(1):21-26, September-November 2006.
Leahy, M. "Primary Angioplasty for Acute ST-Elevation Myocardial Infarction," *Nursing Standard* 21(12):48-56, November-December 2006.
Vorchheimer, D.A., and Becker, R. "Platelets in Atherothrombosis," *Mayo Clinic Proceedings* 81(1):59-68, January 2006.

(continued)

Treating myocardial infarction

This flowchart shows how treatments can be applied to myocardial infarction at various stages.

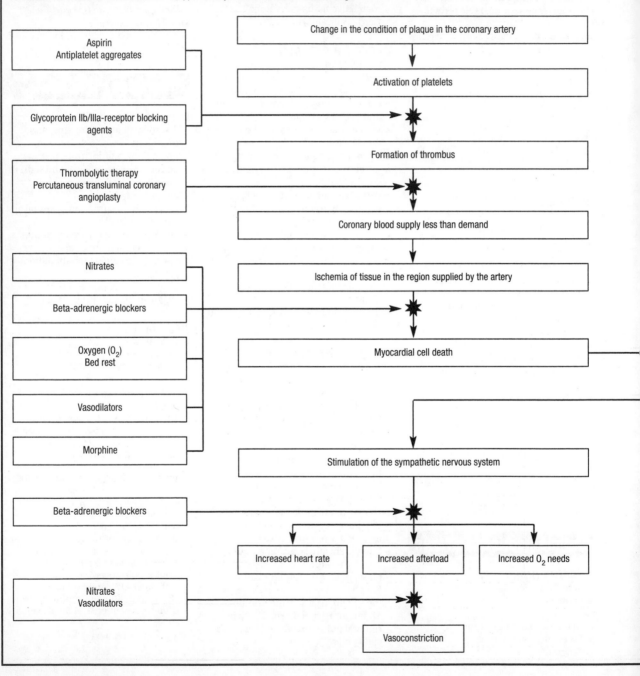

Aspirin Antiplatelet aggregates	Change in the condition of plaque in the coronary artery
	↓
	Activation of platelets
Glycoprotein IIb/IIIa-receptor blocking agents → ✳	
	↓
Thrombolytic therapy Percutaneous transluminal coronary angioplasty → ✳	Formation of thrombus
	↓
	Coronary blood supply less than demand
Nitrates	↓
Beta-adrenergic blockers → ✳	Ischemia of tissue in the region supplied by the artery
	↓
Oxygen (O₂) Bed rest	Myocardial cell death
Vasodilators	
Morphine	Stimulation of the sympathetic nervous system
Beta-adrenergic blockers → ✳	
	Increased heart rate / Increased afterload / Increased O₂ needs
Nitrates Vasodilators → ✳	Vasoconstriction

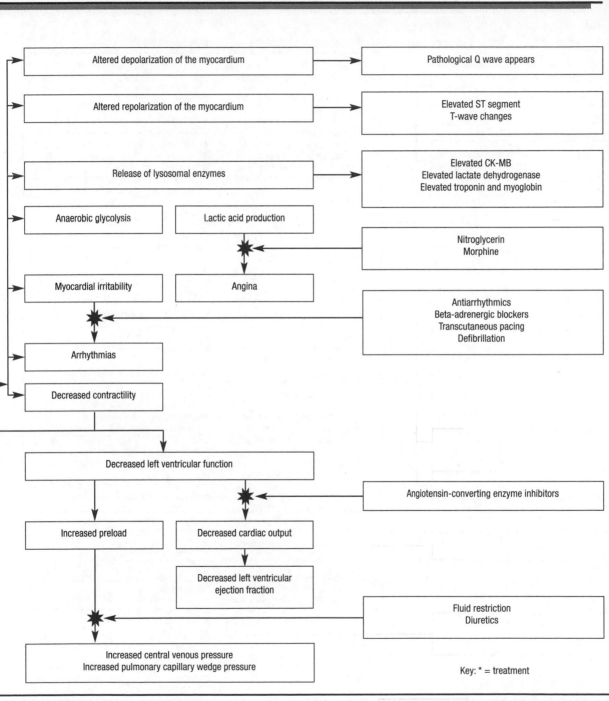

Altered depolarization of the myocardium → Pathological Q wave appears

Altered repolarization of the myocardium → Elevated ST segment
T-wave changes

Release of lysosomal enzymes → Elevated CK-MB
Elevated lactate dehydrogenase
Elevated troponin and myoglobin

Anaerobic glycolysis   Lactic acid production

Nitroglycerin
Morphine

Myocardial irritability   Angina

Antiarrhythmics
Beta-adrenergic blockers
Transcutaneous pacing
Defibrillation

Arrhythmias

Decreased contractility

Decreased left ventricular function

Angiotensin-converting enzyme inhibitors

Increased preload   Decreased cardiac output

Decreased left ventricular
ejection fraction

Fluid restriction
Diuretics

Increased central venous pressure
Increased pulmonary capillary wedge pressure

Key: * = treatment

(continued)

Disorders affecting management of MI

This chart highlights disorders that affect the management of myocardial infarction (MI).

DISORDER	SIGNS AND SYMPTOMS	DIAGNOSTIC TEST RESULTS	TREATMENT AND CARE
Cardiac arrhythmias (complication)	◆ May be asymptomatic ◆ Dizziness ◆ Hypotension ◆ Syncope ◆ Weakness ◆ Cool, clammy skin ◆ Altered level of consciousness (LOC) ◆ Reduced urine output ◆ Shortness of breath ◆ Chest pain	◆ Electrocardiography (ECG) detects arrhythmias and ischemia and infarction that may result in arrhythmias. ◆ Laboratory testing may reveal electrolyte abnormalities, acid-base abnormalities, or drug toxicities that may cause arrhythmias. ◆ Holter monitoring, event monitoring, and loop recording can detect arrhythmias and effectiveness of drug therapy during a patient's daily activities. ◆ Exercise testing may detect exercise-induced arrhythmias. ◆ Electrophysiologic testing identifies the mechanism of an arrhythmia and the location of accessory pathways and assesses the effectiveness of antiarrhythmics, radiofrequency ablation, and implanted cardioverter-defibrillators.	◆ When life-threatening arrhythmias develop, rapidly assess LOC, respirations, and pulse rate. ◆ Initiate cardiopulmonary resuscitation, if indicated. ◆ Evaluate cardiac output. ◆ If the patient develops heart block, prepare for cardiac pacing. ◆ Administer antiarrhythmics, as ordered. ◆ Prepare to assist with medical procedures, if indicated. ◆ Assess intake and output every hour. ◆ Document arrhythmias in the monitored patient, and assess for possible causes and effects. ◆ If the patient's pulse is abnormally rapid, slow, or irregular, watch for signs of hypoperfusion, such as hypotension and diminished urine output. ◆ Monitor for predisposing factors, such as fluid and electrolyte imbalance, or possible drug toxicity.
Cardiogenic shock (complication)	◆ Tachycardia and bounding pulse ◆ Restlessness, irritability, and hypoxia ◆ Tachypnea ◆ Reduced urinary output ◆ Cool, pale skin that progresses to cyanosis ◆ Hypotension ◆ Narrowed pulse pressure ◆ Weak, rapid, thready pulse ◆ Shallow respirations ◆ Reduced urinary output ◆ Unconsciousness and absent reflexes (in irreversible stages) ◆ Rapidly falling blood pressure with decompensation ◆ Anuria	◆ Coagulation studies may detect coagulopathy from disseminated intravascular coagulation (DIC). ◆ White blood cell count and erythrocyte sedimentation rate may be increased. ◆ Blood urea nitrogen and creatinine are elevated due to reduced renal perfusion. ◆ Serum lactate may be increased secondary to anaerobic metabolism. ◆ Serum glucose may be elevated in early stages. ◆ Cardiac enzymes and proteins may be elevated, indicating MI as the cause. ◆ Arterial blood gas (ABG) analysis may reveal respiratory alkalosis in early shock or respiratory acidosis in later stages. ◆ Urine specific gravity may be high. ◆ Chest X-rays may be normal in early stages; pulmonary congestion may be seen in later stages. ◆ Hemodynamic monitoring may reveal characteristic patterns of intracardiac pressures and cardiac output. ◆ ECG determines heart rate and detects arrhythmias, ischemic changes, and MI. ◆ Echocardiography determines left ventricular function and reveals valvular abnormalities.	◆ Assist in identifying and treating the underlying cause. ◆ Maintain a patent airway; prepare for intubation and mechanical ventilation if respiratory distress develops. ◆ Provide supplemental oxygen to increase oxygenation. ◆ Use continuous cardiac monitoring to detect changes in heart rate and rhythm; administer antiarrhythmics, as necessary. ◆ Monitor vital signs every 15 minutes, and assess hemodynamic parameters, as indicated. ◆ Initiate and maintain at least two I.V. lines with large-gauge needles for fluid and drug administration. ◆ Administer I.V. fluids, crystalloids, colloids, blood products, inotropic drugs, or vasodilators, as ordered. ◆ Monitor intake and output and daily weight. Administer diuretics to reduce preload if the patient has fluid volume overload. ◆ Initiate intra-aortic balloon pump (IABP) therapy to reduce the work of left ventricle by decreasing systemic vascular resistance. Monitor the patient carefully. ◆ Monitor the patient receiving thrombolytic therapy or coronary artery revascularization per facility protocol. ◆ Prepare for emergency surgery if the papillary muscle ruptures or if a ventricular septal defect is present. ◆ Monitor the patient with a ventricular assist device.

DISORDER	SIGNS AND SYMPTOMS	DIAGNOSTIC TEST RESULTS	TREATMENT AND CARE
Coagulation defects (complication)	◆ Signs and symptoms of shock if bleeding is severe (tachycardia, hypotension, and tachypnea) ◆ Bleeding (such as from endotracheal tube, wound, or I.V. sites)	◆ Coagulation studies may detect coagulopathy from DIC. ◆ Urinalysis may show red blood cells. ◆ Hemoglobin, hematocrit, and platelet count may be decreased.	◆ Avoid I.M. injections and unnecessary I.V. sticks. ◆ Monitor the patient for signs of bleeding. ◆ Handle the patient gently to avoid bruising. ◆ Test all urine and stool for occult blood. ◆ Monitor vital signs and LOC; report changes. ◆ Administer blood products, as ordered, and monitor for their effects. ◆ If patient is having a reaction to heparin, make sure heparin isn't given, especially in an arterial or pulmonary artery line.
Coronary aneurysm (complication)	◆ Tachycardia and bounding pulse ◆ Restlessness and irritability ◆ Tachypnea ◆ Reduced urinary output ◆ Cool, pale skin ◆ Hypotension as compensatory mechanisms fail ◆ Narrowed pulse pressure ◆ Weak, rapid, thready pulse ◆ Shallow respirations ◆ Reduced urinary output as poor renal perfusion continues ◆ Anuria	◆ Cardiac enzymes and proteins may be elevated, indicating MI as the cause. ◆ ABG analysis may reveal respiratory alkalosis in early shock or respiratory acidosis in later stages. ◆ Urine specific gravity may be high. ◆ Chest X-rays may be normal in early stages; pulmonary congestion may be seen in later stages. ◆ Hemodynamic monitoring may reveal characteristic patterns of intracardiac pressures and cardiac output. ◆ ECG determines heart rate and detects arrhythmias, ischemic changes, and MI. ◆ Echocardiography determines left ventricular function and reveals valvular abnormalities.	◆ Administer supplemental oxygen to increase oxygenation. ◆ Institute continuous cardiac monitoring to detect changes in heart rate and rhythm; administer antiarrhythmics, as necessary. ◆ Monitor blood pressure, pulse rate, peripheral pulses, and other vital signs every 15 minutes; notify physician of changes. ◆ Monitor central venous pressure, pulmonary artery wedge pressure, and cardiac output, as ordered; report changes. ◆ Initiate and maintain at least two I.V. lines with large-gauge needles for fluid and drug administration. ◆ Administer I.V. fluids, crystalloids, colloids, or blood products, as necessary, to maintain intravascular volume. ◆ Administer inotropic drugs, such as dopamine, dobutamine, and epinephrine, to increase heart contractility and cardiac output; monitor peripheral pulses and circulation and report changes. ◆ Administer vasodilators, such as nitroglycerin or nitroprusside, with a vasopressor to reduce the left ventricle's workload. ◆ Monitor intake and output and daily weight. Administer diuretics to reduce preload if the patient has fluid volume overload. ◆ Initiate IABP therapy to reduce the work of left ventricle by decreasing systemic vascular resistance. Monitor the patient carefully. ◆ Monitor the patient receiving thrombolytic therapy or coronary artery revascularization per facility protocol. ◆ Prepare for emergency surgery if repair is required.

(continued)

DISORDER	SIGNS AND SYMPTOMS	DIAGNOSTIC TEST RESULTS	TREATMENT AND CARE
Diabetes mellitus (coexisting)	◆ Polyuria and polydypsia ◆ Anorexia or polyphagia ◆ Weight loss ◆ Headaches, fatigue, lethargy, reduced energy levels, and impaired performance ◆ Muscle cramps ◆ Irritability; emotional imbalance ◆ Vision changes such as blurring ◆ Numbness and tingling ◆ Abdominal discomfort and pain ◆ Nausea, diarrhea, or constipation ◆ Slowly healing skin infections or wounds; itching of skin ◆ Recurrent monilial infections of the vagina or anus	◆ Two-hour postprandial blood glucose shows a level of 200 mg/dl or above. ◆ Fasting blood glucose level is 126 mg/dl or higher after at least an 8-hour fast.	◆ Expect to administer two or more drugs, which are usually necessary to achieve target blood pressure of less than 130 mm Hg. ◆ Administer thiazide diuretics, angiotensin-converting enzyme inhibitors, beta-adrenergic blockers, angiotensin receptor blockers, or calcium channel blockers, as ordered. ◆ Monitor the patient's blood glucose level because beta-adrenergic blockers can cause hyperglycemia. ◆ Watch for signs of diabetic neuropathy (numbness or pain in the hands and feet, footdrop, impotence, neurogenic bladder), infection (increased temperature), cardiac distress (chest pain, palpitations, dyspnea, confusion), changes in vision, peripheral numbness or tingling, constipation, anorexia, and blisters or skin openings, particularly on the feet. ◆ Because thiazide and loop diuretic promote potassium excretion, monitor serum potassium levels for patients receiving diuretics. ◆ Monitor intake and output, and watch for signs of dehydration. ◆ Review foods that are high and low in sodium and potassium with the patient.
Thyroid disease (coexisting)	◆ Tachycardia ◆ Hypertension ◆ Diaphoresis ◆ Irritability ◆ Nervousness	◆ Thyroid hormone levels are altered. ◆ ECG may show arrhythmias.	◆ Monitor vital signs and administer antihypertensives and beta-adrenergic blockers; monitor the patient for effects. ◆ Monitor thyroid levels and the patient's response to thyroid medication. ◆ If the patient is on a low-iodine diet, teach him about avoiding products containing iodine (such as salt).
Valvular heart disease (complication)	*With mitral stenosis or insufficiency* ◆ Dyspnea on exertion ◆ Paroxysmal nocturnal dyspnea ◆ Orthopnea ◆ Weakness and fatigue ◆ Palpitations ◆ Peripheral edema ◆ Jugular vein distention ◆ Acites ◆ Hepatomegaly ◆ Crackles ◆ Atrial fibrillation ◆ Signs of systemic emboli ◆ Loud first heart sound (S_1) or opening snap and diastolic murmur at apex	◆ Cardiac catheterization can differentiate mitral stenosis or mitral insufficiency from aortic stenosis or aortic insufficiency. ◆ Chest X-rays show left atrial and ventricular enlargement, enlarged pulmonary arteries, and mitral valve calcification in mitral valve problems; and left ventricular enlargement, pulmonary congestion, and valvular calcification in aortic valve problems. ◆ Echocardiography shows thickened valve leaflets. ◆ ECG reveals arrhythmias.	◆ Administer oxygen in acute situations to increase oxygenation. ◆ Monitor vital signs and effects of digoxin on heart rate. ◆ Instruct the patient on how to maintain a low-sodium diet. ◆ Monitor the effects of diuretics; record input and output and daily weights. ◆ Monitor the effects of antiarrhythmics and vasodilators. ◆ Monitor the patient taking anticoagulants for bleeding. ◆ Monitor the patient for signs of heart failure or pulmonary edema and for adverse effects of drug therapy. ◆ Administer nitroglycerin to relieve angina, as ordered. ◆ Prepare for cardioversion if patient has atrial fibrillation.

Disorders affecting management of MI *(continued)*

DISORDER	SIGNS AND SYMPTOMS	DIAGNOSTIC TEST RESULTS	TREATMENT AND CARE
Valvular heart disease (complication) *(continued)*	*With aortic stenosis or insufficiency* ◆ Dyspnea ◆ Cough ◆ Fatigue ◆ Palpitations ◆ Angina ◆ Syncope ◆ Pulmonary congestion ◆ Left-sided heart failure ◆ Pulsating nail beds ◆ Rapidly rising and collapsing pulses ◆ Cardiac arrhythmias ◆ Widened pulse pressure ◆ Third heart sound (S_3) and diastolic blowing murmur at left sternal border ◆ Palpation and visualization of apical impulse (in chronic disease)		◆ If the patient requires surgery, monitor for hypotension, arrhythmias, and thrombus formation. Monitor vital signs, ABG values, intake and output, daily weight, blood chemistries, chest X-rays, and pulmonary artery catheter readings.

Near drowning

- Victim surviving physiologic effects of submersion
- Hypoxemia and acidosis primary problems
- "Dry" near drowning: fluid not aspirated; respiratory obstruction or asphyxia
- "Wet" near drowning: fluid aspirated; asphyxia or secondary changes from fluid aspiration
- "Secondary" near drowning: recurrence of respiratory distress
- Most common cause of injury and death in children ages 1 month to 14 years
- Incidence is greater in males

CAUSES

- Blow to the head while in the water
- Boating accident
- Dangerous water conditions
- Decompression sickness from deep-water diving
- Excessive alcohol consumption before swimming
- Inability to swim
- Panic in the water while swimming
- Sudden acute illness
- Suicide attempt
- Venomous stings from aquatic animals

PATHOPHYSIOLOGY

- Submersion stimulates hyperventilation.
- Voluntary apnea occurs.
- Laryngospasm develops.
- Hypoxemia develops, which may lead to brain damage and cardiac arrest.
- Other consequences depend on the type of water aspirated; for example, saltwater aspiration is considered more serious than freshwater aspiration because saltwater contains more disease-causing bacteria. (See *Pathophysiologic changes in near drowning*.)

CARDIOVASCULAR SYSTEM

- Cold water submersion (exposure to temperatures below 69.8° F [21° C]) may lead to a protective effect (most pronounced in children and may be due to the large ratio of body surface area to mass). Rapid body cooling results in cardiac arrest and decreased tissue oxygen demand.
- Hypothermia may occur because water rapidly conducts heat away from the body.

NEUROLOGIC SYSTEM

- The patient's level of consciousness (LOC) may be altered due to hypoxemia.
- The release of catecholamines leads to vasoconstriction, decreasing cerebral oxygen consumption.
- Submersion in cold water leads to decreased central blood flow and cooling of the blood that flows to the brain, resulting in mental confusion.

RESPIRATORY SYSTEM

- In freshwater aspiration, water is absorbed across the alveolar capillary membrane, resulting in destruction of surfactant and subsequent alveolar instability, atelectasis, and decreased compliance.
- In saltwater aspiration, surfactant washout occurs and protein-rich exudates rapidly move into the alveoli and pulmonary interstitium. The hypertonicity of seawater pulls fluid from pulmonary capillaries into the alveoli. The resulting intrapulmonary shunt causes hypoxemia. The pulmonary capillary membrane may be injured, leading to pulmonary edema.
- In wet and secondary near drowning, pulmonary edema and hypoxemia occur secondary to aspiration.
- Aspiration of such contaminants as chlorine, mud algae, and weeds can occur, leading to obstruction, aspiration pneumonia, and pulmonary fibrosis. (See *Disorders affecting management of near drowning*, page 339.)

HISTORY

- Victim found in water

PHYSICAL FINDINGS

- Fever or hypothermia
- Rapid, slow, or absent pulse
- Shallow, gasping, or absent respirations
- Altered LOC
- Seizures
- Cyanosis or pink, frothy sputum, or both
- Abdominal distention
- Crackles, rhonchi, wheezing, or apnea
- Tachycardia
- Irregular heartbeat

DIAGNOSTIC TEST RESULTS

- Arterial blood gas (ABG) analysis shows degree of hypoxia, intrapulmonary shunt, and acid-base balance.
- Electrolyte levels are imbalanced.
- Blood urea nitrogen and creatinine levels reveal impaired renal function.
- Cervical spine X-ray may show evidence of fracture.
- Serial chest X-rays may show pulmonary edema.
- Electrocardiography may show myocardial ischemia, infarct, or cardiac arrhythmias.

TREATMENT

GENERAL
◆ Stabilizing neck with cervical collar
◆ Establishing airway and providing ventilation

◆ Correcting abnormal laboratory values
◆ Warming measures, if hypothermic

DIET
◆ Nothing by mouth until swallowing ability has returned

ACTIVITY
◆ Based on extent of injury and success of resuscitation

MEDICATIONS
◆ Bronchodilators
◆ Cardiac drug therapy, if appropriate
◆ Prophylactic antibiotics

UP CLOSE

Pathophysiologic changes in near drowning

The flowchart below shows the primary cellular alterations that occur during near drowning. Separate pathways are shown for saltwater and freshwater incidents. Hypothermia presents a separate pathway that may preserve neurologic function by decreasing the metabolic rate. All pathways lead to diffuse pulmonary edema.

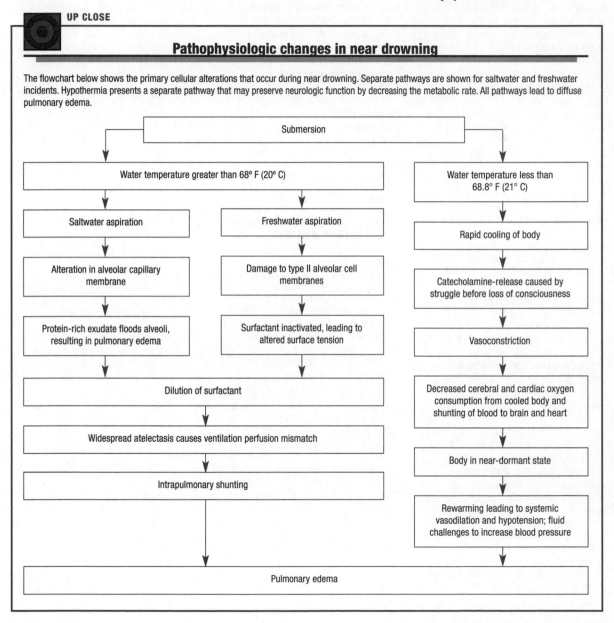

(continued)

NURSING CONSIDERATIONS

NURSING DIAGNOSES
- Anxiety
- Decreased cardiac output
- Hypothermia
- Impaired gas exchange
- Ineffective airway clearance
- Ineffective breathing pattern
- Ineffective coping
- Risk for aspiration
- Risk for infection

EXPECTED OUTCOMES
The patient will:
- express feelings of decreased anxiety
- maintain adequate cardiac output
- maintain a normal body temperature
- maintain adequate ventilation and oxygenation
- maintain a patent airway
- maintain an effective breathing pattern
- develop effective coping mechanisms
- show no signs of aspiration
- remain free from signs and symptoms of infection.

NURSING INTERVENTIONS
- Perform cardiopulmonary resuscitation, as indicated.
- Perform active external rewarming and passive rewarming measures for mild hypothermia (93.2° to 96.8° F [34° to 36° C]); active external rewarming of truncal areas only and passive rewarming measures for moderate hypothermia (86° to 93.2° F [30° to 34° C]); and active internal rewarming measures for severe hypothermia (less than 86° F [30° C]).
- Protect the cervical spine.
- Give prescribed drugs.
- Provide emotional support.
- Monitor electrolyte and ABG measurement results.
- Observe continuous cardiac rhythm for changes.
- Monitor vital signs, core body temperature, neurologic status, and respiratory status.

PATIENT TEACHING

Be sure to cover:
- injury, diagnostic testing, and treatment
- need to avoid using alcohol or drugs before swimming
- water safety measures (such as the "buddy system")
- available water safety courses given by the Red Cross, YMCA, or YWCA
- available psychological counseling or resource and support services, if appropriate.

RESOURCES
Organizations
American Academy of Neurology: *www.aan.com*
Brain Injury Association of America: *www.biausa.org*
Harborview Injury Prevention and Research Center: *www.depts.washington.edu/hiprc*
National Center for Injury Prevention and Control: *www.cdc.gov/ncipc*

Selected references
Burford, A.E., et al. "Drowning and Near-Drowning in Children and Adolescents: A Succinct Review for Emergency Physicians and Nurses," *Pediatric Emergency Care* 21(9):610-16, September 2005.

Day, M.P. "Hypothermia: A Hazard for all Seasons," *Nursing* 36(12):44-47, December 2006.

Garzoni, C., and Garbino, J. "Long-Term Risk of Atypical Fungal Infection after Near-Drowning Episodes," *Pediatrics* 119(2):417-18, February 2007.

Ross, J.L. "Summer Injuries: Near Drowning," *RN* 68(7):36-38, July 2005.

Disorders affecting management of near drowning

This chart highlights disorders that affect the management of near drowning.

DISORDER	SIGNS AND SYMPTOMS	DIAGNOSTIC TEST RESULTS	TREATMENT AND CARE
Acute respiratory distress syndrome (ARDS) (complication)	◆ Dyspnea on exertion ◆ Diminished breath sounds ◆ Tachypnea, tachycardia ◆ Increasing respiratory distress with use of accessory muscles ◆ Restlessness, apprehension ◆ Dry cough or frothy sputum ◆ Cool, clammy skin that progresses to pallor and cyanosis ◆ Basilar crackles, rhonchi ◆ Decreased mental status ◆ Arrhythmias such as premature ventricular contractions ◆ Labile blood pressure	◆ Arterial blood gas (ABG) analysis initially shows decreased partial pressure of arterial oxygen, despite oxygen supplementation, and decreased partial pressure of arterial carbon dioxide ($Paco_2$), causing an increase in blood pH. As ARDS worsens, $Paco_2$ increases and pH decreases as the patient becomes acidotic. ◆ Initially, chest X-rays may be normal. Basilar infiltrates begin to appear in about 24 hours. In later stages, lung fields have a ground glass appearance and, eventually, white patches appear. ◆ Pulmonary artery wedge pressure is 18 mm Hg or lower.	◆ Assess the patient's cardiopulmonary status, including lung sounds, heart rate, and blood pressure at least every 2 hours, or more often if indicated. Note respiratory rate, rhythm, and depth, reporting dyspnea and accessory muscle use. Be alert for inspiratory retractions. ◆ Administer oxygen, assess oxygen saturation continuously, and monitor serial ABG levels. ◆ Institute continuous cardiac monitoring and watch for arrhythmias. ◆ Monitor the patient's level of consciousness, noting confusion or mental sluggishness. ◆ Be alert for signs of treatment-induced complications, including arrhythmias, disseminated intravascular coagulation, GI bleeding, infection, malnutrition, paralytic ileus, pneumothorax, pulmonary fibrosis, renal failure, thrombocytopenia, and tracheal stenosis. ◆ Administer anti-infectives if the underlying cause is sepsis or an infection. ◆ Place the patient in a comfortable position that maximizes air exchange, such as semi-Fowler's or high Fowler's position. ◆ Evaluate the patient's serum electrolyte levels frequently. ◆ Monitor urine output hourly to ensure adequate renal function. Measure intake and output. Weigh the patient daily. ◆ Record caloric intake. Administer tube feedings and parenteral nutrition.
Hypothermia (complication)	*Mild hypothermia* ◆ Severe shivering, slurred speech, and amnesia *Moderate hypothermia* ◆ Unresponsiveness ◆ Peripheral cyanosis ◆ Muscle rigidity *Severe hypothermia* ◆ No palpable pulse or heart sounds ◆ Dilated pupils ◆ State of rigor mortis ◆ Ventricular fibrillation	◆ Technetium-99m pertechnetate scanning shows perfusion defects and deep tissue damage. ◆ Doppler and plethysmographic studies help determine pulses and the extent of frostbite after thawing. ◆ Laboratory studies determine the extent of tissue and organ damage.	◆ Assess airway, breathing, and circulation. ◆ Institute cardiopulmonary resuscitation until the patient's core body temperature increases to at least 86° F (30° C.) ◆ Assist in rewarming techniques; provide supportive measures, such as mechanical ventilation and heated, humidified therapy to maintain tissue oxygenation, and I.V. fluids that have been warmed with a warming coil. ◆ Insert an indwelling urinary catheter and assess urine output hourly. ◆ Continuously monitor core body temperature and other vital signs during and after initial rewarming. Monitor cardiac status with continuous cardiac monitoring for evidence of arrhythmias. ◆ If the patient's core temperature is below 89.6° F (32° C), use internal and external warming methods to raise the patient's body core and surface temperatures 1° to 2° F (0.6° to 1.1° C) per hour. ◆ If the patient's temperature is 86° F to 93° F (30° C to 33.9° C), limit active rewarming to the neck, axilla, or groin areas. Using these techniques in peripheral areas can contribute to a continued drop in core temperature as cold blood from the periphery is mobilized. ◆ If using a hyperthermia blanket, discontinue the warming when core body temperature is within 1° to 2° F of the desired temperature. The patient's temperature will continue to rise even with the device turned off. ◆ If the patient has been hypothermic for longer than 45 to 60 minutes, administer additional fluids to compensate for the expansion of vascular space that occurs during vasodilation in rewarming. Monitor heart rate and hemodynamic parameters closely to evaluate fluid needs and response to treatment. ◆ Monitor serum electrolyte levels closely, especially potassium. Be alert for signs and symptoms of hyperkalemia.

Necrotizing fasciitis

- Progressive, rapidly spreading inflammatory infection of the deep fascia
- Carries a mortality rate of 70% to 80%
- Three times more likely to occur in men than in women
- Rarely occurs in children, except in countries with poor hygiene practices
- Mean age of individuals diagnosed 38 to 44
- Increased risk for disease in elderly or immunocompromised patients and those with chronic illnesses or using steroids
- Most commonly called *flesh-eating bacteria*
- Also called *hemolytic streptococcal gangrene, acute dermal gangrene, suppurative fasciitis,* and *synergistic necrotizing cellulitis*

CAUSES

- Group A streptococci (GAS) and *Staphylococcus aureus,* alone or together, as the most common primary infecting bacteria (Epidemiology of GAS infections is complex because of the more than 80 types of the causative bacteria, *Streptococcus pyogenes.*)

- Infecting bacteria enter the host through a local tissue injury or a breach in a mucous membrane barrier.
- Organisms proliferate in an environment of tissue hypoxia caused by trauma, recent surgery, or a medical condition that compromises the patient.
- Necrosis of the surrounding tissue results, accelerating the disease process by creating a favorable environment for organisms to proliferate.
- The fascia and fat tissues are destroyed, resulting in secondary necrosis of subcutaneous tissue.

INTEGUMENTARY SYSTEM

- Area of injury begins with erythema and progresses to dusky skin discoloration as tissue hypoxia advances.
- Massive undermining of the skin and subcutaneous tissue occurs.
- Tissue necrosis follows, with progression to myositis or myonecrosis if treatment isn't initiated.

RESPIRATORY SYSTEM

- Bacterial invasion results in increased capillary permeability in the pulmonary vasculature that affects gas exchange as septic shock occurs.
- Fluid shifting leads to pulmonary edema, alveolar damage, and alveolar collapse.
- The release of histamine from endotoxins further damages the alveolar capillary membrane, leading to increased fluid shifting.

CARDIOVASCULAR SYSTEM

- The body's defense system activates chemical mediators and low systemic vascular resistance, and increased cardiac output occurs.
- Blood flow is unevenly distributed in the microcirculation and plasma leaks from the capillaries, causing functional hypovolemia.
- Hypovolemia leads to decreased cardiac output and poor tissue perfusion.

URINARY SYSTEM

- Endotoxin production promotes vasoconstriction, impairing blood flow to the kidneys.
- Glomerular membrane damage and increased capillary permeability, along with decreased tissue perfusion results in altered kidney function and may lead to acute renal failure. (See *Disorders affecting management of necrotizing fasciitis,* page 343.)

HISTORY
- Pain
- Tissue injury

PHYSICAL FINDINGS
- Rapidly progressing erythema at the site of insult
- Fluid-filled blisters and bullae (indicate rapid progression of the necrotizing process)
- Large areas of gangrenous skin by days 4 and 5
- Extensive necrosis of the subcutaneous tissue by days 7 to 10
- Fever
- Hypovolemia
- Hypotension
- Respiratory insufficiency
- Deterioration in level of consciousness
- Signs of sepsis

DIAGNOSTIC TEST RESULTS
- Results of biopsy of tissue show infiltration of the deep dermis, fascia, and muscular planes with bacteria and polymorphonuclear cells, and necrosis of fatty and muscular tissue.
- Results of cultures of microorganisms from the periphery of the spreading infection or from deeper tissues during surgical debridement identify the causative organism.
- Results of Gram stain and culture of biopsied tissue identify the causative organism.
- Radiographic study results may pinpoint the presence of subcutaneous gases.
- Computed tomography scan results may show the anatomic site of involvement by locating the area of necrosis.
- Magnetic resonance imaging results show areas of necrosis and areas that require surgical debridement.

GENERAL
- Wound care
- Hyperbaric oxygen therapy

DIET
- High-protein, high-calorie
- Increased fluid intake

ACTIVITY
- Bed rest until treatment effective

MEDICATIONS
- Antimicrobials
- Analgesics

SURGERY
- Immediate surgical debridement, fasciectomy, or amputation

NURSING DIAGNOSES
- Acute pain
- Decreased cardiac output
- Deficient fluid volume
- Hyperthermia
- Impaired tissue integrity
- Ineffective tissue perfusion: Cardiopulmonary, peripheral

EXPECTED OUTCOMES
The patient will:
- express feeling of increased comfort and decreased pain
- maintain adequate cardiac output
- maintain adequate fluid volume
- remain afebrile
- receive adequate blood supply to the wound
- maintain collateral circulation and hemodynamic stability.

NURSING INTERVENTIONS
- Provide supportive care and supplemental oxygen, as appropriate.
- Monitor vital signs and mental status.
- Give prescribed drugs.
- Provide emotional support.
- Observe for signs and symptoms of complications.
- Assess wound and provide wound care, as directed.
- Assess pain level, administer analgesics, as prescribed, and evaluate effect.

(continued)

Be sure to cover:

◆ disorder, diagnostic testing, and treatment
◆ medication administration, dosage, and possible adverse effects
◆ importance of strict sterile technique and proper hand-washing technique for wound care
◆ importance of follow-up care
◆ available rehabilitation programs, if indicated
◆ contact information for education and support, such as for the National Necrotizing Fasciitis Foundation.

RESOURCES

Organizations

Centers for Disease Control and Prevention: *www.cdc.gov*

Harvard University Consumer Health Information: *www.intelihealth.com*

National Institute of Allergy and Infectious Diseases: *www.niaid.nih.gov*

National Necrotizing Fasciitis Foundation: *www.nnff.org*

Selected references

Bresett, J. "Would You Suspect this Skin-Eating Infection?" *RN* 69(3):31-34, March 2006.

Kasper, D.L., et al., eds. *Harrison's Principles of Internal Medicine,* 16th ed. New York: McGraw-Hill Book Co., 2005.

Rodriguez, R.M., et al. "A Pilot Study of Cytokine Levels and White Blood Cell Counts in the Diagnosis of Necrotizing Fasciitis," *American Journal of Emergency Medicine* 24(1):58-61, January 2006.

Ruth-Sahd, L., and Gonzales, M. "Multiple Dimensions of Caring for a Patient with Acute Necrotizing Fasciitis," *Dimensions of Critical Care Nursing* 25(1):15-21, January-February 2006.

Young, M.H., et al. "Therapies for Necrotising Fasciitis," *Expert Opinion on Biological Therapy* 6(2):155-65, February 2006.

Disorders affecting management of necrotizing fasciitis

This chart highlights disorders that affect the management of necrotizing fasciitis.

DISORDER	SIGNS AND SYMPTOMS	DIAGNOSTIC TEST RESULTS	TREATMENT AND CARE
Acute renal failure (complication)	◆ Urine output less than 400 ml/day followed by diuresis of up to 5 L/day ◆ Lethargy ◆ Altered mental status ◆ Headache ◆ Costovertebral pain ◆ Numbness around the mouth ◆ Tingling extremities ◆ Anorexia ◆ Restlessness ◆ Weight gain ◆ Nausea and vomiting ◆ Pallor ◆ Diarrhea	◆ Blood urea nitrogen (BUN) and serum creatinine are increased. ◆ Potassium levels are increased. ◆ Hematocrit, blood pH, bicarbonate, and hemoglobin levels are decreased. ◆ Urine casts and cellular debris are present; specific gravity is decreased.	◆ Treat the underlying cause. ◆ Monitor fluid balance status, including skin turgor, peripheral edema, and intake and output. Monitor urine output hourly and assess daily weight. ◆ Monitor central venous and pulmonary artery pressures. ◆ Insertion of a temporary dialysis catheter may be necessary for hemodialysis or continuous renal replacement therapy. ◆ Monitor vital signs and laboratory values, especially BUN, creatinine, and electrolytes.
Sepsis (complication)	◆ Agitation ◆ Anxiety ◆ Altered level of consciousness ◆ Tachycardia ◆ Hypotension ◆ Rapid, shallow respirations ◆ Fever ◆ Urine output less than 25 ml/hour	◆ Blood cultures are positive for invading organism. ◆ Complete blood count shows increased white blood count and reveals whether anemia, neutropenia, or thrombocytopenia are present. ◆ Arterial blood gas (ABG) studies show metabolic acidosis. ◆ BUN and creatinine levels are increased. ◆ Electrocardiography shows ST-segment depression, inverted T waves, and arrhythmias.	◆ Locate and treat the underlying cause. ◆ Monitor vital signs, cardiac rhythm, pulse oximetry, and intake and output. ◆ Administer antibiotics, vasopressors, drotrecogin alfa (Xigris), and I.V. fluids, as ordered. ◆ Assess respiratory status, and provide supplemental oxygen and mechanical ventilation, as indicated. ◆ Monitor laboratory results and ABG studies.

Obesity

- Excess of body fat, generally 20% above ideal body weight
- Body mass index (BMI) of 30 or greater (see *BMI measurements*)
- Second-leading cause of preventable deaths
- Affects more than half of Americans
- Affects one in five children

CAUSES

- Excessive caloric intake combined with inadequate energy expenditure
- Theories to explain obesity:
- Abnormal absorption of nutrients
- Environmental factors
- Genetic predisposition
- Hypothalamic dysfunction of hunger and satiety centers
- Impaired action of GI and growth hormones and of hormonal regulators such as insulin
- Psychological factors
- Socioeconomic status

BMI measurements

Use these steps to calculate body mass index (BMI):
- Multiply weight in pounds by 705.
- Divide this number by height in inches.
- Then divide this by height in inches again.
- Compare results to these standards:
- 18.5 to 24.9: normal
- 25 to 29.9: overweight
- 30 to 39.9: obese
- 40 or greater: morbidly obese.

PATHOPHYSIOLOGY

- Fat cells increase in size in response to dietary intake.
- When the cells can no longer expand, they increase in number.
- With weight loss, the size of the fat cells decreases, but the number of cells doesn't.
- Fat distribution affects comorbities: android obesity (high abdominal fat) correlates with higher clinical consequences of obesity than gynecoid obesity (high gluteal fat).
- Excess fat cells and weight affect different body systems and the way they function.

CARDIOVASCULAR SYSTEM

- High-fat diet results in atherosclerotic plaques and development of coronary artery disease.
- Narrowing of the arterioles, as a result of plaques, may result in hypertension. (See *Disorders affecting management of obesity*, page 347.)
- Impaired glucose tolerance by the pancreas may contribute to development of diabetes mellitus, which may increase the risk of hypertension.
- Hypertension causes increased left ventricular volume and wall stress and contributes to the development of left ventricular hypertrophy.
- Increased left ventricular volume may occur with obesity (without hypertension) and increased stroke volume and cardiac output occurs, as well as diastolic dysfunction, resulting in dilated cardiomyopathy.
- Left ventricular hypertrophy also leads to right ventricular dysfunction and results in heart failure.

ENDOCRINE SYSTEM

- Studies under investigation regarding the link between diabetes and obesity involve the hormone resistin. It's thought that resistin, secreted by adipose tissue, is involved with endocrine function and is related to insulin resistance. With increased amounts of adipose tissue, resistin also increases, leading to type 2 diabetes.

RESPIRATORY SYSTEM

- Excessive weight against the chest wall and large neck circumference is thought to affect breathing ability while sleeping, resulting in increased levels of carbon dioxide, chronic fatigue, and chronic hypoxia.
- Reduced chest wall compliance and respiratory muscle strength increase the work of breathing and carbon dioxide production.
- Respiratory muscle weakness may result in a diminished cough effect, causing increased incidence of lower respiratory tract infection.
- Chronic hypoventilation results in right ventricular failure.

MUSCULOSKELETAL SYSTEM

- Adipose tissue produces cytokines that destroy the normal cartilage in joints.
- Increased weight causes stress to joints, especially weight-bearing joints of the knees, hips, feet, and spine.
- Degenerative arthritis develops as result of cartilage and joint tissue breakdown.

HISTORY

- Increasing weight
- Complications of obesity

PHYSICAL FINDINGS

- BMI of 30 or greater

DIAGNOSTIC TEST RESULTS

- Comparison of height and weight with a standard table helps determine obesity.
- Measurement of the thickness of subcutaneous fat folds with calipers approximates total body fat. (See *Taking anthropometric arm measurements.*)
- BMI calculation confirms obesity.

TREATMENT

GENERAL

- Hypnosis and behavior modification techniques
- Psychological counseling

DIET

- Reduction in daily caloric intake relative to basal metabolic needs

ACTIVITY

- Increase in daily activity level

SURGERY

- Vertical banded gastroplasty
- Gastric bypass

Taking anthropometric arm measurements

Follow these steps to determine triceps skin-fold thickness, midarm circumference, and midarm muscle circumference.

TRICEPS SKIN-FOLD THICKNESS

- Find the midpoint circumference of the arm by placing the tape measure halfway between the axilla and the elbow. Grasp the patient's skin with your thumb and forefinger, about ⅜" (1 cm) above the midpoint, as shown below.
- Place calipers at the midpoint, and squeeze for 3 seconds.
- Record the measurement to the nearest millimeter.
- Take two more readings, and use the average.

MIDARM CIRCUMFERENCE AND MIDARM MUSCLE CIRCUMFERENCE

- At the midpoint, measure the midarm circumference, as shown below. Record the measurement in centimeters.
- Calculate the midarm muscle circumference by multiplying the triceps skin-fold thickness —measured in millimeters—by 3.14.
- Subtract this number from the midarm circumference.

RECORDING THE MEASUREMENTS

Record all three measurements as a percentage of the standard measurements (see table below), using this formula:

$$\frac{\text{Actual measurement}}{\text{Standard measurement}} \times 100\%$$

Remember, a measurement less than 90% of the standard indicates caloric deprivation. A measurement over 90% indicates adequate or more-than-adequate energy reserves.

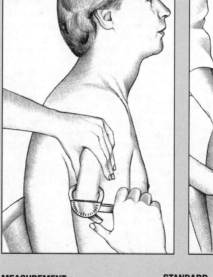 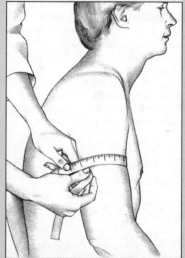

MEASUREMENT	STANDARD	90%
Triceps skin-fold thickness	Men: 12.5 mm Women: 16.5 mm	Men: 11.3 mm Women: 14.9 mm
Midarm circumference	Men: 29.3 cm Women: 28.5 cm	Men: 26.4 cm Women: 25.7 cm
Midarm muscle circumference	Men: 25.3 cm Women: 23.3 cm	Men: 22.8 cm Women: 20.9 cm

(continued)

NURSING CONSIDERATIONS

NURSING DIAGNOSES
◆ Chronic low self-esteem
◆ Disturbed body image
◆ Imbalanced nutrition: More than body requirements
◆ Ineffective coping
◆ Sedentary lifestyle

EXPECTED OUTCOMES
The patient will:
◆ voice feelings related to improved self-esteem
◆ express positive feelings about self
◆ safely reduce weight and reduce BMI to an appropriate level
◆ demonstrate effective coping mechanisms to deal with long-term compliance
◆ state the need to increase activity level.

NURSING INTERVENTIONS
◆ Obtain an accurate diet history to identify the patient's eating patterns.
◆ Promote increased physical activity, as appropriate.
◆ Monitor dietary intake.
◆ Monitor vital signs.
◆ Establish schedule for weight and BMI measurements.

PATIENT TEACHING

Be sure to cover:
◆ need for long-term maintenance after desired weight is achieved
◆ dietary guidelines
◆ safe weight-loss practices
◆ available weight-reduction and exercise programs
◆ contact information for local support groups or services.

RESOURCES
Organizations
American Obesity Association: *www.obesity.org*
Obesity Help, Inc.: *www.obesityhelp.com*
The Obesity Society: *www.naaso.org*

Selected references
Brown, I. "Nurses' Attitudes Towards Adult Patients Who Are Obese: Literature Review," *Journal of Advanced Nursing* 53(2):221-32, January 2006.

Gabriel, S., and Garguilo, H. "Bariatric Surgery Basics: Getting to the Heart of a Weighty Matter," *Nursing Made Incredibly Easy!* 4(1):42-50, January-February 2006.

Groth, S. "Adolescent Gestational Weight Gain; Does It Contribute to Obesity?" *MCN* 31(2):101-105, March-April 2006.

Harrell, J., et al. "Changing our Future: Obesity and the Metabolic Syndrome in Children and Adolescents," *Journal of Cardiovascular Nursing* 21(4):322-30, July-August, 2006.

Ziglar, M., and Bennett, V. "Case Studies: Obesity and the Trauma Patient: Challenges and Guidelines for Care," *Journal of Trauma Nursing* 13(1):22-27, January-March 2006.

Disorders affecting management of obesity

This chart highlights disorders that affect the management of obesity.

DISORDER	SIGNS AND SYMPTOMS	DIAGNOSTIC TEST RESULTS	TREATMENT AND CARE
Diabetes mellitus (complication)	◆ Weight loss despite voracious hunger ◆ Weakness ◆ Vision changes ◆ Frequent skin and urinary tract infections ◆ Dry, itchy skin ◆ Poor skin turgor ◆ Dry mucous membranes ◆ Dehydration ◆ Decreased peripheral pulses ◆ Cool skin temperature ◆ Decreased reflexes ◆ Orthostatic hypotension ◆ Muscle wasting ◆ Loss of subcutaneous fat ◆ Fruity breath odor from ketoacidosis	◆ Fasting blood glucose level is 126 mg/dl or greater, or a random blood glucose level is 200 mg/dl or greater on at least two occasions. ◆ Blood glucose level is 200 mg/dl or greater 2 hours after ingestion of 75 g of oral dextrose. ◆ Ophthalmic examination may reveal diabetic retinopathy.	◆ Monitor glucose level. ◆ Encourage lifestyle modifications or change, especially weight loss, diet, and exercise. ◆ Monitor for hyperglycemia or hypoglycemia and signs of cardiovascular or renal complications. ◆ Administer medications. ◆ Provide skin care and monitor wounds for healing.
Hypertension (complication)	◆ Usually asymptomatic ◆ Elevated blood pressure readings on at least two consecutive occasions ◆ Occipital headache ◆ Epistaxis ◆ Bruits ◆ Dizziness ◆ Confusion ◆ Fatigue ◆ Blurry vision ◆ Nocturia	◆ Serial blood pressure measurements reveal elevations of 140/90 mm Hg or greater on two or more separate occasions. ◆ Urinalysis may show protein, casts, red blood cells, or white blood cells. ◆ Blood urea nitrogen and serum creatinine levels may be elevated. ◆ Electrocardiogram may reveal ventricular hypertrophy or ischemia. ◆ Echocardiography may reveal left ventricular hypertrophy.	◆ Monitor blood pressure readings, response to antihypertensives, and laboratory results. ◆ Encourage lifestyle modifications or change, especially weight loss and exercise programs. ◆ Monitor for complications, such as stroke, myocardial infarction, and renal disease. ◆ Administer medications as ordered.
Obstructive sleep apnea-hypopnea syndrome (complication)	◆ Edema ◆ Body mass index greater than 30 ◆ Loud snoring ◆ Witnessed periods of apnea while sleeping ◆ Restless sleep ◆ Morning headache ◆ Excessive daytime sleepiness ◆ Neck circumference greater than 17″ (43 cm) in men and 15″ (37 cm) in women ◆ Enlarged tonsils	◆ Polysomnography (sleep study) analyzes breathing patterns during sleep and identifies type of apnea or hypopnea. ◆ Pulse oximetry readings decrease by 4% during apneic periods while sleeping. ◆ Apnea-hypopnea index (total number of apneas and hypopneas divided by total sleep time) identifies severity of sleep apnea. ◆ Multiple sleep latency test evaluates degree of excessive daytime sleepiness.	◆ Apply nasal continuous positive airway pressure device before sleep at night. ◆ Monitor for periods of apnea and pulse oximetry readings. ◆ Monitor cardiac rhythm while sleeping. ◆ Note episodes of daytime sleepiness. ◆ Encourage lifestyle modification or changes, such as weight loss and exercise programs. ◆ Administer tricyclic antidepressants and nonamphetamine central nervous system stimulants, as ordered, and evaluate effect.

Paget's disease

- Slow, progressive bone disorder that causes an irregular bone formation
- Affects one or several skeletal areas (spine, pelvis, femur, and skull)
- Causes malignant bone changes in about 5% of patients
- May be fatal, particularly when associated with heart failure, bone sarcoma, or giant cell tumors
- More common after age 40
- Affects men and women equally
- Also known as *osteitis deformans*
- Paget's disease of the breast, a form of breast cancer, is a different disorder from Paget's disease. (See *Paget's disease of the breast.*)

CAUSES

- Exact cause unknown
- Thought to be caused by a slow or dormant viral infection (possibly mumps)

PATHOPHYSIOLOGY

- In the initial phase (osteoclastic phase), excessive bone resorption occurs.
- The second phase (osteoblastic phase) involves excessive abnormal bone formation.
- Chronic accelerated remodeling eventually enlarges and softens the affected bones.
- The new bone structure, which is chaotic, fragile, and weak, causes painful deformities of both external contour and internal structure. Repeated episodes of accelerated osteoclastic resorption of spongy bone occur.

CARDIOVASCULAR SYSTEM

- The widespread nature of Paget's disease and extreme vascularity of the newly formed bone increase metabolic demand, thus creating a continuous need for high cardiac output.
- Increased metabolic demand and high cardiac output can lead to heart failure. (See *Disorders affecting management of Paget's disease,* pages 350 and 351.)

MUSCULOSKELETAL SYSTEM

- The trabeculae diminish, and vascular fibrous tissue replaces marrow. This activity is followed by short periods of rapid, abnormal bone formation.
- The collagen fibers in the new bone are disorganized, and glycoprotein levels in the matrix decrease.
- The partially resorbed trabeculae thicken and enlarge because of excessive bone formation, and the bone becomes soft and weak.
- Impingement of abnormal bone on the spinal cord or sensory nerve root leads to pain and impaired mobility. Pain may also result from the constant inflammation accompanying cell breakdown.
- Pelvic softening may occur, leading to a waddling gait.
- The legs may bow if the femurs or tibias are affected.

- Occasionally, malignant osteosarcoma can occur in the deformed bone.

NEUROLOGIC SYSTEM

- With skull involvement, characteristic cranial enlargement over the frontal and occipital areas can produce headaches, sensory abnormalities, and impaired motor function, depending on the sensory areas affected. For example, blindness and hearing loss with tinnitus and vertigo may result from bony impingement on the cranial nerves.
- Kyphosis may develop as a result of compression fractures of the vertebrae.
- Permanent paralysis can occur if the soft bone of the vertebrae fractures and puts pressure on the spinal cord.

RENAL SYSTEM

- Because of the constant osteoclastic and osteoblastic activity, phosphates and calcium are released and reabsorbed.
- Phosphates and calcium may then accumulate in the renal pelvis, resulting in renal calculi.
- Hypercalcemia and gout may also occur.

RESPIRATORY SYSTEM

- Chronic accelerated remodeling eventually enlarges and softens the affected bones.
- Thoracic deformities may impair respiration, eventually leading to respiratory failure.

Paget's disease of the breast

Commonly misdiagnosed as a dermatologic problem, this rare type of breast cancer appears as a red, scaly crust on the nipple, causing itchiness and burning. Biopsy confirms the diagnosis. Treatment should be started to prevent spread of malignancy to the lymph nodes and other parts of the body.

ASSESSMENT

HISTORY
- Severe, persistent pain
- Impaired mobility
- Pain that worsens with weight bearing
- Increased hat size
- Headaches

PHYSICAL FINDINGS
- Cranial enlargement over frontal and occipital areas
- Kyphosis
- Barrel-shaped chest
- Asymmetrical bowing of the tibia and femur
- Warmth and tenderness over affected sites

DIAGNOSTIC TEST RESULTS
- Red blood cell count shows anemia.
- Serum alkaline phosphatase level is elevated.
- Level of 24-hour urine hydroxyproline is elevated.
- X-ray studies show bone expansion and increased bone density.
- Bone scans clearly show early Pagetic lesions.
- Bone biopsy shows a characteristic mosaic pattern of bone tissue.

TREATMENT

GENERAL
- Heat therapy
- Massage
- Weight management

DIET
- Adequate levels of calcium and vitamin D

ACTIVITY
- As tolerated
- Regular exercise, balanced with appropriate rest periods
- Use of assistive devices such as cane or walker, if needed, to prevent falls

MEDICATIONS
- Calcitonin
- Nonsteroidal anti-inflammatory drugs
- Bisphosphonates
- Calcium supplements
- Vitamin D

SURGERY
- Reduction of pathologic fractures
- Correction of secondary deformities
- Relief of neurologic impairment

NURSING CONSIDERATIONS

NURSING DIAGNOSES
- Chronic pain
- Dressing or grooming self-care deficit
- Impaired physical mobility
- Risk for impaired skin integrity
- Risk for injury

EXPECTED OUTCOMES
The patient will:
- express feelings of increased comfort and decreased pain
- perform activities of daily living to the extent possible
- maintain joint mobility and range of motion
- maintain adequate skin integrity
- remain free from injury.

NURSING INTERVENTIONS
- Take measures to prevent pressure ulcers.
- Instruct the patient with footdrop to wear high-topped sneakers or use a footboard.
- Assess pain level; provide analgesics, as ordered.
- Monitor new areas of pain and new movement restrictions.
- Assess sensory and motor disturbances.
- Monitor serum calcium and alkaline phosphatase levels and intake and output.

(continued)

Be sure to cover:

◆ disorder, diagnostic testing, and treatment
◆ medication administration, dosage, and possible adverse effects
◆ pacing of activities
◆ use of assistive devices
◆ exercise program
◆ use of a firm mattress or a bed board
◆ home safety measures
◆ available community resource and support sources, as appropriate.

RESOURCES
Organizations
Arthritis Foundation: *www.arthritis.org*
National Institutes of Health: *www.nih.gov*
Paget Foundation for Paget's Disease of Bone and Related Disorders: *www.paget.org*

Selected references
Handbook of Pathophysiology, 2nd ed. Philadelphia: Lippincott Williams & Wilkins, 2005.

Hosking, D. "Pharmacological Therapy of Paget's and Other Metabolic Bone Diseases," *Bone* 38(2 Suppl 2):3-7, February 2006.

Langston, A., et al. "Clinical Determinants of Quality of Life in Paget's Disease of the Bone," *Calcified Tissue International* 80(1):1-9, January 2007.

Parvizi, J., et al. "Surgical Management of Paget's Disease of the Bone," *Journal of Bone and Mineral Research* 21(Suppl 2):75-82, December 2006.

Professional Guide to Diseases, 8th ed. Philadelphia: Lippincott Williams & Wilkins, 2005.

Siris, E., et al. "Medical Management of Paget's Disease of the Bone: Indications for Treatment and Review of Current Therapies," *Journal of Bone and Mineral Research* 21(Suppl 2):94-98, December 2006.

Disorders affecting management of Paget's disease

This chart highlights disorders that affect the management of Paget's disease.

DISORDER	SIGNS AND SYMPTOMS	DIAGNOSTIC TEST RESULTS	TREATMENT AND CARE
Heart failure (complication)	*Left-sided heart failure* ◆ Dyspnea ◆ Orthopnea ◆ Paroxysmal nocturnal dyspnea ◆ Fatigue ◆ Nonproductive cough ◆ Crackles ◆ Hemoptysis ◆ Tachycardia ◆ S_3, S_4 ◆ Cool, pale skin ◆ Restlessness and confusion *Right-sided heart failure* ◆ Jugular vein distention ◆ Positive hepatojugular reflex ◆ Right upper quadrant pain ◆ Anorexia ◆ Nausea ◆ Nocturia ◆ Weight gain ◆ Edema ◆ Ascites or anasarca ◆ Typically asymptomatic	◆ Chest X-ray shows increased pulmonary vascular markings, interstitial edema, or pleural effusions and cardiomegaly. ◆ Electrocardiography may reveal hypertrophy, ischemic changes or infarction, tachycardia, and extrasystoles. ◆ Liver function test may be abnormal; blood urea nitrogen (BUN) and creatinine levels may be elevated. ◆ Prothrombin time may be prolonged. ◆ B-type natriuretic peptide (BNP) immunoassay is elevated. ◆ Echocardiography may reveal left ventricular hypertrophy, dilation, and abnormal contractility. ◆ Pulmonary artery pressure, pulmonary artery wedge pressure, and left ventricular end-diastolic pressure are elevated in left-sided heart failure; right atrial or central venous pressure is elevated in right-sided heart failure. ◆ Radionuclide ventriculography may reveal ejection fraction less than 40% in diastolic dysfunction.	◆ Place the patient in Fowler's position and give supplemental oxygen. ◆ Weigh the patient daily, and check for peripheral edema. ◆ Monitor intake and output, vital signs, and mental status. ◆ Auscultate for S_3 and S_4 and adventitious lung sounds such as crackles or rhonchi. ◆ Monitor BUN, creatinine, and serum potassium, sodium, chloride, and magnesium levels. ◆ Institute continuous cardiac monitoring to identify and treat arrhythmias promptly. ◆ Administer angiotensin-converting enzyme (ACE) inhibitors, digoxin, diuretics, beta-adrenergic blockers, human BNP, nitrates, and morphine. ◆ Prepare the patient for possible coronary artery bypass surgery or angioplasty, as appropriate. ◆ Encourage lifestyle modifications to reduce symptoms.

DISORDER	SIGNS AND SYMPTOMS	DIAGNOSTIC TEST RESULTS	TREATMENT AND CARE
Hypertension (complication)	◆ Elevated blood pressure readings on at least two consecutive occasions ◆ Occipital headache ◆ Epistaxis ◆ Bruits ◆ Dizziness ◆ Confusion ◆ Fatigue ◆ Blurred vision ◆ Nocturia ◆ Edema	◆ Urinalysis may show protein, casts, red blood cells, or white blood cells. ◆ Elevated BUN and serum creatinine suggest renal disease. ◆ Complete blood count may reveal polycythemia or anemia. ◆ Excretory urography may reveal renal atrophy. ◆ Electrocardiography may show left ventricular hypertrophy or ischemia. ◆ Chest X-rays may show cardiomegaly. ◆ Echocardiography may reveal left ventricular hypertrophy.	◆ Monitor blood pressure and the patient's response to antihypertensive medications. ◆ Evaluate results of laboratory studies. ◆ Maintain a reduced-sodium diet. ◆ Monitor for complications of hypertension such as signs of stroke, myocardial infarction, and renal disease. ◆ Administer thiazide diuretics, ACE inhibitors, angiotensin-receptor blockers, beta-adrenergic blockers, and calcium channel blockers.
Osteoarthritis (complication)	◆ Deep, aching joint pain ◆ Stiffness in the morning and after exercise ◆ Crepitus or grating of the joint during motion ◆ Heberden's nodes (bony enlargements of the distal interphalangeal joints) ◆ Altered gait from contractures ◆ Decreased range of motion (ROM) ◆ Joint enlargement ◆ Localized headaches	◆ Absence of systemic symptoms rules out an inflammatory joint disorder. ◆ Arthroscopy shows bone spurs and narrowing of joint space. ◆ Erythrocyte sedimentation rate is increased. ◆ X-rays may confirm diagnosis by showing narrowing of joint space or margin, cystlike bony deposits in joint spaces, sclerosis of the subchondral space, joint deformity, bony growths, and joint fusion.	◆ Promote adequate rest, particularly after activity. Plan rest periods during the day. Teach the patient to pace activities and avoid overexertion. ◆ Assist with physical therapy and encourage the patient to perform gentle, isometric ROM exercises. ◆ If the patient needs surgery, provide appropriate preoperative and postoperative care. ◆ Provide emotional support and reassurance. ◆ Assist with care for arthritic joints, such as hot soaks, paraffin dips for the hands, and cervical collar application. ◆ Ensure proper functioning of supportive devices such as canes, braces, crutches, or walkers, and provide instruction for their use. ◆ Instruct the patient to take medications, such as aspirin, and nonsteroidal anti-inflammatory drugs, such as ibuprofen (Motrin), exactly as prescribed.
Renal calculi (complication)	◆ Severe pain ◆ Nausea and vomiting ◆ Fever ◆ Chills ◆ Hematuria ◆ Abdominal distention ◆ Anuria	◆ Kidney-ureter-bladder radiography shows most recent calculi. ◆ Excretory urography confirms diagnosis and determines size and location of calculi. ◆ Kidney ultrasonography helps detect obstructive changes. ◆ Urine culture identifies possible urinary tract infection. ◆ A 24-hour collection of urine reveals calcium oxalate, phosphorus, or uric acid excretion levels; serum calcium and phosphorus levels may be increased.	◆ Maintain 24- to 48-hour record of urine pH. ◆ Encourage the patient to walk, if possible, to aid passage of the stone. ◆ Promote sufficient intake of fluids to maintain a urine output of 2 to 4 qt (2 to 4 L/day). ◆ Record intake and output and strain urine. ◆ Stress the importance of proper diet. ◆ If surgery is required, maintain patency of tubes and monitor for drainage; never irrigate a nephrostomy tube without a physician's order. Check dressings and monitor vital signs. Notify physician of changes. ◆ Monitor for signs of infection.

Peritonitis LIFE-THREATENING DISORDER

OVERVIEW

- Inflammation of the peritoneum
- Commonly decreases intestinal motility and causes intestinal distention with gas
- Fatal in 10% of cases, with bowel obstruction the usual cause of death
- Can be acute or chronic
- More common in men

CAUSES

- Bacterial or chemical inflammation
- GI tract perforation (from appendicitis, diverticulitis, peptic ulcer, or ulcerative colitis)
- Ruptured ectopic pregnancy
- Peritoneal dialysis
- Ascites

PATHOPHYSIOLOGY

- Bacteria invade the peritoneum after inflammation and perforation of the GI tract.
- Fluid containing protein and electrolytes accumulates in the peritoneal cavity; normally transparent, the peritoneum becomes opaque, red, inflamed, and edematous.
- Infection may localize as an abscess rather than disseminate as a generalized infection.
- In some cases, however, such as when the peritoneum becomes weakened or injured, the inflammation and infection spread throughout the peritoneal cavity. The resulting inflammatory response can affect multiple body systems.

CARDIOVASCULAR SYSTEM

- Large amounts of fluid from the intravascular space move into the peritoneal cavity, causing hypovolemia and hemoconcentration, as indicated by cool, clammy skin and pallor.
- If the patient loses excessive fluid, electrolytes, and proteins into the abdominal cavity, dehydration may occur. Hypotension and tachycardia result as the body tries to conserve fluid. (See *Disorders affecting management of peritonitis,* page 355.)

GI SYSTEM

- An inflammatory process causes the release of histamine from the peritonitis.
- Peristaltic action decreases.
- Fibrin formation occurs around the damage, eventually causing adhesions.
- If the inflammation is severe or prolonged, adhesions continue to form, ultimately leading to bowel obstruction.
- The shift in fluid or third-spacing exudate into the peritoneal cavity leads to abdominal distention.
- The increased secretion in the bowel increases intraluminal pressure, commonly resulting in paralytic ileus.

NEUROLOGIC SYSTEM

- The shift in fluid out of the vascular space leads to volume depletion. Impaired blood flow and diminished perfusion of cerebral cells cause changes in the patient's level of consciousness.
- Initial anxiety and restlessness may progress to confusion and lethargy.

RENAL SYSTEM

- The loss of fluid from the intravascular space leads to a drop in blood pressure and, ultimately, decreased perfusion to the kidneys.

RESPIRATORY SYSTEM

- Fluid accumulation in the peritoneal cavity may cause elevation of the diaphragm, leading to an increased respiratory rate.
- Inflammation of the peritoneum can irritate the nerve fibers in the peritoneum and diaphragm. The resulting pain on inspiration may lead to a decrease in the depth of respirations.

ASSESSMENT

HISTORY
Early phase
- If localized, pain over a specific area (usually the inflammation site)
- If generalized, diffuse pain over the abdomen

With progression
- Increasingly severe and constant abdominal pain that increases with movement and respirations
- Possible referral of pain to shoulder or thoracic area
- Anorexia, nausea, and vomiting
- Inability to pass stools and flatus
- Hiccups

PHYSICAL FINDINGS
- Fever
- Tachycardia
- Hypotension
- Shallow breathing
- Signs of dehydration
- Positive bowel sounds (early); absent bowel sounds (later)
- Abdominal rigidity
- General abdominal tenderness
- Rebound tenderness
- Typical patient positioning: lying very still with knees flexed

DIAGNOSTIC TEST RESULTS
- Complete blood count shows leukocytosis.
- Abdominal X-rays show edematous and gaseous distention of the small and large bowel. With perforation of a visceral organ, X-rays show air in the abdominal cavity.
- Chest X-rays may reveal elevation of the diaphragm.
- Computed tomography scanning reveals fluid and inflammation.
- Paracentesis shows the exudate's nature and permits bacterial culture testing.

TREATMENT

GENERAL
- I.V. fluids
- Nasogastric (NG) intubation

DIET
- Nothing by mouth until bowel function returns
- Gradual increase in diet
- Parenteral nutrition, if necessary

ACTIVITY
- Bed rest until condition improves
- Semi-Fowler's position
- Avoidance of lifting for at least 6 weeks postoperatively

MEDICATIONS
- Antibiotics, based on infecting organism
- Electrolytes
- Analgesics

SURGERY
- Dependent on the cause of peritonitis

NURSING CONSIDERATIONS

NURSING DIAGNOSES
- Acute pain
- Anxiety
- Deficient fluid volume
- Fear
- Imbalanced nutrition: Less than body requirements
- Ineffective tissue perfusion: GI

EXPECTED OUTCOMES
The patient will:
- express feelings of increased comfort and decreased pain
- identify strategies to reduce anxiety
- maintain normal fluid volume
- discuss fears and concerns
- maintain adequate caloric intake
- exhibit signs of adequate GI perfusion and regain normal bowel function.

NURSING INTERVENTIONS
- Give prescribed drugs.
- Encourage early postoperative ambulation.
- Encourage the patient to express his feelings.
- Provide emotional support.
- Monitor fluid and nutritional status.
- Assess pain level; administer analgesics, as ordered, and evaluate effect.
- Monitor vital signs.
- Maintain NG tube function and drainage; assess GI status.
- Assess wound site and perform wound care, as directed.
- Observe for signs and symptoms of dehiscence.

WARNING *Watch for signs and symptoms of abscess formation, including persistent abdominal tenderness and fever.*

(continued)

Be sure to cover:
- disorder, diagnostic testing, and treatment
- medication administration, dosage, and possible adverse effects
- preoperative coughing and deep-breathing techniques
- postoperative care procedures
- signs and symptoms of infection
- proper wound care
- dietary and activity limitations (depending on type of surgery).

RESOURCES
Organizations
Digestive Disease National Coalition: *www.ddnc.org*
National Digestive Diseases Information Clearinghouse: *www.niddk.nih.gov/health/digest/nddic.htm*

Selected references
Cole, E., et al. "Assessment of the Patient with Acute Abdominal Pain," *Nursing Standard* 20(38):56-61, May-June 2006.

Courtney, A.E., and Doherty, C.C. "Fulminant Sclerosing Peritonitis Immediately Following Acute Bacterial Peritonitis," *Nephrology Dialysis Transplantation* 21(2):532-34, February 2006.

Kiank, C., et al. "Stress-Induced Immune Conditioning Affects the Course of Experimental Peritonitis," *Shock* 27(3):305-11, March 2007.

McNally, P. *GI/Liver Secrets,* 3rd ed. Philadelphia: Mosby, 2006.

Rosa, N., et al. "Fungal Peritonitis in Peritoneal Dialysis Patients: Is Previous Antibiotic Therapy an Essential Condition?" *Mycoses* 50(1):79-81, January 2007.

Disorders affecting management of peritonitis

This chart highlights disorders that affect the management of peritonitis.

DISORDER	SIGNS AND SYMPTOMS	DIAGNOSTIC TEST RESULTS	TREATMENT AND CARE
Hypovolemic shock (complication)	◆ Depend on the amount of fluid loss *Minimal volume loss (10% to 15%)* ◆ Slight tachycardia ◆ Normal supine blood pressure ◆ Positive postural vital signs, including a decrease in systolic blood pressure greater than 10 mm Hg or an increase in pulse rate greater than 20 beats/minute ◆ Increased capillary refill time (longer than 3 seconds) ◆ Urine output more than 30 ml/hour ◆ Cool, pale skin on arms and legs ◆ Anxiety *Moderate volume loss (about 25%)* ◆ Rapid, thready pulse ◆ Supine hypotension ◆ Cool truncal skin ◆ Urine output of 10 to 30 ml/hour ◆ Severe thirst ◆ Restlessness, confusion, or irritability *Severe volume loss (40% or more)* ◆ Marked tachycardia ◆ Marked hypotension ◆ Weak or absent peripheral pulses ◆ Cold, mottled, or cyanotic skin ◆ Urine output less than 10 ml/hour ◆ Unconsciousness	◆ Complete blood count reveals low hematocrit and decreased hemoglobin level, red blood cell (RBC) count, and platelet counts. ◆ Metabolic studies reveal elevated serum potassium, sodium, lactate dehydrogenase, creatinine, and blood urea nitrogen (BUN) levels. ◆ Urine studies reveal increased urine specific gravity (greater than 1.020) and urine osmolality and urine sodium levels less than 50 mEq/L. ◆ Urine creatinine levels may be decreased. ◆ Arterial blood gas (ABG) studies may reveal decreased pH and partial pressure of arterial oxygen and increased partial pressure of arterial carbon dioxide. ◆ Gastroscopy, X-rays, and aspiration of gastric contents through a nasogastric tube may reveal evidence of frank or occult bleeding. ◆ Coagulation studies may show evidence of coagulopathy.	◆ Assess the patient for the extent of fluid loss and begin fluid replacement. ◆ Obtain a blood type and crossmatch for blood component therapy; administer blood products. ◆ Assess airway, breathing, and circulation, and institute emergency resuscitative measures, as needed. ◆ Administer supplemental oxygen, as indicated, and monitor oxygen saturation. ◆ Monitor vital signs and hemodynamic status continuously for changes. Observe skin color and check capillary refill. ◆ Institute continuous cardiac monitoring to evaluate for possible arrhythmias, myocardial ischemia, or adverse effects of treatment. ◆ Assess neurologic status frequently—about every 30 minutes until the patient stabilizes, and then every 2 to 4 hours. ◆ Monitor urine output at least hourly. ◆ Administer dopamine or norepinephrine I.V., as ordered, to increase cardiac contractility and renal perfusion. ◆ During therapy, assess skin color and temperature and note changes. ◆ Watch for signs of impending coagulopathy (such as petechiae, bruising, and bleeding or oozing from gums or venipuncture sites). ◆ Prepare the patient for surgery, as appropriate.
Sepsis (complication)	◆ Tachycardia and bounding pulse ◆ Restlessness, irritability, and hypoxia ◆ Shallow respirations, tachypnea ◆ Reduced urinary output ◆ Warm, dry skin ◆ Hypotension as compensatory mechanisms fail ◆ Narrowed pulse pressure ◆ Weak, rapid, thready pulse ◆ Reduced urinary output ◆ Cyanosis ◆ Unconsciousness and absent reflexes (in irreversible stages) ◆ Rapidly falling blood pressure with decompensation ◆ Anuria	◆ Blood, urine, or sputum cultures may identify the causative organism. ◆ Coagulation studies may detect coagulopathy from disseminated intravascular coagulation. ◆ White blood cell count and erythrocyte sedimentation rate may be increased. ◆ BUN and creatinine are elevated. ◆ Serum lactate may be increased secondary to anaerobic metabolism. ◆ Serum glucose may be elevated in early stages. ◆ ABG analysis may reveal respiratory alkalosis in early shock or respiratory acidosis in later stages. ◆ Urine specific gravity may be high. ◆ Chest X-rays may be normal in early stages; pulmonary congestion may be seen in later stages. ◆ Hemodynamic monitoring may reveal characteristic patterns of intracardiac pressures and cardiac output.	◆ Assist in identifying and treating underlying cause. ◆ Maintain a patent airway; prepare for intubation and mechanical ventilation if respiratory distress develops. ◆ Administer supplemental oxygen and monitor pulse oximetry. ◆ Perform continuous cardiac monitoring to detect changes in heart rate and rhythm; administer antiarrhythmics, as needed. ◆ Monitor blood pressure, pulse rate, peripheral pulses and other vital signs every 15 minutes; report changes. ◆ Monitor central venous pressure, pulmonary artery wedge pressure, and cardiac output, as ordered. ◆ Administer I.V. fluids, crystalloids, colloids, or blood products, as necessary, to maintain intravascular volume. ◆ Administer antibiotics to eradicate the causative organism. ◆ Administer inotropic drugs, such as dopamine, dobutamine, and epinephrine, to increase heart contractility and cardiac output; monitor blood pressure, cardiac output, peripheral pulses, and circulation; report changes. ◆ Monitor temperature and institute cooling measures, such as using hyperthermia blankets and decreasing room temperature.

Pheochromocytoma

OVERVIEW

- Rare, catecholamine-producing tumor that's typically benign; usually derived from adrenal medullary cells
- Seen in about 0.5% of newly diagnosed hypertensive patients
- Most common cause of adrenal medullary hypersecretion
- Usually produces norepinephrine, with large tumors secreting both epinephrine and norepinephrine
- Potentially fatal, but good prognosis with treatment
- Occurs equally among all races and both sexes
- Occurs in patients ages 30 to 50
- Typically familial
- Also known as *chromaffin tumor*

CAUSES

- May be inherited as an autosomal dominant trait

RISK FACTORS FOR HYPERTENSIVE CRISIS

- Anesthesia
- Medications, such as opiates, cold medicine, dopamine antagonists, tricyclic antidepressants, and cocaine
- Radiographic contrast dye
- Childbirth

PATHOPHYSIOLOGY

- Pheochromocytoma causes excessive catecholamine production from autonomous tumor functioning.
- The tumor stems from a chromaffin cell tumor of the adrenal medulla or sympathetic ganglia (more commonly in the right adrenal gland than in the left).
- Extra-adrenal pheochromocytomas may occur in the abdomen, thorax, urinary bladder, and neck and in association with the 9th and 10th cranial nerves.

CARDIOVASCULAR SYSTEM

- Increased catecholamine (norepinephrine and epinephrine) secretion stimulate alpha-adrenergic receptors and result in elevated blood pressure and increased cardiac contractility.
- Increased heart rate and cardiac contractility also result from stimulation of beta-adrenergic receptors.
- Excessive plasma catecholamine levels may initiate cardiac arrhythmias. (See *Disorders affecting management of pheochromocytoma*, page 359.)

NEUROLOGIC SYSTEM

- Catecholamine-induced hypertensive crisis may precipitate hypertensive encephalopathy, stroke, or intracerebral hemorrhage.

ASSESSMENT

HISTORY

- Unpredictable episodes of hypertensive crisis
- Paroxysmal symptoms, suggesting a seizure disorder or anxiety attack
- Hypertension that responds poorly to conventional treatment
- Hypotension or shock after surgery or diagnostic procedures

During paroxysms or crises

- Throbbing headache
- Palpitations
- Visual blurring
- Nausea and vomiting
- Severe diaphoresis
- Feelings of impending doom
- Precordial or abdominal pain
- Moderate weight loss
- Dizziness or light-headedness when moving to an upright position

PHYSICAL FINDINGS
During paroxysms or crises

- Hypertension
- Tachypnea
- Pallor or flushing
- Profuse sweating
- Tremor
- Seizures
- Tachycardia

DIAGNOSTIC TEST RESULTS

- Levels of vanillylmandelic acid and metanephrine are increased in 24-hour urine specimen.
- Total plasma catecholamine levels are 10 to 50 times higher than normal on direct assay.
- Computed tomography (CT) scan or magnetic resonance imaging of adrenal glands may show intra-adrenal lesions.
- CT scan, chest X-rays, or abdominal aortography may reveal extra-adrenal pheochromocytoma.
- Iodine-131–metaiodobenzylguanidine scan locates or confirms pheochromocytoma.

GENERAL
◆ Measures to control blood pressure

DIET
◆ High-protein with adequate calories

ACTIVITY
◆ Rest during acute attacks

MEDICATIONS
◆ Alpha-adrenergic blockers
◆ Catecholamine-synthesis antagonists
◆ Beta-adrenergic blockers
◆ Calcium channel blockers
◆ Triose kinase inhibitors
◆ I.V. phentolamine or nitroprusside during paroxysms or crises

> **WARNING** *Because severe and, occasionally, fatal paroxysms have been induced by opiates, histamine, and other drugs, all medications should be considered carefully and administered cautiously in patients with known or suspected pheochromocytoma.*

SURGERY
◆ Removal of pheochromocytoma

NURSING DIAGNOSES
◆ Acute pain
◆ Anxiety
◆ Fear
◆ Imbalanced nutrition: Less than body requirements
◆ Ineffective coping
◆ Ineffective tissue perfusion: Cardiopulmonary, renal
◆ Risk for infection

EXPECTED OUTCOMES
The patient will:
◆ express feelings of increased comfort and decreased pain
◆ identify strategies to reduce anxiety
◆ discuss fears and concerns
◆ identify appropriate food choices according to a prescribed diet
◆ demonstrate adaptive coping behaviors
◆ exhibit signs of adequate cardiopulmonary and renal perfusion
◆ remain free from signs and symptoms of infection.

NURSING INTERVENTIONS
◆ Monitor vital signs, noting blood pressure trends.
◆ Give prescribed drugs and evaluate effects.
◆ Watch for signs of hypertensive crisis.
◆ Prepare the patient and family for surgery.
◆ Provide comfort measures.
◆ Consult a dietitian, as needed.
◆ Tell the patient to report symptoms of an acute attack.
◆ Encourage the patient to express his feelings and provide emotional support.
◆ Help the patient develop effective coping strategies.

> **WARNING** *Be aware that postoperative hypertension is common because the stress of surgery, anesthesia, and adrenal gland manipulation stimulate catecholamine secretion.*

◆ Monitor intake and output, serum glucose level, daily weight, and neurologic and cardiovascular status.
◆ Observe for adverse reactions to medications.

After adrenalectomy
◆ Assess GI status.
◆ Assess the incision; provide wound care, as directed.
◆ Observe for signs and symptoms of hemorrhage.
◆ Assess pain level; administer analgesics, as ordered, and evaluate response.

(continued)

Be sure to cover:
- disorder, diagnostic testing, and treatment
- medication administration, dosage, and possible adverse effects
- when to notify the practitioner
- ways to prevent paroxysmal attacks
- signs and symptoms of adrenal insufficiency
- importance of wearing medical identification jewelry
- how to monitor his own blood pressure
- contact information for genetic counseling if autosomal dominant transmission of pheochromocytoma is suspected.

RESOURCES

Organizations

American Association of Clinical Endocrinologists: *www.aace.com*
American Society of Human Genetics: *www.faseb.org/genetics/ashg/ashgmenu.htm*
Endocrine Society: *www.endo-society.org*
Pheochromocytoma Support and Awareness Group: *www.ndrf.org/pheochro.htm*

Selected references

Dahia, P.L. "Evolving Concepts in Pheochromocytoma and Paraganglioma," *Current Opinion in Oncology* 18(1):1-8, January 2006.

Daub, K. "Pheochromocytoma: Challenges in Diagnosis and Nursing Care," *The Nursing Clinics of North America* 42(1):101-11, March 2007.

Disick, G., and Palese, M. "Extra-adrenal Pheochromocytoma: Diagnosis and Management," *Current Urology Reports* 8(1):83-88, January 2007.

Guller, U., et al. "Detecting Pheochromocytoma: Defining the Most Sensitive Test," *Annals of Surgery* 243(1):102-107, January 2006.

Nettina, S.M. *Lippincott Manual of Nursing Practice,* 8th ed. Philadelphia: Lippincott Williams & Wilkins, 2006.

Disorders affecting management of pheochromocytoma

This chart highlights disorders that affect the management of pheochromocytoma.

DISORDER	SIGNS AND SYMPTOMS	DIAGNOSTIC TEST RESULTS	TREATMENT AND CARE
Cardiac arrhythmia (complication)	◆ Palpitations ◆ Chest pain ◆ Dizziness ◆ Weakness, fatigue ◆ Irregular heart rhythm ◆ Hypotension ◆ Syncope ◆ Altered level of consciousness ◆ Diaphoresis, pallor, cold, clammy skin	◆ Electrocardiography identifies specific waveform changes associated with the arrhythmia. ◆ Laboratory testing reveals electrolyte abnormalities, hypoxemia, or acid-base abnormalities. ◆ Electrophysiologic testing identifies the mechanism of an arrhythmia and the location of accessory pathways.	◆ Assess airway, breathing, and circulation if life-threatening arrhythmia develops; follow advanced cardiac life support protocols for treatment. ◆ Monitor cardiac rhythm continuously and obtain serial electrocardiograms (ECGs) to evaluate changes and effects of treatment. ◆ Administer antiarrhythmics and monitor for adverse effects. ◆ Assess cardiovascular system for signs of hypoperfusion; monitor vital signs. ◆ Assist with insertion of temporary pacemaker or apply transcutaneous pacemaker, if appropriate.
Heart failure (complication)	*Left-sided heart failure* ◆ Dyspnea ◆ Orthopnea ◆ Paroxysmal nocturnal dyspnea ◆ Fatigue ◆ Nonproductive cough ◆ Crackles ◆ Hemoptysis ◆ Tachycardia ◆ S_3, S_4 ◆ Cool, pale skin ◆ Restlessness and confusion *Right-sided heart failure* ◆ Jugular vein distention ◆ Positive hepatojugular reflex ◆ Right upper quadrant pain ◆ Anorexia, nausea ◆ Weight gain, edema ◆ Ascites or anasarca	◆ Chest X-ray shows increased pulmonary vascular markings, interstitial edema, or pleural effusions and cardiomegaly. ◆ B-type natriuretic peptide (BNP) immunoassay is elevated. ◆ ECG may reveal hypertrophy, ischemic changes or infarction, tachycardia, and extrasystoles. ◆ Liver function test may be abnormal; blood urea nitrogen (BUN) and creatinine levels may be elevated. ◆ Prothrombin time may be prolonged. ◆ Echocardiography may reveal left ventricular hypertrophy, dilation, and abnormal contractility. ◆ Pulmonary artery pressure, pulmonary artery wedge pressure, and left ventricular end pressure are elevated in left-sided heart failure; right atrial or central venous pressure is elevated in right-sided heart failure. ◆ Radionuclide ventriculography may reveal ejection fraction less than 40% in diastolic dysfunction.	◆ Place the patient in Fowler's position and provide supplemental oxygen. ◆ Weigh the patient daily, and check for peripheral edema. ◆ Monitor intake and output, vital signs, and mental status. ◆ Auscultate for S_3 and S_4 and adventitious lung sounds, such as crackles or rhonchi. ◆ Monitor BUN, creatinine, BNP, serum electrolytes, and magnesium levels. ◆ Monitor cardiac rhythm. ◆ Administer human BNPs, diuretics, nitrates, angiotensin-converting enzyme inhibitors, digoxin, beta-adrenergic blockers, and morphine.
Stroke (complication)	◆ Sudden onset of symptoms ◆ Headache with no known cause ◆ Numbness or weakness of the face, arm, or leg, especially on one side of the body ◆ Confusion, trouble speaking or understanding, facial droop on one side ◆ Trouble seeing or walking, dizziness, and loss of coordination	◆ Computed tomography scan or magnetic resonance imaging shows evidence of thrombosis or hemorrhage ◆ Carotid ultrasound may detect a blockage, stenosis, or reduced blood flow. ◆ Angiography can help pinpoint the site of occlusion or rupture.	◆ Maintain a patent airway and provide oxygen. ◆ Administer thrombolytics if within 3 hours of symptom onset and the patient meets criteria for administration. Administer antihypertensives for elevated blood pressure and antiarrhythmics for cardiac arrhythmia. ◆ Administer antiplatelet drugs to prevent recurrent stroke, benzodiazepines to treat seizures, anticonvulsants to prevent seizures, aspirin or heparin for patient with embolic stroke who isn't a candidate for thrombolytics, stool softeners to prevent straining, corticosteroids to minimize associated cerebral edema, and analgesics for complaints of headache. ◆ Monitor vital signs and neurologic status. Note signs of increasing intracranial pressure. ◆ Assess gag reflex before offering oral fluids. Obtain swallowing evaluation, as indicated. ◆ Promote physical therapy when stable. Provide emotional support.

Polycystic kidney disease

- Growth of multiple, bilateral, grape-like clusters of fluid-filled cysts in the kidneys
- May progress slowly even after renal insufficiency symptoms appear
- Has two distinct forms:
- infantile: Causes stillbirth or early neonatal death; occurs in 1 of 6,000 to 40,000 infants
- adult: Has insidious onset but usually becomes obvious between ages 30 and 50; occurs in 1 of 50 to 1,000 adults; carries a widely varying prognosis
- Usually fatal within 4 years of uremic symptom onset, unless dialysis begins
- Affects both sexes equally
- Also known as *PKD*

CAUSES

- Adult form inherited as an autosomal dominant trait
- Infantile form inherited as an autosomal recessive trait

RISK FACTORS

- Autosomal dominant PKD (ADPKD) in one parent: 50% chance the disease will pass to a child
- Autosomal recessive PKD (ARPKD) if both parents carry the abnormal gene and pass the gene to their child: 1 in 4 chance that disease will pass to a child

PATHOPHYSIOLOGY

- Truncating mutations of genes (PKD1 and PKD2) and inadequate levels of polycystin cause progressive cystic dilation of renal tubules due to renal ciliary dysfunction.
- An abnormality on the short arm of chromosome 16 occurs in 85% to 90% of patients with PKD. An abnormality on the long arm of chromosome 4 occurs in 5% to 15% of patients.

URINARY SYSTEM

- Cysts enlarge the kidneys, compressing and eventually replacing functioning renal tissue.
- Renal deterioration results, but is more gradual in adults than in infants.
- The condition progresses relentlessly to fatal uremia. (See *Disorders affecting management of polycystic kidney disease,* pages 362 and 363.)

GI SYSTEM

- Extrarenal cysts may develop on the liver, resulting in infection. Hepatic cysts occur in 50% of patients.
- As cysts enlarge, nutritional status is affected and abdominal pain occurs.
- Polycystic liver disease may develop.
- With ARPKD, congenital hepatic fibrosis results from the malformation of the developing ductal plate. Portal hypertension may occur.
- Colonic diverticuli develop in approximately 80% of patients, possibly from altered connective tissue.

NEUROLOGIC SYSTEM

- Intracerebral aneurysm is the most serious complication of PKD, possibly resulting in intracerebral bleeding or stroke.
- Stroke may also be caused by uncontrolled severe hypertension.

CARDIOVASCULAR SYSTEM

- Severe hypertension is an early manifestation of PKD, even with normal renal function.
- Mitral valve prolapse, cardiac hypertrophy, and heart failure may occur secondary to uncontrolled hypertension.

HISTORY
Adult form

- Family history
- Polyuria
- Urinary tract infections
- Headaches
- Pain in back or flank area
- Gross hematuria
- Abdominal pain, usually worsened on exertion and eased by lying down

PHYSICAL FINDINGS
Infantile form

- Pronounced epicanthal folds
- Pointed nose
- Small chin
- Floppy, low-set ears (Potter facies)
- Huge, bilateral, symmetrical flank masses that are tense and can't be transilluminated
- Signs of respiratory distress, heart failure and, eventually, uremia and renal failure
- Signs of portal hypertension (bleeding varices)

Adult form

- Hypertension
- Signs of an enlarging kidney mass
- Grossly enlarged kidneys (in advanced stages)

DIAGNOSTIC TEST RESULTS

- Urinalysis may show hematuria or bacteria or protein.
- Creatinine clearance test results may show renal insufficiency or failure.

- Electrolyte study may reveal abnormal sodium level.
- Ultrasonography and radioisotopic scans show kidney enlargement and cysts. Criteria for diagnosis includes one cyst in both kidneys or two or more cysts in one kidney (in patients at risk younger than age 30); two or more cysts in each kidney (in patients at risk ages 30 to 59); and four or more cysts in each kidney (in patients at risk older than age 60).
- Computed tomography scan, and magnetic resonance imaging show multiple areas of cystic damage.

TREATMENT

GENERAL
- Monitoring of renal function
- Dialysis

DIET
- Low-sodium
- Fluid restriction (in renal failure)

ACTIVITY
- Avoidance of contact sports

MEDICATIONS
- Analgesics
- Antibiotics for urinary tract or cyst infection
- Angiotensin-converting enzyme inhibitors for hypertension
- Electrolyte supplements

SURGERY
- Kidney transplantation
- Surgical drainage for cystic abscess or retroperitoneal bleeding

NURSING CONSIDERATIONS

NURSING DIAGNOSES
- Acute pain
- Deficient fluid volume
- Fatigue
- Impaired urinary elimination
- Ineffective coping
- Ineffective tissue perfusion: Renal
- Interrupted family processes
- Risk for infection
- Risk for injury

EXPECTED OUTCOMES
The patient (or family) will:
- report feelings of increased comfort and decreased pain
- maintain fluid balance
- verbalize the importance of balancing activity with adequate rest periods
- demonstrate skill in managing the urinary elimination problem
- demonstrate adaptive coping behaviors
- modify lifestyle to minimize risk of decreased tissue perfusion
- discuss the impact of the patient's condition on the family unit
- remain free from signs and symptoms of infection
- remain free from injury.

NURSING INTERVENTIONS
- Give prescribed drugs.
- Provide supportive care to minimize symptoms.
- Individualize patient care accordingly.
- Assess urine (for blood, cloudiness, calculi, and granules).
- Monitor intake and output, electrolytes, and vital signs.
- Assess dialysis access site for function and signs of infection.

PATIENT TEACHING

Be sure to cover:
- disorder, diagnostic testing, and treatment
- medication administration, dosage, and possible adverse effects
- follow up with the practitioner for severe or recurring headaches
- signs and symptoms of urinary tract infection and prompt notification of the practitioner
- importance of blood pressure control
- possible need for dialysis or transplantation.

RESOURCES
Organizations
American Association of Kidney Patients: *www.aakp.org*
National Institute of Diabetes and Digestive and Kidney Diseases: *www.niddk.nih.gov*
Polycystic Kidney Research Foundation: *www.pkdcure.org*

Selected references
Bisceglia, M., et al. "Renal Cystic Diseases: A Review," *Advances in Anatomic Pathology* 13(1):26-56, January 2006.
Hamer, R., et al. "Polycystic Disease is a Risk Factor for New-Onset Diabetes after Transplantation," *Transplantation* 83(1):36-40, January 2007.
Thivierge, C., et al. "Overexpression of PKD1 Causes Polycystic Kidney Disease," *Molecular and Cellular Biology* 26(4):1538-48, February 2006.
Thomas, M. "Autosomal-Dominant Polycystic Kidney Disease," *Nephrology* 12(Suppl 1):S52-56, February 2007.

(continued)

Disorders affecting management of polycystic kidney disease

This chart highlights disorders that affect the management of polycystic kidney disease.

DISORDER	SIGNS AND SYMPTOMS	DIAGNOSTIC TEST RESULTS	TREATMENT AND CARE
Chronic renal failure (complication)	◆ Muscle twitching ◆ Paresthesia ◆ Bone pain ◆ Pruritus ◆ Decreased urine output ◆ Stomatitis ◆ Lethargy ◆ Seizures ◆ Brittle nails and hair ◆ Kussmaul's respirations ◆ Uremic frost ◆ Ecchymosis ◆ Weight gain	◆ Glomerular filtration rate is decreased; urinalysis shows albuminuria, proteinuria, glycosuria, erythrocytes, and leukocytes. ◆ Serum creatinine may increase by 2 mg/dl or more over a 2-week period. ◆ Blood urea nitrogen (BUN) suddenly increases. ◆ Uric acid is elevated. ◆ Potassium level is elevated. ◆ Arterial blood gas (ABG) analysis may show metabolic acidosis.	◆ Therapeutic goals are to reduce the deterioration of renal function and prevent stroke. ◆ Administer angiotensin-converting enzyme (ACE) inhibitors and angiotensin receptor blockers to achieve target blood pressure of less than 130/80 mg Hg. ◆ Monitor creatinine clearance, BUN, uric acid, potassium levels, and ABG studies. ◆ Be alert for drug toxicity and adverse reactions. ◆ Assist with dialysis, as indicated.
Heart failure (complication)	*Left-sided heart failure* ◆ Dyspnea ◆ Orthopnea ◆ Paroxysmal nocturnal dyspnea ◆ Fatigue ◆ Nonproductive cough ◆ Crackles ◆ Hemoptysis ◆ Tachycardia ◆ S_3, S_4 ◆ Cool, pale skin ◆ Restlessness and confusion *Right-sided heart failure* ◆ Jugular vein distention ◆ Positive hepatojugular reflex ◆ Right upper quadrant pain ◆ Anorexia, nausea ◆ Weight gain, edema ◆ Ascites or anasarca ◆ Usually asymptomatic	◆ Chest X-ray shows increased pulmonary vascular markings, interstitial edema, or pleural effusions and cardiomegaly. ◆ B-type natriuretic peptide (BNP) immunoassay is elevated. ◆ Electrocardiography may reveal hypertrophy, ischemic changes or infarction, tachycardia, and extrasystoles. ◆ Liver function test may be abnormal; BUN and creatinine levels may be elevated. ◆ Prothrombin time may be prolonged. ◆ Echocardiography may reveal left ventricular hypertrophy, dilation, and abnormal contractility. ◆ Pulmonary artery pressure, pulmonary artery wedge pressure, and left ventricular end pressure are elevated in left-sided heart failure; right atrial or central venous pressure is elevated in right-sided heart failure. ◆ Radionuclide ventriculography may reveal ejection fraction less than 40% in diastolic dysfunction.	◆ Place the patient in Fowler's position and provide supplemental oxygen. ◆ Weigh the patient daily, and check for peripheral edema. ◆ Monitor intake and output, vital signs, and mental status. ◆ Auscultate for S_3 and S_4 and adventitious lung sounds, such as crackles or rhonchi. ◆ Monitor BUN, creatinine, BNP, and serum electrolyte and magnesium levels. ◆ Monitor cardiac rhythm. ◆ Administer nesiritide (Natrecor), diuretics, nitrates, ACE inhibitors, digoxin, beta-adrenergic blockers, and morphine. ◆ Monitor blood pressure readings, response to antihypertensives, and laboratory readings.

Disorders affecting management of polycystic kidney disease *(continued)*

DISORDER	SIGNS AND SYMPTOMS	DIAGNOSTIC TEST RESULTS	TREATMENT AND CARE
Hypertension (coexisting and complication)	◆ Elevated blood pressure readings on at least two consecutive occasions ◆ Occipital headache ◆ Epistaxis ◆ Bruits ◆ Dizziness ◆ Confusion ◆ Fatigue ◆ Blurry vision ◆ Nocturia ◆ Edema	◆ Serial blood pressure measurements reveal elevations of 140/90 mm Hg or greater on two or more separate occasions. ◆ Urinalysis may show protein, casts, red blood cells, or white blood cells. ◆ BUN and serum creatinine levels may be elevated. ◆ Electrocardiography may reveal ventricular hypertrophy or ischemia. ◆ Echocardiography may reveal left ventricular hypertrophy.	◆ Encourage lifestyle modifications or change, especially weight loss, diet, and exercise. ◆ Monitor for complications, such as stroke, myocardial infarction, and renal disease. ◆ Administer medications.

Pulmonary embolism LIFE-THREATENING DISORDER

OVERVIEW

- Obstruction of the pulmonary arterial bed that occurs when a mass (such as a dislodged thrombus) lodges in the main pulmonary artery or branch, partially or completely obstructing it
- Usually originates in deep veins of the leg
- Causes rapid death from pulmonary infarction
- Develops in 600,000 to 700,000 people annually
- Affects both sexes equally and is more common with advancing age

CAUSES

- Deep vein thrombosis
- Pelvic, renal, and hepatic vein thrombosis
- Rarely, other types of emboli, such as bone, air, fat, amniotic fluid, tumor cells, or a foreign body
- Right heart thrombus
- Upper extremity thrombosis
- Valvular heart disease

RISK FACTORS

- Various disorders and treatments (see *Who's at risk for pulmonary embolism?*)

PATHOPHYSIOLOGY

- Thrombus formation results from vascular wall damage, venous stasis, or blood hypercoagulability.
- Trauma, clot dissolution, sudden muscle spasm, intravascular pressure changes, or peripheral blood flow changes can cause the thrombus to loosen or fragmentize.
- The thrombus (now an embolus) floats to the heart's right side and enters the lung through the pulmonary artery. There, the embolus may dissolve, continue to fragmentize, or grow.
- If the embolus enlarges, it may occlude most or all of the pulmonary vessels and prevent perfusion to organs or cause death. (See *Disorders affecting management of pulmonary embolism*, page 367.)

CARDIOVASCULAR SYSTEM

- Initially, hypoxia leads to tachycardia and hypertension.
- Right ventricular failure occurs due to the obstruction in outflow. This, in turn, reduces the output from the left ventricle, ultimately leading to hypotension.

RESPIRATORY SYSTEM

- Occlusion of the pulmonary artery limits alveolar surfactant production, leading to alveolar collapse and subsequent atelectasis.
- Inadequate tissue oxygenation leads to an initial increase in the respiratory rate, which may progress to respiratory distress.
- If the pulmonary artery becomes completely occluded, respiratory failure may result. If the embolus enlarges and obstructs most or all pulmonary vessels, death may result.

Who's at risk for pulmonary embolism?

Many disorders and treatments heighten the risk of pulmonary embolism. At particular risk are surgical patients. The anesthetic used during surgery can injure lung vessels, and surgery or prolonged bed rest can promote venous stasis, which compounds the risk.

PREDISPOSING DISORDERS

- Cardiac arrhythmia (especially atrial fibrillation)
- Lung disorders, especially chronic types
- Cardiac disorders
- Infection
- Diabetes mellitus
- History of thromboembolism, thrombophlebitis, or vascular insufficiency
- Sickle cell disease
- Autoimmune hemolytic anemia
- Polycythemia

- Osteomyelitis
- Long-bone fracture
- Manipulation or disconnection of central lines

VENOUS STASIS

- Prolonged bed rest or immobilization
- Obesity
- Older than age 40
- Burns
- Recent childbirth
- Orthopedic casts

VENOUS INJURY

- Surgery, particularly of the legs, pelvis, abdomen, or thorax
- Leg or pelvic fractures or injuries
- I.V. drug abuse
- I.V. therapy

INCREASED BLOOD COAGULABILITY

- Cancer
- Use of high-estrogen hormonal contraceptives

HISTORY

◆ Predisposing risk factor
◆ Shortness of breath for no apparent reason
◆ Pleuritic pain or angina

PHYSICAL FINDINGS

◆ Tachycardia
◆ Low-grade fever
◆ Weak, rapid pulse
◆ Hypotension
◆ Productive cough, possibly with blood-tinged sputum
◆ Warmth, tenderness, and edema of the lower leg
◆ Restlessness
◆ Transient pleural friction rub
◆ Crackles
◆ S_3 and S_4 with increased intensity of the pulmonic component of S_2
◆ With a large embolus, cyanosis, syncope, and distended neck veins

DIAGNOSTIC TEST RESULTS

◆ Arterial blood gas (ABG) values show hypoxemia.
◆ D-dimer level is elevated.
◆ Lung ventilation-perfusion scan shows a ventilation-perfusion mismatch.
◆ Pulmonary angiography shows a pulmonary vessel filling defect or an abrupt vessel ending and reveals the location and extent of pulmonary embolism.
◆ Chest X-rays may show a small infiltrate or effusion.
◆ Spiral chest computed tomography scan may show central pulmonary emboli.
◆ Electrocardiography may reveal right axis deviation and right bundle-branch block; it also may show atrial fibrillation.

GENERAL

◆ Maintenance of adequate cardiovascular and pulmonary function
◆ Mechanical ventilation, if indicated

DIET

◆ Possible fluid restriction

ACTIVITY

◆ Bed rest during the acute phase

MEDICATIONS

◆ Oxygen therapy
◆ Thrombolytics
◆ Anticoagulants
◆ Corticosteroids (controversial)
◆ Diuretics
◆ Antiarrhythmics
◆ Vasopressors (for hypotension)
◆ Antibiotics (for septic embolus)

SURGERY

◆ Vena caval interruption
◆ Vena caval filter placement
◆ Pulmonary embolectomy

NURSING DIAGNOSES

◆ Acute pain
◆ Anxiety
◆ Decreased cardiac output
◆ Fear
◆ Imbalanced nutrition: Less than body requirements
◆ Impaired gas exchange
◆ Ineffective airway clearance
◆ Ineffective coping
◆ Ineffective tissue perfusion: Cardiopulmonary
◆ Risk for injury

EXPECTED OUTCOMES

The patient will:
◆ verbalize feelings of increased comfort and decreased pain
◆ identify strategies to reduce anxiety
◆ maintain adequate cardiac output
◆ discuss fears and concerns
◆ consume required daily caloric intake
◆ maintain adequate ventilation and oxygenation
◆ maintain a patent airway
◆ use support systems to assist with coping
◆ maintain adequate cardiopulmonary perfusion
◆ remain free from injury.

NURSING INTERVENTIONS

◆ Give prescribed drugs.
◆ Avoid I.M. injections.
◆ Encourage active and passive range-of-motion exercises, unless contraindicated.
◆ Avoid massage of the lower legs.
◆ Apply antiembolism stockings.
◆ Provide adequate nutrition.
◆ Assist with ambulation as soon as the patient is stable.
◆ Encourage use of incentive spirometry.
◆ Monitor vital signs, intake and output, pulse oximetry, and ABG values.
◆ Assess respiratory status.
◆ Observe for signs of deep vein thrombosis.

(continued)

- Assess for complications, such as abnormal bleeding.
- Monitor coagulation study results.

PATIENT TEACHING

Be sure to cover:
- disorder, diagnostic testing, and treatment
- medication administration, dosage, and possible adverse effects
- ways to prevent deep vein thrombosis and pulmonary embolism
- signs and symptoms of abnormal bleeding
- prevention of abnormal bleeding
- how to monitor anticoagulant effects
- dietary sources of vitamin K
- when to notify the practitioner.

RESOURCES
Organizations
American Lung Association: *www.lungusa.org*
National Heart, Lung, and Blood Institute: *www.nhlbi.nih.gov*

Selected references
Bonde, P., and Graham, A. "Surgical Management of Pulmonary Embolism," *Journal of Thoracic and Cardiovascular Surgery* 131(2):503-504, February 2006.

Kucher, N., et al. "Massive Pulmonary Embolism," *Circulation* 113(4):577-82, January 2006.

Marchigiano, G., et al. "New Technology Applications: Thrombolysis of Acute Deep Vein Thrombosis," *Critical Care Nursing Quarterly* 29(4):312-23, October-December 2006.

Morrison, R. "Venous Thromboembolism: Scope of the Problem and the Nurse's Role in Risk Assessment and Prevention," *Journal of Vascular Nursing* 24(3):82-90, September 2006.

Roy, P.M., et al. "Appropriateness of Diagnostic Management and Outcomes of Suspected Pulmonary Embolism," *Annals of Internal Medicine* 144(3):157-64, February 2006.

Disorders affecting management of pulmonary embolism

This chart highlights disorders that affect the management of pulmonary embolism.

DISORDER	SIGNS AND SYMPTOMS	DIAGNOSTIC TEST RESULTS	TREATMENT AND CARE
Deep vein thrombophlebitis (coexisting)	◆ Homan's sign elicited ◆ Severe pain in affected leg ◆ Fever, chills ◆ Malaise ◆ Swelling and cyanosis of the affected leg ◆ Affected area possibly warm to touch	◆ Doppler ultrasonography identifies reduced blood flow to the area of the thrombus and any obstruction to venous blood flow. ◆ Plethysmography shows decreased circulation distal to the affected area. ◆ Phlebography (also called *venography*), which usually confirms diagnosis, shows filling defects and diverted blood flow.	◆ Administer anticoagulants and monitor for adverse effects, such as bleeding, dark tarry stools, and coffee ground vomitus. ◆ Assess pulses, skin color, and temperature of the affected leg. ◆ Measure and record the circumference of the affected leg. ◆ Perform range-of-motion exercises with the unaffected leg and turn the patient every 2 hours. ◆ Apply warm soaks to improve circulation and relieve pain and inflammation. ◆ Assess for signs of pulmonary emboli.
Heart failure (complication)	*Left-sided heart failure* ◆ Dyspnea ◆ Orthopnea ◆ Paroxysmal nocturnal dyspnea ◆ Fatigue ◆ Nonproductive cough ◆ Crackles ◆ Hemoptysis ◆ Tachycardia ◆ S_3, S_4 ◆ Cool, pale skin ◆ Restlessness and confusion *Right-sided heart failure* ◆ Jugular vein distention ◆ Positive hepatojugular reflex ◆ Right upper quadrant pain ◆ Anorexia, nausea ◆ Nocturia ◆ Weight gain, edema ◆ Ascites or anasarca	◆ Chest X-ray shows increased pulmonary vascular markings, interstitial edema, or pleural effusions and cardiomegaly. ◆ Electrocardiography may reveal hypertrophy, ischemic changes or infarction, tachycardia, and extrasystoles. ◆ Liver function test may be abnormal; blood urea nitrogen (BUN) and creatinine levels may be elevated. ◆ Prothrombin time may be prolonged. ◆ B-type natriuretic peptide (BNP) immunoassay is elevated. ◆ Echocardiography may reveal left ventricular hypertrophy, dilation, and abnormal contractility. ◆ Pulmonary artery pressure, pulmonary artery wedge pressure, and left ventricular end-diastolic pressure are elevated in the presence of left-sided heart failure; right atrial or central venous pressure is elevated in right-sided heart failure. ◆ Radionuclide ventriculography may reveal ejection fraction less than 40% in diastolic dysfunction.	◆ Place the patient in Fowler's position and give supplemental oxygen. ◆ Weigh the patient daily, and check for peripheral edema. ◆ Monitor intake and output, vital signs, and mental status. ◆ Auscultate for S_3 and S_4 and adventitious lung sounds, such as crackles or rhonchi. ◆ Monitor BUN, creatinine, and serum potassium, sodium, chloride, and magnesium. ◆ Institute continuous cardiac monitoring to identify and treat arrhythmias promptly. ◆ Administer angiotensin-converting enzyme inhibitors, digoxin, diuretics, beta-adrenergic blockers, human BNPs, nitrates, and morphine. ◆ Prepare the patient for possible coronary artery bypass surgery or angioplasty, as appropriate. ◆ Encourage lifestyle modifications to reduce symptoms.
Respiratory failure or acute respiratory distress (complication)	◆ Increased respiratory rate, decreased rate, or normal rate (depending on the cause) ◆ Cyanosis ◆ Crackles, rhonchi, wheezing, and diminished breath sounds ◆ Restlessness, confusion, loss of concentration ◆ Irritability ◆ Coma ◆ Tachycardia ◆ Elevated blood pressure ◆ Arrhythmias	◆ Arterial blood gas (ABG) analysis reveals deteriorating values and a pH below 7.35. ◆ Chest X-rays identify characteristic pulmonary diseases or conditions. ◆ Electrocardiography can demonstrate ventricular arrhythmias or right ventricular hypertrophy. ◆ Pulse oximetry reveals decreased arterial oxygen saturation. ◆ White blood cell count detects underlying infection.	◆ Administer oxygen therapy and monitor for its effectiveness. ◆ Maintain a patent airway, Prepare for endotracheal intubation, if indicated. ◆ In the intubated patient, suction, as needed, after hyperoxygenation. Observe for changes in quantity, consistency, and color of sputum. Provide humidification to liquefy secretions. ◆ Observe closely for respiratory arrest. Auscultate for chest sounds. ◆ Monitor ABG levels and report changes immediately. ◆ Monitor serum electrolyte levels and correct imbalances. ◆ Monitor fluid balance. ◆ Check the cardiac monitor for arrhythmias.

Pulmonary hypertension LIFE-THREATENING DISORDER

OVERVIEW

- Condition in which there's increased pressure in the pulmonary artery
- Occurs in a primary form, which is most common in women ages 20 to 40 (rare); and in secondary form
- In both forms, resting systolic pulmonary artery pressure (PAP) above 30 mm Hg and mean PAP above 20 mm Hg
- More prevalent in people with collagen disease

CAUSES
Primary pulmonary hypertension
- Exact cause unknown
- Associated with portal hypertension
- Possible altered autoimmune mechanisms
- Possible hereditary factors

Secondary pulmonary hypertension
- Lung disease

RISK FACTORS
Secondary pulmonary hypertension
- Chronic obstructive pulmonary disease
- Congenital cardiac defects
- Diffuse interstitial pneumonia
- Hypoventilation syndromes
- Kyphoscoliosis
- Left atrial myxoma
- Malignant metastasis
- Mitral stenosis
- Obesity
- Pulmonary embolism
- Sarcoidosis
- Scleroderma
- Sleep apnea
- Use of some diet drugs
- Vasculitis

PATHOPHYSIOLOGY

- In primary pulmonary hypertension, the intimal lining of the pulmonary arteries thickens for no apparent reason. This narrows the artery and impairs distensibility, increasing vascular resistance. (See *Disorders affecting management of pulmonary hypertension,* pages 370 and 371.)
- Secondary pulmonary hypertension occurs from hypoxemia caused by conditions involving alveolar hypoventilation, vascular obstruction, or left-to-right shunting.

RESPIRATORY SYSTEM
- Changes to the pulmonary artery endothelium as a result of chronic hypoxia can cause ventilation-perfusion mismatch.
- Increased vascular resistance impairs gas exchange and can result in chronic hypoxia.

CARDIOVASCULAR SYSTEM
- Unresolved pulmonary hypertension causes hypertrophy in the medial smooth muscle layer of the arterioles. The larger arteries stiffen, and hypertension progresses.
- Pulmonary pressures begin to equal systemic blood pressure, causing right ventricular hypertrophy and, eventually, cor pulmonale.
- Pulmonary artery distention and right ventricular ischemia causes mitral stenosis and results in anginal pain.
- Right ventricular failure may occur and result in systemic venous hypertension.

ASSESSMENT

HISTORY
- Shortness of breath upon exertion
- Weakness, fatigue
- Pain during breathing
- Near-syncope

PHYSICAL FINDINGS
- Ascites
- Jugular vein distention
- Peripheral edema
- Restlessness and agitation
- Mental status changes
- Decreased diaphragmatic excursion
- Apical impulse displaced beyond mid-clavicular line
- Right ventricular lift
- Reduced carotid pulse
- Hepatomegaly
- Tachycardia
- Systolic ejection murmur
- Widely split S_2
- S_3 and S_4
- Hypotension
- Decreased breath sounds
- Tubular breath sounds

DIAGNOSTIC TEST RESULTS
- Arterial blood gas (ABG) values show hypoxemia.
- Ventilation-perfusion lung scan may show a ventilation-perfusion mismatch.
- Pulmonary angiography may reveal filling defects in the pulmonary vasculature.
- Electrocardiography may reveal right-axis deviation.
- Pulmonary artery catheterization shows increased PAP, with systolic pressure above 30 mm Hg; increased pulmonary artery wedge pressure; decreased cardiac output; and decreased cardiac index.
- Pulmonary function tests may show decreased flow rates and increased residual volume or reduced total lung capacity.
- Echocardiography may show valvular heart disease or atrial myxoma.
- Lung biopsy may show tumor cells.

TREATMENT

GENERAL
◆ Based on underlying disease
◆ Symptom relief
◆ Smoking cessation

DIET
◆ Low-sodium
◆ Fluid restriction (with right-sided heart failure)

ACTIVITY
◆ Bed rest during acute phase

MEDICATIONS
◆ Oxygen therapy
◆ Cardiac glycosides
◆ Diuretics
◆ Vasodilators
◆ Calcium channel blockers
◆ Bronchodilators
◆ Beta-adrenergic blockers
◆ Epoprostenol
◆ Endothelial receptor antagonists
◆ Phosphodiesterase (type 5) enzyme inhibitors
◆ Anticoagulants (if cause is chronic pulmonary emboli)

SURGERY
◆ Heart-lung transplantation, if indicated

NURSING CONSIDERATIONS

NURSING DIAGNOSES
◆ Activity intolerance
◆ Anxiety
◆ Decreased cardiac output
◆ Fatigue
◆ Fear
◆ Impaired gas exchange
◆ Ineffective coping

EXPECTED OUTCOMES
The patient will:
◆ demonstrate skill in conserving energy while carrying out daily activities to tolerance level
◆ verbalize strategies to reduce anxiety
◆ maintain adequate cardiac output
◆ express feelings of energy and decreased fatigue
◆ discuss fears and concerns
◆ maintain adequate ventilation and oxygenation
◆ use support systems to assist with coping.

NURSING INTERVENTIONS
◆ Give prescribed drugs and oxygen.
◆ Implement comfort measures.
◆ Provide adequate rest periods.
◆ Offer emotional support.
◆ Monitor vital signs, intake and output, and daily weight.
◆ Assess respiratory status and observe for signs and symptoms of right-sided heart failure.
◆ Monitor cardiac rhythm, ABG values, and hemodynamic values.

PATIENT TEACHING

Be sure to cover:
◆ disorder, diagnostic testing, and treatment
◆ medication administration, dosage, and possible adverse effects
◆ dietary restrictions
◆ frequent rest periods
◆ signs and symptoms of right-sided heart failure
◆ when to notify the practitioner
◆ contact information for a smoking-cessation program, if indicated.

RESOURCES
Organizations
American Lung Association:
www.lungusa.org
American Thoracic Society:
www.thoracic.org
National Heart, Lung, and Blood Institute: *www.nhlbi.nih.gov*

Selected references
Hoeper, M., and Welte, T. "Systemic Inflammation, COPD, and Pulmonary Hypertension," *Chest* 131(2):634-35, February 2007.
Thistlethwaite, P.A., et al. "Outcomes of Pulmonary Endarterectomy for Treatment of Extreme Thromboembolic Pulmonary Hypertension," *Journal of Thoracic and Cardiovascular Surgery* 131(2):307-13, February 2006.
Verklan, M. "Persistent Pulmonary Hypertension of the Newborn: Not a Honeymoon Anymore," *Journal of Perinatal and Neonatal Nursing* 20(1):108-12, January-March 2006.

(continued)

Disorders affecting management of pulmonary hypertension

This chart highlights disorders that affect the management of pulmonary hypertension.

DISORDER	SIGNS AND SYMPTOMS	DIAGNOSTIC TEST RESULTS	TREATMENT AND CARE
Chronic obstructive pulmonary disease (coexisting)	◆ Dyspnea ◆ Abdominal discomfort ◆ Cyanosis	◆ Pulmonary function tests show increased residual volume lung capacity and decreased vital capacity. ◆ Chest X-ray shows hyperinflation. ◆ Arterial blood gas analysis shows decreased partial pressure of arterial oxygen (Pao_2) and normal or increased partial pressure of arterial ($Paco_2$) (emphysema). ◆ Electrocardiography may show atrial arrhythmias and peaked P waves in leads II, III, and AV_F (chronic bronchitis); tall symmetrical P waves in leads II, III, and AV_F; and vertical QRS axis (emphysema).	◆ Encourage lifestyle changes to adjust to oxygen demands. ◆ Perform chest physiotherapy. ◆ Administer bronchodilators. ◆ Encourage daily activity to maximize lung capacity and promote well-being. ◆ Provide frequent rest periods. ◆ Provide a high-calorie, protein-rich diet.
Heart failure (complication)	*Left-sided heart failure* ◆ Dyspnea ◆ Orthopnea ◆ Paroxysmal nocturnal dyspnea ◆ Fatigue ◆ Nonproductive cough ◆ Crackles ◆ Hemoptysis ◆ Tachycardia ◆ S_3, S_4 ◆ Cool, pale skin ◆ Restlessness and confusion *Right-sided heart failure* ◆ Jugular vein distention ◆ Positive hepatojugular reflex ◆ Right upper quadrant pain ◆ Anorexia, nausea ◆ Weight gain, edema ◆ Ascites or anasarca ◆ Body mass index greater than 30	◆ Chest X-ray shows increased pulmonary vascular markings, interstitial edema, or pleural effusions and cardiomegaly. ◆ B-type natriuretic peptide (BNP) immunoassay is elevated. ◆ Electrocardiography may reveal hypertrophy, ischemic changes or infarction, tachycardia, and extrasystoles. ◆ Liver function test may be abnormal; blood urea nitrogen (BUN) and creatinine levels may be elevated. ◆ Prothrombin time may be prolonged. ◆ Echocardiography may reveal left ventricular hypertrophy, dilation, and abnormal contractility. ◆ Pulmonary artery pressure, pulmonary artery wedge pressure, and left ventricular end pressure are elevated in left-sided heart failure; right atrial or central venous pressure is elevated in right-sided heart failure. ◆ Radionuclide ventriculography may reveal ejection fraction less than 40% in diastolic dysfunction.	◆ Place the patient in Fowler's position and provide supplemental oxygen. ◆ Weigh the patient daily, and check for peripheral edema. ◆ Monitor intake and output, vital signs, and mental status. ◆ Auscultate for S_3 and S_4 and adventitious lung sounds, such as crackles or rhonchi. ◆ Monitor BUN, creatinine, BNP, serum electrolytes, and magnesium levels. ◆ Monitor cardiac rhythm. ◆ Administer nesiritide (Natrecor), diuretics, nitrates, angiotensin-converting enzyme (ACE) inhibitors, digoxin, beta-adrenergic blockers, and morphine, as ordered.

Disorders affecting management of pulmonary hypertension *(continued)*

DISORDER	SIGNS AND SYMPTOMS	DIAGNOSTIC TEST RESULTS	TREATMENT AND CARE
Obstructive sleep apnea-hypopnea syndrome (complication)	◆ Loud snoring ◆ Witnessed periods of apnea while sleeping ◆ Restless sleep ◆ Morning headache ◆ Excessive daytime sleepiness ◆ Neck circumference greater than 17″ (43 cm) in men and 15″ (37 cm) in women ◆ Enlarged tonsils	◆ Polysomnography (sleep study) analyzes breathing patterns during sleep and identifies type of apnea or hypopnea. ◆ Pulse oximetry readings decrease by 4% during apneic periods while sleeping. ◆ Apnea-hypopnea index (total number of apneas and hypopneas divided by total sleep time) identifies severity of sleep apnea. ◆ Multiple sleep latency test evaluates degree of excessive daytime sleepiness.	◆ Apply nasal continuous positive airway pressure device before sleep at night. ◆ Monitor for periods of apnea and pulse oximetry readings. ◆ Monitor cardiac rhythm while sleeping. ◆ Note episodes of daytime sleepiness. ◆ Encourage lifestyle modification or changes, such as weight loss and exercise programs. ◆ Administer tricyclic antidepressants and non-amphetamine central nervous system stimulants, as ordered, and evaluate effect.

Radiation exposure

OVERVIEW

- Exposure to excessive radiation that causes tissue damage
- Damage dependent on amount of body area exposed, length of exposure, dosage absorbed, distance from the source, and presence of protective shielding
- May result from cancer radiotherapy, working in a radiation facility, or other exposure to radioactive materials
- Can be acute or chronic
- Incidence unknown

CAUSES

- Exposure to radiation through inhalation, ingestion, or direct contact

RISK FACTORS

- Cancer treatment
- Employment in a radiation facility

PATHOPHYSIOLOGY

- Ionization occurs in the molecules of living cells.
- Electrons are removed from atoms. Charged atoms or ions form and react with other atoms to cause cell damage.
- Rapidly dividing cells are the most susceptible to radiation damage. Highly differentiated cells are more resistant to radiation.

CARDIOVASCULAR SYSTEM

- Exposure to more than 40 grays (Gy), which is equivalent to 4,000 rad, may result in pericarditis, myocardial ischemia, and (later) fibrous scars.
- Conduction defects may occur.

GI SYSTEM

- Exposure to more than 5 to 12 Gy causes intestinal mucosal stem cell destruction.
- New stem cell growth is inhibited, and GI tract denudation occurs.

HEMATOLOGIC SYSTEM

- Exposure to 2 to 5 Gy of radiation causes apoptosis, resulting in lymphocyte destruction.
- Precursor cells are destroyed in the bone marrow, preventing new leukocyte and platelet production. (See *Disorders affecting management of radiation exposure,* page 375.)

INTEGUMENTARY SYSTEM

- Localized radiation exposure causes damage to cutaneous cells and results in erythema, blistering, and ulceration.

NEUROLOGIC SYSTEM

- Exposure to more than 30 Gy produces vascular damage, resulting in cerebral edema.
- Neurologic and cardiovascular collapse cause death.

ASSESSMENT

HISTORY

Acute hematologic radiation toxicity

- Bleeding from the skin, genitourinary tract, and GI tract due to thrombocytopenia (initial response)
- Pancytopenia with no apparent signs and symptoms (latent period)
- Nosebleeds, hemorrhage, and increased susceptibility to infection (after latent period)

Cardiovascular radiation toxicity

- Chest pain
- Irregular heartbeat

Cerebral radiation toxicity

- Nausea, vomiting, and diarrhea
- Lethargy

GI radiation toxicity

- Intractable nausea, vomiting, and diarrhea

PHYSICAL FINDINGS

Generalized radiation exposure

- Signs of hypothyroidism
- Cataracts
- Skin dryness, erythema, atrophy, and malignant lesions
- Alopecia
- Brittle nails

Acute hematologic radiation toxicity

- Petechiae
- Pallor
- Weakness
- Oropharyngeal abscesses

Cardiovascular radiation toxicity

- Cardiac arrhythmia
- Hypotension
- Signs of cardiogenic shock

Cerebral radiation toxicity

- Tremors
- Seizures
- Confusion
- Coma and death

GI radiation toxicity
◆ Mouth and throat ulcers and infection
◆ Circulatory collapse and death

DIAGNOSTIC TEST RESULTS
◆ White blood cell, platelet, and lymphocyte counts are decreased.
◆ Serum potassium and chloride levels are decreased.
◆ X-rays may reveal bone necrosis.
◆ Bone marrow studies may show blood dyscrasia.
◆ Geiger counter helps determine if radioactive material was ingested or inhaled and evaluates the amount of radiation in open wounds.
◆ Electrocardiography reveals cardiac arrhythmia or cardiac damage.

TREATMENT

GENERAL
◆ Management of life-threatening injuries
◆ Symptomatic and supportive treatment
◆ Based on the type and extent of radiation injury

DIET
◆ High-protein, high-calorie

ACTIVITY
◆ As tolerated

MEDICATIONS
◆ Chelating agents
◆ Potassium iodide
◆ Aluminum phosphate gel
◆ Barium sulfate

NURSING CONSIDERATIONS

NURSING DIAGNOSES
◆ Anxiety
◆ Decreased intracranial adaptive capacity
◆ Deficient fluid volume
◆ Imbalanced nutrition: Less than body requirements
◆ Impaired oral mucous membrane
◆ Impaired skin integrity
◆ Risk for infection

EXPECTED OUTCOMES
The patient will:
◆ verbalize feelings of anxiety and fear
◆ remain oriented to person, place, and time
◆ maintain normal fluid volume
◆ maintain an acceptable weight
◆ remain free from complications related to trauma to oral mucous membranes
◆ experience skin healing without complications
◆ remain free from signs and symptoms of infection.

NURSING INTERVENTIONS
◆ Implement appropriate respiratory and cardiac support measures.
◆ Give prescribed I.V. fluids and electrolytes.
◆ For skin contamination, wash the patient's body thoroughly with mild soap and water.
◆ Debride and irrigate open wounds.
◆ For ingested radioactive material, perform gastric lavage and whole-bowel irrigation, and administer activated charcoal.
◆ Dispose of contaminated clothing properly.
◆ Dispose of contaminated excrement and body fluids according to facility policy.
◆ Use strict sterile technique.
◆ Monitor intake and output, fluid and electrolyte balance, and vital signs.
◆ Observe for signs and symptoms of hemorrhage.
◆ Monitor nutritional status.

(continued)

Be sure to cover:
- injury, diagnostic testing, and treatment
- effects of radiation exposure
- how to prevent a recurrence
- skin and wound care
- importance of follow-up care
- contact information for resource and support services or genetic counseling resources.

RESOURCES
Organizations
Environmental Protection Agency: *www.epa.gov/radiation*
National Center for Injury Prevention and Control: *www.cdc.gov/ncipc*
National Institutes of Health: *www.nih.gov*
United States Nuclear Regulatory Commission—Radiation Exposure Information and Reporting System (REIRS) for Radiation Workers: *www.reirs.com*

Selected references
Donaldson, L. "Reducing Harm from Radiotherapy," *British Medical Journal* 334(7588):272, February 2007.
McQuestion, M. "Evidence-based Skin Care Management in Radiation Therapy," *Seminars in Oncology Nursing* 22(3):163-73, August 2006.
Thieden, E., et al. "Ultraviolet Radiation Exposure Pattern in Winter Compared with Summer Based on Time-stamped Personal Dosimeter Readings," *British Journal of Dermatology* 154(1):133-38, January 2006.

Disorders affecting management of radiation exposure

This chart highlights disorders that affect the management of radiation exposure.

DISORDER	SIGNS AND SYMPTOMS	DIAGNOSTIC TEST RESULTS	TREATMENT AND CARE
Anemia (complication)	◆ Possibly asymptomatic early; signs and symptoms developing as anemia becomes more severe ◆ Dyspnea on exertion ◆ Fatigue ◆ Listlessness, inability to concentrate ◆ Pallor, irritability ◆ Tachycardia ◆ Brittle, thinning nails	◆ Total iron binding capacity is elevated and serum iron levels are decreased. ◆ Bone marrow aspiration reveals reduced iron stores and reduced production of red blood cell (RBC) precursors. ◆ Complete blood count (CBC) reveals decreased hemoglobin and hematocrit and low mean corpuscular hemoglobin. ◆ RBC indices reveal decreased cells that are microcytic and hypochromic.	◆ Assess for decreased perfusion to vital organs, including heart and lungs; monitor for dyspnea, chest pain, and dizziness. ◆ Administer oxygen therapy to prevent hypoxemia. ◆ Monitor vital signs for changes. ◆ Administer iron replacement therapy. ◆ Administer blood products if anemia is severe. ◆ Allow for frequent rest periods. ◆ Monitor laboratory studies.
Hemorrhage (complication)	◆ Evidence of bleeding ◆ Fatigue, weakness ◆ Altered level of consciousness ◆ Tachycardia ◆ Hypotension	◆ CBC shows decreased hematocrit and hemoglobin levels. ◆ Computed tomography scan or magnetic resonance imaging shows areas of bleeding. ◆ Endoscopy identifies GI sites of bleeding.	◆ Administer blood products, as ordered, and monitor for reaction. ◆ Monitor CBC for changes. ◆ Note sites of bleeding and amount. ◆ Monitor vital signs and pulse oximetry. ◆ Administer hematopoietic growth factor, as ordered.
Leukemia (complication)	◆ Sudden onset of high fever ◆ Abnormal bleeding ◆ Fatigue and weakness ◆ Tachycardia, palpitations ◆ Pallor ◆ Lymph node enlargement ◆ Liver or spleen enlargement	◆ CBC shows thrombocytopenia and neutropenia, and a white blood cell (WBC) differential shows the cell type. ◆ Bone marrow aspiration shows a proliferation of immature WBCs.	◆ Infuse blood products, as ordered, and monitor for reaction. ◆ Monitor CBC for changes. ◆ Provide frequent rest periods. ◆ Administer prescribed medications. ◆ Encourage verbalization of feelings and provide comfort.

Respiratory acidosis LIFE-THREATENING DISORDER

OVERVIEW

- Acid-base disturbance that's characterized by reduced alveolar ventilation
- Impaired carbon dioxide clearance leading to hypercapnia (partial pressure of arterial carbon dioxide [$Paco_2$] greater than 45 mm Hg) and acidosis (pH less than 7.35)
- May be acute (due to a sudden failure in ventilation) or chronic (due to long-term pulmonary disease)

CAUSES

- Neuromuscular dysfunction
- Depression of the respiratory center in the brain
- Airway obstruction

RISK FACTORS

- Use of certain drugs (opioids, general anesthetics, hypnotics, and sedatives)
- Severe alcohol intake
- Trauma
- Cardiac arrest
- Sleep apnea
- Ventilation therapy
- Neuromuscular diseases
- Lung disease or illness

PATHOPHYSIOLOGY

- A compromise in any of the three essential parts of breathing—ventilation, perfusion, and diffusion—may result in respiratory acidosis. (See *What happens in respiratory acidosis.*)
- Although it initially affects the respiratory system, respiratory acidosis can affect other body systems, placing the patient at risk for numerous complications. (*Disorders affecting management of respiratory acidosis,* pages 378 and 379.)

CARDIOVASCULAR SYSTEM

- Cardiovascular deterioration occurs when blood pH is less than 7.15.
- The movement of hydrogen ions into cells overwhelms compensatory mechanisms.
- Changes in electrolyte concentrations affect cardiac contractility.
- Anaerobic metabolism produces lactic acid, which depresses the myocardium, leading to shock and cardiac arrest.

NEUROLOGIC SYSTEM

- Carbon dioxide and hydrogen ions dilate cerebral blood vessels and increase blood flow to the brain, causing cerebral edema and depressing central nervous system (CNS) activity.
- Profound CNS deterioration occurs as a result of a dangerously low blood pH (less than 7.15).

RENAL SYSTEM

- As respiratory mechanisms fail, rising $Paco_2$ stimulates the kidneys to retain bicarbonate and sodium ions and excrete hydrogen ions, leading to greater availability of sodium bicarbonate ($NaHCO_3^-$) to buffer free hydrogen ions.

RESPIRATORY SYSTEM

- Decreased pulmonary ventilation leads to increased $Paco_2$, and the carbon dioxide level rises in all tissues (including the medulla) and in all fluids (including cerebrospinal fluid).
- Retained carbon dioxide combines with water to form carbonic acid (H_2CO_3), which dissociates to release free hydrogen and bicarbonate (HCO_3^-) ions.
- Increased $Paco_2$ and free hydrogen ions stimulate the medulla to increase respiratory drive and expel carbon dioxide.
- As pH falls, 2,3-diphosphoglycerate (2,3-DPG) accumulates in red blood cells, where it alters hemoglobin and releases oxygen. This activity reduces hemoglobin, which is strongly alkaline; picks up hydrogen ions and carbon dioxide; and removes them from the serum.

ASSESSMENT

HISTORY

- Clinical features dependent on the underlying disease, the presence of hypoxemia, and the cause, severity, and duration of respiratory acidosis

PHYSICAL FINDINGS

- Headache
- Altered level of consciousness
- Dyspnea
- Diaphoresis
- Nausea and vomiting
- Warm, flushed skin
- Papilledema
- Depressed reflexes
- Fine or flapping tremor (asterixis)
- Tachycardia
- Hypertension
- Atrial and ventricular arrhythmias
- Hypotension with vasodilation
- Rapid, shallow respirations
- Diminished or absent breath sounds over the affected area
- Cyanosis (late sign)

DIAGNOSTIC TEST RESULTS

- Arterial blood gas (ABG) analysis shows $Paco_2$ greater than 45 mm Hg, pH less than 7.35, and normal HCO_3^- in the acute stage (confirms the diagnosis).

- Chest X-ray commonly shows causes, such as heart failure, pneumonia, chronic obstructive pulmonary disease (COPD), and pneumothorax.
- Serum potassium level is usually greater than 5 mEq/L.
- Serum chloride level is low.

- Urine pH is acidic as the kidneys excrete hydrogen ions to return blood pH to normal.
- Drug screening may confirm suspected drug overdose.

TREATMENT

GENERAL
- Airway and ventilation support
- Treatment of underlying cause
- Bronchoscopy

UP CLOSE

What happens in respiratory acidosis

This series of illustrations shows how respiratory acidosis develops at the cellular level.

When pulmonary ventilation decreases, retained carbon dioxide (CO_2) combines with water (H_2O) to form carbonic acid (H_2CO_3) in larger-than-normal amounts. The carbonic acid dissociates to release free hydrogen ions (H^+) and bicarbonate ions (HCO_3^-). The excessive carbonic acid causes a drop in pH. Look for a partial pressure of arterial carbon dioxide ($Paco_2$) level above 45 mm Hg and a pH level below 7.35.

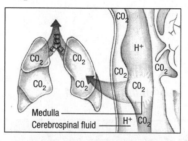

As the pH level falls, 2,3-diphosphoglycerate (2,3-DPG) increases in the red blood cells and causes a change in hemoglobin (Hb) that makes Hb release oxygen (O_2). The altered Hb, now strongly alkaline, picks up H^+ and CO_2, thus eliminating some of the free H^+ and excess CO_2. Look for decreased arterial oxygen saturation.

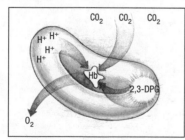

Whenever $Paco_2$ increases, CO_2 builds up in all tissues and fluids, including cerebrospinal fluid and the respiratory center in the medulla.

The CO_2 reacts with water to form carbonic acid, which then breaks into free H^+ and bicarbonate ions. The increased amount of CO_2 and free H^+ stimulate the respiratory center to increase the respiratory rate. An increased respiratory rate expels more CO_2 and helps to reduce the CO_2 level in blood and tissues. Look for rapid, shallow respirations and a decreasing $Paco_2$.

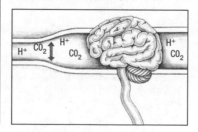

Medulla
Cerebrospinal fluid

Eventually, CO_2 and H^+ cause cerebral blood vessels to dilate, which increases blood flow to the brain. That increased flow can cause cerebral edema and depress central nervous system activity. Look for headache, confusion, lethargy, nausea, and vomiting.

As respiratory mechanisms fail, the increasing $Paco_2$ stimulates the kidneys to conserve bicarbonate and sodium ions and to excrete H^+,

some in the form of ammonium (NH_4). The additional HCO_3^- and sodium combine to form extra sodium bicarbonate ($NaHCO_3^-$), which is then able to buffer more free H^+. Look for increased acid content in the urine, increased serum pH and HCO_3^- levels, and shallow, depressed respirations.

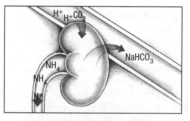

As the concentration of H^+ overwhelms the body's compensatory mechanisms, the H^+ moves into the cells, and potassium (K) ions move out. A simultaneous lack of oxygen causes an increase in the anaerobic production of lactic acid, which further skews the acid-base balance and critically depresses neurologic and cardiac functions. Look for hyperkalemia, arrhythmias, increased $Paco_2$, decreased partial pressure of arterial oxygen, decreased pH, and decreased level of consciousness.

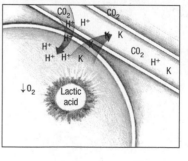

(continued)

DIET
◆ Nothing by mouth until acidosis resolves

ACTIVITY
◆ Bed rest until stable

MEDICATIONS
◆ Oxygen
◆ Antibiotics
◆ Bronchodilators
◆ Sodium bicarbonate

NURSING CONSIDERATIONS

NURSING DIAGNOSES
◆ Disturbed thought processes
◆ Impaired gas exchange
◆ Ineffective airway clearance
◆ Ineffective breathing pattern

EXPECTED OUTCOMES
The patient will:
◆ communicate effectively with appropriate thought process
◆ maintain adequate ventilation and oxygenation
◆ maintain a patent airway
◆ exhibit adequate breathing patterns.

NURSING INTERVENTIONS
◆ Assess respiratory and neurologic status; provide respiratory support, as indicated.
◆ Provide treatment for underlying cause, as indicated.
◆ Administer ordered medications and note response.
◆ Monitor vital signs, pulse oximetry, cardiac rhythm, and intake and output.
◆ Monitor results of ABG analysis and electrolyte therapy.
◆ Perform tracheal suctioning, incentive spirometry, and postural drainage.
◆ Encourage coughing and deep-breathing exercises, as indicated.
◆ Provide safety measures.

PATIENT TEACHING

Be sure to cover:
◆ disorder, diagnostic testing, and treatment
◆ medication administration, dosage, and possible adverse effects
◆ follow-up care for underlying cause.

RESOURCES
Organizations
American Lung Association:
www.lungusa.org
American Thoracic Society:
www.thoracic.org

Selected references
Broccard, A. "Respiratory Acidosis and Acute Respiratory Distress Syndrome: Time to Trade in a Bull Market?" *Critical Care Medicine* 34(1):229-31, January 2006.
Frangiosa, A., et al. "Acid-base Balance in Heart Failure," *Journal of Nephrology* 19(Suppl 9):S115-20, March-April 2006.
Nagler, J., et al. "End-tidal Carbon dioxide as a Measure of Acidosis Among Children with Gastroenteritis," *Pediatrics* 118(1):260-67, July 2006.
Strategies for Managing Multisystem Disorders. Philadelphia: Lippincott Williams & Wilkins, 2006.

Disorders affecting management of respiratory acidosis

This chart highlights disorders that affect the management of respiratory acidosis.

DISORDER	SIGNS AND SYMPTOMS	DIAGNOSTIC TEST RESULTS	TREATMENT AND CARE
Cardiac arrhythmia (complication)	◆ May be asymptomatic ◆ Dizziness ◆ Hypotension ◆ Syncope ◆ Weakness ◆ Cool, clammy skin ◆ Altered level of consciousness (LOC) ◆ Reduced urine output ◆ Shortness of breath	◆ Electrocardiography detects arrhythmias as well as ischemia and infarction that may result in arrhythmias. ◆ Laboratory testing may reveal electrolyte abnormalities, acid-base abnormalities, or drug toxicities that may cause arrhythmias.	◆ When life-threatening arrhythmias develop, rapidly assess LOC, respirations, and pulse rate. ◆ Initiate cardiopulmonary resuscitation, if indicated. ◆ Evaluate cardiac output resulting from arrhythmias. ◆ If the patient develops heart block, prepare for cardiac pacing. ◆ Administer antiarrhythmics, as ordered. ◆ Prepare to assist with medical procedures, if indicated. ◆ Assess intake and output every hour; insert an indwelling urinary catheter, as indicated, to ensure accurate urine measurement. ◆ Document arrhythmias in a monitored patient and assess for possible causes and effects. ◆ If the patient's pulse is abnormally rapid, slow, or irregular, watch for signs of hypoperfusion, such as hypotension and diminished urine output. ◆ Monitor for predisposing factors, such as fluid and electrolyte imbalance or possible drug toxicity.

DISORDER	SIGNS AND SYMPTOMS	DIAGNOSTIC TEST RESULTS	TREATMENT AND CARE
Hyperkalemia (complication)	◆ Abdominal cramping ◆ Diarrhea ◆ Chest pain ◆ Hypotension ◆ Irregular pulse rate; tachycardia changing to bradycardia ◆ Irritability ◆ Muscle weakness, especially of the lower extremities ◆ Nausea ◆ Paresthesia	◆ Serum potassium level is greater than 5 mEq/L. ◆ Electrocardiography reveals changes (first noted as a tall, tented T wave; widened QRS complex; prolonged PR interval; flattened or absent P wave; and depressed ST-segment). ◆ Arterial blood gas (ABG) analysis reveals decreased pH and metabolic acidosis.	◆ Assess vital signs. Anticipate cardiac monitoring if the patient's serum potassium level exceeds 6 mEq/L. ◆ Monitor the patient's intake and output and report an output of less than 30 ml/hour. ◆ Administer a slow calcium gluconate I.V. infusion to counteract the myocardial depressant effects of hyperkalemia. ◆ For a patient receiving repeated insulin and glucose treatments, check for signs and symptoms of hypoglycemia, including muscle weakness, syncope, hunger, and diaphoresis. ◆ Administer sodium polystyrene sulfonate and monitor serum sodium levels, which may rise; assess for signs of heart failure. Encourage the patient to retain sodium polystyrene sulfonate enemas for 30 to 60 minutes. Monitor the patient for hypokalemia when administering the drug on 2 or more consecutive days. ◆ Monitor bowel sounds and the number and character of bowel movements. ◆ Monitor serum potassium level and related laboratory test results. ◆ Begin continuous cardiac monitoring if serum potassium level exceeds 6 mEq/L. ◆ If the patient has acute hyperkalemia that doesn't respond to other treatments, prepare for dialysis. ◆ If the patient has muscle weakness, implement safety measures. ◆ Assess for signs of hypokalemia after treatment.
Shock (coexisting)	◆ Tachycardia and bounding pulse ◆ Restlessness and hypoxia ◆ Restlessness and irritability ◆ Tachypnea ◆ Reduced urinary output or anuria ◆ Cool, pale skin ◆ Hypotension ◆ Narrowed pulse pressure ◆ Reduced stroke volume ◆ Weak, rapid, thready pulse ◆ Shallow respirations ◆ Cyanosis ◆ Unconsciousness and absent reflexes in irreversible stages	◆ Coagulation studies may detect coagulopathy from disseminated intravascular coagulation. ◆ White blood cell count and erythrocyte sedimentation rate may be increased. ◆ Blood urea nitrogen and creatinine are elevated. ◆ Serum lactate may be increased. ◆ Serum glucose may be elevated in early stages. ◆ Cardiac enzymes and proteins may be elevated. ◆ ABG analysis may reveal respiratory alkalosis in early shock or respiratory acidosis in later stages. ◆ Chest X-rays may be normal in early stages; pulmonary congestion may be seen in later stages. ◆ Electrocardiography determines heart rate and detects arrhythmias, ischemic changes, and myocardial infarction. ◆ Echocardiography determines left ventricular function and reveals valvular abnormalitiies.	◆ Assist in identifying and treating the underlying cause. ◆ Maintain a patent airway; prepare for intubation and mechanical ventilation if respiratory distress develops. ◆ Administer supplemental oxygen. ◆ Use continuous cardiac monitoring to detect changes in heart rate and rhythm; administer antiarrhythmics, as necessary. ◆ Monitor blood pressure, pulse rate, peripheral pulses, and other vital signs every 15 minutes; report changes. ◆ Monitor central venous pressure, pulmonary artery wedge pressure, and cardiac output, as ordered, and report changes. ◆ Initiate and maintain at least two I.V. lines with large-gauge needles for fluid and drug administration. ◆ Administer I.V. fluids, crystalloids, colloids, or blood products, as necessary, to maintain intravascular volume. ◆ Administer inotropic drugs, such as dopamine, dobutamine, and epinephrine, to increase heart contractility and cardiac output. ◆ Administer vasodilators, such as nitroglycerin or nitroprusside, with a vasopressor to reduce the left ventricle's workload. ◆ Monitor intake and output and daily weight. Administer diuretics to reduce preload if patient has fluid volume overload. ◆ Initiate intra-aortic balloon pump therapy to reduce the work of the left ventricle by decreasing systemic vascular resistance. Monitor the patient carefully. ◆ Monitor the patient receiving thrombolytic therapy or coronary artery revascularization per facility protocol. ◆ Prepare for emergency surgery if repair of a ruptured papillary muscle is required or if a ventricular septal defect is present. ◆ Monitor the patient with a ventricular assist device.

Respiratory alkalosis

OVERVIEW

- Acid-base disturbance that's characterized by a partial pressure of arterial carbon dioxide ($Paco_2$) less than 35 mm Hg and blood pH greater than 7.45
- Hypocapnia (below normal $Paco_2$) occurring when the lungs eliminate more carbon dioxide (CO_2) than the cells produce
- Most common acid-base disturbance in patients who are critically ill and, when severe, have a poor prognosis

CAUSES
Pulmonary
- Severe hypoxemia
- Pneumonia
- Interstitial lung disease
- Pulmonary vascular disease
- Acute asthma
- Mechanical overventilation

Nonpulmonary
- Anxiety
- Fever
- Aspirin toxicity
- Metabolic acidosis
- Central nervous system (CNS) inflammation or tumor
- Sepsis
- Hepatic failure
- Pregnancy

PATHOPHYSIOLOGY

- Increased pulmonary ventilation leads to excessive exhalation of CO_2, resulting in hypocapnia.
- Chemical reduction of carbonic acid occurs, along with excretion of hydrogen and bicarbonate ions and elevated pH. (See *What happens in respiratory alkalosis.*)
- Respiratory alkalosis can affect other body systems, placing the patient at risk for numerous complications. (See *Disorders affecting management of respiratory alkalosis*, pages 382 and 383.)

CARDIOVASCULAR SYSTEM
- Hypocapnia stimulates the carotid and aortic bodies and the medulla, increasing the heart rate (which hypokalemia can further aggravate) without increasing blood pressure. Stimulation can also alter the excitability of the myocardium, leading to arrhythmias.
- The risk for arrhythmias is further compounded by the shift of potassium into the cells, which can lead to hypokalemia and the inhibition of calcium ionization, ultimately leading to hypocalcemia.
- Continued low $Paco_2$ increases vasoconstriction, ultimately impairing blood flow to the peripheral tissues.
- Eventually, alkalosis overwhelms the heart's ability to function.

NEUROLOGIC SYSTEM
- Hypocapnia causes cerebral vasoconstriction, which prompts a reduction in cerebral blood flow. It also overexcites the medulla, pons, and other parts of the autonomic nervous system, resulting in anxiety and dizziness.
- Continued low $Paco_2$ and the resulting vasoconstriction increases cerebral and peripheral hypoxia.
- Severe alkalosis inhibits calcium ionization, thus nerves and muscles become progressively more excitable. Hypocalcemia can occur.

- Eventually, alkalosis overwhelms the CNS, resulting in a decreased level of consciousness (LOC), hyperreflexia, carpopedal spasms, tetany, seizures, and coma.

RENAL SYSTEM
- If hypocapnia lasts more than 6 hours, the kidneys increase secretion of bicarbonate and reduce secretion of hydrogen, leading to low pH.

RESPIRATORY SYSTEM
- Hypocapnia occurs in respiratory alkalosis regardless of the underlying cause. The rate and depth of respirations increase in an attempt to retain CO_2 and decrease pH.
- Increasing serum pH causes hydrogen ions to shift from cells to the blood in exchange for potassium ions. The hydrogen ions combine with available bicarbonate ions in the blood to form carbonic acid, resulting in decreased pH.

ASSESSMENT

HISTORY
- An increase in the rate and depth of respirations
- Muscle weakness or difficulty breathing

PHYSICAL FINDINGS
- Deep, rapid respirations
- CNS and neuromuscular disturbances (cardinal sign) including anxiety, restlessness, confusion or syncope, tingling in fingers and toes, progressive decrease in LOC, seizures, and coma
- Diaphoresis
- Agitation
- Light-headedness or dizziness
- Tachycardia
- Alternating periods of apnea and hyperventilation
- Hyperreflexia
- Carpopedal spasm
- Tetany
- Arrhythmias

◆ Arterial blood gas (ABG) analysis shows PaCO_2 less than 35 mm Hg, elevated pH in proportion to the decrease in PaCO_2 in the acute stage that decreases toward normal in the chronic stage, and normal bicarbonate in the acute stage but less than normal in the chronic stage.

◆ Serum electrolyte studies detect metabolic disorders causing compensatory respiratory alkalosis; serum chloride levels may be low in severe respiratory alkalosis.

◆ Electrocardiography reveals changes that may indicate cardiac arrhythmias.

◆ Toxicology screening reveals possible salicylate poisoning.

◆ Urine pH is basic as kidneys excrete bicarbonate to raise blood pH.

UP CLOSE

What happens in respiratory alkalosis

This series of illustrations shows how respiratory alkalosis develops at the cellular level. When pulmonary ventilation increases above the amount needed to maintain normal carbon dioxide (CO_2) levels, excessive amounts of CO_2 are exhaled. This causes hypocapnia (a fall in PaCO_2), which leads to a reduction in carbonic acid (H_2CO_3) production, a loss of hydrogen (H^+) ions and bicarbonate (HCO_3^-) ions, and a subsequent rise in pH. Look for a pH level above 7.45, a PaCO_2 level below 35 mm Hg, and an HCO_3^- level below 22 mEq/L.

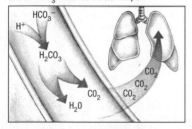

In defense against the rising pH, H^+ ions are pulled out of the cells and into the blood in exchange for potassium (K) ions. The H^+ ions entering the blood combine with HCO_3^- ions to form carbonic acid, which lowers pH. Look for a further decrease in HCO_3^- levels, a fall in pH, and a fall in serum potassium levels (hypokalemia).

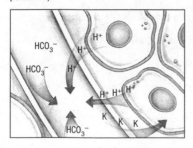

Hypocapnia stimulates the carotid and aortic bodies and the medulla, which causes an increase in heart rate without an increase in blood pressure. Look for angina, electrocardiogram changes, restlessness, and anxiety.

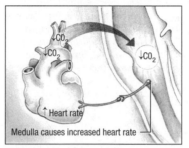

Medulla causes increased heart rate

Simultaneously, hypocapnia produces cerebral vasoconstriction, which prompts a reduction in cerebral blood flow. Hypocapnia also overexcites the medulla, pons, and other parts of the autonomic nervous system. Look for increasing anxiety, diaphoresis, dyspnea, alternating periods of apnea and hyperventilation, dizziness, and tingling in the fingers or toes.

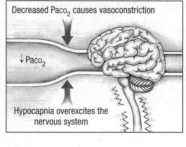

Decreased PaCO_2 causes vasoconstriction

↓PaCO_2

Hypocapnia overexcites the nervous system

When hypocapnia lasts more than 6 hours, the kidneys increase secretion of HCO_3^- and reduce excretion of H^+. Periods of apnea may result if the pH remains high and the PaCO_2 remains low. Look for slowed respiratory rate, hypoventilation, and Cheyne-Stokes respirations.

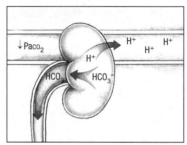

Continued low PaCO_2 increases cerebral and peripheral hypoxia from vasoconstriction. Severe alkalosis inhibits calcium (Ca) ionization, which in turn causes increased nerve excitability and muscle contractions. Eventually, the alkalosis overwhelms the central nervous system and the heart. Look for decreasing level of consciousness, hyperreflexia, carpopedal spasm, tetany, arrhythmias, seizures, and coma.

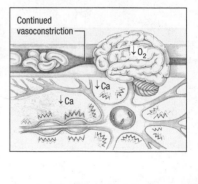

Continued vasoconstriction

↓O_2
↓Ca

(continued)

GENERAL
◆ Airway and ventilation support
◆ Treatment of underlying cause
◆ Bronchoscopy

DIET
◆ Nothing by mouth until stable

ACTIVITY
◆ Bedrest until stable

MEDICATIONS
◆ Oxygen
◆ Sedatives
◆ Electrolyte replacement therapy
◆ Antibiotics

NURSING CONSIDERATIONS

NURSING DIAGNOSES
◆ Anxiety
◆ Disturbed thought processes
◆ Impaired gas exchange
◆ Ineffective breathing pattern

EXPECTED OUTCOMES
The patient will:
◆ identify strategies to reduce anxiety
◆ communicate effectively with appropriate thought process
◆ maintain adequate ventilation and oxygenation
◆ exhibit an effective breathing pattern.

NURSING INTERVENTIONS
◆ Monitor vital signs, pulse oximetry, cardiac rhythm, and intake and output.
◆ Assess neurologic, respiratory, and cardiovascular status.
◆ Monitor ABG values and serum electrolyte levels.
◆ Reassure the patient and maintain a quiet, calm environment.

WARNING *For hyperventilation caused by severe anxiety, have the patient breathe into a paper bag, which forces him to breathe exhaled carbon dioxide, thereby raising the CO_2 level.*

◆ Institute seizure precautions and safety measures.

PATIENT TEACHING

Be sure to cover:
◆ disorder, diagnostic testing, and treatment
◆ medication administration, dosage, and possible adverse effects
◆ anxiety-reducing techniques.

RESOURCES
Organizations
American Lung Association:
www.lungusa.org
American Thoracic Society:
www.thoracic.org

Selected references
Ahya, S., et al. "Acid-base and Potassium Disorders in Liver Disease," *Seminars in Nephrology* 26(6):466-70, November 2006.
Frangiosa, A., et al. "Acid-Base Balance in Heart Failure," *Journal of Nephrology* 19(Suppl 9):S115-20, March-April 2006.
Mazarati, A.M. "Respiratory Alkalosis: 'Basic' Mechanism of Febrile Seizures?" *Epilepsy Currents* 7(1):25-27, January-February 2007.
Strategies for Managing Mulitsystem Disorders. Philadelphia: Lippincott Williams & Wilkins, 2006.

Disorders affecting management of respiratory alkalosis

This chart highlights disorders that affect the management of respiratory alkalosis.

DISORDER	SIGNS AND SYMPTOMS	DIAGNOSTIC TEST RESULTS	TREATMENT AND CARE
Cardiac arrhythmia (complication)	◆ Palpitations ◆ Chest pain ◆ Dizziness ◆ Weakness, fatigue ◆ Irregular heart rhythm ◆ Hypotension ◆ Syncope ◆ Altered level of consciousness (LOC) ◆ Diaphoresis ◆ Pallor ◆ Cold, clammy skin	◆ Electrocardiography identifies waveform changes associated with the arrhythmia. ◆ Laboratory testing reveals hyperkalemia, electrolyte abnormalities, hypoxemia, or acid-base abnormalities.	◆ Evaluate the monitored patient's electrocardiogram (ECG) regularly for arrhythmias and assess hemodynamic parameters, as indicated. Document arrhythmias and notify the physician immediately. ◆ Assess an unmonitored patient for rhythm disturbances. If the patient's pulse rate is abnormally rapid, slow, or irregular, watch for signs of hypoperfusion, such as hypotension and diminished urine output. ◆ As ordered, obtain an ECG tracing in an unmonitored patient to confirm and identify the type of arrhythmia present. ◆ Administer medications such as antiarrhythmic agents, as ordered, and monitor the patient for adverse effects. ◆ If a life-threatening arrhythmia develops, rapidly assess the patient's LOC, pulse and respiratory rates, and hemodynamic parameters. Be alert for trends. Monitor EGG continuously. Be prepared to initiate cardiopulmonary resuscitation or cardioversion, if indicated.

DISORDER	SIGNS AND SYMPTOMS	DIAGNOSTIC TEST RESULTS	TREATMENT AND CARE
Hypocalcemia (complication)	◆ Anxiety ◆ Irritability ◆ Twitching around the mouth ◆ Laryngospasm ◆ Seizures ◆ Muscle cramps ◆ Paresthesia of the face, fingers, or toes ◆ Tetany ◆ Positive Chvostek's and Trousseau's signs ◆ Hypotension ◆ Arrhythmias ◆ Hyperactive deep tendon reflexes	◆ Serum calcium level is less than 8.5 mg/dl. ◆ Ionized calcium level is usually below 4.5 mg/dl. ◆ Platelet count is decreased. ◆ EGG shows lengthened QT interval, prolonged ST segment, and arrhythmias. ◆ Serum protein levels may reveal changes because half of serum calcium is bound to albumin.	◆ Assess cardiovascular status and neurologic status for changes; monitor vital signs frequently. ◆ Monitor respiratory status, including rate, depth, and rhythm. Watch for stridor, dyspnea, and crowing. ◆ Keep a tracheotomy tray and a handheld resuscitation bag at the bedside in case laryngospasm occurs. ◆ Institute cardiac monitoring, and evaluate for changes in heart rate and rhythm. ◆ Assess for Chvostek's sign or Trousseau's sign. ◆ Ensure the patency of the I.V. line because infiltration can cause tissue necrosis and sloughing; give oral replacements, as ordered. Give calcium supplements 1 to 1½ hours after meals. If GI upset occurs, give the supplement with milk. ◆ Monitor pertinent laboratory test results, including calcium, albumin, and magnesium levels and those of other electrolytes. Remember to check the ionized calcium level after every 4 units of blood transfused. ◆ Institute seizure precautions and safety measures to prevent injury.
Hypokalemia (complication)	◆ Dizziness ◆ Hypotension ◆ Arrhythmias ◆ Cardiac arrest ◆ Nausea, vomiting ◆ Anorexia ◆ Diarrhea ◆ Decreased peristalsis ◆ Abdominal distention ◆ Muscle weakness ◆ Fatigue ◆ Leg cramps	◆ Serum potassium is less than 3.5 mEq/L. ◆ Arterial blood gas analysis reveals metabolic alkalosis. ◆ EGG changes include flattened T waves, elevated U waves, and a depressed ST segment.	◆ Monitor vital signs, especially pulse and blood pressure; check heart rate and rhythm and ECG tracings in patients with a serum potassium level less than 3 mEq/L. ◆ Assess the patient's respiratory rate, depth, and pattern. Keep a manual resuscitation bag at the bedside of a patient with severe hypokalemia. ◆ Monitor serum potassium levels. ◆ Monitor and document fluid intake and output, especially when administering I.V. potassium replacement. Urine volume should be greater than 30 ml/hour to prevent rebound hyperkalemia. ◆ Check for signs of hypokalemia-related metabolic alkalosis, including irritability and paresthesia. ◆ Insert and maintain patent I.V. access. ◆ Administer I.V. potassium replacement solutions, as prescribed. Administer I.V. potassium infusions cautiously. Make sure that infusions are diluted and mixed thoroughly in adequate amounts of fluid. Use premixed potassium solutions when possible. ◆ Continuously monitor heart rate and rhythm and ECG tracings of patients receiving potassium infusions of more than 5 mEq/hour or a concentration of more than 40 mEq/L of fluid. ◆ Monitor the patient for signs and symptoms of hyperkalemia that may result due to potassium replacement. ◆ To prevent gastric irritation, administer oral supplements in at least 4 oz (118 ml) of fluid or with food; never crush slow-release oral potassium supplement tablets. The patient could experience a rapid rise in potassium levels. ◆ Check for signs of constipation, such as abdominal distention and decreased bowel sounds. Although medication may be prescribed to combat constipation, avoid laxatives that promote potassium loss.

Rheumatic fever and rheumatic heart disease

OVERVIEW

- Systemic inflammatory disease of childhood that occurs 2 to 6 weeks after an inadequately treated upper respiratory tract infection with group A streptococci (GAS)
- Principally involves the heart, joints, central nervous system, skin, and subcutaneous tissues
- In rheumatic heart disease, early acute phase that may affect endocardium, myocardium, or pericardium, possibly followed later by chronic valvular disease
- Commonly recurs
- In the United States, incidence most common in the northern states
- Worldwide, 15 to 20 million new cases each year

CAUSES

- Group A beta-hemolytic streptococcal pharyngitis

PATHOPHYSIOLOGY

- Rheumatic fever appears to be a hypersensitivity reaction in which antibodies produced to combat streptococci react and produce lesions at specific tissue sites.
- Antigens of GAS bind to receptors in the heart, muscle, brain, and synovial joints, causing an autoimmune response.
- Because the antigens are similar to the body's own cells, antibodies may attack healthy body cells by mistake.

CARDIOVASCULAR SYSTEM

- Carditis may affect the endocardium, myocardium, or pericardium.
- Pericarditis produces a serofibrinous effusion.
- Myocarditis produces characteristic lesions called *Aschoff's bodies* in the interstitial tissue of the heart as well as cellular swelling and fragmentation of interstitial collagen that lead to fibrotic nodule and interstitial scar formation.
- Endocarditis causes leaflet swelling, erosion along the lines of the leaflet closure, and blood, platelet, and fibrin deposits, which form beadlike growths and eventually cause scarring. (See *Disorders affecting the management of rheumatic fever and rheumatic heart disease*, page 387.)

MUSCULOSKELETAL SYSTEM

- Inflammation of the joints causes polyarthritis.

ASSESSMENT

HISTORY

- Recent streptococcal infection
- Recent history of low-grade fever spiking to at least 100.4° F (38° C) in late afternoon, along with unexplained epistaxis and abdominal pain
- Migratory joint pain (polyarthritis)

PHYSICAL FINDINGS

- Swelling, redness, and signs of effusion, most commonly in the knees, ankles, elbows, and hips
- With pericarditis, sharp, sudden pain that usually starts over the sternum and radiates to the neck, shoulders, back, and arms; increases with deep inspiration and decreases when the patient sits up and leans forward
- With heart failure caused by severe rheumatic carditis, dyspnea, right upper quadrant pain, and a hacking, nonproductive cough
- Skin lesions, such as erythema marginatum, typically on the trunk and extremities
- Subcutaneous nodules, 3 mm to 2 cm in diameter, that are firm, movable, and nontender occurring near tendons or bony prominences of joints and persisting for several days to weeks
- With left-sided heart failure, edema and tachypnea, bibasilar crackles, and ventricular or atrial gallop
- Transient chorea up to 6 months after original streptococcal infection
- Pericardial friction rub
- Heart murmurs and gallops

DIAGNOSTIC TEST RESULTS

- Jones criteria are met for rheumatic heart disease. (See *Jones criteria for diagnosing rheumatic fever.*)
- During acute phase, white blood cell count and erythrocyte sedimentation rate are elevated.
- During inflammation, complete blood count shows slight anemia.
- C-reactive protein test is positive, especially during acute phase.
- In severe carditis, cardiac enzyme levels are increased.

- Antistreptolysin-O titer is elevated in 95% of patients within 2 months of onset.
- Throat cultures show GAS.
- Chest X-rays show normal heart size (except with myocarditis, heart failure, and pericardial effusion).
- Echocardiography helps evaluate valvular damage, chamber size, and ventricular function and detects pericardial effusion.
- Electrocardiography reveals no diagnostic changes, but 20% of patients show a prolonged PR interval.
- Cardiac catheterization evaluates valvular damage and left ventricular function in severe cardiac dysfunction.

TREATMENT

GENERAL
- Symptomatic

DIET
- Sodium restriction, if indicated

ACTIVITY
- Bed rest during acute phase
- Gradual activity increase, as tolerated

MEDICATIONS
- Antibiotics
- Anti-inflammatories

SURGERY
- Commissurotomy, valvuloplasty, or heart valve replacement

NURSING CONSIDERATIONS

NURSING DIAGNOSES
- Activity intolerance
- Acute pain
- Anxiety
- Decreased cardiac output
- Deficient diversional activity
- Fatigue
- Impaired gas exchange
- Ineffective role performance
- Risk for infection

EXPECTED OUTCOMES
The patient will:
- carry out activities of daily living without weakness or fatigue
- express feelings of increased comfort and decreased pain
- cope with medical condition without demonstrating severe signs of anxiety
- maintain hemodynamic stability, have no arrhythmias, and maintain adequate cardiac output
- identify appropriate diversionary activities to partake in while on bed rest
- verbalize the importance of balancing activity with adequate rest periods
- maintain adequate ventilation and oxygenation
- express feelings about diminished capacity to perform usual roles
- remain free from signs and symptoms of infection.

NURSING INTERVENTIONS
- Monitor vital signs and cardiac rhythm.
- Assess heart and breath sounds.
- Provide analgesics and oxygen, as needed.
- Give prescribed antibiotics on time.
- Stress the importance of bed rest. Provide a bedside commode.
- Position the patient upright.
- Allow the patient to express feelings and concerns.

Jones criteria for diagnosing rheumatic fever

The Jones criteria are used to standardize the diagnosis of rheumatic fever. Diagnosis requires that the patient have either two major criteria *or* one major criterion and two minor criteria, plus evidence of a previous streptococcal infection.

MAJOR CRITERIA
- Carditis
- Migratory polyarthritis
- Sydenham's chorea
- Subcutaneous nodules
- Erythema marginatum

MINOR CRITERIA
- Fever
- Arthralgia
- Elevated acute phase reactants
- Prolonged PR interval

(continued)

Be sure to cover:
◆ disorder, diagnostic testing, and treatment
◆ importance of frequent rest periods
◆ importance of reporting early signs and symptoms of left-sided heart failure
◆ keeping the child away from people with respiratory tract infections
◆ transient nature of chorea
◆ compliance with prolonged antibiotic therapy and follow-up care
◆ need for prophylactic antibiotics before any dental work or invasive procedures.

RESOURCES
Organizations
American Heart Association: *www.americanheart.org*
National Heart, Lung, and Blood Institute: *www.nhlbi.nih.gov*

Selected references
Cilliers, A. "Rheumatic Fever and Its Management," British Medical Journal 333(7579):1153-56, December 2006.

Lee, G.M., and Wessels, M.R. "Changing Epidemiology of Acute Rheumatic Fever in the United States," *Clinical Infectious Diseases* 42(4):448-50, February 2006.

The Merck Manual of Diagnosis & Therapy, 18th ed., Whitehouse Station, N.J.: Merck & Co., Inc., 2006.

Odemis, E., et al. "Assessment of Cardiac Function and Rheumatic Heart Disease in Children with Adenotonsillar Hypertrophy," *Journal of the National Medical Association* 98(12): 1973-76, December 2006.

Disorders affecting management of rheumatic fever and rheumatic heart disease

This chart highlights disorders that affect the management of rheumatic fever and rheumatic heart disease.

DISORDER	SIGNS AND SYMPTOMS	DIAGNOSTIC TEST RESULTS	TREATMENT AND CARE
Heart failure (complication)	*Left-sided heart failure* ◆ Dyspnea ◆ Orthopnea ◆ Paroxysmal nocturnal dyspnea ◆ Fatigue ◆ Nonproductive cough ◆ Crackles ◆ Hemoptysis ◆ Tachycardia ◆ S_3, S_4 ◆ Cool, pale skin ◆ Restlessness and confusion *Right-sided heart failure* ◆ Jugular vein distention ◆ Positive hepatojugular reflex ◆ Right upper quadrant pain ◆ Anorexia, nausea ◆ Weight gain, edema ◆ Ascites or anasarca	◆ Chest X-ray shows increased pulmonary vascular markings, interstitial edema, or pleural effusions and cardiomegaly. ◆ B-type natriuretic peptide (BNP) immunoassay is elevated. ◆ Electrocardiography may reveal hypertrophy, ischemic changes or infarction, tachycardia, and extrasystoles. ◆ Liver function test may be abnormal; blood urea nitrogen (BUN) and creatinine levels may be elevated. ◆ Prothrombin time may be prolonged. ◆ Echocardiography may reveal left ventricular hypertrophy, dilation, and abnormal contractility. ◆ Pulmonary artery pressure, pulmonary artery wedge pressure (PAWP), and left ventricular end pressure are elevated in left-sided heart failure; right atrial or central venous pressure is elevated in right-sided heart failure. ◆ Radionuclide ventriculography may reveal ejection fraction less than 40% in diastolic dysfunction.	◆ Place the patient in Fowler's position and provide supplemental oxygen. ◆ Weigh the patient daily, and check for peripheral edema. ◆ Monitor intake and output, vital signs, and mental status. ◆ Auscultate for S_3 and S_4 and adventitious lung sounds, such as crackles or rhonchi. ◆ Monitor BUN, creatinine, BNP, serum electrolytes, and magnesium levels. ◆ Monitor cardiac rhythm. ◆ Administer nesiritide (Natrecor), diuretics, nitrates, angiotensin-converting enzyme inhibitors, digoxin, beta-adrenergic blockers, and morphine.
Mitral insufficiency (complication)	◆ Orthopnea and dyspnea ◆ Fatigue ◆ Angina, palpitations, and tachycardia ◆ Peripheral edema ◆ Jugular vein distention and hepatomegaly (right-sided heart failure) ◆ Crackles ◆ Holosystolic murmur at apex	◆ Echocardiography reveals abnormal valve leaflet motion and left atrial enlargement. ◆ Cardiac catheterization reveals mitral insufficiency with increased left ventricular end-diastolic volume and pressure, increased atrial pressure and PAWP, and decreased cardiac output.	◆ Monitor vital signs, pulse oximetry, cardiac rhythm, and intake and output. ◆ Promote measures to reduce activity level and decrease myocardial oxygen demand. ◆ Place the patient in an upright position to decrease dyspnea and administer oxygen, if indicated. ◆ Administer medications for heart failure, if present, as well as nitrates for anginal pain. ◆ Provide preoperative and postoperative care for valvular surgery, if appropriate.
Pericarditis (complication)	◆ Sharp and sudden chest pain ◆ Pericardial friction rub ◆ Shallow, rapid respirations ◆ Dyspnea, orthopnea, and tachycardia ◆ Muffled, distant heart sounds ◆ Pallor, clammy skin, hypotension	◆ Echocardiography may show an echo-free space between the ventricular wall and the pericardium. ◆ Computed tomography scan and magnetic resonance imaging reveal pericardial thickness. ◆ Electrocardiography shows initial ST-elevation across the pericardium. ◆ White blood cell count is elevated, especially in infectious pericarditis.	◆ Administer analgesics and oxygen to decrease chest pain. ◆ Administer antibiotics, as ordered. ◆ Place the patient in an upright position and maintain bedrest to reduce metabolic needs. ◆ Monitor for signs of cardiac tamponade and assist with pericardiocentesis, if indicated. ◆ Monitor vital signs, pulse oximetry, cardiac rhythm, and intake and output.

Rheumatoid arthritis

OVERVIEW

- Chronic, systemic, symmetrical inflammatory disease
- Primarily attacks peripheral joints and surrounding muscles, tendons, ligaments, and blood vessels
- Marked by spontaneous remissions and unpredictable exacerbations
- Potentially crippling
- Strikes three times as many women as men
- Can occur at any age, with peak onset between ages 35 and 50

CAUSES

- Exact cause unknown
- Possible link to viral or bacterial infection, hormonal factors, and lifestyle

PATHOPHYSIOLOGY

- An autoimmune response causes inflammation in one or more joints.
- The resulting cartilage damage triggers additional immune responses, including complement activation.
- Polymorphonuclear leukocytes, macrophages, and lymphocytes are attracted to the area of inflammation.
- The immune complexes formed by the rheumatoid factor (RF) aggregation are destroyed or disintegrated by the leukocytes and macrophages. Subsequently, lysosomal enzymes are released, which cause destruction of the joint cartilage.
- This destruction sets up an inflammatory response, which draws more lymphocytes and plasma cells to the area, ultimately causing a continuous cycle of events.
- Continued inflammation results in hyperplasia of the cells in the synovial space and tissues. Increased capillary permeability secondary to the inflammatory response leads to swelling; vasodilation and resultant increased blood flow lead to redness and warmth.

- Although typically thought of as a disorder of the musculoskeletal system, the inflammatory response can extend beyond the joints, affecting other body systems. (See *Disorders affecting management of rheumatoid arthritis,* page 391.)

CARDIOVASCULAR SYSTEM

- Vasculitis results from an inflammatory response in the small and medium arterioles. Ischemia and necrosis of the affected areas can occur, ultimately leading to skin breakdown or myocardial tissue ischemia and necrosis.
- Immune complex invasion and subsequent ischemia and necrosis of the myocardial tissue can lead to pericarditis.

MUSCULOSKELETAL SYSTEM

- If not arrested, the inflammatory process in the joints occurs in four stages: synovitis, pannus, fibrous ankylosis, and calcification.
- *Synovitis* develops from congestion and edema of the synovial membrane and joint capsule. Infiltration by lymphocytes, macrophages, and neutrophils continues the local inflammatory response. These cells, as well as fibroblast-like synovial cells,

---

Visualizing joint changes

Inflammatory changes in the joint are characteristic of rheumatoid arthritis. The joint inflammation progresses through four stages: synovitis, pannus formation, fibrous ankylosis, and joint fixation. These illustrations highlight the inflammatory changes of the knee, hand and wrist, and hip joints.

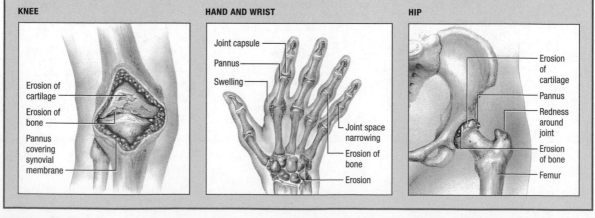

KNEE

- Erosion of cartilage
- Erosion of bone
- Pannus covering synovial membrane

HAND AND WRIST

- Joint capsule
- Pannus
- Swelling
- Joint space narrowing
- Erosion of bone
- Erosion

HIP

- Erosion of cartilage
- Pannus
- Redness around joint
- Erosion of bone
- Femur

produce enzymes that help to degrade bone and cartilage.

– *Pannus*—thickened layers of granulation tissue—covers and invades cartilage and eventually destroys the joint capsule and bone.
– *Fibrous ankylosis*—fibrous invasion of the pannus and scar formation—occludes the joint space; bone atrophy and misalignment causes visible deformities and disrupts the articulation of opposing bones, leading to muscle atrophy and imbalance and, possibly, partial dislocations (subluxations) or compression fractures. (See *Visualizing joint changes.*)
– *Calcification* of fibrous tissue occurs, resulting in bony ankylosis and total immobility.

♦ As the disease progresses, the inflammation and destruction that occurs results in decreased joint mobility and pain.
♦ Osteoporosis and compression fractures can occur secondary to weakening of the joint.
♦ Disorders, such as Sjögren's syndrome, can develop because of the underlying autoimmune processes.

NEUROLOGIC SYSTEM

♦ Immune complex invasion can affect the tissue of the eyes and peripheral nerves.
♦ Scleritis and peripheral neuropathy may occur, leading to numbness or tingling in the feet and loss of sensation in the fingers.

RESPIRATORY SYSTEM

♦ Immune complex formation and the resultant inflammatory response can cause pulmonary tissue damage and necrosis, leading to pulmonary nodules or fibrosis and pleuritis.

ASSESSMENT

HISTORY

♦ Insidious onset of nonspecific symptoms, including fatigue, malaise, anorexia, persistent low-grade fever, weight loss, and vague articular symptoms
♦ Later, more specific localized articular symptoms, commonly in the fingers
♦ Bilateral and symmetrical symptoms, which may extend to the wrists, elbows, knees, and ankles
♦ Stiff joints
♦ Stiff, weak, or painful muscles
♦ Numbness or tingling in the feet or weakness or loss of sensation in the fingers
♦ Pain on inspiration
♦ Shortness of breath

PHYSICAL FINDINGS

♦ Joint deformities and contractures
♦ Painful, red, swollen arms
♦ Foreshortened hands
♦ Boggy wrists
♦ Rheumatoid nodules
♦ Leg ulcers
♦ Eye redness
♦ Joints that are warm to the touch
♦ Pericardial friction rub
♦ Positive Babinski's sign

DIAGNOSTIC TEST FINDINGS

♦ RF test is positive in 75% to 80% of patients, as indicated by a titer of 1:160 or higher.
♦ Synovial fluid analysis shows increased volume and turbidity but decreased viscosity and complement (C3 and C4) levels, with white blood cell count possibly exceeding 10,000/μl.
♦ Serum globulin levels are elevated.
♦ Erythrocyte sedimentation rate is elevated.
♦ Complete blood count shows moderate anemia and slight leukocytosis.
♦ In early stages, X-rays show bone demineralization and soft-tissue swelling. Later, they help determine the extent of cartilage and bone de-

struction, erosion, subluxations, and deformities and show the characteristic pattern of these abnormalities.
♦ Magnetic resonance imaging and computed tomography scan may show the extent of damage.
♦ Synovial tissue biopsy shows inflammation.

TREATMENT

GENERAL

♦ Moist heat application
♦ Adequate sleep
♦ Splinting

ACTIVITY

♦ Range-of-motion (ROM) exercises and carefully individualized therapeutic exercises
♦ Frequent rest periods

MEDICATIONS

♦ Salicylates
♦ Nonsteroidal anti-inflammatory drugs
♦ Antimalarials (hydroxychloroquine)
♦ Gold salts
♦ Penicillamine
♦ Corticosteroids
♦ Antineoplastics
♦ Monoclonal antibody therapy, such as infliximab (Remicade)

SURGERY

♦ Metatarsal head and distal ulnar resectional arthroplasty and insertion of Silastic prosthesis between the metacarpophalangeal and proximal interphalangeal joints
♦ Arthrodesis (joint fusion)
♦ Synovectomy
♦ Osteotomy
♦ Repair of ruptured tendon
♦ In advanced disease, joint reconstruction or total joint arthroplasty

(continued)

NURSING CONSIDERATIONS

NURSING DIAGNOSES
- Activity intolerance
- Bathing or hygiene self-care deficit
- Chronic pain
- Energy field disturbance
- Fatigue
- Hopelessness
- Impaired physical mobility
- Ineffective health maintenance
- Ineffective role performance
- Ineffective tissue perfusion: Peripheral
- Powerlessness
- Risk for impaired skin integrity
- Risk for infection

EXPECTED OUTCOMES
The patient will:
- verbalize the importance of balancing activity, as tolerated, with rest
- participate in activities of daily living to the fullest extent possible
- express feelings of increased comfort and decreased pain
- express an increased sense of well-being
- express feelings of increased energy
- make decisions on own behalf
- attain the highest degree of mobility possible within the confines of the disease
- continue to receive treatments that promote relaxation and inner well-being
- recognize limitations imposed by the illness and express feelings about these limitations
- maintain adequate peripheral perfusion, as evidenced by palpable pulses and warm extremities
- express feelings of control over condition
- maintain skin integrity
- remain free from signs or symptoms of infection.

NURSING INTERVENTIONS
- Give prescribed analgesics, and monitor effects.
- Perform meticulous skin care.
- Supply adaptive devices, such as a zipper-pull, easy-to-open beverage cartons, lightweight cups, and unpackaged silverware.

After total knee or hip arthroplasty
- Give prescribed blood products and antibiotics.
- Have the patient perform active dorsiflexion; immediately report inability to do so.
- Supervise isometric exercises every 2 hours.
- After total hip arthroplasty, check traction for pressure areas and keep head of bed raised 30 to 45 degrees.
- Change or reinforce dressings, as needed, using sterile technique.
- Have the patient turn, cough, and breathe deeply every 2 hours.
- After total knee arthroplasty, keep the leg extended and slightly elevated.
- After total hip arthroplasty, keep the hip in abduction. Watch for and immediately report inability to rotate the hip or bear weight on it, increased pain, or a leg that appears shorter.
- Assist patient in activities, keeping the weight on the unaffected side.
- Assess joint mobility and skin integrity.
- Assess pain level; administer analgesics, and evaluate response.
- Monitor vital signs, daily weight, serum electrolytes, hematocrit, and hemoglobin levels.
- Observe activity tolerance.

PATIENT TEACHING

Be sure to cover:
- disorder, diagnostic testing, and treatment
- chronic nature of rheumatoid arthritis and possible need for major lifestyle changes
- importance of a balanced diet and weight control
- importance of adequate sleep
- sexual concerns.

   If the patient requires total knee or hip arthroplasty, be sure to cover:
- preoperative and surgical procedures
- postoperative exercises
- deep-breathing and coughing exercises to perform after surgery
- performing frequent ROM leg exercises after surgery
- use of a constant-passive-motion device after total knee arthroplasty, or placement of an abduction pillow between the legs after total hip arthroplasty
- how to use a trapeze to move about in bed
- medication administration, dosage, and possible adverse effects
- contact information for the Arthritis Foundation.

RESOURCES
Organizations
Arthritis Foundation: *www.arthritis.org*
The Arthritis Society: *www.arthritis.ca*
Johns Hopkins Arthritis Center: *www.hopkins-arthritis.som.jhmi.edu*
National Institute of Arthritis and Musculoskeletal and Skin Diseases: *www.nih.gov/niams/healthinfo*

Selected references
Bathon, J.M., et al. "Safety and Efficacy of Etanercept Treatment in Elderly Subjects with Rheumatoid Arthritis," *Journal of Rheumatology* 33(2):234-43, February 2006.
Firestein, G.S. "Inhibiting Inflammation in Rheumatoid Arthritis," *New England Journal of Medicine* 354(1):80-82, January 2006.
Leff, L. "Emerging New Therapies in Rheumatoid Arthritis; What's Next for the Patient?" *Journal of Infusion Nursing* 29(6):326-37, November-December 2006.
Professional Guide to Pathophysiology, 2nd ed. Philadelphia: Lippincott Williams & Wilkins, 2007.

Disorders affecting management of rheumatoid arthritis

This chart highlights disorders that affect the management of rheumatoid arthritis.

DISORDER	SIGNS AND SYMPTOMS	DIAGNOSTIC TEST RESULTS	TREATMENT AND CARE
Carpal tunnel syndrome (complication)	◆ Weakness, pain, burning, numbness, or tingling that occurs in one or both hands ◆ Paresthesia that worsens at night and in the morning ◆ Pain that spreads to the forearm and, in severe cases, as far as the shoulder ◆ Pain that's relieved by shaking the hands vigorously or dangling the arms at sides ◆ Inability to make a fist	◆ Electromyography shows a median nerve motor conduction delay of more than 5 milliseconds ◆ Digital electrical stimulation shows median nerve compression by measuring the length and intensity of stimulation from the fingers to the median nerve in the wrist.	◆ Assist the patient in applying a splint to the wrist. ◆ Administer nonsteroidal anti-inflammatory drugs or corticosteroids, as ordered. ◆ Provide preoperative and postoperative care, as appropriate.
Osteoporosis (complication)	◆ Vertebral collapse ◆ Backache with pain that radiates around the trunk ◆ Increased deformity of the spine ◆ Kyphosis ◆ Loss of height ◆ Markedly aged appearance	◆ X-rays show typical degeneration in the lower thoracic and lumbar vertebrae. The vertebral bodies may appear flattened and may look denser than normal. ◆ Bone mineral density shows demineralization. Loss of bone mineral becomes evident in later stages. ◆ Dual- or single-photon absorptiometry allows measurement of bone mass, which helps to assess the extremities, hips, and spine. ◆ Serum calcium, phosphorus, and alkaline phosphatase levels are all within normal limits, but parathyroid hormone level may be elevated. ◆ Bone biopsy shows thin, porous, but otherwise normal-looking bone.	◆ Carefully position the patient. ◆ Assist in ambulation and prescribed exercises. ◆ Check skin for redness, warmth, and new sites of pain, which may indicate new fracture. ◆ Perform passive range-of-motion exercises, or encourage the patient to perform active exercise. ◆ Institute safety precautions and help prevent fractures. ◆ Provide a balanced diet high in nutrients that support skeletal metabolism, such as vitamin D, calcium, and protein. ◆ Administer an analgesic and use heat to relieve pain. ◆ Teach the patient about the drug regimen, bracing (if indicated), and proper body mechanics.
Sjögren's syndrome (complication)	◆ Confirmed rheumatoid arthritis and a history of slowly developing Sjögren's syndrome (in about 50% of patients) ◆ Oral dryness, redness, burning, difficulty swallowing, ulcers, dental caries ◆ Difficulty talking ◆ Altered sense of taste, smell or both ◆ Photosensitivity, eye fatigue, itching, and mucoid discharge ◆ Dyspareunia and pruritus ◆ Generalized itching ◆ Fatigue ◆ Recurrent low-grade fever ◆ Arthralgia or myalgia and extraglandular findings, such as pneumonitis, nephritis, arthritis, neuropathy, and vasculitis	◆ A patient with Sjögren's syndrome has at least two of these conditions: Xerophthalmia, xerostomia, and an associated autoimmune or lymphoproliferative disorder. ◆ Antinuclear antibody testing is positive.	◆ Advise the patient to avoid drugs that decrease saliva production, such as atropine derivatives, antihistamines, anticholinergics, and antidepressants. ◆ Suggest high-protein, high-calorie liquid supplements to prevent malnutrition when mouth ulcers are painful. ◆ Encourage good oral hygiene. ◆ Suggest use of sunglasses to protect eyes. ◆ Encourage humidification in the home to prevent dryness of nasal passages. ◆ Advise to avoid prolonged hot showers and baths and to use moisturizing lotions to help ease dry skin.
Spinal compression fractures (complication)	◆ Muscle spasms and back pain that worsens with movement ◆ Point tenderness with cervical fractures ◆ Pain radiating to other body areas with dorsal and lumbar fractures ◆ Mild paresthesia to quadriplegia and shock (if injury involves the spinal cord)	◆ Computed tomography scan, magnetic resonance imaging, and X-rays locate fracture.	◆ Suspect cord damage until proven otherwise. ◆ Immobilize the patient on a firm surface. ◆ Prepare for surgical correction as necessary. ◆ Institute traction, as ordered, and assess circulation and effects of traction. ◆ Assist the patient with turning, log rolling, deep breathing, and coughing to prevent complications. ◆ Monitor vital signs and neurologic status; report changes. ◆ Assess respiratory function and effort.

Sarcoidosis

OVERVIEW

- Multisystemic, granulomatous disorder that characteristically produces lymphadenopathy, pulmonary infiltration, and skeletal, liver, eye, or skin lesions
- May be acute (usually resolves within 2 years) or chronic
- Chronic, progressive sarcoidosis (uncommon) associated with pulmonary fibrosis and progressive pulmonary disability
- Most common in people ages 20 to 40
- In United States, occurs predominantly among blacks
- Affects twice as many women as men
- Slightly higher incidence in families, suggesting genetic predisposition

CAUSES

- Exact cause unknown
- Possible causes:
- Hypersensitivity response to atypical mycobacteria, fungi, and pine pollen
- Chemicals
- T-cell abnormalities
- Lymphokine production abnormalities

PATHOPHYSIOLOGY

- Monocyte-macrophages accumulate in the target tissue where they induce the inflammatory process.
- $CD4^+$ T-lymphocytes and sensitized immune cells form a ring around the inflamed area.
- Fibroblasts, mast cells, collagen fibers, and proteoglycans encase the inflammatory and immune cells, causing granuloma formation.

RESPIRATORY SYSTEM

- An excessive inflammatory process begins in the alveoli, bronchioles, and blood vessels of the lungs.
- Inflammation results in exertional oxygen desaturation, bilateral hilar lymphadenopathy, pulmonary infiltrates, and fibrosis. (See *Disorders affecting management of sarcoidosis*, page 395.)

INTEGUMENTARY SYSTEM

- Granulomatous skin lesions develop and often cause erythema nodosum.

CARDIOVASCULAR SYSTEM

- Changes in lung movement and gas exchange indirectly affect cardiac vasculature and muscle function.
- Heart block and sudden death may occur.

NEUROLOGIC SYSTEM

- Accumulation of T lymphocytes, mononuclear phagocytes, and non-secreting epithelial granulomas distort normal tissue architecture.
- Depending on the distribution of the granulomas, muscle involvement may result in myositis and nerve involvement may result in a neuropathy.
- Cranial nerve palsies, hypothalamic or pituitary dysfunction, or lymphocytic meningitis may result.

ASSESSMENT

HISTORY

- Pain in the wrists, ankles, and elbows
- General fatigue and malaise
- Unexplained weight loss
- Breathlessness and dyspnea
- Nonproductive cough
- Substernal pain

PHYSICAL FINDINGS

- Erythema nodosum
- Punched out lesions on the fingers and toes
- Cranial or peripheral nerve palsies
- Extensive nasal mucosal lesions
- Anterior uveitis
- Glaucoma and blindness occasionally in advanced disease
- Bilateral hilar and paratracheal lymphadenopathy
- Splenomegaly
- Arrhythmias

DIAGNOSTIC TEST RESULTS

- Arterial blood gas (ABG) analysis shows a decreased partial pressure of arterial oxygen and increased carbon dioxide levels.
- Chest X-rays show bilateral hilar and right paratracheal adenopathy, with or without diffuse interstitial infiltrates.
- Kveim test shows granuloma development at the injection site in 2 to 4 weeks when positive.
- Lymph node, skin, or lung biopsy shows noncaseating granulomas with negative cultures for mycobacteria and fungi.
- Pulmonary function tests show decreased total lung capacity and compliance and reduced diffusing capacity.

TREATMENT

GENERAL
- None needed for sarcoidosis that produces no symptoms
- Protection from sunlight

DIET
- Low-calcium for hypercalcemia
- Reduced-sodium, high-calorie
- Adequate fluids

ACTIVITY
- As tolerated

MEDICATIONS
- Corticosteroids
- Nonsteroidal anti-inflammatory drugs
- Antimetabolites
- Antimalarials

SURGERY
- Lung transplantation

NURSING CONSIDERATIONS

NURSING DIAGNOSES
- Activity intolerance
- Anxiety
- Complicated grieving
- Fear
- Imbalanced nutrition: Less than body requirements
- Impaired gas exchange
- Risk for infection

EXPECTED OUTCOMES
The patient will:
- perform activities of daily living within confines of the illness
- identify strategies to reduce anxiety
- use support systems to assist with coping
- discuss fears and concerns
- maintain adequate nutrition and hydration
- maintain adequate ventilation and oxygenation
- remain free from signs and symptoms of infection.

NURSING INTERVENTIONS
- Give prescribed drugs and monitor response.
- Administer supplemental oxygen.
- Provide a nutritious, high-calorie diet.
- Encourage oral fluid intake.
- Provide a low-calcium diet for hypercalcemia.
- Provide comfort measures and emotional support.
- Include the patient in care decisions whenever possible.
- Monitor vital signs, cardiac rhythm, intake and output, and daily weight.
- Assess respiratory status, sputum production, and ABG results.
- Monitor blood glucose levels.

WARNING *Because corticosteroids may induce or worsen diabetes mellitus, test the patient's blood by fingersticks for glucose and acetone at least every 12 hours at the beginning of corticosteroid therapy. Also, watch for other adverse effects, such as fluid retention, electrolyte imbalance (especially hypokalemia), moon face, hypertension, and personality changes.*

(continued)

Be sure to cover:
- disorder, diagnostic testing, and treatment
- medication administration, dosage, and possible adverse effects
- when to notify the practitioner
- steroid therapy
- need for regular follow-up examinations
- importance of wearing a medical identification bracelet
- measures to prevent infection
- contact information for community support and resource groups such as the National Sarcoidosis Resource Center.

RESOURCES
Organizations
American Lung Association:
www.lungusa.org
American Thoracic Society:
www.thoracic.org
National Sarcoidosis Resource Center:
www.nsrc-global.net
Sarcoidosis Center:
www.sarcoidcenter.com

Selected references
Caca, I., et al. "Conjunctival Deposits as the First Sign of Systemic Sarcoidosis in a Pediatric Patient," *European Journal of Ophthalmology* 16(1):168-70, January-February 2006.

Choi, H.J., et al. "Papular Sarcoidosis Limited to the Knees: A Clue for Systemic Sarcoidosis," *International Journal of Dermatology* 45(2):169-70, February 2006.

Doughan, A.R., and Williams, B.R. "Cardiac Sarcoidosis," *Heart* 92(2):282-88, February 2006.

Nicholson, B., and Mills, S. "Sarcoidosis of the Breast: An Unusual Presentation of a Systemic Disease," *The Breast Journal* 13(1):99-100, January-February 2007.

Sullivan, M., and Mason, L. "Slowly Dying from Sarcoidosis: A Patient's Story of Hanging on and Letting Go," *Journal of Palliative Care* 22(2):119-23, Summer 2006.

Disorders affecting management of sarcoidosis

This chart highlights disorders that affect the management of sarcoidosis.

DISORDER	SIGNS AND SYMPTOMS	DIAGNOSTIC TEST RESULTS	TREATMENT AND CARE
Acute respiratory failure (complication)	◆ Tachypnea ◆ Cyanosis ◆ Crackles, rhonchi, wheezing ◆ Diminished breath sounds ◆ Restlessness ◆ Altered mental status ◆ Tachycardia ◆ Increased cardiac output ◆ Increased blood pressure ◆ Cardiac arrhythmias	◆ Arterial blood gas (ABG) values show deteriorating values and a pH below 7.35. ◆ Chest X-ray shows pulmonary disease or condition. ◆ Electrocardiography may show cardiac arrhythmia or right ventricular hypertrophy. ◆ Pulse oximetry shows decreasing arterial oxygen saturation.	◆ Monitor ABG values and pulse oximetry. ◆ Monitor vital signs and intake and output. ◆ Monitor cardiac rhythm for arrhythmias. ◆ Administer antibiotics, bronchodilators, corticosteroids, positive inotropic agents, diuretics, vasopressors, or antiarrhythmics.
Cor pulmonale (complication)	◆ Progressive dyspnea worsening on exertion ◆ Tachycardia and bounding pulse ◆ Tachypnea and orthopnea ◆ Dependent edema ◆ Weakness ◆ Distended jugular veins ◆ Enlarged, tender liver and enlarged spleen	◆ Echocardiography or angiography indicates right ventricular enlargement. ◆ Pulmonary artery pressure (PAP) measurement shows increased right ventricular pressure. ◆ Chest X-ray shows right ventricular enlargement. ◆ Electrocardiography may show cardiac arrhythmia.	◆ Administer oxygen therapy and monitor respiratory status; assist with endotracheal intubation and mechanical ventilation, if necessary. ◆ Assess breath sounds and note changes.
Pulmonary hypertension (complication)	◆ Dyspnea on exertion ◆ Weakness, fatigue ◆ Pain during breathing ◆ Near-syncopal episodes ◆ Peripheral edema ◆ Jugular vein distention ◆ Hepatomegaly ◆ Tachycardia and hypotension ◆ Widely split S_2, presence of S_3 and S_4, and systolic ejection murmur ◆ Decreased breath sounds	◆ ABG values show hypoxia. ◆ Ventilation-perfusion lung scan may show a ventilation-perfusion mismatch. ◆ Pulmonary angiography may reveal filling defects in the pulmonary vasculature. ◆ Pulmonary artery catheterization shows increased PAP, with systolic pressures above 30 mm Hg; increased pulmonary artery wedge pressure; decreased cardiac output; and decreased cardiac index ◆ Pulmonary function tests may show decreased flow rates and increased residual volume or reduced total lung capacity.	◆ Encourage bed rest to reduce myocardial oxygen demands. ◆ Administer digoxin, antibiotics or pulmonary artery vasodilators, such as diazoxide, nitroprusside, hydralazine, angiotensin-converting enzyme inhibitors, calcium channel blockers, or prostaglandins to reduce pulmonary hypertension. ◆ Provide oxygen therapy and suctioning and encourage deep breathing and coughing. ◆ Monitor vital signs, pulse oximetry, intake and output, and laboratory values.

■ Septic shock LIFE-THREATENING DISORDER

OVERVIEW

◆ Probable response to infections that release microbes or an immune mediator
◆ Causes a low systemic vascular resistance and an elevated cardiac output

CAUSES

◆ Any pathogenic organism
◆ Gram-negative bacteria, such as *Escherichia coli, Klebsiella pneumoniae, Serratia, Enterobacter,* and *Pseudomonas,* most common causes (up to 70% of cases)

RISK FACTORS

◆ Young or old age
◆ Impaired immunity
   WARNING About two-thirds of septic shock cases occur in hospitalized patients, most of whom have underlying diseases. Those at high risk for septic shock include patients with burns, diabetes mellitus, immunosuppression, malnutrition, stress, and chronic cardiac, hepatic, or renal disorders. Also at risk are patients who have undergone invasive diagnostic or therapeutic procedures, surgery, traumatic wounds, or excessive antibiotic therapy.

PATHOPHYSIOLOGY

◆ Endotoxins released by bacteria trigger an immune response in which macrophages secrete immune mediators such as tumor necrosis factor (TNF) or interleukin-1.
◆ The immune mediators cause increased release of platelet-activating factor (PAF), prostaglandins, leukotrienes, thromboxane A2, kinins, and complement.
◆ Eventually, cardiac output decreases, and poor tissue perfusion and hypotension cause multisystem dysfunction syndrome and death.

CARDIOVASCULAR SYSTEM

◆ As the body's defense system activates chemical mediators, low systemic vascular resistance and increased cardiac output results. Blood flow is unevenly distributed in the microcirculation and plasma leaks from the capillaries, causing functional hypovolemia. Eventually, hypovolemia leads to decreased cardiac output and poor tissue perfusion and hypotension, causing multisystem organ dysfunction syndrome and, ultimately, death.

HEMATOLOGIC SYSTEM

◆ The release of TNF and endotoxins activates the clotting cascade, damaging tissue.
◆ The mediators involved in the inflammatory process upset the balance of coagulation and fibrinolysis, which may lead to disseminated intravascular coagulation.

INTEGUMENTARY SYSTEM

◆ Vasodilation of peripheral vessels and decreased systemic vascular resistance cause the patient's skin to appear flushed.
◆ Later, peripheral vasoconstriction occurs and systemic vascular resistance increases, leading to pallor and cyanosis.

NEUROLOGIC SYSTEM

◆ Vasodilation and vasoconstriction affect the cerebral blood vessels, leading to changes in levels of consciousness (LOC).

RESPIRATORY SYSTEM

◆ Increased capillary permeability in the pulmonary vasculature affects gas exchange.
◆ Fluid shifting leads to pulmonary edema, alveolar damage, and alveolar collapse.
◆ The release of histamine from endotoxins further damages the alveolar capillary membrane, leading to increased fluid shifting.
◆ Continued pulmonary edema and inflammation can lead to fibrosis and acute respiratory distress syndrome (ARDS).

RENAL SYSTEM

◆ Endotoxin production promotes vasoconstriction, impairing blood flow to the kidneys.
◆ Glomerular membrane damage and increased capillary permeability can lead to renal failure. (See *Disorders affecting management of septic shock,* pages 399 to 401.)

HISTORY

◆ Possible disorder or treatment that can cause immunosuppression
◆ Possibly, previous invasive tests or treatments, surgery, or trauma
◆ Possible fever and chills (although 20% of patients possibly hypothermic)

PHYSICAL FINDINGS

Hyperdynamic (or warm) phase
◆ Peripheral vasodilation
◆ Skin possibly pink and flushed or warm and dry
◆ Altered mental status
◆ Respirations rapid and shallow
◆ Urine output below normal
◆ Rapid, full, bounding pulse
◆ Blood pressure normal or slightly elevated

Hypodynamic (or cold) phase
◆ Peripheral vasoconstriction and inadequate tissue perfusion
◆ Pale skin and possible cyanosis
◆ Decreased LOC; possible obtundation and coma
◆ Respirations possibly rapid and shallow
◆ Urine output possibly less than 25 ml/hour or absent
◆ Rapid, weak, thready pulse
◆ Irregular pulse if arrhythmias are present
◆ Cold, clammy skin
◆ Hypotension
◆ Crackles or rhonchi if pulmonary congestion is present

DIAGNOSTIC TEST RESULTS

◆ Blood cultures are positive for the causative organism.
◆ Complete blood count shows severe or absent neutropenia, and usually thrombocytopenia.
◆ Blood urea nitrogen and creatinine levels are increased, and creatinine clearance is decreased.
◆ Prothrombin time and partial thromboplastin time are abnormal.

◆ Serum lactate dehydrogenase levels are elevated (with metabolic acidosis).
◆ Urine studies show increased specific gravity (more than 1.02), increased osmolality, and decreased sodium levels.
◆ Arterial blood gas (ABG) analysis demonstrates increased blood pH, decreased partial pressure of arterial oxygen and decreased partial pressure of arterial carbon dioxide (with respiratory alkalosis in early stages).
◆ Invasive hemodynamic monitoring shows:
– increased cardiac output and decreased systemic vascular resistance in warm phase
– decreased cardiac output and increased systemic vascular resistance in cold phase.

GENERAL

◆ Removal or replacement of I.V., intra-arterial, or urinary drainage catheters whenever possible
◆ In patients immunosuppressed from drug therapy, drugs discontinued or reduced, if possible
◆ Mechanical ventilation if respiratory failure occurs
◆ Fluid volume replacement

DIET

◆ Possible parenteral nutrition or tube feedings

ACTIVITY

◆ Bed rest

MEDICATIONS

◆ Antimicrobials
◆ Granulocyte transfusions
◆ Colloid or crystalloid infusions
◆ Oxygen
◆ Diuretics
◆ Vasopressors
◆ Antipyretics
◆ Drotrecogin alfa (Xigris)
◆ I.V. fluids

(continued)

NURSING CONSIDERATIONS

NURSING DIAGNOSES
- Anxiety
- Decreased cardiac output
- Deficient fluid volume
- Disabled family coping
- Impaired gas exchange
- Ineffective tissue perfusion: Cardiopulmonary, renal
- Risk for imbalanced body temperature
- Risk for infection
- Risk for injury

EXPECTED OUTCOMES
The patient (or family) will:
- verbalize strategies to reduce anxiety
- maintain adequate cardiac output and hemodynamic stability
- maintain adequate fluid volume
- express feelings and develop adequate coping mechanisms
- maintain adequate ventilation and oxygenation
- maintain adequate cardiopulmonary and renal perfusion
- maintain a normal body temperature
- remain free from signs and symptoms of infection
- remain free from injury.

NURSING INTERVENTIONS
- Remove or replace I.V., intra-arterial, or urinary drainage catheters, and send them to the laboratory to culture for the presence of the causative organism.
- Give prescribed I.V. fluids and blood products.

 WARNING *A progressive drop in blood pressure with a thready pulse usually signals inadequate cardiac output from reduced intravascular volume. Notify the practitioner immediately, and increase the infusion rate.*

WARNING *Be alert for signs and symptoms of possible fluid overload, such as dyspnea, tachypnea, crackles, peripheral edema, jugular vein distention, and increased pulmonary artery pressures.*

- Administer appropriate antimicrobial I.V. drugs.
- Notify the practitioner if urine output is less than 30 ml/hour.
- Administer prescribed oxygen.
- Provide emotional support to the patient and his family.
- Document the occurrence of a nosocomial infection, and report it to the infection control practitioner.
- Monitor ABG levels and pulse oximetry.
- Monitor intake and output, vital signs, and hemodynamic parameters.

WARNING *Temperature is usually elevated in the early stages of septic shock, and the patient commonly experiences shaking chills. As shock progresses, temperature typically drops and the patient experiences diaphoresis. If the patient's systolic blood pressure drops below 80 mm Hg, increase the oxygen flow rate, and notify the physician immediately. Systolic blood pressure below 80 mm Hg usually results in inadequate coronary artery blood flow, cardiac ischemia, arrhythmias, and further complications of low cardiac output.*

- Observe continuous cardiac rhythm.
- Assess heart and breath sounds regularly.

PATIENT TEACHING

Be sure to cover:
- disorder, diagnostic testing, and treatment
- medication administration, dosage, and possible adverse effects
- risks associated with blood transfusions
- possible complications.

RESOURCES
Organizations
American Heart Association: *www.americanheart.org*
National Heart, Lung, and Blood Institute: *www.nhlbi.nih.gov*

Selected references
Clayson. L. "Identifying Sepsis," *Nursing Standards* 21(8):59, November 2006.
Hernandez, G., et al. "Implementation of a Norepinephrine-Based Protocol for Management of Septic Shock: A Pilot Feasibility Study," *Journal of Trauma—Injury, Infection and Critical Care* 60(1):77-81, January 2006.
Kleinpell, R., et al. "Incidence, Pathogenesis, and Management of Sepsis; An Overview," *AACN Advanced Critical Care* 17(4):385-93, October-December 2006.
Nettina, S.M. *Lippincott Manual of Nursing Practice*, 8th ed. Philadelphia: Lippincott Williams & Wilkins, 2006.
Rivers, E.P. "Early Goal-Directed Therapy in Severe Sepsis and Septic Shock: Converting Science to Reality," *Chest* 129(2):217-18, February 2006.
Sutherland, A.M., et al. "Are Vasopressin Levels Increased or Decreased in Septic Shock?" *Critical Care Medicine* 34(2):542-43, February 2006.

Disorders affecting management of septic shock

This chart highlights disorders that affect the management of septic shock.

DISORDER	SIGNS AND SYMPTOMS	DIAGNOSTIC TEST RESULTS	TREATMENT AND CARE
Acute renal failure (complication)	◆ Oliguria, azotemia and, rarely, anuria ◆ Electrolyte imbalance, metabolic acidosis ◆ Anorexia, nausea, vomiting, diarrhea or constipation, stomatitis, bleeding, hematemesis, dry mucous membranes, and uremic breath ◆ Headache, drowsiness, irritability, confusion, peripheral neuropathy, seizures, and coma ◆ Skin dryness, pruritus, pallor, purpura and, rarely, uremic frost ◆ Hypotension (early), hypertension, arrhythmias, fluid overload, heart failure, systemic edema, anemia, and altered clotting mechanisms (later) ◆ Pulmonary edema ◆ Kussmaul's respirations	◆ Blood studies show elevated blood urea nitrogen (BUN), serum creatinine, and potassium levels; decreased bicarbonate level, hematocrit, and hemoglobin levels; and low blood pH. ◆ Urine studies show casts, cellular debris, and decreased specific gravity. ◆ Creatinine clearance test measures glomerular filtration rate and reflects the number of remaining functioning nephrons. ◆ Electrocardiography shows tall, peaked T waves; widening QRS complex; and disappearing P waves if hyperkalemia is present.	◆ Measure and record intake and output, including body fluids. Weigh the patient daily. ◆ Anticipate fluid restriction to minimize edema. ◆ Assess hemoglobin levels and hematocrit and replace blood components. ◆ Monitor vital signs. Watch for and report signs of pericarditis (pleuritic chest pain, tachycardia pericardial friction rub), inadequate renal perfusion (hypotension) and acidosis. ◆ Maintain proper electrolyte balance. Strictly monitor potassium levels. ◆ Administer medications as ordered. ◆ Prepare for hemodialysis or peritoneal dialysis to correct electrolyte and fluid imbalances. ◆ Assess the patient frequently, especially during emergency treatment to lower potassium levels. ◆ Maintain nutritional status. Provide a high-calorie, low-protein, low-sodium diet with vitamin supplements. ◆ Encourage frequent coughing and deep breathing and perform passive range-of-motion exercises. ◆ Provide good mouth care frequently.
Acute respiratory distress syndrome (ARDS) (complication)	◆ Dyspnea on exertion ◆ Diminished breath sounds ◆ Tachypnea, tachycardia ◆ Increased respiratory distress with use of accessory muscles ◆ Restlessness, apprehension ◆ Dry cough or frothy sputum ◆ Cool, clammy skin that progresses to pallor and cyanosis ◆ Basilar crackles, rhonchi ◆ Decreased mental status ◆ Arrhythmias such as premature ventricular contractions ◆ Labile hypotension	◆ Arterial blood gas (ABG) analysis initially shows decreased partial pressure of arterial oxygen despite oxygen supplementation; partial pressure of arterial carbon dioxide ($Paco_2$) is decreased, causing an increase in blood pH; as ARDS worsens, $Paco_2$ increases and pH decreases as the patient becomes acidotic. ◆ Initially, chest X-rays may be normal. Basilar infiltrates begin to appear in about 24 hours. In later stages, lung fields have a ground-glass appearance; and, as fluid fills the alveoli, white patches appear. ◆ Pulmonary artery wedge pressure is 18 mm Hg or lower.	◆ Assess the patient's respiratory status, including lung sounds, heart rate, and blood pressure at least every 2 hours, or more often if indicated. Note respiratory rate, rhythm, and depth, reporting dyspnea and accessory muscle use. Be alert for inspiratory retractions. If the patient has injuries that affect his lungs, watch for adverse respiratory changes, especially in the first few days after the injury, when his condition may appear to be improving. ◆ Administer oxygen; assess oxygen saturation continuously; and monitor serial ABG levels. ◆ Check ventilator settings frequently. Assess hemodynamic parameters if a pulmonary catheter is inserted. ◆ Institute continuous cardiac monitoring and watch for arrhythmias. ◆ Monitor the patient's level of consciousness, noting confusion or mental sluggishness. ◆ Be alert for signs of treatment-induced complications, including arrhythmias, disseminated intravascular coagulation (DIC), GI bleeding, infection, malnutrition, paralytic ileus, pneumothorax, pulmonary fibrosis, renal failure, thrombocytopenia, and tracheal stenosis. ◆ Give sedatives to reduce restlessness. Administer sedatives and analgesics at regular intervals if the patient is receiving neuromuscular blocking agents.

(continued)

DISORDER	SIGNS AND SYMPTOMS	DIAGNOSTIC TEST RESULTS	TREATMENT AND CARE
Acute respiratory distress syndrome (ARDS) (complication) *(continued)*			◆ Administer anti-infective agents, as ordered, if the underlying cause is sepsis or an infection. ◆ Place the patient in a comfortable position that maximizes air exchange such as semi-Fowler's or high-Fowler's position. ◆ Evaluate the patient's serum electrolyte levels frequently. ◆ Monitor urine output hourly to ensure adequate renal function. Weigh the patient daily. ◆ Record caloric intake. Administer tube feedings and parenteral nutrition.
Disseminated intravascular coagulation (complication)	◆ Abnormal bleeding without a history of a hemorrhagic disorder ◆ Bleeding into the skin, such as cutaneous oozing, petechiae, ecchymoses, and hematomas ◆ Bleeding from surgical or invasive procedure sites such as incisions or venipuncture sites ◆ Nausea, vomiting ◆ Severe muscle, back, and abdominal pain or chest pain ◆ Hemoptysis, epistaxis ◆ Seizures ◆ Oliguria ◆ Diminished peripheral pulses ◆ Hypotension ◆ Mental status changes, including confusion	◆ Platelet count is decreased. ◆ Fibrinogen level is less than 150 mg/dl. ◆ Prothrombin time is longer than 15 seconds. ◆ Partial thromboplastin time is longer than 60 seconds. ◆ Fibrin degradation products are increased, commonly greater than 45 mcg/ml. ◆ D-dimer test is positive at less than 1:8 dilutions. ◆ Fibrin monomers are positive; levels of factors V and VIII are diminished with fragmentation of red blood cells. ◆ Hemoglobin level is less than 10 g/dl. ◆ Urine studies reveal BUN greater than 25 mg/dl. ◆ Serum creatinine level is greater than 1.3 mg/dl.	◆ Ensure a patent airway and assess breathing and circulation. Monitor vital signs, cardiac and respiratory status closely, at least every 30 minutes—or more frequently—depending on the patient's condition. ◆ Observe skin color and check peripheral circulation, including color, temperature, and capillary refill. ◆ Administer supplemental oxygen and monitor oxygen saturation with continuous pulse oximetry and serial ABG studies; anticipate the need for endotracheal intubation and mechanical ventilation should the patient's respiratory status deteriorate. ◆ Assess neurologic status at least every hour—or more often, if indicated—for changes. ◆ Assess extent of blood loss and begin fluid replacement. Obtain a type and cross match for blood component therapy, and administer. ◆ If hypotension occurs, administer vasoactive drugs. ◆ Assess hemodynamic parameters, as indicated. ◆ Institute continuous cardiac monitoring to evaluate for possible arrhythmias, myocardial ischemia, or adverse effects of treatment. ◆ Administer medications, including I.V. heparin in low doses, antifibrinolytics, vitamin K, and folate. ◆ Assess urine output hourly. ◆ Check all stools and drainage for occult blood. ◆ Inspect skin and mucous membranes for signs of bleeding; assess all invasive insertion sites and dressings for evidence of frank bleeding or oozing. Weigh the dressings that are wet or saturated to aid in determining extent of blood loss. Watch for bleeding from the GI and genitourinary tracts. ◆ Institute bleeding precautions. Limit all invasive procedures, such as venipunctures and I.M. injections, as much as possible. Apply pressure for 3 to 5 minutes over venous insertion sites and 10 to 15 minutes over arterial sites. ◆ Institute safety precautions to minimize the risk of injury.

DISORDER	SIGNS AND SYMPTOMS	DIAGNOSTIC TEST RESULTS	TREATMENT AND CARE
Multiple organ dysfunction syndrome (complication)	◆ Tachycardia ◆ Increased respiratory rate; hyperventilation ◆ Oliguria or anuria ◆ Petechiae and purpura (with skin infection) ◆ Jaundice ◆ Confusion ◆ Coma ◆ Profound depression in mental status ◆ Poor distal perfusion, cool skin, cool extremities, delayed capillary refill ◆ Inflamed or swollen tympanic membranes, sinus tenderness, pharyngeal exudates, stridor, cervical lymphadenopathy (if patient has head and neck infection) ◆ Tenderness, guarding or rebound, rectal tenderness or swelling (if GI infection present) ◆ Costovertebral angle tenderness, pelvic tenderness, cervical motion pain, adnexal tenderness (with pelvic and genitourinary infections) ◆ Localized crackles or evidence of consolidation (if chest and pulmonary infection present) ◆ Regurgitant valvular murmur (with cardiac infection) ◆ Diminished bowel sounds	◆ Microbiologic studies show occult bacterial infection or bacteremia in sepsis and can indicate the specific microbial etiology. ◆ Platelet count decreases at onset of serious stress and falls with persistent sepsis; DIC may develop. ◆ White blood cell count is greater than 15,000 cells/µl or neutrophil band count is greater than 1,500 cells/µl, indicating bacterial infection. ◆ Serum creatinine and BUN are elevated if renal system is involved. ◆ Serum transaminase and bilirubin levels are increased. ◆ Alkaline phosphate and alanine aminotransferase are altered, indicating hepatic involvement. ◆ ABG analysis may show elevated serum lactate levels—evidence of tissue hypoperfusion. Higher serum lactate indicates a worse degree of shock and higher mortality. ◆ Altered prothrombin time and partial thromboplastin time show evidence of coagulopathy, as in DIC. ◆ Urinalysis and urine culture may show infecting organism in urinary tract infection. ◆ Tissue stain and culture from sites of potential infection may be positive for the causative organism. ◆ Chest X-ray may show infiltrates. ◆ Abdominal X-rays (supine and upright or lateral decubitus) may show source of intra-abdominal sepsis. ◆ Computed tomography (CT) scan may help diagnosis intra-abdominal abscess or retroperitoneal source of infection. CT scan of the head in patients with increased intracranial pressure or in patients undergoing lumbar puncture may show focal defects, sinusitis, or otitis (if meningitis is suspected). ◆ X-ray of the area of suspected involvement may show presence of soft tissue gas and spread of infection beyond disease site; surgical exploration may be required. ◆ Lumbar puncture may show evidence of meningitis. ◆ Pulmonary artery catheterization shows evidence of altered cardiac output and tissue oxygenation.	◆ Support respiratory and circulatory function with mechanical ventilation, supplemental oxygen, hemodynamic monitoring, and fluid volume therapy. ◆ Closely monitor renal function, including hourly urine output measurements and serial laboratory tests, for trends indicating renal failure. ◆ Prepare the patient for dialysis if indicated. ◆ Give drugs, such as antimicrobials, vasopressors (such as dopamine and norepinephrine), isotonic crystalloid solutions (such as normal saline and lactated Ringer's solution), and colloids (such as albumin).

Sickle cell anemia

OVERVIEW

- Congenital hemolytic disease that results from a defective hemoglobin (Hb) molecule (Hb S) that causes red blood cells (RBCs) to become sickle-shaped
- Impairs circulation, resulting in chronic ill health (fatigue, dyspnea on exertion, swollen joints), periodic crises, long-term complications, and premature death
- Most common in tropical Africans and in people of African descent
- About 1 in 10 blacks carrying the abnormal gene; if two such carriers have offspring, each child having a 1 in 4 chance of developing disease
- Affects 1 in every 500 blacks in the United States
- Also occurs in Puerto Rico, Turkey, India, the Middle East, and the Mediterranean area

CAUSES

- Homozygous inheritance of the Hb S-producing gene (defective Hb gene from each parent)

PATHOPHYSIOLOGY

- Sickle cell anemia results from substitution of the amino acid valine for glutamic acid in the Hb S gene encoding the beta chain of Hb.
- Abnormal Hb S in the RBCs becomes insoluble during hypoxia. As a result, these cells become rigid, rough, and elongated, forming a crescent or sickle shape. (See *Characteristics of sickled cells.*)
- The sickling produces hemolysis. The altered cells accumulate in the capillaries and smaller blood vessels, increasing the viscosity of the blood. Normal circulation is impaired, causing pain, tissue infarctions, and swelling.
- Each patient with sickle cell anemia has a different hypoxic threshold and particular factors that trigger a sickle cell crisis. Illness, exposure to cold, stress, acidotic states, or a pathophysiologic process that pulls water out of the sickle cells can precipitate sickle cell crisis. (See *Sickle cell crisis.*)
- The obstructions lead to anoxic changes that cause additional sick-ling and blockage and can affect multiple organs. (See *Disorders affecting management of sickle cell anemia,* pages 406 and 407.)

CARDIOVASCULAR SYSTEM

- Sickled cells accumulate in the heart and blood vessels, obstructing blood flow.
- Oxygen delivery to the heart and organs supplied by the blood vessels is diminished, causing ischemia and, possibly, necrosis.
- Obstruction and ischemia, when coupled with the already sluggish blood flow and chronic anemia, can lead to heart failure, cardiomegaly, and systolic murmurs.

GENITOURINARY SYSTEM

- The blood vessels supplying the kidneys can become obstructed by sickle cells, which can lead to decreased renal perfusion that, in turn, affects the capillary permeability of the glomerulus and may lead to renal failure.
- Plasma proteins, such as albumin, can be lost, leading to hyperprotein-

---

Characteristics of sickled cells

Normal red blood cells (RBCs) and sickled cells vary in shape, life span, oxygen-carrying capacity, and the rate at which they're destroyed. These illustrations show normal and sickled cells and list their major differences.

NORMAL RBCS

- 120-day life span
- Hemoglobin (Hb) has normal oxygen-carrying capacity
- 12 to 14 g/ml of Hb
- RBCs destroyed at normal rate

SICKLED CELLS

- 30- to 40-day life span
- Hb has decreased oxygen-carrying capacity
- 6 to 9 g/ml of Hb
- RBCs destroyed at accelerated rate

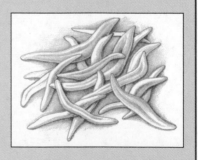

uria and hypoalbuminemia, which may progress to nephrotic syndrome.

IMMUNE SYSTEM

◆ Obstruction of blood flow to the spleen by sickled cells leads to ischemia, impairing the spleen's filtering capability. Functioning cells are gradually replaced with fibrotic tissue.
◆ Impaired splenic function places the patient at high risk for infections.

NEUROLOGIC SYSTEM

◆ Sickle cells accumulate in cerebral vessels, obstructing the blood flow to the brain and leading to decreased cerebral perfusion and cerebral ischemia. Stroke may occur.

ASSESSMENT

HISTORY

◆ Signs and symptoms usually not apparent until after age 6 months
◆ Chronic fatigue
◆ Unexplained dyspnea or dyspnea on exertion
◆ Joint swelling
◆ Aching bones
◆ Chest pain
◆ Ischemic leg ulcers
◆ Increased susceptibility to infection
◆ Pulmonary infarctions and cardiomegaly

Sickle cell crisis

Infection, exposure to cold, high altitudes, overexertion, or other situations that cause cellular oxygen deprivation may trigger a sickle cell crisis. The deoxygenated, sickle-shaped red blood cells stick to the capillary wall and each other, blocking blood flow and causing cellular hypoxia. The crisis worsens as tissue hypoxia and acidic waste products cause more sickling and cell damage. With each new crisis, organs and tissues are slowly destroyed; the spleen and kidneys are particularly prone to damage.

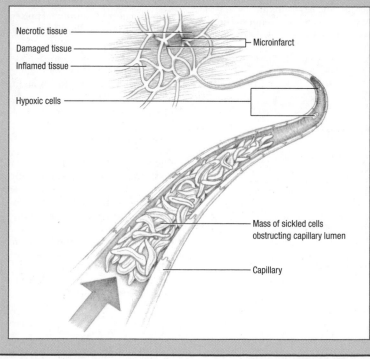

Necrotic tissue
Damaged tissue
Inflamed tissue
Microinfarct
Hypoxic cells
Mass of sickled cells obstructing capillary lumen
Capillary

PHYSICAL FINDINGS

◆ Jaundice or pallor
◆ Small in stature for age
◆ Delayed growth and puberty
◆ Spiderlike body build (narrow shoulders and hips, long extremities, curved spine, and barrel chest) in adult
◆ Tachycardia
◆ Hepatomegaly and, in children, splenomegaly
◆ Systolic and diastolic murmurs
◆ Sleepiness, with difficulty awakening
◆ Hematuria
◆ Pale lips, tongue, palms, and nail beds
◆ Body temperature greater than 104° F (40° C) or a temperature of 100° F (37.8° C) that persists for 2 or more days

In painful crisis

◆ Most common crisis and the hallmark of the disease; usually appears periodically after age 5, characterized by severe abdominal, thoracic, muscle, or bone pain and, possibly, increased jaundice, dark urine, and a low-grade fever

In aplastic crisis

◆ Pallor, lethargy, sleepiness, dyspnea, possible coma, markedly decreased bone marrow activity, and RBC hemolysis

In acute splenic sequestration crisis

◆ Occurs in infants between ages 8 months and 2 years; causes lethargy and pallor and, if untreated, progresses to hypovolemic shock and death

In hemolytic crisis

◆ Liver congestion and hepatomegaly

DIAGNOSTIC TEST RESULTS

◆ Stained blood smear shows sickle cells; Hb electrophoresis shows Hb S. (Electrophoresis should be done on umbilical cord blood samples of all neonates at risk to provide sickle cell disease screening at birth.)

(continued)

- RBC counts are decreased, white blood cell and platelet counts are elevated, erythrocyte sedimentation rate is decreased, and serum iron levels are increased.
- RBC survival is decreased, and reticulocytosis is present; Hb levels are normal or low.
- A lateral chest X-ray detects the characteristic "Lincoln log" deformity. (This spinal abnormality develops in many adults and in some adolescents with sickle cell anemia, leaving the vertebrae resembling logs that form the corner of a cabin.)
- Ophthalmoscopic examination reveals corkscrew-shaped or comma-shaped vessels in the conjunctivae.

TREATMENT

GENERAL
- Avoidance of extreme temperatures
- Avoidance of stress

DIET
- Well-balanced
- Adequate amounts of folic acid–rich foods
- Adequate fluid intake

ACTIVITY
- Bed rest in crisis
- As tolerated

MEDICATIONS
- Vaccines, such as polyvalent pneumococcal vaccine and *Haemophilus influenzae* type B vaccine
- Anti-infectives
- Analgesics
- Iron supplements
- Transfusion of packed RBCs, if Hb level decreases suddenly or if condition deteriorates rapidly
- Sedation and administration of analgesics, blood transfusion, oxygen therapy, and large amounts of oral or I.V. fluids, in an acute sequestration crisis

NURSING CONSIDERATIONS

NURSING DIAGNOSES
- Acute pain
- Delayed growth and development
- Disturbed body image
- Fatigue
- Hyperthermia
- Impaired gas exchange
- Impaired tissue integrity
- Ineffective tissue perfusion: Peripheral
- Risk for deficient fluid volume

EXPECTED OUTCOMES
The patient will:
- express feelings of increased comfort and decreased pain
- demonstrate age-appropriate skills and behaviors to the extent possible
- verbalize feelings about changed body image
- express feelings of energy and decreased fatigue
- remain afebrile
- exhibit adequate ventilation and oxygenation
- maintain normal skin color and temperature
- maintain normal peripheral pulses
- maintain balanced fluid volume in which input equals output.

NURSING INTERVENTIONS
- Encourage the patient to talk about his fears and concerns.
- Ensure that the patient receives adequate amounts of folic acid–rich foods, such as green, leafy vegetables.
- Encourage adequate fluid intake.
- Apply warm compresses, warmed thermal blankets, and warming pads or mattresses to painful areas of the patient's body, unless he has neuropathy.
- Administer analgesics and antipyretics, as necessary.
- When culture specimens demonstrate the presence of infection, give prescribed antibiotics.

- Give prescribed prophylactic antibiotics.
- Use strict sterile technique when performing treatments.
- Encourage bed rest, with the head of the bed elevated to decrease tissue oxygen demand.
- Administer oxygen, as needed.
- Administer blood transfusions.
- Monitor vital signs, intake and output, and complete blood count and other laboratory study results.

PATIENT TEACHING

Be sure to cover:
- disorder, diagnostic testing, and treatment
- medication administration, dosage, and possible adverse effects
- conditions that provoke hypoxia, such as strenuous exercise, use of vasoconstrictors, cold temperatures, unpressurized aircraft, and high altitude
- importance of normal childhood immunizations, meticulous wound care, good oral hygiene, regular dental checkups, and a balanced diet
- need for prompt treatment of infection
- need to increase fluid intake to prevent dehydration
- symptoms of vaso-occlusive crisis
- need to inform all health care providers about the disorder before patient undergoes any treatment, especially major surgery
- effect on pregnancy
- information about genetic counseling
- birth control counseling for women with sickle cell anemia.

RESOURCES
Organizations
Sickle Cell Disease Association of America: *www.sicklecelldisease.org*
U.S. Food and Drug Administration: *www.fda.gov*

Selected references

Sibinga, E., et al. "Pediatric Patients with Sickle Cell Disease: Use of Complementary and Alternative Therapies," *Journal of Complementary and Alternative Medicine* 12(3):291-98, April 2006.
Strategies for Managing Multisystem Disorders. Philadelphia: Lippincott Williams & Wilkins, 2006.
Thomas, V., and Cohn, T. "Communication Skills and Cultural Awareness Courses for Healthcare Professionals Who Care for Patients with Sickle Cell Disease," *Journal of Advanced Nursing* 53(4):480-48, February 2006.
Westfold, F. "Sickle Cell Disorders," *Nursing Standard* 20(38):67, May-June 2006.

(continued)

Disorders affecting management of sickle cell anemia

This chart highlights disorders that affect the management of sickle cell anemia.

DISORDER	SIGNS AND SYMPTOMS	DIAGNOSTIC TEST RESULTS	TREATMENT AND CARE
Acute renal failure (complication)	◆ Oliguria, azotemia and, rarely, anuria ◆ Electrolyte imbalance, metabolic acidosis ◆ Anorexia, nausea, vomiting, diarrhea or constipation, stomatitis, bleeding, hematemesis, dry mucous membranes, and uremic breath ◆ Headache, drowsiness, irritability, confusion, peripheral neuropathy, seizures, and coma ◆ Skin dryness, pruritus, pallor, purpura and, rarely, uremic frost ◆ Hypotension (early); hypertension, arrhythmias, fluid overload, heart failure, systemic edema, anemia, and altered clotting mechanisms (later) ◆ Pulmonary edema ◆ Kussmaul's respirations	◆ Blood studies show elevated blood urea nitrogen (BUN), serum creatinine, and potassium levels; decreased bicarbonate level, hematocrit, and hemoglobin levels; and low blood pH. ◆ Urine studies show casts, cellular debris, and decreased specific gravity; urine sodium level is more than 40 mEq/L. ◆ Creatinine clearance test measures glomerular filtration rate and reflects the number of remaining functioning nephrons. ◆ Electrocardiography shows tall, peaked T waves; widening QRS complex; and disappearing P waves if hyperkalemia is present.	◆ Measure and record intake and output, including body fluids. Weigh the patient daily. ◆ Anticipate fluid restriction to minimize edema. ◆ Assess hemoglobin levels and hematocrit and replace blood components. ◆ Monitor vital signs. Watch for and report signs of pericarditis (pleuritic chest pain, tachycardia, pericardial friction rub), inadequate renal perfusion (hypotension), and acidosis. ◆ Maintain proper electrolyte balance. Strictly monitor potassium levels. ◆ Administer medications such as diuretic therapy to treat oliguric phase; sodium polystyrene sulfonate by mouth or enema to reverse hyperkalemia; and hypertonic glucose, insulin, and sodium bicarbonate I.V. for more severe hyperkalemic symptoms. ◆ Prepare for hemodialysis or peritoneal dialysis to correct electrolyte and fluid imbalances. ◆ Assess the patient frequently, especially during emergency treatment to lower potassium levels. If the patient receives hypertonic glucose and insulin infusions, monitor potassium and glucose levels. If sodium polystyrene sulfonate is used rectally, make sure the patient doesn't retain it and become constipated. Doing so prevents bowel perforation. ◆ Maintain nutritional status. Give the anorexic patient small, frequent meals. ◆ Encourage frequent coughing and deep breathing and perform passive range-of-motion exercises. ◆ Provide frequent mouth care.
Heart failure (complication)	*Left-sided heart failure* ◆ Dyspnea ◆ Orthopnea ◆ Paroxysmal nocturnal dyspnea ◆ Fatigue ◆ Nonproductive cough ◆ Crackles ◆ Hemoptysis ◆ Tachycardia ◆ S_3, S_4 ◆ Cool, pale skin ◆ Restlessness and confusion *Right-sided heart failure* ◆ Jugular vein distention ◆ Positive hepatojugular reflex ◆ Right upper quadrant pain ◆ Anorexia, nausea ◆ Nocturia ◆ Weight gain, edema ◆ Ascites or anasarca	◆ Chest X-ray shows increased pulmonary vascular markings, interstitial edema, or pleural effusions and cardiomegaly. ◆ Electrocardiography may reveal hypertrophy, ischemic changes or infarction, tachycardia, and extrasystoles. ◆ Liver function test may be abnormal; BUN and creatinine levels may be elevated. ◆ Prothrombin time may be prolonged. ◆ B-type natriuretic peptide (BNP) immunoassay is elevated. ◆ Echocardiography may reveal left ventricular hypertrophy, dilation, and abnormal contractility. ◆ Pulmonary artery pressure, pulmonary artery wedge pressure, and left ventricular end-diastolic pressure are elevated in left-sided heart failure; right atrial or central venous pressure is elevated in right-sided heart failure. ◆ Radionuclide ventriculography may reveal ejection fraction less than 40% in diastolic dysfunction.	◆ Place the patient in Fowler's position and give supplemental oxygen. ◆ Weigh the patient daily, and check for peripheral edema. ◆ Monitor intake and output, vital signs, and mental status. ◆ Auscultate for S_3 and S_4 and adventitious lung sounds such as crackles or rhonchi. ◆ Monitor BUN, creatinine, and serum potassium, sodium, chloride, and magnesium. ◆ Institute continuous cardiac monitoring to identify and treat arrhythmias promptly. ◆ Administer angiotensin-converting enzyme inhibitors, digoxin, diuretics, beta-adrenergic blockers, human BNPs, nitrates, and morphine. ◆ Encourage lifestyle modifications, as appropriate.

Disorders affecting management of sickle cell anemia *(continued)*

DISORDER	SIGNS AND SYMPTOMS	DIAGNOSTIC TEST RESULTS	TREATMENT AND CARE
Stroke (complication)	◆ Headache with no known cause ◆ Numbness or weakness of the face, arm, or leg, especially on one side of the body ◆ Confusion, trouble speaking or understanding ◆ Trouble seeing or walking, dizziness, and loss of coordination	◆ Magnetic resonance imaging or a computed tomography scan shows evidence of thrombosis or hemorrhage. ◆ Brain scan reveals ischemia (may not be positive for up to 2 weeks after the stroke). ◆ Lumbar puncture may reveal blood in the cerebrospinal fluid (if hemorrhagic). ◆ Carotid ultrasound may detect a blockage, stenosis, or reduced blood flow. ◆ Angiography can help pinpoint the site of occlusion or rupture. ◆ EEG may help localize the area of damage.	◆ Administer medications such as antiplatelet agents to prevent recurrent stroke (but not in hemorrhagic stroke); benzodiazepines to treat seizures; anticonvulsants to treat or prevent seizures after the patient's condition has stabilized; thrombolytics, such as alteplase, for emergency treatment of embolic stroke (typically within 3 hours of onset), aspirin or heparin for patients with embolic or thrombotic stroke who aren't candidates for alteplase, stool softeners to prevent straining; antihypertensives and antiarrhythmics to reduce risks associated with recurrent stroke; corticosteroids to minimize associated cerebral edema, and analgesics to relieve headache following a hemorrhagic stroke. ◆ Maintain a patent airway and provide oxygen. If unconscious, the patient may aspirate saliva. Place the patient in lateral position to promote drainage, or suction as needed. ◆ Insert an artificial airway and start mechanical ventilation or supplemental oxygen if needed. ◆ Check the patient's vital signs and neurologic status. Record observations and report significant changes, such as changes in pupil dilation, signs of increased intracranial pressure, and nuchal rigidity or flaccidity. ◆ Monitor blood pressure, level of consciousness, motor function (voluntary and involuntary movements), sensory reflexes, speech, skin color, and temperature. ◆ Assess gag reflex before offering oral fluids. Maintain fluid intake orally or with I.V. therapy as appropriate.

Spinal injury

- Fractures, contusions, dislocations, or compressions of the spine
- Most common sites: C5, C6, C7, T12, and L1 vertebrae
- Most common between ages 15 and 35

CAUSES
- Trauma to the spine

RISK FACTORS
- Diving into shallow water
- Fall
- Gunshot and related wound
- Motor vehicle accident
- Improper lifting of heavy object
- Neoplastic lesion
- Osteoporosis

PATHOPHYSIOLOGY

- Spinal cord injury results from acceleration, deceleration, or other deforming forces, usually applied from a distance. Mechanisms involved with spinal cord injury include:
- hyperextension from acceleration-deceleration forces and sudden reduction in the anteroposterior diameter of the spinal cord
- hyperflexion from sudden and excessive force, propelling the neck forward or causing an exaggerated movement to one side
- vertical compression from force applied from the top of the cranium along the vertical axis through the vertebra
- rotational forces from twisting, which adds shearing forces.

NEUROLOGIC SYSTEM
- Injury causes microscopic hemorrhages in the gray matter and pia arachnoid.
- The hemorrhages gradually increase in size until all of the gray matter is filled with blood, which causes necrosis.

- From the gray matter, the blood enters the white matter, where it impedes the circulation within the spinal cord.
- Ensuing edema causes compression and decreases the blood supply; thus, the spinal cord loses perfusion and becomes ischemic; edema and hemorrhage are greatest approximately two segments above and below the injury.
- Edema temporarily adds to the patient's dysfunction by increasing pressure and compressing the nerves.
- In the gray matter, an inflammatory reaction prevents restoration of circulation. Phagocytes appear at the injury site within 36 to 48 hours after the injury, macrophages engulf degenerating axons, and collagen replaces the normal tissue. Scarring and meningeal thickening leaves the nerves in the area blocked or tangled.

RESPIRATORY SYSTEM
- If near the 3rd to 5th cervical vertebrae, edema and hemorrhage may interfere with phrenic nerve impulse transmission to the diaphragm, inhibiting respiratory function. (See *Disorders affecting management of spinal cord injury,* pages 412 and 413.)

HISTORY
- Muscle spasm
- Back or neck pain
- In cervical fractures, point tenderness
- Predisposing risk factors

PHYSICAL FINDINGS
- Level of injury and any spinal cord damage located by neurologic assessment (see *Types of spinal cord injury,* pages 410 and 411)
- Limited movement and activities that cause pain
- Surface wounds
- Pain location
- Loss of sensation below the level of injury
- Deformity

DIAGNOSTIC TEST RESULTS
- Spinal X-rays, myelography, computed tomography scans, and magnetic resonance imaging can indicate the location of the fracture and the site of the compression.

TREATMENT

GENERAL
- Spine stabilized through immobilization before surgery
- Hemodynamic support
- Application of a hard cervical collar
- Wound care, if appropriate
- Radiation for neoplastic lesion
- Aspiration precautions
- Skeletal traction with skull tongs
- Rotation bed with cervical traction, if appropriate
- Splinting, using thoracic lumbar sacral orthotics
- Intubation and mechanical ventilation, if indicated

ACTIVITY
- Bed rest on a firm surface
- Physical therapy, as appropriate

MEDICATIONS
- Corticosteroids
- Analgesics
- Muscle relaxants
- Chemotherapy for neoplastic lesion
- Oxygen therapy

SURGERY
- Decompression of spinal cord
- Stabilization of spinal column

NURSING CONSIDERATIONS

NURSING DIAGNOSES
- Acute pain
- Anxiety
- Autonomic dysreflexia
- Deficient diversional activity
- Deficient fluid volume
- Disturbed body image
- Dressing or grooming self-care deficit
- Hopelessness
- Impaired physical mobility
- Ineffective airway clearance
- Ineffective breathing pattern
- Ineffective coping
- Risk for aspiration
- Risk for disuse syndrome
- Risk for impaired skin integrity
- Risk for infection
- Risk for posttrauma syndrome

EXPECTED OUTCOMES
The patient will:
- express feelings of increased comfort and decreased pain
- express feelings of decreased anxiety
- show no signs or symptoms of autonomic dysreflexia
- participate in interests and activities unrelated to the illness or confinement
- maintain adequate fluid volume
- express positive feelings about self
- participate in self-care activities at the highest level possible within the confines of the injury
- recognize choices and alternatives and make decisions on own behalf
- attain the highest degree of mobility possible within the confines of the injury
- maintain a patent airway

- maintain adequate ventilation and oxygenation
- develop effective coping mechanisms
- show no signs of aspiration
- maintain muscle strength and joint range of motion (ROM) to the highest degree possible within the confines of the injury
- maintain skin integrity with no signs or symptoms of breakdown
- remain free from signs or symptoms of infection
- express feelings and fears about the traumatic event.

NURSING INTERVENTIONS
- Apply a hard cervical collar.
- Immobilize the patient.
- Perform ROM exercises of the extremities, as appropriate.
- Comfort and reassure the patient.
- Give prescribed drugs.
- Provide wound care, if appropriate.
- Provide diversionary activities.
- Assess for neurologic or respiratory changes.
- Observe changes in skin sensation and loss of muscle strength.
- Reposition every 2 hours, provide skin care, and assess skin integrity.
- Monitor hydration and nutritional status.
- Assess pain level, administer analgesics, and evaluate effect.

PATIENT TEACHING

Be sure to cover:
- injury, diagnostic testing, and treatment
- traction methods used
- exercises to maintain physical mobility
- medication administration, dosage, and possible adverse effects
- prescribed home care regimen
- importance of follow-up examinations
- contact information for resource and support services.

RESOURCES
Organizations
American Academy of Neurology: *www.aan.com*
American Spinal Injury Association: *www.asia-spinalinjury.org*
Christopher and Dana Reeve Foundation: *www.christopherreeve.org*
National Spinal Cord Injury Association: *www.spinalcord.org*

Selected references
Demir, S., et al. "Spinal Cord Injury Associated with Thoracic Osteoporotic Fracture," *American Journal of Physical Medicine and Rehabilitation* 86(3):242-46, March 2007.
McKinley, W., et al. "Incidence, Etiology, and Risk Factors for Fever Following Spinal Cord Injury," *Journal of Spinal Cord Medicine* 29(5):501-506, 2006.
Professional Guide to Pathophysiology, 2nd ed. Philadelphia: Lippincott Williams & Wilkins. 2007.
Wilson, J.B., et al. "Spinal Injuries in Contact Sports," *Current Sports Medicine Reports* 5(1):50-55, February 2006.

(continued)

Types of spinal cord injury

Injury to the spinal cord can be classified as complete or incomplete. An incomplete spinal injury may be an anterior cord syndrome, central cord syndrome, or Brown-Séquard's syndrome, depending on the area of the cord affected. This chart highlights the characteristic signs and symptoms of each.

TYPE	DESCRIPTION	SIGNS AND SYMPTOMS

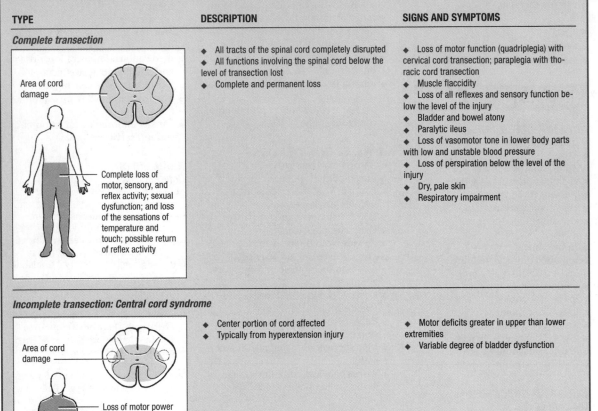

Complete transection

Area of cord damage

Complete loss of motor, sensory, and reflex activity; sexual dysfunction; and loss of the sensations of temperature and touch; possible return of reflex activity

Description
- All tracts of the spinal cord completely disrupted
- All functions involving the spinal cord below the level of transection lost
- Complete and permanent loss

Signs and symptoms
- Loss of motor function (quadriplegia) with cervical cord transection; paraplegia with thoracic cord transection
- Muscle flaccidity
- Loss of all reflexes and sensory function below the level of the injury
- Bladder and bowel atony
- Paralytic ileus
- Loss of vasomotor tone in lower body parts with low and unstable blood pressure
- Loss of perspiration below the level of the injury
- Dry, pale skin
- Respiratory impairment

Incomplete transection: Central cord syndrome

Area of cord damage

Loss of motor power and sensation

Incomplete loss

Description
- Center portion of cord affected
- Typically from hyperextension injury

Signs and symptoms
- Motor deficits greater in upper than lower extremities
- Variable degree of bladder dysfunction

TYPE	DESCRIPTION	SIGNS AND SYMPTOMS

Incomplete transection: Anterior cord syndrome

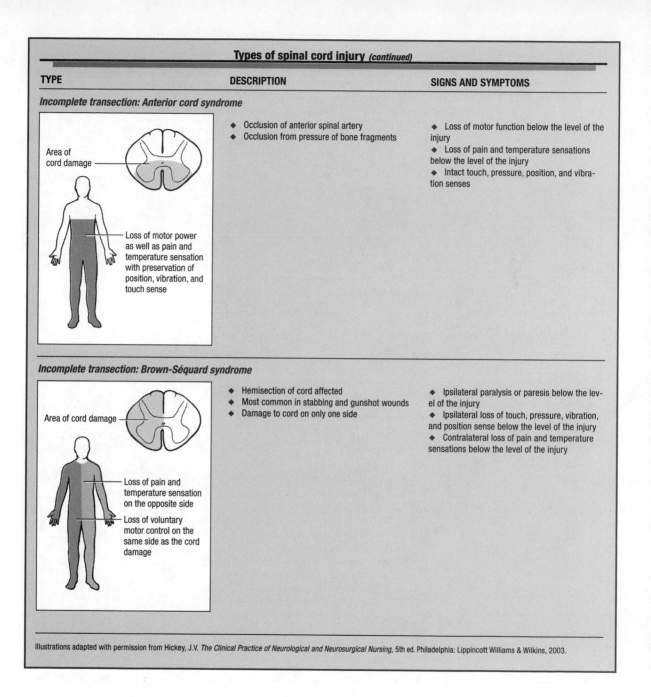

Area of cord damage

Loss of motor power as well as pain and temperature sensation with preservation of position, vibration, and touch sense

- Occlusion of anterior spinal artery
- Occlusion from pressure of bone fragments

- Loss of motor function below the level of the injury
- Loss of pain and temperature sensations below the level of the injury
- Intact touch, pressure, position, and vibration senses

Incomplete transection: Brown-Séquard syndrome

Area of cord damage

Loss of pain and temperature sensation on the opposite side

Loss of voluntary motor control on the same side as the cord damage

- Hemisection of cord affected
- Most common in stabbing and gunshot wounds
- Damage to cord on only one side

- Ipsilateral paralysis or paresis below the level of the injury
- Ipsilateral loss of touch, pressure, vibration, and position sense below the level of the injury
- Contralateral loss of pain and temperature sensations below the level of the injury

Illustrations adapted with permission from Hickey, J.V. *The Clinical Practice of Neurological and Neurosurgical Nursing*, 5th ed. Philadelphia: Lippincott Williams & Wilkins, 2003.

(continued)

Disorders affecting management of spinal cord injury

This chart highlights disorders that affect the management of spinal cord injury.

DISORDER	SIGNS AND SYMPTOMS	DIAGNOSTIC TEST RESULTS	TREATMENT AND CARE
Autonomic dysreflexia (complication)	◆ Bradycardia ◆ Hypertension ◆ Severe, pounding headache ◆ Cold or goose-fleshed skin below the lesion ◆ Diaphoresis, flushed feeling, and flushing of skin above the level of the lesion ◆ Pallor below the level of the lesion ◆ Chills	◆ None; diagnosis is primarily based on signs and symptoms. ◆ Tests support evidence of spinal cord trauma above level T6.	◆ Elevate the head of the bed. ◆ Monitor blood pressure and heart rate every 3 to 5 minutes. ◆ Determine the underlying stimulus for the event, such as a blocked catheter, fecal impaction, or urinary tract infection; remove or correct it. ◆ Administer antihypertensives.
Depression (complication)	◆ Difficulty sleeping ◆ Difficulty concentrating or thinking clearly ◆ Profound loss of pleasure in all activities ◆ Change in eating patterns ◆ Agitation ◆ Psychomotor retardation ◆ Recent weight loss or gain ◆ Use of prescription, over-the-counter, or recreational drugs	◆ Psychiatric evaluation identifies symptoms meeting *DSM-IV-TR* criteria for major depression. ◆ Toxicology screening suggests drug use. ◆ Beck Depression Inventory shows the onset, severity, duration, and progression of depressive symptoms.	◆ Encourage participation in activities of daily living. ◆ Encourage verbalization of feelings. ◆ Encourage interaction with others. ◆ Administer medications and observe for adverse effects. ◆ Provide a structured routine. ◆ Identify support systems and encourage interaction. ◆ Assess for suicidal ideation and provide surveillance, if appropriate.
Neurogenic shock (complication)	◆ Orthostatic hypotension ◆ Bradycardia ◆ Inability to sweat below the level of the injury	◆ None; diagnosis is primarily based on signs and symptoms. ◆ Tests support evidence of spinal cord trauma.	◆ Minimize abrupt changes in position. ◆ Monitor blood pressure frequently when the patient is lying, sitting, and standing, if appropriate. ◆ Assess heart rate frequently; administer medications to promote cardiac function. ◆ Avoid excessive bed covers and extremes in room temperature.

DISORDER	SIGNS AND SYMPTOMS	DIAGNOSTIC TEST RESULTS	TREATMENT AND CARE
Respiratory failure (complication)	◆ Diminished chest movement ◆ Restlessness, irritability, and confusion ◆ Decreased level of consciousness ◆ Pallor, possible cyanosis of skin and mucous membranes ◆ Tachypnea, tachycardia (strong and rapid initially, but thready and irregular in later stages) ◆ Cold, clammy skin and frank diaphoresis, especially around the forehead and face ◆ Diminished breath sounds; possible adventitious breath sounds ◆ Possible cardiac arrhythmias	◆ Arterial blood gas (ABG) analysis indicates early respiratory failure when partial pressure of arterial oxygen is low (usually less than 70 mm Hg), partial pressure of arterial carbon dioxide is greater than 45 mm Hg, and the bicarbonate level is normal. ◆ Serial vital capacity reveals readings less than 800 ml. ◆ Electrocardiography may indicate arrhythmias. ◆ Pulse oximetry reveals a decreased oxygen saturation level. Levels less than 50% indicate impaired tissue oxygenation.	◆ Institute oxygen therapy immediately to optimize oxygenation of pulmonary blood. ◆ Prepare for endotracheal (ET) intubation and mechanical ventilation, if necessary; anticipate the need for high-frequency or pressure ventilation to force airways open. ◆ Administer drug therapy, such as bronchodilators, to open airways, corticosteroids to reduce inflammation, continuous I.V. solutions of positive inotropic agents (which increase cardiac output) and vasopressors (which induce vasoconstriction) to maintain blood pressure, and diuretics to reduce fluid overload and edema. ◆ Assess the patient's respiratory status at least every 2 hours, or more often as indicated. Observe for a positive response to oxygen therapy, such as improved breathing, color, and oximetry and ABG values. Provide assisted coughing. ◆ Position the patient for optimal breathing effort. ◆ Maintain a normothermic environment to reduce the patient's oxygen demand. ◆ Monitor vital signs, heart rhythm, and fluid intake and output. ◆ If the patient is intubated, auscultate the lungs to check for accidental intubation of the esophagus or the mainstem bronchus. Be alert for aspiration, broken teeth, nosebleeds, and vagal reflexes causing bradycardia, arrhythmias, and hypotension. Perform suctioning using strict aseptic technique. ◆ Monitor oximetry and capnography values to detect changes in the patient's condition. ◆ Note the amount and quality of lung secretions and look for changes in the patient's status. ◆ Check cuff pressure on the ET tube to prevent erosion from an overinflated cuff. Normal cuff pressure is about 20 mm Hg. ◆ Implement measures to prevent nasal tissue necrosis. Position and maintain the nasotracheal tube midline in the nostrils and reposition daily. Tape the tube securely but use skin protection measures and nonirritating tape to prevent skin breakdown. ◆ Provide a means of communication for patients who are intubated and alert.

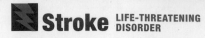

- Sudden impairment of blood circulation to the brain
- Classified as ischemic or hemorrhagic (see *Types of stroke*)
- Third most common cause of death in the United States
- Affects 500,000 people each year, causing death in half
- Most common cause of neurologic disability
- About 50% of stroke survivors permanently disabled
- Recurrences possible within weeks, months, or years
- Mostly affects older adults but can strike at any age
- More common in men than in women
- Affects Blacks and Hispanics more commonly than other groups
- Also known as *cerebrovascular accident* or *brain attack*

CAUSES
Cerebral thrombosis
- Most common cause of stroke
- Obstruction of a blood vessel in the extracerebral vessels
- Site possibly intracerebral

Cerebral embolism
- Second most common cause of stroke
- Cardiac arrhythmias
- Endocarditis
- History of rheumatic heart disease
- Open heart surgery
- Posttraumatic valvular disease

Cerebral hemorrhage
- Third most common cause of stroke
- Arteriovenous malformation
- Cerebral aneurysms
- Chronic hypertension

RISK FACTORS
- History of transient ischemic attack
- Heart disease
- Smoking
- Familial history
- Obesity
- Alcohol use
- Cardiac arrhythmias

- Diabetes mellitus
- Hypertension
- Use of hormonal contraceptives in conjunction with smoking and hypertension
- High red blood cell count
- Elevated cholesterol and triglycerides levels.

- Deprivation of oxygen and nutrients occurs from obstruction or hemorrhage.
- If the compensatory mechanisms become overworked or if cerebral blood flow remains impaired for more than a few minutes, oxygen deprivation leads to infarction of brain tissue.
- The brain cells cease to function because they can't store glucose or glycogen for use and they can't engage in anaerobic metabolism.
- Loss of neurologic function can affect organ function. (See *Disorders affecting management of stroke*, pages 418 and 419.)

Types of stroke

Strokes are typically classified as ischemic or hemorrhagic depending on the underlying cause. This chart describes the major types of strokes.

TYPE	DESCRIPTION
Ischemic: Thrombotic	◆ Most common type of stroke ◆ Frequently the result of atherosclerosis; also associated with hypertension, smoking, and diabetes ◆ Thrombus in extracranial or intracranial vessel that blocks blood flow to the cerebral cortex ◆ Carotid artery most commonly affected extracranial vessel ◆ Common intracranial sites: bifurcation of carotid arteries, distal intracranial portion of vertebral arteries, and proximal basilar arteries ◆ May occur during sleep or shortly after awakening, during surgery, or after a myocardial infarction
Ischemic: Embolic	◆ Second most common type of stroke ◆ Embolus from heart or extracranial arteries that floats into cerebral bloodstream and lodges in middle cerebral artery or branches ◆ Embolus commonly originating during atrial fibrillation ◆ Typically occurs during activity ◆ Develops rapidly
Ischemic: Lacunar	◆ Subtype of thrombotic stroke ◆ Hypertension creating cavities deep in white matter of the brain, affecting the internal capsule, basal ganglia, thalamus, and pons ◆ Lipid-coated lining of the small penetrating arteries thickens and weakens wall, causing microaneurysms and dissections
Hemorrhagic	◆ Third most common type of stroke ◆ Typically caused by hypertension or rupture of aneurysm ◆ Diminished blood supply to area supplied by ruptured artery and compression by accumulated blood

NEUROLOGIC SYSTEM

Pathophysiologic processes vary depending on the type of stroke.

Thrombotic or embolic stroke

◆ A thrombotic or embolic stroke causes ischemia. Some of the neurons served by the occluded vessel die from lack of oxygen and nutrients.

◆ Neuron death results in cerebral infarction, in which tissue injury triggers an inflammatory response that increases intracranial pressure (ICP).

◆ Injury to surrounding cells disrupts metabolism and leads to changes in ionic transport, localized acidosis, and free radical formation.

◆ Calcium, sodium, and water accumulate in the injured cells, and excitatory neurotransmitters are released.

◆ Consequent continued cellular injury and swelling set up a vicious cycle of further damage.

Hemorrhagic stroke

◆ Impaired cerebral perfusion causes infarction, and the blood itself acts as a space-occupying mass, exerting pressure on the brain tissues.

◆ The brain's regulatory mechanisms attempt to maintain equilibrium by increasing blood pressure to maintain cerebral perfusion pressure.

◆ The increased ICP forces cerebrospinal fluid (CSF) out, thus restoring the balance. If the hemorrhage is small, the patient may live with only minimal neurologic deficits. If the bleeding is heavy, ICP increases rapidly and perfusion stops. Even if the pressure returns to normal, many brain cells die.

◆ Initially, the ruptured cerebral blood vessels may constrict to limit the blood loss.

◆ This vasospasm further compromises blood flow, leading to more ischemia and cellular damage.

◆ If a clot forms in the vessel, decreased blood flow promotes ischemia.

◆ If the blood enters the subarachnoid space, meningeal irritation occurs.

◆ Blood cells that pass through the vessel wall into the surrounding tissue may break down and block the arachnoid villi, causing hydrocephalus.

CARDIOVASCULAR SYSTEM

◆ Cerebral ischemia and infarction can ultimately affect the autonomic nervous system, which can alter blood vessel constriction and dilation, heart rate, blood pressure, and cardiac contractility.

◆ Cardiovascular effects are increasingly problematic if the patient has an underlying disorder, such as heart disease or hypertension.

MUSCULOSKELETAL SYSTEM

◆ Cerebral infarction can lead to a disturbance in impulse transmission via the cranial and peripheral nerves, altering motor and sensory function.

◆ Changes in sensation or mobility can lead to pressure areas, especially with prolonged bed rest or limited activity. In addition, the ability of the blood vessels to constrict and dilate as necessary may be altered, increasing the risk of impaired blood flow to the area. Subsequently, pressure ulcers may develop.

RESPIRATORY SYSTEM

◆ If infarction resulting from increased ICP and decreased perfusion involves the respiratory center in the medulla, respiration—including the depth and rate—can be affected because nerve impulse transmission via the phrenic nerves to the diaphragm and intercostal nerves to the intercostal muscles is interrupted.

◆ If the pons (the location for apneustic and pneumotaxic centers) is affected, breathing patterns become altered and impulse transmission via the cranial nerves may be interrupted.

◆ If the glossopharyngeal (CN IX) and vagus nerves (CN X) are affected, impaired swallowing and possible aspiration may occur.

HISTORY

◆ Varying clinical features, depending on artery affected, severity of damage, and extent of collateral circulation (see *Assessment findings in stroke*, page 416)

◆ One or more risk factors present

◆ Sudden onset of hemiparesis or hemiplegia

◆ Gradual onset of dizziness, mental disturbances, or seizures

◆ Loss of consciousness or sudden aphasia

PHYSICAL FINDINGS

◆ With stroke in left hemisphere, signs and symptoms on right side

◆ With stroke in right hemisphere, signs and symptoms on left side

◆ With stroke that causes cranial nerve damage, signs and symptoms on same side

◆ Change in level of consciousness

◆ With conscious patient, anxiety along with communication and mobility difficulties

◆ Urinary incontinence

◆ Loss of voluntary muscle control

◆ Hemiparesis or hemiplegia on one side of the body

◆ Decreased deep tendon reflexes

◆ Hemianopsia on the affected side of the body

◆ With left-sided hemiplegia, problems with visuospatial relations

◆ Sensory losses

DIAGNOSTIC TEST RESULTS

◆ Laboratory tests, including anticardiolipin antibodies, antiphospholipid, factor V mutation, antithrombin III, protein S, and protein C, may show increased thrombotic risk.

◆ Magnetic resonance imaging and angiography allow for evaluation of the location and size of the lesion.

◆ Cerebral angiography details the disruption of cerebral circulation and is the test of choice for examining the entire cerebral blood flow.

◆ Computed tomography scan detects structural abnormalities.

(continued)

Assessment findings in stroke

A stroke can leave one patient with mild hand weakness and another with complete unilateral paralysis. In both patients, the functional loss reflects damage to the brain area normally perfused by the occluded or ruptured artery. In general, assessment findings associated with a stroke may include:

◆ unilateral limb weakness
◆ speech difficulties
◆ numbness on one side

◆ headache
◆ vision disturbances (diplopia, hemianopsia, ptosis)
◆ vertigo
◆ anxiety
◆ altered level of consciousness (LOC).

Typical assessment findings based on the artery affected are highlighted in the chart below.

AFFECTED ARTERY	ASSESSMENT FINDINGS
Middle cerebral artery	◆ Aphasia ◆ Dysphasia ◆ Visual field deficits ◆ Hemiparesis of affected side (more severe in the face and arm than in the leg)
Carotid artery	◆ Weakness ◆ Paralysis ◆ Numbness ◆ Sensory changes ◆ Vision disturbances on the affected side ◆ Altered LOC ◆ Bruits ◆ Aphasia ◆ Ptosis
Vertebrobasilar artery	◆ Weakness on the affected side ◆ Numbness around lips and mouth ◆ Visual field deficits ◆ Diplopia ◆ Poor coordination, slurred speech ◆ Dysphagia ◆ Vertigo ◆ Nystagmus ◆ Amnesia ◆ Ataxia
Anterior cerebral artery	◆ Confusion ◆ Weakness ◆ Numbness, especially in the leg on the affected side ◆ Incontinence ◆ Loss of coordination ◆ Impaired motor and sensory functions ◆ Personality changes
Posterior cerebral artery	◆ Visual field deficits (homonymous hemianopsia) ◆ Sensory impairment ◆ Dyslexia ◆ Perseveration (abnormally persistent replies to questions) ◆ Coma ◆ Cortical blindness ◆ Absence of paralysis (usually)

◆ Positron-emission tomography provides data on cerebral metabolism and on cerebral blood flow changes.
◆ Transcranial Doppler studies evaluate the velocity of blood flow.
◆ Carotid Doppler measures flow through the carotid arteries.
◆ Two-dimensional echocardiography evaluates the heart for dysfunction.
◆ Cerebral blood flow studies measure blood flow to the brain.
◆ Electrocardiography evaluates electrical activity in cortical infarction.

TREATMENT

GENERAL
- Careful blood pressure management
- Physical, speech, and occupational rehabilitation
- Supportive, symptomatic treatment

DIET
- Pureed dysphagia diet or tube feedings, if indicated

MEDICATIONS
- Tissue plasminogen activator when the cause isn't hemorrhagic (emergency care within 3 hours of onset of the symptoms) (see *Fibrinolytic therapy contraindications*)
- Anticonvulsants
- Stool softeners
- Anticoagulants
- Analgesics
- Antidepressants
- Antiplatelets
- Lipid-lowering agents
- Antihypertensives

SURGERY
- Craniotomy
- Endarterectomy
- Extracranial intracranial bypass
- Ventricular shunts

Fibrinolytic therapy contraindications

Criteria that exclude a patient from receiving fibrinolytics for ischemic stroke include:
- evidence of intracranial hemorrhage during pretreatment evaluation
- suspicion of subarachnoid hemorrhage during pretreatment
- history of recent (within 3 months) intracranial or intraspinal surgery, serious head trauma, or previous stroke
- history of intracranial bleeding
- uncontrolled hypertension at time of treatment
- seizure at stroke onset
- active internal bleeding
- intracranial neoplasm, arteriovenous malformation, or aneurysm
- known bleeding diathesis, including but not limited to current use of an anticoagulant such as warfarin, international normalized ratio greater than 1.7, or prothrombin time greater than 15 seconds; use of heparin within 48 hours before the onset of stroke with elevation of partial thromboplastin time or platelet count less than 100,000/µl.

NURSING CONSIDERATIONS

NURSING DIAGNOSES
- Anxiety
- Bathing or hygiene self-care deficit
- Disturbed sensory perception: Tactile
- Dressing or grooming self-care deficit
- Impaired gas exchange
- Impaired physical mobility
- Impaired verbal communication
- Ineffective airway clearance
- Ineffective coping
- Ineffective tissue perfusion: Cerebral
- Powerlessness
- Risk for aspiration
- Risk for disuse syndrome
- Risk for impaired skin integrity
- Risk for infection
- Risk for injury
- Situational low self-esteem
- Toileting self-care deficit
- Total urinary incontinence

EXPECTED OUTCOMES
The patient (or family) will:
- identify strategies to reduce anxiety
- perform bathing and hygiene activities to the fullest extent possible
- report signs and symptoms of impaired sensation
- perform dressing and grooming activities to the fullest extent possible
- maintain adequate ventilation and oxygenation
- achieve maximum mobility possible
- effectively communicate needs verbally or through an alternate means of communication
- maintain a patent airway
- develop adequate coping mechanisms and support systems
- exhibit signs of adequate cerebral perfusion
- express feelings of control over health and well-being
- remain free from signs of aspiration
- maintain joint mobility and range of motion
- maintain intact skin with no signs of breakdown
- remain free from signs or symptoms of infection and injury
- verbalize feelings about self-esteem

(continued)

- perform toileting needs to the fullest extent possible.

NURSING INTERVENTIONS
- Maintain a patent airway and oxygenation.
- Offer urinal or bedpan every 2 hours.
- Insert an indwelling urinary catheter, if necessary.
- Ensure adequate nutrition.
- Follow the physical therapy program, and assist the patient with exercise.
- Establish and maintain patient communication.
- Provide psychological support.
- Set realistic, short-term goals.
- Protect the patient from injury and complications.
- Provide careful positioning to prevent aspiration and contractures.
- Give prescribed drugs.
- Monitor neurologic, GI, and respiratory status.
- Monitor vital signs, fluid, electrolyte, and nutritional intake.
- Assess for development of deep vein thrombosis and pulmonary embolus.

PATIENT TEACHING

Be sure to cover:
- disorder, diagnostic testing, and treatment
- medication administration, dosage, and possible adverse effects
- occupational and speech therapy programs
- dietary and drug regimens
- stroke prevention
- contact information for community resource and support services.

RESOURCES
Organizations
American Academy of Neurology: *www.aan.com*
American Heart Association: *www.americanheart.org*
American Neurological Association: *www.aneuroa.org*
American Stroke Association: *www.strokeassociation.org*
National Aphasia Association: *www.aphasia.org*
National Stroke Association: *www.stroke.org*

Selected references
Edwards, G. "The Training and Education of Nurses Working in Stroke Care," *British Journal of Nursing* 15(21):1180-84, November-December 2006.
Sauerbeck, L. "Primary Stroke Prevention," *AJN* 106(11):40-49, November 2006.
Smithard, D. et al. "Long-Term Outcome After Stroke: Does Dysphagia Matter?" *Age and Ageing* 36(1):90-94, January 2007.
Strategies for Managing Multisystem Disorders. Philadelphia: Lippincott Williams & Wilkins, 2006.
Yeung, S., et al. "Family Carers in Stroke Care: Examining the Relationship Between Problem-Solving, Depression, and General Health," *Journal of Clinical Nursing* 16(2):344-52, February 2007.

Disorders affecting management of stroke

This chart highlights disorders that affect the management of stroke.

DISORDER	SIGNS AND SYMPTOMS	DIAGNOSTIC TEST RESULTS	TREATMENT AND CARE
Aspiration pneumonia (complication)	- Fever - Crackles - Dyspnea - Hypertension initially (as a compensatory mechanism), then hypotension - Tachycardia - Cough with blood-tinged or yellow or green sputum - Cyanosis	- Chest X-ray reveals infiltrates. - Sputum for Gram stain and culture and sensitivity may reveal inflammatory cells and possible secondary bacterial infection. - Bronchoscopy or transtracheal aspiration reveals possible secondary bacterial infection.	- Maintain a patent airway and oxygenation. Place the patient in Fowler's position to maximize chest expansion and give supplemental oxygen as ordered. Monitor oxygen saturation and arterial blood gas levels as ordered. - Assess carbon dioxide levels closely to prevent increased intracranial pressure (ICP) and decreased cerebral perfusion pressure. - Assess respiratory status often, at least every 2 hours. Auscultate the lungs for abnormal breath sounds. If respiratory status deteriorates, anticipate the need for intubation and mechanical ventilation. - Encourage coughing and deep breathing. - Adhere to standard precautions and institute appropriate transmission-based precautions, depending on the causative organism associated with secondary bacterial infection. - Institute cardiac monitoring to detect arrhythmias secondary to hypoxemia. - Reposition the patient to maximize chest expansion, allow rest, and reduce discomfort and anxiety. - Administer drug therapy, such as bronchodilators and antimicrobials.

DISORDER	SIGNS AND SYMPTOMS	DIAGNOSTIC TEST RESULTS	TREATMENT AND CARE
Hydrocephalus (complication)	◆ Distended scalp veins ◆ Thin, shiny, fragile-looking scalp skin ◆ Projectile vomiting ◆ Decreased level of consciousness ◆ Ataxia ◆ Incontinence ◆ Headache ◆ Blurred vision ◆ Papilledema ◆ Downward deviation of eyes (setting sun sign) ◆ Impaired intellect	◆ Skull X-rays may show thinning of the skull. ◆ Angiography shows vessel abnormalities caused by stretching. ◆ Computed tomography scan and magnetic resonance imaging reveal variations in tissue density and possible fluid in the ventricular system. ◆ Lumbar puncture reveals normal or increased fluid pressure. ◆ Ventriculography shows ventricular dilation with excess fluid.	◆ Position the patient on his side to prevent aspiration. ◆ Handle the head gently and pad the area under head. ◆ Prepare for insertion of a shunt, ventriculostomy, or ICP monitoring as indicated. ◆ Administer medications, such as osmotic diuretics and corticosteroids. ◆ Monitor neurologic status for evidence of increasing pressure and deterioration.
Pressure ulcers (complication)	◆ Blanching erythema (first clinical sign): Varying from pink to bright red depending on the patient's skin color (in dark-skinned people, purple discoloration or a darkening of normal skin color); area whitens with application of pressure, but color returns within 1 to 3 seconds if capillary refill is good ◆ Pain at the site and surrounding area ◆ Localized edema ◆ Increased body temperature (in more severe cases, cool skin due to more severe damage or necrosis) ◆ Nonblanching erythema (more severe cases) ranging from dark red to purple or cyanotic, indicating deeper dermal involvement ◆ Blisters, crusts, or scaling as the skin deteriorates and the ulcer progresses ◆ Dusky-red, possibly mottled, lesion that doesn't bleed easily (in cases of deep ulcer originating at the bony prominence below the skin surface) ◆ Possible foul-smelling, purulent drainage from ulcerated lesion ◆ Eschar tissue on and around the lesion	◆ Physical examination shows presence of the ulcer. ◆ Wound culture with exudate suggests infection. ◆ White blood cell count may be elevated with infection. ◆ Total serum protein and serum albumin levels show severe hypoproteinemia.	◆ Frequently inspect the skin for possible changes in color, turgor, temperature, and sensation. Examine an existing ulcer for changes in size or degree of damage. ◆ Assess the patient for pain. ◆ Reposition the patient at least every 2 hours around the clock. ◆ Perform passive range-of-motion exercises, or encourage the patient to do active exercises, if possible. ◆ Use pressure relief aids on the patient's bed. ◆ Provide meticulous skin care. Keep the skin clean and dry without the use of harsh soaps. ◆ Change bedding frequently, as indicated. ◆ Perform wound care using strict sterile technique. ◆ Assist with debridement, as needed. ◆ Encourage adequate nutritional intake; consult with the dietitian to develop a diet to promote granulation of new tissue.

Subarachnoid hemorrhage LIFE-THREATENING DISORDER

OVERVIEW

- Bleeding into the subarachnoid space between the pial and arachnoid membranes
- Most commonly occurs from rupture of a cerebral, or intracranial, aneurysm or arteriovenous malformation
- Most cerebral aneurysms are berry aneurysms—saclike outpouchings in cerebral arteries; usually arise at an arterial junction in the circle of Willis—the circular anastomosis forming the major cerebral arteries at the base of the brain
- Slightly higher incidence in women than in men
- May occur at any age, but most commonly between ages 40 and 65
- Fatal in approximately 50% of all patients who suffer a subarachnoid hemorrhage, 40% in the first 24 hours after occurrence

CAUSES
- Congenital defect
- Degenerative process

RISK FACTORS FOR ANEURYSM FORMATION
- Smoking
- Heavy alcohol use
- Hypertension

RISK FACTORS FOR RUPTURE
- Trauma
- Pregnancy
- Hyperdynamic stress

PATHOPHYSIOLOGY

- Hydrostatic pressure from blood flow exerts force against a weakened arterial wall, stretching it.
- Increased tension on the aneurysm wall causes rupture, and blood extravasates into the subarachnoid space and spreads to the cerebrospinal fluid (CSF).
- Intracranial pressure (ICP) increases, and meningeal irritation occurs.

ENDOCRINE SYSTEM
- Bleeding causes dilation of the third ventricle, which exerts mechanical pressure on the hypothalamus, causing progressive loss of nerve tissue, ultimately leading to hypothalamic dysfunction.
- Hypothalamic dysfunction leads to impaired synthesis and transport, or release of antidiuretic hormone (ADH).
- ADH doesn't respond to changes in plasma osmolarity, and the kidneys are unable to reabsorb water in the distal and collecting tubules, which leads to excretion of large amounts of dilute urine. (See *Disorders affecting management of subarachnoid hemorrhage,* pages 422 and 423.)

NEUROLOGIC SYSTEM
- Bleeding causes increased pressure on the surrounding structures, such as the cranial nerves.
- Blood in the subarachnoid space and CSF causes increased ICP.
- Clot formation may also cause potentially fatal ICP and brain tissue damage.
- Clots in the basal cisterns are believed to undergo hemolysis, causing a release of substances that initiate spasms of the cerebral blood vessels.

RESPIRATORY SYSTEM
- Increased ICP causes pressure on the respiratory center in the medulla.
- Interrupted nerve impulse transmission from the phrenic nerves to the diaphragm and from the intercostal nerves to the intercostal muscles alter the depth and rate of respirations.
- If the pons (the location of the apneustic and pneumotaxic centers) is affected, breathing patterns become altered.
- Interruption in nerve impulse transmission to the diaphragm can lead to respiratory failure.

Hunt-Hess classification for subarachnoid hemorrhage

The severity of symptoms accompanying subarachnoid hemorrhage varies from patient to patient, depending on the site and the amount of bleeding. The Hunt-Hess classification identifies five grades that characterize a subarachnoid hemorrhage from a ruptured cerebral aneurysm:

- Grade I (minimal bleeding)—The patient is alert and oriented without symptoms.
- Grade II (mild bleeding)—The patient is alert and oriented, with a mild to severe headache and nuchal rigidity.
- Grade III (moderate bleeding)—The patient is lethargic and confused or drowsy, with nuchal rigidity and, possibly, a mild focal deficit such as hemiparesis.
- Grade IV (severe bleeding)—The patient is stuporous, with nuchal rigidity and, possibly, moderate to severe focal deficits, hemiplegia, early decerebrate rigidity, and vegetative disturbances.
- Grade V (moribund; often fatal)—If the rupture is nonfatal, the patient is in a deep coma, with such severe neurological deficits as decerebrate rigidity and moribund appearance.

HISTORY

◆ Aneurysm or arteriovenous malformation (AVM) commonly asymptomatic until rupture

PHYSICAL FINDINGS

◆ Severity of subarachnoid hemorrhage graded according to the patient's signs and symptoms (see *Hunt-Hess classification for subarachnoid hemorrhage*)

Oozing aneurysm

◆ Headache
◆ Intermittent nausea
◆ Nuchal rigidity
◆ Stiff back and legs

Rupture of aneurysm or AVM

◆ Sudden, severe headache
◆ Nausea and projectile vomiting
◆ Altered level of consciousness (LOC), including deep coma, depending on the severity and location of bleeding
◆ Signs of meningeal irritation, such as nuchal rigidity, back and leg pain, fever, restlessness, irritability, occasional seizures, photophobia, and blurred vision
◆ Motor and sensory defects

DIAGNOSTIC TEST RESULTS

◆ Cerebral angiography reveals altered cerebral blood flow, vessel lumen dilation, and differences in arterial filling.
◆ Computed tomography (CT) scan identifies evidence of aneurysm and possible hemorrhage; it may also identify hydrocephalus, areas of infarction, and the extent of blood spillage within the cisterns around the brain.
◆ Magnetic resonance imaging may help locate the aneurysm and the bleeding.
◆ Positron-emission tomography shows the chemical activity of the brain and the extent of tissue damage.

◆ Electrocardiography commonly shows flattened or depressed T waves.
◆ Lumbar puncture (LP) and CSF analysis reveal blood in CSF; elevated CSF pressure, protein, and white blood cell count; and decreased glucose level.

WARNING *Because LP increases the risk for herniation and rebleeding in patients with subarachnoid hemorrhage and increased ICP, the procedure is performed only if the results of the CT scan are inconclusive.*

GENERAL

◆ Supportive (maintaining airway and ventilation)
◆ Interventional radiology in conjunction with endovascular balloon therapy
◆ Transluminal balloon angioplasty to treat arterial vasospasm
◆ ICP monitoring

◆ Aneurysm and seizure precautions (see *Aneurysm precautions*)

DIET

◆ Avoidance of coffee and other stimulants

ACTIVITY

◆ Bedrest in a darkened room

MEDICATIONS

◆ Analgesics (codeine)
◆ Antihypertensives
◆ Corticosteroids
◆ Sedatives
◆ Calcium channel blockers
◆ Anticonvulsants
◆ Stool softeners

SURGERY

◆ Surgery within 1 to 3 days for grade III or higher anterior circulation aneurysms
◆ Aneurysm clipping, ligation, or wrapping
◆ Craniotomy

Aneurysm precautions

Aneurysm precautions are measures to help prevent increased intracranial pressure and reduce the risk of rebleeding by minimizing increases in blood pressure. Although the specific precautions may vary among facilities, the following general guidelines are helpful.

◆ Place the patient on immediate and complete bed rest in a dimly lit, quiet, nonstressful environment.
◆ Keep the head of the patient's bed flat or slightly elevated (15 to 30 degrees).
◆ Avoid hyperflexion, hyperextension, or hyperrotation of the neck (minimizes jugular venous compression).
◆ Have the patient avoid activities involving isometric muscle contraction, such as pulling or pushing on the side rails or against the foot of the bed. Provide passive range-of-motion exercises.
◆ Administer stool softeners to prevent straining. Advise the patient to avoid bearing down with bowel movements (Valsalva's maneuver); encourage him to exhale slowly when defecating or voiding.

◆ Avoid rectal temperature measurement, suppositories, enemas, or digital impaction removal.
◆ Urge the patient to avoid coughing; administer antitussives, if ordered.
◆ Administer antiemetics, as ordered, to prevent or manage vomiting.
◆ Eliminate coffee, tea, or other caffeinated beverages from the patient's intake.
◆ Assist with personal care and activities of daily living to prevent exertion.
◆ Eliminate exposure to external stimuli, such as television, radio, and books.
◆ Restrict visitors to family; encourage visitors to talk quietly with the patient, avoiding stressful topics as much as possible.

(continued)

NURSING CONSIDERATIONS

NURSING DIAGNOSES
- ◆ Acute pain
- ◆ Decreased cardiac output
- ◆ Decreased intracranial adaptive capacity
- ◆ Grieving (family)
- ◆ Impaired gas exchange
- ◆ Ineffective breathing pattern
- ◆ Ineffective tissue perfusion: Cerebral

EXPECTED OUTCOMES
The patient will:
- ◆ express feelings of increased comfort and decreased pain
- ◆ maintain adequate cardiac output
- ◆ maintain neurologic stability
- ◆ utilize available support systems and exhibit appropriate coping behaviors
- ◆ exhibit adequate ventilation and oxygenation
- ◆ maintain effective breathing pattern
- ◆ exhibit signs of adequate cerebral perfusion.

NURSING INTERVENTIONS
- ◆ Assess neurologic and respiratory systems; provide respiratory support, as appropriate.

 WARNING *Development of cerebral hypoxia, along with hypox-*emia and hypercapnia, can lead to increased cerebral vasodilation, subsequently increasing cerebral edema and ICP.

- ◆ Monitor vital signs, pulse oximetry, intake and output, ICP readings, and neurologic status.
- ◆ Administer medications, as ordered, and evaluate response.
- ◆ Maintain aneurysm and seizure precautions.
- ◆ Apply sequential compression stockings.
- ◆ Provide emotional support

PATIENT TEACHING

Be sure to cover:
- ◆ disorder, diagnostic testing, and treatment
- ◆ medication administration, dosage, and possible adverse effects
- ◆ end-of-life care
- ◆ available support services.

RESOURCES
Organizations
American Academy of Neurology: *www.aan.com*
American Neurological Association: *www.aneuroa.org*
National Institute of Neurological Disorders and Stroke: *www.ninds.nih.gov*

Selected references
Blissitt, P. "Hemodynamic Monitoring in the Care of the Critically Ill Neuroscience Patient," *AACN Advanced Critical Care* 17(3):327-40, July-September 2006.
Edlow, J. "Diagnosis of Subarachnoid Hemorrhage: Are We Doing Better?" *Stroke* 38:1129-31, April 2007.
Fernandez, A., et al. "Fever After Subarachnoid Hemorrhage; Risk Factors and Impact on Outcome," *Neurology* 68(13):1013-19, March 2007.
Professional Guide to Pathophysiology, 2nd ed. Philadelphia: Lippincott Williams & Wilkins, 2007.
Rizzolo, D. "Subarachnoid Hemorrhage," *JAAPA* 20(2):76, February, 2007.

Disorders affecting management of subarachnoid hemorrhage

This chart highlights disorders that affect the management of subarachnoid hemorrhage.

DISORDER	SIGNS AND SYMPTOMS	DIAGNOSTIC TEST RESULTS	TREATMENT AND CARE
Diabetes insipidus (complication)	◆ Extreme polyuria—usually 4 to 6 L/day of dilute urine but sometimes as much as 30 L/day, with a low specific gravity (less than 1.005) ◆ Polydipsia, particularly for cold, iced drinks ◆ Nocturia ◆ Fatigue (in severe cases) ◆ Dehydration, characterized by weight loss, poor tissue turgor, dry mucous membranes, constipation, muscle weakness, dizziness, tachycardia, and hypotension	◆ Urinalysis reveals almost colorless urine of low osmolality (less than 200 mOsm/kg) and low specific gravity (less than 1.005). ◆ A water deprivation test confirms the diagnosis by demonstrating renal inability to concentrate urine (evidence of antidiuretic hormone deficiency). ◆ If the patient has central diabetes insipidus, subcutaneous injection of 5 units of vasopressin produces decreased urine output with increased specific gravity.	◆ Anticipate using thiazide diuretics to reduce urine volume by creating mild salt depletion. ◆ Record fluid intake and output carefully; monitor daily weights. ◆ Watch for signs of hypovolemic shock, and monitor blood pressure and heart and respiratory rates regularly, especially during the water deprivation test. ◆ Monitor urine specific gravity between doses. ◆ Watch for decreased specific gravity with increased urine output, indicating an inability to concentrate urine and the need for the next dose or a dosage increase. ◆ Provide meticulous skin and mouth care, and apply a lubricant to cracked or sore lips. ◆ Make sure caloric intake is adequate and the meal plan is low in sodium.

DISORDER	SIGNS AND SYMPTOMS	DIAGNOSTIC TEST RESULTS	TREATMENT AND CARE
Respiratory failure (complication)	◆ Diminished chest movement ◆ Restlessness, irritability, and confusion ◆ Decreased level of consciousness (LOC) ◆ Pallor, possible cyanosis of skin and mucous membranes ◆ Tachypnea, tachycardia (strong and rapid initially, but thready and irregular in later stages) ◆ Cold, clammy skin and frank diaphoresis ◆ Diminished breath sounds; possible adventitious breath sounds ◆ Possible cardiac arrhythmias	◆ Arterial blood gas (ABG) analysis indicates early respiratory failure when partial pressure of arterial oxygen is low (usually less than 70 mm Hg), partial pressure of arterial carbon dioxide is greater than 45 mm Hg, and the bicarbonate level is normal. ◆ Serial vital capacity reveals readings less than 800 ml. ◆ Electrocardiography may indicate arrhythmias. ◆ Pulse oximetry reveals a decreasing oxygen saturation level. Levels less than 50% indicate impaired tissue oxygenation.	◆ Institute oxygen therapy immediately to optimize oxygenation of pulmonary blood. ◆ Prepare for endotracheal (ET) intubation and mechanical ventilation if necessary; anticipate the need for high-frequency or pressure ventilation to force airways open. ◆ Administer drug therapy, such as bronchodilators, to open airways, corticosteroids to reduce inflammation, continuous I.V. solutions of positive inotropic agents (which increase cardiac output) and vasopressors (which induce vasoconstriction) to maintain blood pressure, and diuretics to reduce fluid overload and edema. ◆ Assess the patient's respiratory status at least every 2 hours, or more often as indicated. Observe for a positive response to oxygen therapy, such as improved breathing, color, and oximetry and ABG values. ◆ Position the patient for optimal breathing effort. ◆ Maintain a normothermic environment to reduce the patient's oxygen demand. ◆ Monitor vital signs, heart rhythm, and fluid intake and output. ◆ If the patient is intubated, auscultate the lungs to check for accidental intubation of the esophagus or the mainstem bronchus. Be alert for aspiration, broken teeth, nosebleeds, and vagal reflexes causing bradycardia, arrhythmias, and hypotension. Perform suctioning, as ordered, using strict aseptic technique. Check cuff pressure on the ET tube to prevent erosion from an overinflated cuff. Normal cuff pressure is about 20 mm Hg. ◆ Monitor oximetry and capnography values to detect changes in the patient's condition. ◆ Note the amount and quality of lung secretions and look for changes in the patient's status. ◆ Implement measures to prevent nasal tissue necrosis with a nasotracheal tube. ◆ Provide a means of communication for patients who are intubated and alert.
Vasospasm (complication)	◆ Intense headache ◆ Decreased LOC; increased confusion ◆ Increased blood pressure ◆ Aphasia ◆ Partial paralysis	◆ Cerebral angiography reveals altered cerebral blood flow, vessel lumen dilation, and differences in arterial filling. ◆ Computed tomography scan identifies evidence of aneurysm and possible hemorrhage; it may also identify hydrocephalus, areas of infarction, and the extent of blood spillage within the cisterns around the brain. ◆ Magnetic resonance imaging may help locate the aneurysm and the bleeding. ◆ Positron-emission tomography shows the chemical activity of the brain and the extent of tissue damage. ◆ Electrocardiography commonly shows flattened or depressed T waves. ◆ Lumbar puncture and CSF analysis reveal blood in CSF; elevated CSF pressure, protein, and white blood cell count; and decreased glucose level.	◆ Anticipate the use of hypervolemic hemodilution therapy, such as administration of normal saline, whole blood, packed red blood cells, albumin, plasma protein fraction (increase circulating volume to reverse or prevent ischemia secondary to vasospasm) and crystalloid solution (to decrease blood viscosity). ◆ Monitor closely for signs and symptoms of increased intracranial pressure (ICP). ◆ Monitor the patient's blood pressure and ICP continuously. ◆ Assess closely for signs and symptoms of fluid overload. ◆ Monitor urine output every hour. ◆ Auscultate lungs for crackles; observe for jugular vein distention; and monitor central venous pressure and pulmonary artery pressure for increases.

Syndrome of inappropriate antidiuretic hormone LIFE-THREATENING DISORDER

OVERVIEW

- Disease of the posterior pituitary marked by excessive release of antidiuretic hormone (ADH) (vasopressin)
- Prognosis dependent on underlying disorder and response to treatment
- Common cause of hospital-acquired hyponatremia
- Also known as *SIADH*

CAUSES

- Central nervous system disorders
- Drugs
- Miscellaneous conditions, such as myxedema and psychosis
- Neoplastic diseases
- Oat cell carcinoma of the lung
- Pulmonary disorders

PATHOPHYSIOLOGY

- Excessive ADH secretion occurs in the absence of normal physiologic stimuli for its release.
- Excessive water reabsorption from the distal convoluted tubule and collecting ducts results in hyponatremia and normal to slightly increased extracellular fluid volume. (See *Understanding SIADH*.)

NEUROLOGIC SYSTEM

- Intracellular fluid shifts, causing cerebral edema, which leads to increased intracranial pressure (ICP).
- Cerebral perfusion pressure falls and cerebral blood flow decreases.
- Ischemia leads to cellular hypoxia, which initiates vasodilation of cerebral blood vessels in an attempt to increase cerebral blood flow. Unfortunately, this causes the ICP to increase further.
- As pressure continues to rise, compression of brain tissue and cerebral vessels further impairs cerebral blood flow. (See *Disorders affecting*

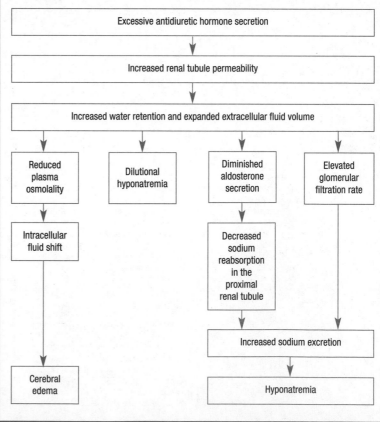

UP CLOSE

Understanding SIADH

The flowchart below highlights the events that produce syndrome of inappropriate antidiuretic hormone (SIADH).

Excessive antidiuretic hormone secretion

↓

Increased renal tubule permeability

↓

Increased water retention and expanded extracellular fluid volume

↓

| Reduced plasma osmolality | Dilutional hyponatremia | Diminished aldosterone secretion | Elevated glomerular filtration rate |

Reduced plasma osmolality → Intracellular fluid shift → Cerebral edema

Diminished aldosterone secretion → Decreased sodium reabsorption in the proximal renal tubule → Increased sodium excretion → Hyponatremia

Elevated glomerular filtration rate → Increased sodium excretion → Hyponatremia

management of SIADH, pages 426 and 427.)

- With the continued rise in ICP, the brain begins to shift under the extreme pressure and may herniate to an area of lesser pressure.
- When the herniating brain tissue's blood supply is compromised, cerebral ischemia and hypoxia worsen. The herniation increases pressure in the area where the pressure was lower, thus impairing its blood supply.
- As ICP approaches systemic blood pressure, cerebral perfusion slows even more, ceasing when ICP equals systemic blood pressure.

CARDIOVASCULAR SYSTEM
- Excessive water reabsorption causes increased extracellular fluid that may result in heart failure, especially with the coexistence of cardiovascular disease.

ASSESSMENT

HISTORY
- Possible clue to the cause
- Cerebrovascular disease
- Cancer
- Pulmonary disease
- Recent head injury
- Anorexia, nausea, vomiting
- Weight gain
- Lethargy, headaches, emotional and behavioral changes

PHYSICAL FINDINGS
- Tachycardia
- Disorientation
- Seizures and coma
- Sluggish deep tendon reflexes
- Muscle weakness

DIAGNOSTIC TEST RESULTS
- Serum osmolality levels are less than 280 mOsm/kg.
- Serum sodium levels are less than 123 mEq/L.
- Urine sodium levels are more than 20 mEq/L without diuretics.
- Renal function tests are normal.

TREATMENT

GENERAL
- Based primarily on symptoms
- Correction of the underlying cause

DIET
- Restricted water intake (500 to 1,000 ml/day)
- High-salt, high-protein or urea supplements to enhance water excretion

ACTIVITY
- As tolerated

MEDICATIONS
- Demeclocycline (Declomycin) or lithium (Eskalith)
- Loop diuretics
- 3% sodium chloride solution
- Conivaptan (Vaprisol)

SURGERY
- To treat underlying cause such as cancer

(continued)

NURSING CONSIDERATIONS

NURSING DIAGNOSES
◆ Anxiety
◆ Excess fluid volume
◆ Fear
◆ Risk for injury

EXPECTED OUTCOMES
The patient will:
◆ identify strategies to reduce anxiety
◆ maintain adequate fluid balance
◆ discuss fears and concerns
◆ remain free from injury.

NURSING INTERVENTIONS
◆ Restrict fluids, providing comfort measures for thirst.
◆ Reduce unnecessary environmental stimuli.
◆ Reorient, as needed.
◆ Provide a safe environment.
◆ Institute seizure precautions, as needed.
◆ Give prescribed drugs.
◆ Monitor vital signs, intake and output, daily weight, and serum electrolyte levels, especially sodium.
◆ Evaluate response to treatment.

◆ Assess breath and heart sounds, and perform neurologic checks regularly.
◆ Observe for changes in level of consciousness.

WARNING *Watch closely for signs and symptoms of heart failure, which may occur because of fluid overload.*

PATIENT TEACHING

Be sure to cover:
◆ disorder, diagnostic testing, and treatment
◆ medication administration, dosage, and possible adverse effects
◆ fluid restriction
◆ methods to decrease discomfort from thirst
◆ self-monitoring techniques for fluid retention such as daily weight
◆ signs and symptoms that require immediate medical intervention.

RESOURCES
Organizations
American Cancer Society: *www.cancer.org*
Endocrine and Metabolic Diseases Information Service: *www.endocrine.niddk.nih.gov*
Endocrine Society: *www.endo-society.org*

Selected references
Diseases: A Nursing Process Approach to Excellent Care, 4th ed. Philadelphia: Lippincott Williams & Wilkins, 2006.
Huang, E.A., et al. "Oral Urea for the Treatment of Chronic Syndrome of Inappropriate Antidiuresis in Children," *Journal of Pediatrics* 148(1):128-31, January 2006.
Nakazato, Y., et al. "Unpleasant Sweet Taste: A Symptom of SIADH Caused by Lung Cancer," *Journal of Neurology, Neurosurgery, and Psychiatry* 77(3): 405-406, March 2006.
Rottmann, C. "SSRIs and the Syndrome of Inappropriate Antidiuretic Hormone Secretion," *AJN* 107(1):51-58, January 2007.

Disorders affecting management of SIADH

This chart highlights disorders that affect the management of syndrome of inappropriate antidiuretic hormone (SIADH).

DISORDER	SIGNS AND SYMPTOMS	DIAGNOSTIC TEST RESULTS	TREATMENT AND CARE
Brain herniation (complication)	◆ Drowsiness ◆ Confusion ◆ Dilation of one or both pupils ◆ Nuchal rigidity ◆ Bradycardia ◆ Changes in respiratory patterns including Cheyne-Stokes respirations or hyperventilation ◆ Decorticate or decerebrate posturing	◆ Computed tomography scan may reveal the area of herniation.	◆ Check vital signs, level of consciousness (LOC), and pupil size every 15 minutes. ◆ Establish and maintain a patent airway; anticipate endotracheal intubation and mechanical ventilation, if necessary. ◆ Observe for cerebrospinal fluid (CSF) drainage from the patient's ears, nose, or mouth. Check pillows for CSF and look for a halo sign; test drainage for glucose with reagent strip. If the patient's nose is draining CSF, wipe it—don't let him blow it. If an ear is draining, cover it lightly with sterile gauze; don't pack it. ◆ Take seizure precautions. ◆ Speak in a calm voice and touch the patient gently. Don't make sudden, unexpected moves. ◆ Restrict total fluid intake to 1,200 to 1,500 ml/day to reduce fluid volume and intracellar swelling.

DISORDER	SIGNS AND SYMPTOMS	DIAGNOSTIC TEST RESULTS	TREATMENT AND CARE
Heart failure (complication)	*Left-sided heart failure* ◆ Dyspnea ◆ Othopnea ◆ Paroxysmal nocturnal dyspnea ◆ Fatigue ◆ Nonproductive cough ◆ Crackles ◆ Hemoptysis ◆ Tachycardia ◆ S_3, S_4 ◆ Cool, pale skin ◆ Restlessness and confusion *Right-sided heart failure* ◆ Jugular vein distention ◆ Positive hepatojugular reflex ◆ Right upper quadrant pain ◆ Anorexia, nausea ◆ Weight gain, edema ◆ Ascites or anasarca	◆ Chest X-ray shows increased pulmonary vascular markings, interstitial edema, or pleural effusions and cardiomegaly. ◆ B-type natriuretic peptide (BNP) immunoassay is elevated. ◆ Electrocardiography may reveal hypertrophy, ischemic changes or infarction, tachycardia, and extrasystoles. ◆ Liver function test may be abnormal; blood urea nitrogen (BUN) and creatinine levels may be elevated. ◆ Prothrombin time may be prolonged. ◆ Echocardiography may reveal left ventricular hypertrophy, dilation, and abnormal contractility. ◆ Pulmonary artery pressure, pulmonary artery wedge pressure, and left ventricular end pressure are elevated in left-sided heart failure; right atrial or central venous pressure is elevated in right-sided heart failure. ◆ Radionuclide ventriculography may reveal ejection fraction less than 40% in diastolic dysfunction.	◆ Place the patient in Fowler's position and provide supplemental oxygen. ◆ Weigh the patient daily, and check for peripheral edema. ◆ Monitor intake and output, vital signs, and mental status. ◆ Auscultate for S_3 and S_4 and adventitious lung sounds, such as crackles or rhonchi. ◆ Monitor BUN, creatinine, BNP, and serum electrolyte and magnesium levels. ◆ Monitor cardiac rhythm. ◆ Administer nesiritide (Natrecor), diuretics, nitrates, angiotensin-converting enzyme inhibitors, digoxin, beta-adrenergic blockers, and morphine.
Hyponatremia (severe) (complication)	◆ Headache, nausea, or abdominal cramps ◆ Muscle twitching, tremors, or weakness ◆ Changes in LOC possibly starting as a shortened attention span, lethargy, or confusion and progressing to stupor and even coma ◆ Seizures ◆ Hypovolemia with poor skin turgor and dry, cracked mucous membranes ◆ Weak, rapid pulse ◆ Hypotension, orthostatic hypotension ◆ Possibly decreased CVP, PAP, and PAWP	◆ Serum osmolality is less than 280 mOsm/kg (dilute blood). ◆ Serum sodium level is less than 135 mEq/L; if severe, less than 110 mEq/L. ◆ Urine specific gravity is elevated and urine sodium levels are above 20 mEq/L. ◆ Hematocrit and plasma protein levels are elevated.	◆ Administer isotonic or hypertonic saline solution (such as 3% or 5% saline) with an infusion pump, as ordered. ◆ Monitor the patient carefully during the infusion for signs of circulatory overload or worsening neurologic status. A hypertonic saline solution causes water to shift out of cells, which may lead to intravascular volume overload and serious brain damage (osmotic demyelination), especially in the pons. ◆ Accurately measure and record intake and output; obtain daily weights. ◆ Monitor for extreme changes in serum sodium levels and accompanying serum chloride levels. Also monitor other test results such as urine specific gravity and serum osmolality. ◆ Institute safety measures and seizure precautions, as indicated.
Seizure (complication)	◆ Aura ◆ Loss of consciousness ◆ Dyspnea ◆ Fixed and dilated pupils ◆ Incontinence	◆ EEG slows abnormal wave patterns and the focus of the seizure activity. ◆ Magnetic resonance imaging may show pathologic changes. ◆ Brain mapping identifies seizure areas.	◆ Ensure patient safety; initiate seizure precautions. ◆ Monitor neurologic and respiratory status. ◆ Observe and document the seizure activity (body movement, respiratory pattern, duration of seizure, loss of consciousness, incontinence, and papillary changes). ◆ Administer medications. ◆ Monitor vital signs, intake and output, and laboratory values.

Thyrotoxic crisis

- Acute manifestation of hyperthyroidism, a condition in which thyroid hormone overproduction results in a metabolic imbalance (see *Types of hyperthyroidism*)
- Usually occurs in patients with pre-existing (though commonly unrecognized) hyperthyroidism
- Medical emergency that can lead to life-threatening cardiac, hepatic, or renal failure; if left untreated, invariably fatal
- Also known as *thyroid storm* or *thyrotoxicosis*

CAUSES

- Genetic and immunologic factors
- Stressful event such as trauma, surgery, or infection
- Insulin-induced hypoglycemia or diabetic ketoacidosis
- Stroke
- Myocardial infarction
- Pulmonary embolism

- Sudden discontinuation of antithyroid drug therapy
- Initiation of radioactive iodine (^{131}I) therapy
- Subtotal thyroidectomy with excess intake of synthetic thyroid hormone

PATHOPHYSIOLOGY

- Triiodothyronine and thyroxine (T_3 and T_4) are hormones secreted by the thyroid gland.
- Overproduction of T_3 and T_4 causes an increase in systemic adrenergic activity, which leads to overproduction of epinephrine.
- Severe hypermetabolism leads to cardiac and sympathetic nervous system decompensation.

CARDIOPULMONARY SYSTEM

- Hypermetabolism causes increases in ventilation, blood volume, and cardiac output.
- Heart rate and myocardial contractility increase to compensate for the increased cardiac output, possibly leading to arrhythmias, especially atrial fibrillation. (See *Disorders affecting management of thyrotoxic crisis,* pages 430 and 431.)
- Heart failure and respiratory failure may occur if hypermetabolism is prolonged.

NEUROLOGIC SYSTEM

- The overproduction of epinephrine leads to decompensation of the central nervous system, resulting in signs of irritability, restlessness, and tremors.

ASSESSMENT

HISTORY

- Recent acute physical or emotional stress
- Family or personal history of Graves' disease
- Menstrual abnormalities

PHYSICAL FINDINGS

- Marked tachycardia, vomiting, and stupor
- Difficulty concentrating, nervousness, irritability, and restlessness
- Vision disturbances, such as diplopia
- Angina or palpitations
- Shortness of breath, dyspnea on exertion (and possibly at rest)
- Cough
- Swollen extremities
- Fine tremors of the fingers and tongue, shaky handwriting, and clumsiness
- Emotional instability or lability and mood swings (occasional outbursts to overt psychosis)
- Flushed skin, diaphoresis
- Premature graying, increased hair loss, and fine, soft hair
- Fragile nails, possible onycholysis (distal nail is separated from the nail bed)
- Pretibial myxedema over the dorsum of the legs or feet, which produces raised, thickened skin that may be itchy and hyperpigmented
- Plaquelike or nodular lesions

Types of hyperthyroidism

Other forms of hyperthyroidism include toxic adenoma, thyrotoxicosis factitia, functioning metastatic thyroid carcinoma, thyroid-stimulating hormone (TSH)–secreting pituitary tumor, and subacute thyroiditis.

TOXIC ADENOMA

The second most common cause of hyperthyroidism, toxic adenoma is a small, benign nodule in the thyroid gland that secretes thyroid hormone. The cause of toxic adenoma is unknown; its incidence is highest in elderly people. Clinical effects are similar to those of Graves' disease except that toxic adenoma doesn't induce ophthalmopathy, pretibial myxedema, or acropachy (clubbing of fingers or toes). A radioactive iodine (^{131}I) uptake and a thyroid scan show a single hyperfunctioning nodule suppressing the rest of the gland. Treatment includes ^{131}I therapy or surgery to remove the adenoma after antithyroid drugs restore normal gland function.

THYROTOXICOSIS FACTITIA

Thyrotoxicosis factitia results from chronic ingestion of thyroid hormone for TSH suppression in patients with thyroid carcinoma. It may also result from thyroid hormone abuse by people trying to lose weight.

FUNCTIONING METASTATIC THYROID CARCINOMA

This rare disease causes excess production of thyroid hormone.

TSH-SECRETING PITUITARY TUMOR

This form of hyperthyroidism causes excess production of thyroid hormone.

SUBACUTE THYROIDITIS

A virus-induced granulomatous inflammation of the thyroid, subacute thyroiditis produces transient hyperthyroidism associated with fever, pain, pharyngitis, and tenderness of the thyroid gland.

- Generalized or localized muscle atrophy and acropachy (soft-tissue swelling with underlying bone changes where new bone formation occurs)
- Infrequent blinking, characteristic stare, lid lag, exophthalmos, reddened conjunctiva and cornea, possible impaired upward gaze, convergence, and strabismus
- Asymmetrical, lobular, and enlarged thyroid gland
- Possibly enlarged liver
- Warm and moist skin with a velvety texture
- Hyperreflexia
- Paroxysmal supraventricular tachycardia and atrial fibrillation (especially in elderly patients) and, occasionally, a systolic murmur at the left sternal border
- Wide pulse pressures
- Increased bowel sounds
- In Graves' disease, an audible bruit over the thyroid gland
- High temperature, typically above 100.4° F (38° C) that begins insidiously and rises rapidly to a lethal level

DIAGNOSTIC TEST RESULTS

Thyrotoxic crisis occurs only in patients with hyperthyroidism. The following laboratory test results confirm the diagnosis of hyperthyroidism.
- Radioimmunoassay shows increased serum T_3 and T_4 concentrations.
- Thyroid scan reveals increased uptake of ^{131}I.
- Thyrotropin-releasing hormone (TRH) stimulation test indicates hyperthyroidism if TSH level fails to rise within 30 minutes after administration of TRH.
- Other supportive test results show increased serum protein-bound iodine and decreased serum cholesterol and total lipid levels.

TREATMENT

GENERAL
- Supportive measures (airway and ventilation)
- Fluid resuscitation
- Cooling methods

DIET
- Nothing by mouth during acute episode

ACTIVITY
- Bedrest during acute episode

MEDICATIONS
- Antithyroid drugs (propylthiouracil [PTU])
- Beta-adrenergic blockers
- Corticosteroids
- Iodides
- Antipyretics

WARNING *Don't administer aspirin to patients with thyrotoxic crisis because it increases circulating thyroid hormones, thus exacerbating the patient's already hyperthyroid state.*

WARNING *If PTU and iodide are ordered, give iodide at least 1 hour after giving PTU to enhance effectiveness.*

SURGERY
- Partial thyroidectomy (to treat underlying disorder)

NURSING CONSIDERATIONS

NURSING DIAGNOSES
- Deficient knowledge (disorder and treatment)
- Disturbed thought processes
- Hyperthermia
- Impaired gas exchange
- Ineffective breathing pattern

EXPECTED OUTCOMES
The patient will:
- verbalize understanding of underlying disorder and treatment plan
- exhibit appropriate thought processes
- achieve and maintain a normal temperature
- exhibit adequate ventilation and oxygenation
- maintain effective breathing pattern.

NURSING INTERVENTIONS
- Assess neurologic, respiratory, and cardiovascular systems.
- Provide supportive respiratory measures, if indicated.
- Institute cooling measures.
- Monitor vital signs, temperature, pulse oximetry, cardiac rhythm, and intake and output.
- Monitor for symptoms of hypothyroidism, such as weakness, fatigue, sensitivity to cold, weight gain, decreased level of consciousness, and bradycardia.
- Monitor laboratory values and blood glucose levels.

WARNING *When thyroid hormones are excessive, glycogenolysis increases and insulin levels decrease, placing the patient at risk for hyperglycemia. Insulin therapy may be necessary.*

(continued)

Be sure to cover:
♦ disorder, diagnostic testing, and treatment
♦ medication administration, dosage, and possible adverse effects
♦ when to notify the physician
♦ signs and symptoms of thyroid crisis
♦ signs and symptoms of hyperthyroidism and hypothyroidism
♦ importance of wearing or carrying medical identification
♦ need for follow-up care.

RESOURCES
Organizations
American Thyroid Association: *www.thyroid.org*
Endocrine and Metabolic Diseases Information Service: *www.endocrine.niddk.nih.gov*
Endocrine Society: *www.endo-society.org*
Thyroid Foundation of America: *www.tsh.org*

Selected references
Azizi, F. "Treatment of Post-partum Thyrotoxicosis," *Journal of Endocrinological Investigation* 29(3):244-47, March 2006.
Erdem, F., et al. "Autoimmune Thyroiditis during Thalidomide Treatment," *American Journal of Hematology* 81(2):152, February 2006.
Goldani, L.Z., et al. "Fungal Thyroiditis: An Overview," *Mycopathologia* 161(3):129-39, March 2006.
Liel, Y. "The Survivor: Association of an Autonomously Functioning Thyroid Nodule and Subacute Thyroiditis," *Thyroid* 17(2):183-84, February 2007.
Strategies for Managing Multisystem Disorders. Philadelphia: Lippincott Williams & Wilkins, 2006.

Disorders affecting management of thyrotoxic crisis

This chart highlights disorders that affect the management of thyrotoxic crisis.

DISORDER	SIGNS AND SYMPTOMS	DIAGNOSTIC TEST RESULTS	TREATMENT AND CARE
Atrial fibrillation (complication)	♦ Irregularly irregular pulse rhythm with normal or abnormal heart rate ♦ Radial pulse rate slower than apical pulse rate ♦ Palpable peripheral pulse with stronger contractions ♦ Evidence of decreased cardiac output, such as hypotension and light-headedness, with new-onset atrial fibrillation and a rapid ventricular rate	♦ Electrocardiography reveals no clear P waves, irregularly irregular ventricular response and uneven baseline fibrillation waves, and wide variation in R-R intervals resulting in loss of atrial kick. Atrial fibrillation may be preceded by premature atrial contractions. ♦ Transesophageal electrocardiography rules out the presence of thrombi in the atria.	♦ Focus interventions on reducing the ventricular response rate to less than 100 beats/minute, establishing anticoagulation, and restoring and maintaining sinus rhythm. ♦ Administer drug therapy, such as calcium channel blockers or beta-adrenergic blockers, or expect to combine electrical cardioversion and drug therapy; administer anticoagulant therapy as ordered to prevent atrial thrombi. ♦ If the patient is hemodynamically unstable, perform synchronized electrical cardioversion. It's most successful if done within 48 hours after atrial fibrillation starts. ♦ Prepare for possible transesophageal echocardiogram before cardioversion to rule out the presence of thrombi in the atria. ♦ If drug therapy is used, monitor serum drug levels and observe the patient for evidence of toxicity. ♦ Tell the patient to report changes in pulse rate, dizziness, feeling faint, chest pain, and signs of heart failure, such as dyspnea and peripheral edema. ♦ Monitor the patient's peripheral and apical pulses; watch for evidence of decreased cardiac output and heart failure. If the patient isn't on a cardiac monitor, be alert for an irregular pulse and differences in the radial and apical pulse rates.

DISORDER	SIGNS AND SYMPTOMS	DIAGNOSTIC TEST RESULTS	TREATMENT AND CARE
Heart failure (complication)	*Left-sided heart failure* ◆ Dyspnea ◆ Orthopnea ◆ Paroxysmal nocturnal dyspnea ◆ Fatigue ◆ Nonproductive cough ◆ Crackles ◆ Hemoptysis ◆ Tachycardia ◆ S_3, S_4 ◆ Cool, pale skin ◆ Restlessness and confusion *Right-sided heart failure* ◆ Jugular vein distention ◆ Positive hepatojugular reflex ◆ Right upper quadrant pain ◆ Anorexia ◆ Nausea ◆ Nocturia ◆ Weight gain ◆ Edema ◆ Ascites or anasarca	◆ Chest X-ray shows increased pulmonary vascular markings, interstitial edema, or pleural effusions and cardiomegaly. ◆ Electrocardiography may reveal hypertrophy, ischemic changes or infarction, tachycardia, and extrasystoles. ◆ Liver function test may be abnormal; blood urea nitrogen (BUN) and creatinine levels may be elevated. ◆ Prothrombin time may be prolonged. ◆ B-type natriuretic peptide (BNP) immunoassay is elevated. ◆ Echocardiography may reveal left ventricular hypertrophy, dilation, and abnormal contractility. ◆ Pulmonary artery pressure, pulmonary artery wedge pressure, and left ventricular end-diastolic pressure are elevated in left-sided heart failure; right atrial or central venous pressure is elevated in right-sided heart failure. ◆ Radionuclide ventriculography may reveal ejection fraction less than 40% in diastolic dysfunction.	◆ Place the patient in Fowler's position and give supplemental oxygen. ◆ Weigh the patient daily, and check for peripheral edema. ◆ Monitor intake and output, vital signs, and mental status. ◆ Auscultate for S_3 and S_4 and adventitious lung sounds such as crackles or rhonchi. ◆ Monitor BUN, creatinine, and serum potassium, sodium, chloride, and magnesium. ◆ Institute continuous cardiac monitoring to identify and treat arrhythmias promptly. ◆ Administer angiotensin-converting enzyme inhibitors, digoxin, diuretics, beta-adrenergic blockers, human BNPs, nitrates, or morphine. ◆ Encourage lifestyle modifications, as appropriate.
Hyperthyroidism (coexisting)	◆ Nervousness ◆ Heat intolerance ◆ Weight loss despite increased appetite ◆ Sweating ◆ Diarrhea ◆ Palpitations ◆ Emotional instability and mood swings ◆ Fertility problems ◆ Tremor ◆ Tachycardia at rest ◆ Arrhythmias, especially atrial fibrillation ◆ Dyspnea ◆ Wide pulse pressure and possible systolic murmur ◆ Hypertension	◆ Radioimmunoassay shows increased serum T_4 and triiodothyronine (T_3) concentrations. ◆ Thyroid scan reveals increased uptake of radioactive iodine. ◆ Thyroid-stimulating hormone levels are decreased. ◆ Ultrasonography confirms subclinical ophthalmopathy. ◆ Antithyroglobin antibody is positive in Graves' disease.	◆ Monitor vital signs, cardiac rhythm, and cardiopulmonary status. ◆ Give antithyroid drugs, such as propylthiouracil (PTU), or beta-adrenergic blockers or corticosteroids and iodide. ◆ Observe for signs and symptoms of thyroid crisis. ◆ Provide preoperative and postoperative care, as appropriate.

Traumatic brain injury

OVERVIEW

- Insult to the brain resulting in physical, cognitive, or vocational impairment
- Classified as closed (most common) or open, depending on whether the cranial vault is breached
- Children ages 6 months to 2 years, those between ages 15 to 24, and elderly people at highest risk
- Affects twice as many men as women

CAUSES

- Transportation or motor vehicle accidents (number one cause)
- Falls
- Sports-related accidents
- Assault

PATHOPHYSIOLOGY

CLOSED TRAUMA

- Forceful impact occurs between the head and a stationary object.
- The brain strikes the skull (coup), injuring cranial tissues near the point of contact, and residual force causes the brain to rebound, driving it against the opposite side of the skull (contrecoup).
- Contusions and lacerations may occur as brain tissues slide over the rough bone of the cranial cavity.
- Diffuse axonal injury (or shearing) causes damage and severing of connections between neurons.

OPEN TRAUMA

- Typically associated with skull fractures, the cranial vault and dura are breached and brain tissues are exposed, which may result from impact or penetration.
- Bone fragments commonly cause hematomas and meningeal tears with consequent loss of cerebrospinal fluid (CSF).

> **WARNING** *All patients with head injuries must be presumed to have spine injury until X-rays have shown otherwise.*

NEUROLOGIC SYSTEM

- Inflammation impairs the vascular tone of cerebral blood vessels.
- Capillary permeability increases, disrupting the blood-brain barrier.
- Edema leads to increased intracranial pressure (ICP), which impairs the flow of oxygen and nutrients to the brain as well as to other body tissues.
- Increased ICP causes distortion of blood vessels and displacement of brain tissue, ultimately leading to herniation. (See *Disorders affecting management of traumatic brain injury,* page 437.)

RESPIRATORY SYSTEM

- Increased ICP disrupts nerve impulse transmissions to the diaphragm and intercostal muscles, affecting respiratory depth and rate.
- Interruption in nerve impulse transmission to the diaphragm can lead to respiratory failure.

HISTORY

◆ History of traumatic injury to the head
◆ Altered level of consciousness (LOC) ranging from drowsy or easily disturbed by any form of stimulation, such as noise or light, to unconsciousness

PHYSICAL FINDINGS

◆ Assessment findings based on the type and location of the head injury (see *Types of brain injury,* pages 435 and 436)

DIAGNOSTIC TEST RESULTS

◆ Skull X-rays locate a fracture, if present, unless the fracture occurs in the cranial vault.
◆ Cerebral angiography locates vascular disruptions from internal pressure or injuries due to cerebral contusion or skull fracture.
◆ Computed tomography scan shows intracranial hemorrhage from ruptured blood vessels, ischemic or necrotic tissue, cerebral edema, areas of petechial hemorrhage, a shift in brain tissue, and subdural, epidural, and intracerebral hematomas.
◆ Magnetic resonance imaging and a radioisotope scan may also disclose intracranial hemorrhage from ruptured blood vessels in a patient with a skull fracture.

GENERAL

◆ Supportive (airway and ventilation management)
◆ Spine immobilization until cervical injury ruled out

DIET

◆ Nothing by mouth if severe injury or altered LOC

ACTIVITY

◆ Bed rest if severe injury

MEDICATIONS

◆ Analgesics (codeine)
◆ Corticosteroids
◆ Diuretics
◆ Anticonvulsants

SURGERY

◆ Evacuation of hematoma
◆ Craniotomy
◆ Cervical stabilization

NURSING DIAGNOSES

◆ Acute pain
◆ Anxiety
◆ Disturbed thought processes
◆ Impaired physical mobility
◆ Risk for posttrauma syndrome

EXPECTED OUTCOMES

The patient will:
◆ express feelings of increased comfort and decreased pain
◆ identify strategies to reduce anxiety
◆ communicate effectively with logical thought process
◆ attain or maintain highest degree of mobility possible
◆ express feelings and concerns regarding injury.

NURSING INTERVENTIONS

◆ Assess neurologic and respiratory status; provide respiratory support, if indicated.
   WARNING *Abnormal respirations could indicate a breakdown in the brain's respiratory center and, possibly, impending tentorial herniation—a neurologic emergency.*
◆ Provide spinal immobilization until cervical spinal injury is ruled out.
◆ Monitor vital signs, pulse oximetry, ICP readings, and intake and output.
◆ Observe for signs and symptoms of increased ICP.
◆ Administer medications and evaluate response.
◆ Provide safety measures; initiate seizure precautions.
◆ Provide wound care, as indicated.
◆ Observe for CSF leakage.
   WARNING *If the patient has CSF leakage or is unconscious, elevate the head of the bed to 30 degrees and keep his head aligned to reduce the risk of jugular compression and elevated ICP.*
◆ Apply sequential compression stockings and observe for signs if deep vein thrombosis.
◆ Provide emotional support.

(continued)

PATIENT TEACHING

Be sure to cover:
◆ disorder, diagnostic testing, and treatment
◆ medication administration, dosage, and possible adverse effects
◆ activity restrictions
◆ signs and symptoms of complications
◆ importance of follow-up care
◆ available community support and resource groups.

RESOURCES
Organizations
American Academy of Neurology: *www.aan.com*
American Academy of Orthopaedic Surgeons: *www.aaos.org*
Brain Injury Association of America: *www.biausa.org*

Selected references
Denson, K., et al. "Incidence of Venous Thromboembolism in Patients with Traumatic Brain Injury," *American Journal of Surgery* 193(3):380-83, March 2007.

Peiffer, K. "Brain Death and Organ Procurement: Nursing Management of Adults with Brain Injury is Crucial to the Viability of Donor Organs," *AJN* 107(3):58-67, March 2007.

Professional Guide to Pathophysiology, 2nd ed. Philadelphia: Lippincott Williams & Wilkins. 2007.

Servadei, F., et al. "The Role of Surgery in Traumatic Brain Injury," *Current Opinion in Critical Care* 13(2):163-68, April 2007.

Thompson, H., et al. "Intensive Care Unit Management of Fever Following Traumatic Brain Injury," *Intensive Critical Care Nurse* 23(2):91-96, April 2007.

Types of brain injury

TYPE	DESCRIPTION	SIGNS AND SYMPTOMS	DIAGNOSTIC TEST RESULTS
Concussion (closed head injury)	◆ A blow to the head hard enough to cause the brain hit the skull but not hard enough to cause a cerebral contusion causes temporary neural dysfunction. ◆ Recovery is usually complete within 24 to 48 hours. ◆ Repeated injuries exact a cumulative toll on the brain.	◆ Short-term loss of consciousness secondary to disruption of reticular activating system (RAS), possibly due to abrupt pressure changes in the areas responsible for consciousness, changes in polarity of the neurons, ischemia, or structural distortion of neurons ◆ Vomiting from localized injury and compression ◆ Anterograde and retrograde amnesia (patient can't recall events immediately after the injury or events that led up to the traumatic incident) correlating with severity of injury; all related to disruption of RAS ◆ Irritability or lethargy from localized injury and compression ◆ Behavior out of character due to focal injury ◆ Complaints of dizziness, nausea, or severe headache due to focal injury and compression	◆ Computed tomography (CT) scan reveals no sign of fracture, bleeding, or other nervous system lesion.
Epidural hematoma	◆ Acceleration-deceleration or contrecoup injuries disrupt normal nerve functions in bruised area. ◆ Injury is directly beneath the site of impact when the brain rebounds against the skull from the force of a blow (a beating with a blunt instrument, for example), when the force of the blow drives the brain against the opposite side of the skull, or when the head is hurled forward and stopped abruptly (as in an automobile accident when a driver's head strikes the windshield). ◆ Brain continues moving and slaps against the skull (acceleration), then rebounds (deceleration). Brain may strike bony prominences inside the skull (especially the sphenoidal ridges), causing intracranial hemorrhage or hematoma that may result in tentorial herniation.	◆ Brief period of unconsciousness after injury reflecting the concussive effects of head trauma, followed by a lucid interval varying from 10 to 15 minutes to hours or, rarely, days ◆ Severe headache ◆ Progressive loss of consciousness and deterioration in neurologic signs resulting from expanding lesion and extrusion of medial portion of temporal lobe through tentorial opening ◆ Compression of brain stem by temporal lobe causing clinical manifestations of intracranial hypertension ◆ Deterioration in level of consciousness resulting from compression of brainstem reticular formation as temporal lobe herniates on its upper portion ◆ Respirations, initially deep and labored, becoming shallow and irregular as brain stem is impacted ◆ Contralateral motor deficits reflecting compression of corticospinal tracts that pass through the brainstem ◆ Ipsilateral (same-side) pupillary dilation due to compression of third cranial nerve ◆ Seizures possible from increased intracranial pressure (ICP) ◆ Continued bleeding leading to progressive neurologic degeneration, evidenced by bilateral pupillary dilation, bilateral decerebrate response, increased systemic blood pressure, decreased pulse, and profound coma with irregular respiratory patterns	◆ CT scan or magnetic resonance imaging (MRI) identifies abnormal masses or structural shifts within the cranium.

(continued)

TYPE	DESCRIPTION	SIGNS AND SYMPTOMS	DIAGNOSTIC TEST RESULTS
Intracerebral hematoma	◆ Subacute hematomas have better prognosis because venous bleeding tends to be slower. ◆ Traumatic or spontaneous disruption of cerebral vessels in brain parenchyma cause neurologic deficits, depending on site and amount of bleeding. ◆ Shear forces from brain movement frequently cause vessel laceration and hemorrhage into the parenchyma. ◆ Frontal and temporal lobes are common sites. Trauma is associated with few intracerebral hematomas; most caused by result of hypertension.	◆ Unresponsive immediately or experiencing a lucid period before lapsing into a coma from increasing ICP and mass effect of hemorrhage ◆ Possible motor deficits and decorticate or decerebrate responses from compression of corticospinal tracts and brain stem	◆ CT scan or cerebral arteriography identifies bleeding site. Cerebrospinal fluid (CSF) pressure is elevated; fluid may appear bloody or xanthochromic (yellowish) from hemoglobin breakdown.
Skull fracture	◆ There are four types of skull fractures: linear, comminuted, depressed, and basilar. A blow to the head causes one or more of the types. May not be problematic unless brain is exposed or bone fragments are driven into neural tissue. ◆ Fractures of the anterior and middle fossae are associated with severe head trauma and are more common than those of the posterior fossa.	◆ Possibly asymptomatic, depending on underlying brain trauma ◆ Discontinuity and displacement of bone structure with severe fracture ◆ Motor sensory and cranial nerve dysfunction with associated facial fractures ◆ Persons with anterior fossa basilar skull fractures may have periorbital ecchymosis ("raccoon eyes"), anosmia (loss of smell due to first cranial nerve involvement), and pupil abnormalities (second and third cranial nerve involvement) ◆ CSF rhinorrhea (leakage through nose), CSF otorrhea (leakage from the ear), and hemotympanium (blood accumulation at the tympanic membrane) ◆ Signs of medullar dysfunction such as cardiovascular and respiratory failure (posterior fossa basilar skull fracture)	◆ CT scan and MRI reveal intracranial hemorrhage from ruptured blood vessels and swelling. ◆ Skull X-ray may reveal fracture. ◆ Lumbar puncture contraindicated by expanding lesions.
Subdural hematoma	◆ Meningeal hemorrhages, resulting from accumulation of blood in subdural space (between dura mater and arachnoid) are most common. ◆ It may be acute, subacute, or chronic; unilateral or bilateral. ◆ Usually associated with torn connecting veins in cerebral cortex; rarely from arteries. ◆ Acute hematomas are a surgical emergency.	◆ Similar to epidural hematoma but significantly slower in onset because bleeding typically originates in veins	◆ CT scan, X-rays, and arteriography reveal mass and altered blood flow in the area, confirming hematoma. ◆ CT scan or MRI reveals evidence of masses and tissue shifting. ◆ CSF is yellow and has relatively low protein (chronic subdural hematoma).

Disorders affecting management of traumatic brain injury

This chart highlights disorders that affect the management of traumatic brain injury.

DISORDER	SIGNS AND SYMPTOMS	DIAGNOSTIC TEST RESULTS	TREATMENT AND CARE
Brain herniation (complication)	◆ Drowsiness ◆ Confusion ◆ Dilation of one or both pupils ◆ Hyperventilation ◆ Nuchal rigidity ◆ Bradycardia ◆ Decorticate or decerebrate posturing ◆ Changes in respiratory patterns, including Cheyne-Stokes respirations or hyperventilation	◆ Computed tomography scan may reveal the area of herniation.	◆ Check vital signs, level of consciousness (LOC), and pupil size every 15 minutes. ◆ Establish and maintain a patent airway; anticipate endotracheal (ET) intubation and mechanical ventilation if necessary. ◆ Observe for cerebrospinal fluid (CSF) drainage from the patient's ears, nose, or mouth. Check pillows for a CSF leak and look for a halo sign. If the patient's nose is draining CSF, wipe it—don't let him blow it. If an ear is draining, cover it lightly with sterile gauze, don't pack it. ◆ Take seizure precautions but don't restrain the patient. Agitated behavior may be due to hypoxia or increased intracranial pressure. ◆ Speak in a calm voice and touch the patient gently. Don't make any sudden, unexpected movements. ◆ Restrict total fluid intake to 1,200 to 1,500 ml/day to reduce fluid volume and intracellular swelling.
Respiratory failure (complication)	◆ Diminished chest movement ◆ Restlessness, irritability, and confusion ◆ Decreased LOC ◆ Pallor, possible cyanosis of skin, mucous membranes, lips, and nail beds ◆ Tachypnea, tachycardia (strong and rapid initially, but thready and irregular in later stages) ◆ Cold, clammy skin and frank diaphoresis are apparent, especially around the forehead and face ◆ Diminished breath sounds; possibly adventitious breath sounds ◆ Possibly cardiac arrhythmias	◆ Arterial blood gas (ABG) analysis indicates early respiratory failure when partial pressure of arterial oxygen is low (usually less than 70 mm Hg). ◆ Partial pressure of arterial carbon dioxide is greater than 45 mm Hg; bicarbonate level is normal. ◆ Serial vital capacity shows readings less than 800 ml. ◆ Electrocardiography may demonstrate arrhythmias. ◆ Pulse oximetry reveals a decreased oxygen saturation level; oxygen levels less than 50% indicate impaired tissue oxygenation.	◆ Institute oxygen therapy immediately to optimize oxygenation of pulmonary blood. ◆ Prepare for ET intubation and mechanical ventilation if necessary; anticipate the need for high-frequency or pressure ventilation to force airways open. ◆ Administer drug therapy, such as bronchodilators, to open airways; corticosteroids to reduce inflammation, continuous I.V. solutions of positive inotropic agents (which increase cardiac output), and vasopressors (which induce vasoconstriction) to maintain blood pressure; and diuretics to reduce fluid overload and edema, as ordered. ◆ Assess the patient's respiratory status at least every 2 hours, or more often as indicated. Observe for a positive response to oxygen therapy, such as improved breathing, color, and oximetry and ABG values. ◆ Maintain a normothermic environment to reduce the patient's oxygen demand. ◆ Monitor vital signs, heart rhythm, and fluid intake and output. ◆ If intubated, auscultate the lungs to check for accidental intubation of the esophagus or the mainstem bronchus. Be alert for aspiration, broken teeth, nosebleeds, and vagal reflexes causing bradycardia, arrhythmias, and hypotension. Perform suctioning, as ordered, using strict aseptic technique. ◆ Monitor oximetry and capnography values to detect important indicators of changes in the patient's condition. ◆ Check cuff pressure on the ET tube to prevent erosion from an overinflated cuff. Normal cuff pressure is about 20 mm Hg. ◆ Implement measures to prevent nasal tissue necrosis from nasotracheal tube if used.

i refers to an illustration; t refers to a table.

i refers to an illustration; t refers to a table.

i refers to an illustration; t refers to a table.

i refers to an illustration; t refers to a table.

i refers to an illustration; t refers to a table.

i refers to an illustration; t refers to a table.

i refers to an illustration; t refers to a table.